REVIEW OF MEDICAL MICROBIOLOGY

9
Edition

review of
MEDICAL
MICROBIOLOGY

ERNEST JAWETZ, Ph D, MD
Professor of Microbiology and Chairman
Department of Microbiology
Professor of Medicine, Lecturer in Pediatrics
University of California School of Medicine
San Francisco

JOSEPH L. MELNICK, Ph D
Professor of Virology and Epidemiology
Baylor University College of Medicine
Houston, Texas

EDWARD A. ADELBERG, Ph D
Professor of Microbiology and of Molecular Biophysics
Director, Division of Biological Sciences
Yale University

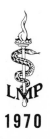

Lange Medical Publications
Los Altos, California

1970

Spanish Edition: *El Manual Moderno, S.A., Mexico, D.F.*
German Edition: *Springer-Verlag, Heidelberg, Germany*
Italian Edition: *Piccin Editore, Padua, Italy*
Turkish Edition: *Hacettepe University, Ankara, Turkey*
Portuguese Edition: *Editora Guanabara Koogan S.A., Rio de Janeiro, Brazil*
Serbo-Croatian Edition: *Skolska Knjiga, Zagreb, Yugoslavia*

International Standard Book Number: *0−87041−050−4*
Library of Congress Catalogue Card Number: *60−11336*

A Concise Medical Library for Practitioner and Student

Current Diagnosis & Treatment, 1970 H. Brainerd, M.A. Krupp, M.J. Chatton, S. Margen, Editors	$11.00
Review of Physiological Chemistry, 12th Edition, 1969 H.A. Harper	$7.00
Review of Medical Physiology, 4th Edition, 1969 W.F. Ganong	$7.50
Review of Medical Microbiology, 9th Edition, 1970 E. Jawetz, J.L. Melnick, E.A. Adelberg	$7.50
Review of Medical Pharmacology, 2nd Edition, 1970 F.H. Meyers, E. Jawetz, A. Goldfien	$8.50
General Urology, 6th Edition, 1969 D.R. Smith	$8.00
General Ophthalmology, 5th Edition, 1968 D. Vaughan, R. Cook, T. Asbury	$6.50
Correlative Neuroanatomy & Functional Neurology, 14th Edition, 1970 J.G. Chusid	
Principles of Clinical Electrocardiography, 7th Edition, 1970 M.J. Goldman	$7.00
Handbook of Psychiatry, 1969 P. Solomon, V.D. Patch, Editors	$7.00
Handbook of Surgery, 4th Edition, 1969 J.L. Wilson, Editor	$6.00
Handbook of Obstetrics & Gynecology, 3rd Edition, 1968 R.C. Benson	$5.50
Physician's Handbook, 16th Edition, 1970 M.A. Krupp, N.J. Sweet, E. Jawetz, E.G. Biglieri	$6.00
Handbook of Medical Treatment, 12th Edition, 1970 M.J. Chatton, S. Margen, H. Brainerd, Editors	$6.50
Handbook of Pediatrics, 8th Edition, 1969 H.K. Silver, C.H. Kempe, H.B. Bruyn	$6.00
Handbook of Poisoning: Diagnosis & Treatment, 6th Edition, 1969 R.H. Dreisbach	$6.00
Current Medical References, 6th Edition, 1970 M.J. Chatton, P.J. Sanazaro, Editors	$12.00

Preface

The authors' intention in preparing this Review has been to make available a brief, accurate, up-to-date presentation of those aspects of medical microbiology which are of particular significance in the fields of clinical infections and chemotherapy. The book is directed primarily at the medical student, house officer, and practicing physician. However, because the necessity for a clear understanding of microbiologic principles has increased in recent years as a result of important developments in biochemistry, virology, chemotherapy, and other fields of direct medical significance, a considerable portion of this Review has been devoted to a discussion of basic science. It is to be expected that the inclusion of these sections will extend the book's usefulness to students in introductory microbiology courses as well. In general, details of technic and procedure, as well as certain materials of a controversial nature, have been excluded.

With the appearance of the Ninth Edition the authors are pleased to report that Spanish, German, Italian, Portuguese, Turkish, and Serbo-Croatian translations have proved successful.

The authors wish to reaffirm their gratitude to everyone who assisted them with the preparation of this edition and to all those whose comments and criticisms have helped to keep the biennial revisions of this Review accurate and up to date. We are especially grateful to the following for their help: Stephen Cohen, Robert M. McCombs, F. Blaine Hollinger, William E. Rawls, Nilambar Biswal, Janet S. Butel, Satvir S. Tevethia, and Matilda Benyesh-Melnick.

Ernest Jawetz
Joseph L. Melnick
Edward A. Adelberg

San Francisco
July, 1970

Table of Contents

Notice

In keeping with the decision of several scientific societies to employ a uniform system of metric nomenclature, this edition of *Review of Medical Microbiology* has been converted to such a uniform system. Equivalents of present and past measurements are listed below.

Present Unit	Symbol	Equivalents	Past Unit	Symbol
Meter	m	. . .	Meter	m
Millimeter	mm	10^{-3} m	Millimeter	mm
Micrometer	μm	10^{-6} m	Micron	μ
Nanometer	nm	10^{-9} m	Millimicron	mμ
. . .	. . .	10^{-10} m	Angstrom	A

1...

The Microbial World

Before the discovery of microorganisms, all known living things were believed to be either plant or animal; no transitional types were thought to exist. During the 19th century, however, it became clear that the microorganisms combine plant and animal properties in all possible combinations. It is now generally accepted that they have evolved, with relatively little change, from the common ancestors of plants and animals.

The compulsion of biologists to categorize all organisms in one of the 2 "kingdoms," plant or animal, has resulted in a number of absurdities. The fungi, for example, were classified as plants because they are largely nonmotile, although they have few other plant-like properties and show strong phylogenetic affinities with the protozoa.

In order to avoid the arbitrary assignment of transitional groups to one or the other kingdom, Haeckel proposed in 1866 that microorganisms be placed in a separate kingdom, the **Protista**. Members of the kingdom Protista are distinguished from true plants and animals by their simple organization: They are unicellular, or, if multicellular, their tissues show little differentiation. The Protista can be subdivided as follows:*

I. Higher protists: Cell structure similar to that of plants and animals.
    A. Algae (except blue-green)
    B. Protozoa
    C. Fungi
    D. Slime molds
II. Lower protists: Cell structure greatly simplified (see Chapter 2).
    A. Bacteria
    B. Blue-green algae

The bacteria include the organisms called **rickettsiae**, which differ from other bacteria only in being somewhat smaller (0.2–0.5 μm in diameter) and in being obligate intracellular parasites. They were formerly thought to represent a transitional group between the bacteria and the viruses. It is now clear, however, that **viruses** are sharply differentiated from all cellular organisms, including rickettsiae and other bacteria. A viral particle consists of a nucleic acid molecule, either DNA or RNA, enclosed in a protein

*The classification proposed by Stanier, Doudoroff, & Adelberg in: *The Microbial World*, 2nd ed. Prentice-Hall, 1963.

coat or **capsid**. The capsid serves only to protect the nucleic acid and to facilitate attachment and penetration of the virus into the host cell. Viral nucleic acid is the infectious principle; inside the host cell it behaves like host genetic material in that it is replicated by the host's enzymatic machinery and also governs the formation of specific (viral) proteins. Maturation consists of assemblage of newly synthesized nucleic acid and protein subunits into mature viral particles; these are liberated into the extracellular environment.

Animal viruses pathogenic for man are described in Chapter 27. Bacterial viruses are described in Chapter 9.

Higher Protists

The higher protists share with true plants and animals the type of cell construction called **eucaryotic** ("possessing a true nucleus"). In such cells the nucleus contains a set of chromosomes which are separated, following replication, by an elaborate mitotic apparatus. The cytoplasm of the cell contains mitochondria and vacuoles, and the nuclear membrane is continuous with the ramifying endoplasmic reticulum. Motility organelles (cilia or flagella) are complex multistranded elements.

In contrast, the lower protists exhibit a much simpler cell construction, called **procaryotic**. A detailed comparison of eucaryotic and procaryotic cell structure is given in Chapter 2.

A. Algae: The term "algae" refers in general to chlorophyll-containing higher protists. Four general properties are constant enough within related series of algae to be used as a basis for classification (Table 1–1).

TABLE 1–1. Classification of algae. *Example:* **Green algae (Chlorophyta).**

Chemical nature of the food reserve	Starch
Array of photosynthetic and other pigments	Same as that found in true plants
Structure of the motile cell	Two or 4 anterior flagella of equal length
Specialized features	Form gametes in unicellular sex organs

On this basis, the algae of the higher protists may be divided into 6 phylogenetic groups. The names of the algal groups are recorded in Fig 1–1. For descriptions the reader is referred to Smith, G.M.: *Cryptogamic Botany*, 2nd ed. Vol 1: *Algae and Fungi.* McGraw-Hill, 1955.

B. Protozoa: In Smith's classification of algae, several types of photosynthetic, flagellated, unicellular forms are included which many textbooks class with the protozoa. These include members of Volvocales in Chlorophyta, members of Euglenophyta, the dinoflagellates in Pyrrophyta, and some of the golden-browns in Chrysophyta. These have not been classified as algae arbitrarily but because definite phylogenetic series are recognized which link them to typical algal forms.

On the other hand, these photosynthetic flagellates probably represent transitional forms between algae and protozoa; according to this view, the protozoa have evolved from various algae by loss of chlorophyll. They thus have a polyphyletic origin (ancestors in many different groups). Indeed, mutations of flagellates from green to colorless have been observed in the laboratory. The resulting forms are indistinguishable from certain protozoa.

The most primitive protozoa are thus the flagellated forms. "Protozoa" are unicellular, nonphotosynthetic higher protists. From the flagellated forms appear to have evolved the ameboid and the ciliated types; intermediate types are known which have flagella at one stage in the life cycle and pseudopodia (characteristic of the ameba) at another stage. The simplest classification of protozoa would be the following:

Phylum: Protozoa
  Sub-phylum I: Sarcomastigophora. Includes two major groups: Sarcodina (amebas) and Mastigophora (flagellates).
  Sub-phylum II: Sporozoa. Parasites with complex life cycles which include a resting or spore stage.
  Sub-phylum III: Ciliophora. Motility by cilia; high degree of internal organization.

C. Fungi: Those who argue that fungi have evolved from the algae point to similarities between the most primitive fungi (the phycomycetes) and members of the Chlorophyceae (in the Chlorophyta). However, the latter always store starch as their food reserve, and their motile cells are always multiflagellate; the most primitive fungi generally store glycogen (never starch), and the motile cells in the aquatic forms are usually uniflagellate. It thus appears more reasonable to trace their origin from the protozoa. (Note: The fungi show no evolutionary link with the mycelial bacteria called "actinomycetes.")

The fungi are nonphotosynthetic microorganisms growing as a mass of branching, interlacing filaments ("hyphae") known as a mycelium. Although the hyphae exhibit cross-walls, the cross-walls are perfo-

rated and allow the free passage of nuclei and cytoplasm. The entire organism is thus a coenocyte (a multinucleate mass of continuous cytoplasm) confined within a series of branching tubes. These tubes, made of the polysaccharide chitin, are homologous with cell walls. The mycelial forms are called molds; a few types, yeasts, do not form a mycelium but are easily recognized as fungi by the nature of their sexual reproductive processes and by the presence of transitional forms. The fungi differ from bacteria, including the filamentous actinomycetes, in being eucaryotic. They are subdivided as follows:

Class I: Phycomycetae. Mycelium usually nonseptate, asexual spores produced in indefinite numbers within a structure called a sporangium. Sexual fusion results in formation of a resting, thick-walled cell termed a zygote. **Example:** The black mold *Rhizopus nigricans.* **Pathogens:** Coccidioides (taxonomy uncertain).
Class II: Ascomycetae. Sexual fusion results in formation of a sac or ascus containing the meiotic products as 2, 4, or 8 spores (ascospores). Asexual spores (conidia) are borne externally at the tips of hyphae. **Examples:** Yeasts with known sexual life cycles (eg, *Saccharomyces cerevisiae*); species of Penicillium and Aspergillus with known sexual life cycles.
Class III: Basidiomycetae. Sexual fusion results in formation of a club-shaped organ called a basidium, on the surface of which are borne the 4 meiotic products (basidiospores). Asexual spores (conidia) are borne externally at the tips of hyphae. **Example:** *Psalliota campestris (Agaricus campestris),* the common mushroom.
Class IV: Fungi imperfecti. This is not a true phylogenetic group but merely a "taxonomic dumpheap" onto which are thrown all forms in which the sexual process has not yet been observed. Most of them resemble ascomycetes morphologically. **Pathogens:** Dermatophytes (Trichophyton, Epidermophyton, and Microsporum), probably related to ascomycetes; Blastomyces; Histoplasma; Sporotrichum; Cryptococcus (a yeast-like fungus); Candida (a yeast-like fungus).

The evolution of the ascomycetes from the phycomycetes is seen in the transitional Protoascomycetae, members of which form a zygote but then transform this directly into an ascus. The basidiomycetes are believed to have evolved in turn from the ascomycetes.

While the fungi are classified on the basis of their sexual processes, the sexual stages are difficult to induce and are rarely observed. Descriptions of species thus deal principally with various asexual structures, including the following: (See Figs 22–1 to 22–6 for drawings of some of these structures.)

1. Sporangiospores—Asexual spores borne internally inside a sac known as a sporangium. The sporangium is borne at the tip of a filament called a sporangiophore. These structures are characteristic of the phycomycetes.

2. Conidia—Asexual spores borne externally (not enclosed in a sac). The hyphae which bear them are called conidiophores. Conidia are formed by abstriction of the conidiophore; some species of fungi produce 2 types of conidia of differing size, in which case they are designated microconidia and macroconidia.

3. Thallospores—This term denotes actively reproducing cells which are formed by segmentation of the mycelium. Once formed, thallospores may reproduce by fission, by budding, or by growth into a new mycelium. There are 2 types: (1) arthrospores (oidia), produced by disarticulation of a filament of a septate mycelium into separate cells, and (2) blastospores, produced by budding from the ends or sides of the mycelial filaments. Blastospores are also known as "yeast-like cells."

4. Chlamydospores—Thick-walled, enlarged, resting spores formed (like thallospores) by segmentation of the mycelium. The chlamydospores remain as part of the mycelium, surviving after the remainder of the mycelium has died and disintegrated.

D. Slime Molds: These organisms are characterized by the presence, as a stage in the life cycle, of an ameboid multinucleate mass of cytoplasm called a plasmodium. The creeping plasmodium, which reaches macroscopic size, gives rise to walled spored which germinate to produce naked uniflagellate swarm spores or, in some cases, naked nonflagellated amebas ("myxamoebae"). These usually undergo sexual fusion before growing into typical plasmodia again.

The plasmodium of a slime mold is analogous to the mycelium of a true fungus. Both are coenocytes; but in the latter, cytoplasmic flow is confined within the branching network of chitinous tubes, whereas in the former the cytoplasm is free to flow (creep) in all directions. The slime molds are divided into 3 groups:

Class I: Myxomycetae. The vegetative body is a free-living plasmodium. The plasmodium shapes itself into a more or less elaborate fructification, forming spore-containing sporangia or fruiting pillars bearing external spores. **Examples:** Didymium, Physarum, Ceratiomyxa.

Class II: Phytomyxinae. The vegetative body is a plasmodium which is parasitic on plant tissues. The plasmodium breaks up into a mass of spores. **Examples:** *Plasmodiophora brassicae,* the cause of clubroot of cabbage.

Class III: Acrasiae. The plasmodium is formed by the aggregation of a large number of independent myxamoebae. The pseudoplasmodium, as it is actually called, shapes itself

into a sporangium-bearing sporophore. **Example:** Dictyostelium.

These 3 classes may actually have had a polyphyletic origin within the protozoa, although they appear sufficiently similar to justify their classification within a single division.

Lower Protists (Bacteria & Blue-Green Algae)

The bacteria form a heterogeneous group of microorganisms distinguished from higher protists by the following criteria: size range (0.2–2 μm for the smallest diameter); procaryotic cell construction; and a unique system of genetic transfer (see Chapter 4).

The blue-green algae include a variety of procaryotic forms which overlap bacteria and eucaryotic algae in their range of cellular sizes. They are photosynthetic, possessing the same chlorophylls as the eucaryotic algae and oxidizing H_2O to gaseous oxygen in their photosynthesis (see Chapter 5). By these properties they differ from the photosynthetic bacteria, which have specialized chlorophylls and do not produce gaseous oxygen.

Both the blue-green algae and the photosynthetic bacteria contain their photosynthetic pigments in a series of lamellas just under the cell membrane. In some photosynthetic bacteria, these lamellae differentiate under certain environmental conditions into ovoid or spherical particles called chromatophores. In contrast, the eucaryotic algae always contain their photosynthetic pigments in autonomous cytoplasmic organelles called chloroplasts. Chloroplasts are highly complex structures; in some algae they have been found to contain DNA of a unique base composition, as well as a unique ribosomal RNA.

The blue-green algae exhibit a type of motility called "gliding" or "creeping," the mechanism of which is unknown. Many nonphotosynthetic bacteria also possess gliding motility; some of these resemble certain blue-green algae so closely that they are believed to be "colorless blue-greens" which have lost their photosynthetic pigments in the course of evolution.

No further generalizations can be made about the lower protists. The reader is referred instead to the descriptions of the various bacterial groups in Chapter 3.

Summary

The concepts presented above are summarized in Fig 1–1. Listed at the right are the major groups of present-day microorganisms; the horizontal scale indicates time; and the vertical scale indicates relative evolutionary advance. Thus, from an unknown procaryotic ancestral form presumed to have been photosynthetic, the eucaryotic type of cell construction emerged. From this line the various algal groups diverged; some of these, by loss of chlorophyll, gave rise to early forms of protozoa. Our present-day protozoa, fungi, and slime molds, as well as the animal kingdom, are thought to have arisen from these early protozoa.

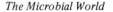

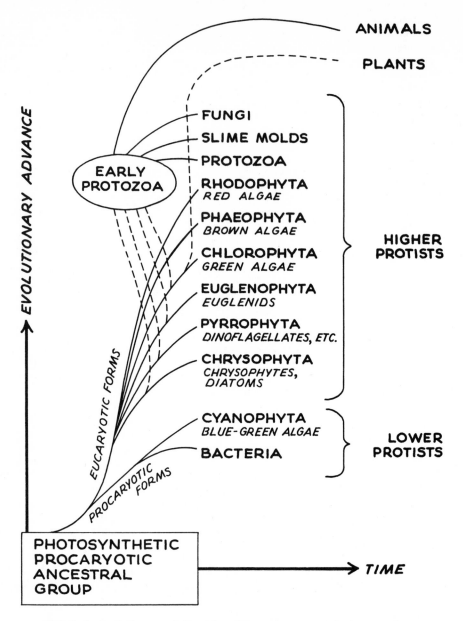

FIG 1–1. Evolutionary relationships of the major groups of microorganisms.

The true plants most likely evolved from early forms of green algae.

Present-day bacteria and blue-green algae represent, by this line of reasoning, forms which have evolved with relatively little change from the earliest procaryotic groups.

•   •   •

General References

Books

Alexopoulos, C.J.: *Introductory Mycology,* 2nd ed. Wiley, 1962.

Brock, T.D. (editor): *Milestones in Microbiology.* Prentice-Hall, 1961.

Bulloch, W.: *The History of Bacteriology.* Oxford, 1960.

Dobell, C.: *Antony van Leeuwenhoek and His "Little Animals."* Staples Press, 1932.

Fritsch, F.E.: *The Structure and Reproduction of the Algae.* Vol 2. Cambridge, 1945.

Large, E.C.: *Advance of the Fungi.* Jonathan Cape, 1940.

Mackinnon, D.L., & R.S. Hawes: *An Introduction to the Study of Protozoa.* Clarendon Press, 1961.

Moulder, J.W.: *The Psittacosis Group as Bacteria.* Wiley, 1964.

Smith, G.M.: *Cryptogamic Botany,* 2nd ed. Vol 1. McGraw-Hill, 1955.

Articles & Reviews

Lwoff, A.: The concept of virus. J Gen Microbiol 17:239–253, 1957.

Van Niel, C.B.: Natural selection in the microbial world. J Gen Microbiol 13:201–217, 1955.

2 . . .

Bacterial Cytology

OPTICAL METHODS

The Light Microscope

The resolving power of the light microscope under ideal conditions is about ½ the wavelength of the light being used. (Resolving power is the distance that must separate 2 point sources of light if they are to be seen as 2 distinct images.) With yellow light of a wavelength of 0.4 μm, the smallest separable diameters are thus about 0.2 μm. The **useful magnification** of a microscope is that magnification that makes visible the smallest resolvable particles. Microscopes used in bacteriology generally employ a 90-power objective lens with a 10-power ocular lens, thus magnifying the specimen 900 times. Particles 0.2 μm in diameter are therefore magnified to about 0.2 mm and so become clearly visible. Further magnification would give no greater resolution of detail and would reduce the visible area (field).

Further improvement in resolving power can be accomplished only by the use of light of shorter wavelengths. The **ultraviolet microscope** uses wavelengths of about 0.2 μm, thus allowing resolution of particles with diameters of 0.1 μm. Such microscopes, employing quartz lenses and photographic systems, are too expensive and complicated for general use.

The Electron Microscope

Using a beam of electrons focused by magnets, the electron microscope can resolve particles 0.001 μm apart. Viruses, with diameters of 0.01–0.2 μm, can be easily resolved.

An important advance in electron microscopy is the technic of "shadowing." This involves depositing a thin layer of metal (such as platinum) on the object by placing it in the path of a beam of metal ions in a vacuum. The beam is directed obliquely, so that the object acquires a "shadow" in the form of an uncoated area on the other side. When an electron beam is then passed through the coated preparation in the electron microscope and a positive print made from the "negative" image, a 3-dimensional effect is achieved (Figs 2–20, 2–21, 2–22).

Other important advances in electron microscopy include the use of ultrathin sections of imbedded material and the method of freeze-drying specimens which prevents the distortion caused by conventional drying procedures. The most recent advance has been negative staining with an electron-dense material such as phosphotungstic acid (Fig 27–31).

Darkfield Illumination

By arranging the condenser lens system so that no light reaches the eye unless reflected from an object on the microscope stage, particles that cannot be resolved can be made visible as points of reflected light. This technic is particularly valuable for observing organisms such as the spirochetes, which have a refractive index so close to that of the medium that they are difficult to observe by transmitted light.

Phase Microscopy

The phase microscope takes advantage of the fact that light waves passing through transparent objects, such as cells, emerge in different phases depending on the properties of the materials through which they pass. A special optical system converts difference in phase into difference in intensity, so that some structures appear darker than others. An important feature is that internal structures are thus differentiated in living cells; with ordinary microscopes, killed and stained preparations must be used.

Autoradiography

If cells which have incorporated radioactive atoms are fixed on a slide, covered with photographic emulsion, and stored in the dark for a suitable period of time, tracks appear in the developed film emanating from the sites of radioactive disintegration. If the cells are labeled with a weak emitter such as tritium, the tracks are sufficiently short to reveal the position in the cell of the radioactive label. This procedure, called autoradiography, has been particularly useful in following the replication of DNA, using tritium-labeled thymidine as a specific tracer (Fig 4–1).

EUCARYOTIC CELL STRUCTURE

The principal features of the eucaryotic cell are shown in the electron micrograph in Fig 2–1. Note the following structures.

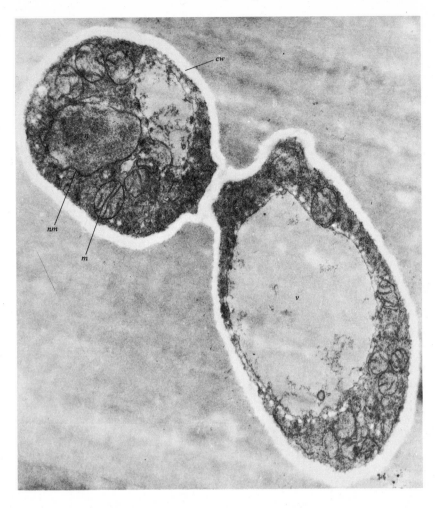

FIG 2–1. Thin section of a eucaryotic cell. A dividing cell of the unicellular yeast, Lipomyces (17,500 X). n = nucleus; **nm** = nuclear membrane; v = vacuole; **m** = mitochondrion; **cw** = cell wall. Electron micrograph taken by Dr. C.F. Robinow. (From Stanier, R.Y., Doudoroff, M., & E.A. Adelberg: *The Microbial World,* 2nd ed. Copyright 1963. By permission of Prentice-Hall, Inc., Englewood Cliffs, N.J.)

Nucleus

The nucleus is bounded by a membrane (**nm**) which is continuous with the endoplasmic reticulum. The chromosomes, embedded in the nuclear matrix, are not distinguishable. The mitotic apparatus is not present at this stage in the division cycle.

Cytoplasmic Structures

The cytoplasm of eucaryotic cells is characterized by the presence of an **endoplasmic reticulum, vacuoles,** and self-reproducing **plastids.** The plastids include the **mitochondria,** which contain the electron transport system of oxidative phosphorylation, and the **chloroplasts** (in photosynthetic organisms), which contain the chlorophylls and other photosynthetic components. The plastids contain their own DNA and multiply by binary fission.

Surface Layers

The cytoplasm is enclosed within a lipoprotein cell membrane. Most animal cells have no other surface layers; many eucaryotic microorganisms, however, have an outer **cell wall** which may be composed of a polysaccharide such as cellulose or chitin, or may be inorganic, as in the silica wall of diatoms.

Motility Organelles

Many eucaryotic cells propel themselves through water by means of contractile appendages called **cilia** or **flagella** (cilia are short; flagella are long). In every case the organelle consists of a bundle of 9 fibrils surrounding 2 central fibrils (Figs 2–2 and 2–3).

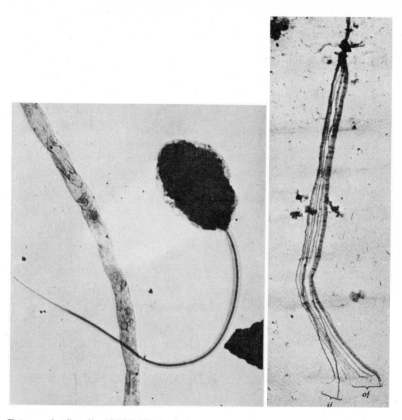

FIG 2–2. Eucaryotic flagella (3000 X). Left: A zoospore of the fungus allomyces, with a single flagellum. **Right:** A partially disintegrated flagellum of allomyces, showing the 2 inner fibrils (**if**) and 9 outer fibrils (**of**). (Courtesy of Manton, I., & others: J Exp Bot 3:204–215, 1952.)

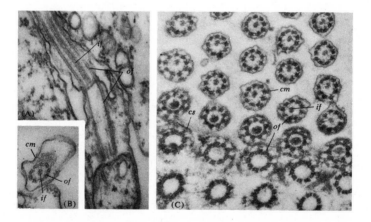

FIG 2–3. Fine structure of eucaryotic flagella and cilia (31,500 X). A: Longitudinal section of a flagellum of Bodo, a protozoon, showing kinetoplast (**k**) from which extend the outer fibrils (**of**). Note the origin of the inner fibrils (**if**) at the cell surface. **B:** Cross-section of same flagellum near the surface of the cell, showing outer fibrils (**of**), inner fibrils (**if**), and extension of cell membrane (**cm**). **C:** Cross-section through surface layer of the ciliate protozoon, Glaucoma, which cuts across a field of cilia just within the cell membrane (lower half) as well as outside the cell membrane (upper half). **cs** = cell surface. Electron micrographs taken by Dr. D. Pitelka. (From Stanier, R.Y., Doudoroff, M., & E.A. Adelberg: *The Microbial World,* 2nd ed. Copyright 1963. By permission of Prentice-Hall, Inc., Englewood Cliffs, N.J.)

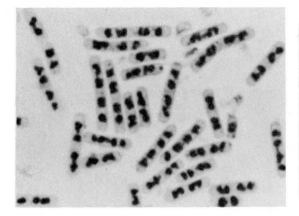

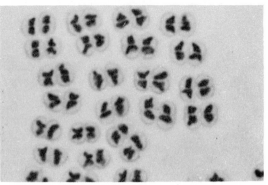

FIG 2–4. Nuclei of *Bacillus cereus* (2500 X). (Courtesy of C. Robinow: Bact Rev 20: 207–242, 1956.)

FIG 2–5. Nuclei of a tetrad-forming coccus; cells hydrolyzed with acid before staining (2500 X). (Courtesy of C. Robinow.)

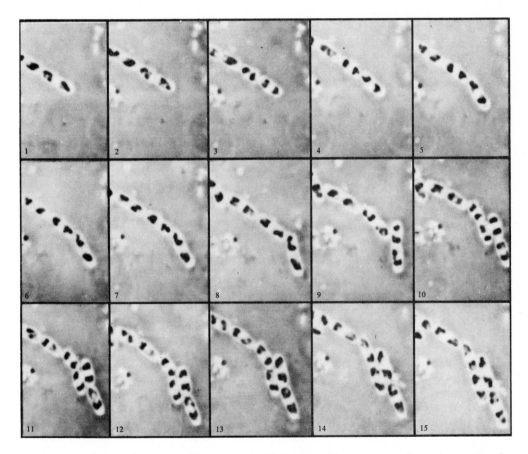

FIG 2–6. **Growth and nuclear division in a bacterium** (1750 X). Successive photomicrographs of a group of cells of *Escherichia coli,* suspended in a concentrated protein solution to enhance the contrast between nuclei and cytoplasm. Sequence represents 78 minutes, or 2.5 generations. Phase contrast photomicrographs taken by Dr. D.J. Mason & Dr. D. Powelson. (Courtesy of Stanier, R.Y., Doudoroff, M., & E.A. Adelberg: *The Microbial World,* 2nd ed. Copyright 1963. By permission of Prentice-Hall, Inc., Englewood Cliffs, N.J.)

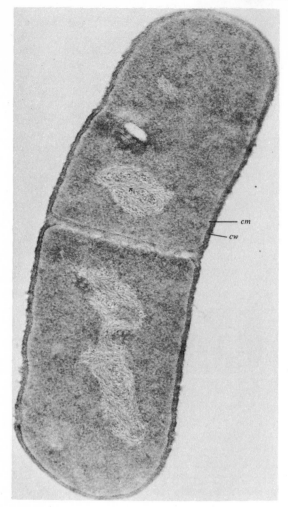

FIG 2—7. **Thin section of a procaryotic cell (42,000 X).** A dividing cell of the unicellular bacterium, *Bacillus subtilis.* n = nucleus; cm = cytoplasmic membrane; cw = cell wall. Electron micrograph taken by Dr. C. Robinow. (From Stanier, R.Y., Doudoroff, M., & E.A. Adelberg: *The Microbial World,* 2nd ed. Copyright 1963. By permission of Prentice-Hall, Inc., Englewood Cliffs, N.J.)

PROCARYOTIC CELL STRUCTURE

The procaryotic cell is simpler than the eucaryotic cell at every level, with one exception: The cell wall may be more complex. The following information has been obtained mostly from work on bacteria, but it is assumed to apply to blue-green algae also.

Nucleus

The procaryotic nucleus can be seen with the light microscope in stained material (Figs 2—4 and 2—5) or by phase contrast microscopy of cells suspended in a medium of appropriate refractive index (Fig 2—6). It is Feulgen positive, indicating the pres-

ence of DNA. The negatively charged DNA is neutralized by small polyamines rather than by basic proteins.

Electron micrographs such as Fig 2—7 reveal the absence of a nuclear membrane and of a mitotic apparatus. The nuclear region is filled with DNA fibrils; the DNA of the bacterial nucleus can be extracted as a single continuous molecule with a molecular weight of approximately 3×10^9 (see Chromosome Structure, Chapter 4). It may thus be considered to be a **single chromosome**, approximately 1 mm long in the unfolded state.

The electron microscopy of serial thin sections through bacterial cells shows that the DNA is attached at one point to a mesosome (see description of mesosomes and Fig 2—11). This attachment plays a key role in the segregation of the 2 sister chromosomes following chromosomal replication (see Cell Division). The genetics and chemistry of the bacterial chromosome are presented in Chapter 4.

Cytoplasmic Structures

Procaryotic cells lack autonomous plastids, such as mitochondria and chloroplasts. The cytochrome enzymes are localized instead in the cell membrane; in photosynthetic organisms, the photosynthetic pigments are localized in **lamellae** underlying the cell membrane (Fig 2—8). In some photosynthetic bacteria, the lamellae may become convoluted and pinch off into discrete particles called **chromatophores** (Fig 2—9).

A structure which may be analogous to the endoplasmic reticulum has been seen in several species of bacteria. Fig 2—10 shows cells of Azotobacter which have been freed of their soluble contents; a dense system of tubules invaginating from the cell membrane can be seen. Fig 2—11 shows another type of invagination, called the **mesosome.** It has been suggested that these invaginations may be the site of the cytochrome enzymes. It also seems possible that the ribosomes, which are densely packed in the bacterial cytoplasm, may be associated with the invaginated membrane, since in vitro protein synthesis takes place most actively in cell fractions rich in membrane fragments.

Bacteria often store reserve materials in the form of insoluble cytoplasmic **granules.** In the absence of a nitrogen source, carbon source material is converted by some bacteria to the polymer **poly-β-hydroxybutyric acid,** and by other bacteria to various glycogen-like polymers of glucose collectively called **granulose** (Fig 2—12). The granules are used as carbon source when protein and nucleic acid synthesis is resumed. Similarly, certain sulfur-oxidizing bacteria convert excess H_2S from the environment into intracellular granules of elemental **sulfur.** Finally, many bacteria accumulate reserves of inorganic phosphate as granules of polymerized metaphosphate, called **volutin.**

Surface Layers

A. Cell Membrane: The bacterial cell membrane can be demonstrated by 4 methods:

1. Plasmolysis—The cytoplasm of a bacterial cell shrinks away from the rigid cell wall when the cell is placed in a hypertonic solution. This phenomenon requires the presence of a semipermeable membrane; the shrinkage is caused by the osmotic loss of water from the cell which compensates for the higher solute concentration outside of the membrane.

2. Staining—"Victoria blue 4R" stains both cell wall and cell membrane. In Fig 2–13, cell contents of *Bacillus megaterium* cells have been caused to shrink slightly from the cell wall by plasmolysis. The stained cell membrane is clearly visible.

3. Isolation—Cell membranes have been isolated from cells of *Bacillus megaterium* by treatment with lysozyme and differential centrifugation. A phase con-

trast photomicrograph of this material is shown in Fig 2–14(c).

4. Ultrathin sections—In Fig 2–15, the membrane (m) is clearly seen as a distinct layer.

The cell membrane serves several major functions: It is the **osmotic barrier** of the cell, impeding the entry of many hydrophilic substances, as well as the **osmotic link**, catalyzing the active transport of other substances into the cell. In addition, the membrane is the site of several enzyme systems, including the following: the cytochrome enzymes, succinic dehydrogenase, lactic dehydrogenase, malic enzyme, malic dehydrogenase, formic dehydrogenase, and acid phosphatase. It thus serves the same function as the mitochondria of higher protists, plants, and animals.

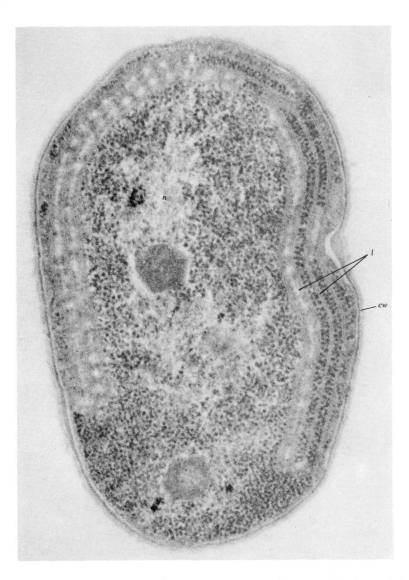

FIG 2–8. Thin section of a procaryotic alga (80,500 ✕). The blue-green alga, Anacystis. l = lamellae bearing photosynthetic pigments; cw = cell wall; n = nuclear region. (Reprinted by permission of the Rockefeller Institute Press, from Ris, H., & R.N. Singh: J Biophys Biochem Cytol 9:63, 1961.)

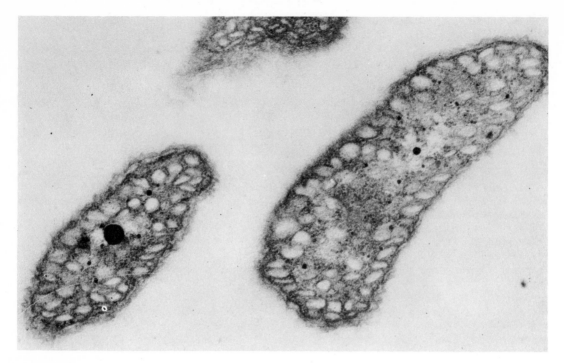

FIG 2–9. Ultrathin section of *Rhodospirillum rubrum,* showing nuclear area and chromatophores. (Courtesy of Vatter, A., & R. Wolfe: J Bact 75:480–488, 1958.)

B. Cell Wall: The existence of a rigid cell wall was inferred in the past from the constant cell form of many bacteria. As with the cell membrane, the inference was confirmed by plasmolysis, by staining, and by direct isolation. Fig 2–13 shows plasmolyzed cells of a bacillus in which the cell membranes and walls have been stained with Victoria blue.

Cell walls can be freed from their contents by boiling or by mechanical disintegration (eg, sonic vibration) and separated by differential centrifugation (Fig 2–16). Analysis of purified cell wall fractions has so far shown the following components to exist:

1. Gram-positive bacteria–The major component, called **mucopeptide,** is a polymer of which the principal subunits are the amino sugars N-acetylglucosamine and N-acetylmuramic acid (muramic acid is 3-O-α-carboxyethylglucosamine), and short peptides containing alanine, glutamic acid, and diaminopimelic acid or lysine. A considerable fraction of the alanine and glutamic acid is in the form of their D-isomers. A segment of mucopeptide polymer is shown in Fig 2–17.

In addition to mucopeptide, which is responsible for the structural integrity of the wall and is the substrate for lysozyme action, the walls of some gram-positive bacteria contain teichoic acids, polymers of ribitol phosphate and of glycerol phosphate. In some species the teichoic acids account for as much as 30% of the dry weight of the cell wall. Still another component of some gram-positive walls is a mucopolysaccharide, composed of amino sugars and simple monosaccharides.

2. Gram-negative bacteria–The walls of gram-negative bacteria appear to consist of 3 layers: a mucopeptide inner layer, and outer layers of lipopolysaccharide and lipoprotein; the protein of the latter contains all of the common amino acids. The teichoic acids are not present. Mucopeptide is apparently bound to the lipid material by glycosidic bonds. Lysozyme weakens the wall of gram-negative bacteria; detergents can degrade the wall by action on the lipid "cementing" substance.

Fig 2–15 shows an ultrathin section of a phage-infected cell of *Escherichia coli;* the wall (**w**) is seen to be a multilayered structure.

The internal environment of bacterial cells has a very high osmotic strength, equivalent to 10–20% sucrose; in ordinary media, only the rigid cell wall prevents the cell from bursting. The enzyme lysozyme, which cleaves the mucopeptide polymer, can be used to dissolve the cell walls of gram-positive bacteria, causing them to lyse. If the cells are first suspended in a medium containing 10–20% sucrose, however, the dissolution of the rigid cell wall simply causes the remaining structure (the **protoplast)** to assume a spherical shape.

As long as such protoplasts are kept in a medium isotonic with respect to their internal milieu, they will remain viable and capable of normal metabolic functions, including growth (Fig 2–18).

Fig 2–14 shows cells of *Bacillus megaterium* before and after removal of the cell walls by treatment with the enzyme lysozyme. The freed protoplasts have

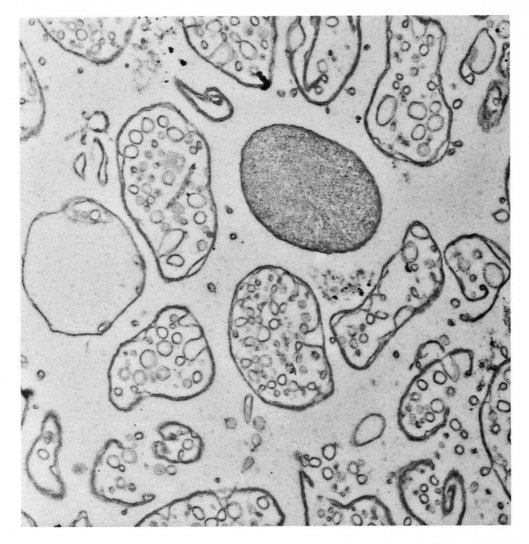

FIG 2–10. **Section of cells of** *Azotobacter agilis* (30,000 X). The cells were disrupted by brief shaking with glass beads, permitting leakage of cytoplasmic material. One cell has escaped disruption. Note system of tubules ramifying from the cell membrane. Electron micrograph. (Courtesy of Pangborn, J., Marr, A., & S. Robrish: J Bact 84:669–678, 1962.)

assumed a spherical shape, which demonstrates the role of the cell wall in determining cell morphology. Its principal function, however, is to serve as a corseting structure, protecting the cell from osmotic lysis.

C. Capsule: The capsule consists of excreted slime, usually polysaccharide, although in one case (*Bacillus anthracis*) it consists of a polypeptide of D-glutamic acid. Fig 2–19 shows encapsulated cells.

Mutations affecting capsule production are easily demonstrated, since encapsulated cells form "smooth" or "mucoid" colonies while nonencapsulated cells produce "rough" colonies. Nongenetic variation is also easily demonstrated, since most capsule formers only do so under special environmental conditions such as

the presence of high sugar concentrations, blood serum, or growth in a living host organism.

Flagella

Bacterial flagella are thread-like appendages composed entirely of protein, about 0.013 μm in thickness. They are the organs of locomotion for the forms that possess them. Three types of arrangement are known: **monotrichous** (single polar flagellum), **lophotrichous** (tuft of polar flagella), or **peritrichous** (flagella distributed over the entire cell). The 3 types are illustrated in Figs 2–20, 2–21, and 2–22.

Experiments in which the cell wall has been dissolved by lysozyme, leaving flagellated protoplasts (Fig 2–23), have proved that flagella originate in the protoplast and not in the cell wall. The existence of a basal

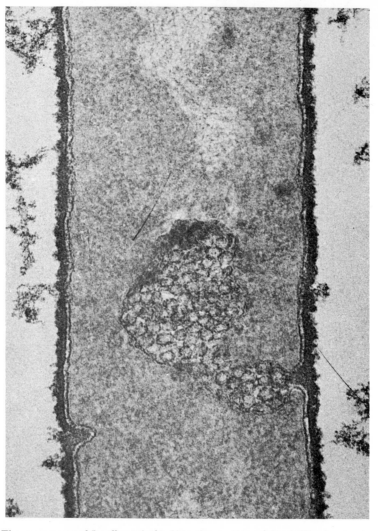

FIG 2–11. The mesosome of *Bacillus subtilis.* Ultrathin section of *B subtilis,* showing invagination of the membrane called the "mesosome." Electron micrograph taken by Dr. W. van Iterson. (From Roger Y. Stanier, Michael Doudoroff, & Edward A. Adelberg: *The Microbial World,* 2nd ed. Copyright 1963. By permission of Prentice-Hall, Inc., Englewood Cliffs, N.J.)

granule at the point of insertion has been inferred from electron micrographs like that shown in Fig 2–22.

Flagella have been removed from bacterial cells by rapid shaking and purified by differential centrifugation. Chemical analysis and x-ray diffraction studies on suspensions of purified flagella show them to be elastic proteins similar to hair and muscle fibers.

A bacterial flagellum is made up of a single kind of subunit, called flagellin; the flagellum is formed by the aggregation of subunits to form a hollow cylindric structure. If flagella are removed by mechanically agitating a suspension of bacteria, new flagella are rapidly formed by the synthesis, aggregation, and extrusion of flagellin subunits; motility is restored within 3–6 minutes. The flagellins of different bacterial species presumably differ from one another in primary structure.

The motion of the flagella can be observed in the larger bacteria by darkfield illumination, and less directly by observing the agitation of India ink particles in the vicinity of cells enmeshed in agar. The motions observed suggest that flagella propel the organism by means of waves passing along their lengths rather than by a lashing action.

Pili (Fimbriae)

Many gram-negative bacteria possess surface appendages called pili (Latin "hairs") or fimbriae (Latin "fringes"). They are shorter and finer than flagella; like flagella, they are composed of protein subunits. Their function is unknown, although in one case (sex pili) they play an essential role in the attachment of conjugating cells to each other. Pili are illustrated in Fig 2–24, in which the sex pili have been

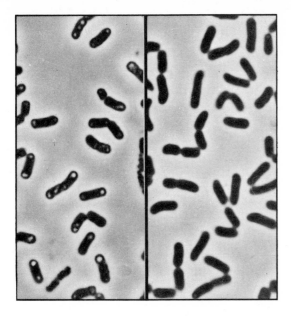

FIG 2–12. **Poly-β-hydroxybutyric acid granules (1900 X).** Formation and utilization of the polymer by *Bacillus megaterium.* Left: Cells grown on glucose plus acetate, showing granules (light areas). **Right:** Cells from the same culture after 24 hours' further incubation in the presence of a nitrogen source but without an exogenous carbon source. The polymer has been completely metabolized. Phase contrast photomicrograph taken by Dr. J.F. Wilkinson. (From Stanier, R.Y., Doudoroff, M., & E.A. Adelberg: *The Microbial World,* 2nd ed. Copyright 1963. By permission of Prentice-Hall, Inc., Englewood Cliffs, N.J.)

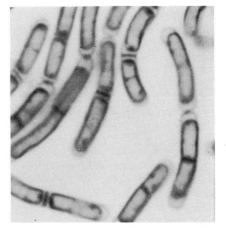

FIG 2–13. **Cell wall and membrane in *Bacillus megaterium* (3600 X).** (See text for explanation.) (Courtesy of C. Robinow.)

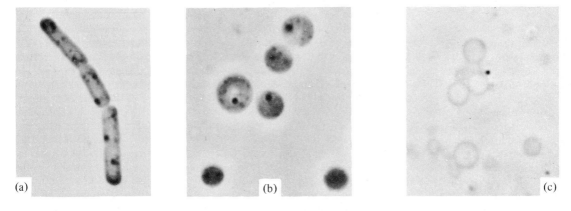

(a) (b) (c)

FIG 2–14. *Bacillus megaterium* **phase contrast photomicrographs (3000 X). (a)** Before treatment. **(b)** After treatment with lysozyme and sucrose (protoplasts). **(c)** After treatment with lysozyme alone; the empty structures are cytoplasmic membranes. (Courtesy of C. Weibull: J Bact 66:688–695, 1953.)

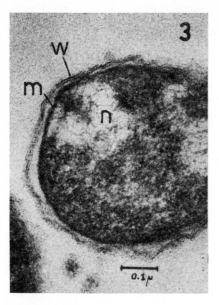

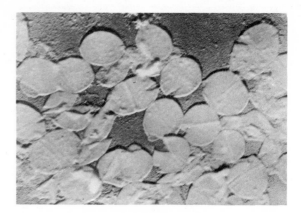

FIG 2–16. Cell walls of *Streptococcus faecalis,* removed from protoplasts by mechanical disintegration and differential centrifugation (11,000 ✕). (Courtesy of Salton, M., & R. Horne: Biochim Biophys Acta 7:177–197, 1951.)

FIG 2–15. **Ultrathin section of *E coli* cell infected with T2 phage,** showing double layered wall (**w**) and cell membrane (**m**) (100,000 ✕). (**n**) refers to plasma of vegetative phage DNA. (Courtesy of Kellenberger, E., & A. Ryter: J Biophys Biochem Cytol 4:323–326, 1958.)

coated with phage particles for which they serve as specific receptors.

Spores

Members of the genera Bacillus, Clostridium, and Sporosarcina characteristically form endospores (internal spores) under certain environmental conditions. One cell generally gives rise to one spore, which may be located centrally, terminally, or subterminally, according to the species.

While in general it can be stated that spores are formed when conditions are unfavorable for growth, the specific environmental condition that triggers sporulation is still unknown. When conditions are again favorable for growth, the spore germinates to produce one vegetative cell again (Fig 2–25).

Electron micrographs and photomicrographs of sectioned bacterial spores show the presence of a spore coat, a cortex, and a core containing a chromatinic structure (nucleus) (Fig 2–26).

The bacterial endospore was first thought to be metabolically inert, but more refined measurements show that it possesses a large number of active enzymes, including those necessary for conversion of carbohydrate to pyruvate by a nonglycolytic shunt; a particulate pyruvate oxidizing system, including the tricarboxylic acid cycle; an electron transport system, involving flavoprotein; alanine racemase; catalase; and glutamine synthetase.

Germination of endospores requires the presence in the medium of an amino acid (L-alanine is required for many species), a metabolizable carbon source, and a precursor of nucleic acids. Germination is characterized by the loss of heat resistance and the release of cell wall mucopeptide components plus dipicolinic acid. The latter is found only in spores, and may have a role in the inactivation of the normal cell enzymes that reappear after germination.

STAINING

Stains combine chemically with the bacterial protoplasm; if the cell is not already dead, the staining process itself will kill it. The process is thus a drastic one and may produce artefacts.

The commonly used stains are salts. **Basic** stains consist of a colored cation with a colorless anion (eg, methylene blue[+] chloride[−]); **acidic** stains are the reverse (eg, sodium[+] eosinate[−]). Bacterial cells are rich in nucleic acid, bearing negative charges as phosphate groups. These combine with the positively charged basic dyes. Acidic dyes do not stain bacterial cells and hence can be used to stain background material a contrasting color (see Negative Staining, below).

The basic dyes stain bacterial cells uniformly unless the cytoplasmic nucleic acid is destroyed first. Special staining technics can be used, however, to differentiate flagella, capsules, cell walls, cell membranes, granules, nuclei, and spores.

Gram's Stain

An important taxonomic characteristic of bacteria is their response to Gram's stain. The Gram staining property appears to be a fundamental one, since the Gram reaction is correlated with many other morphologic properties in phylogenetically related

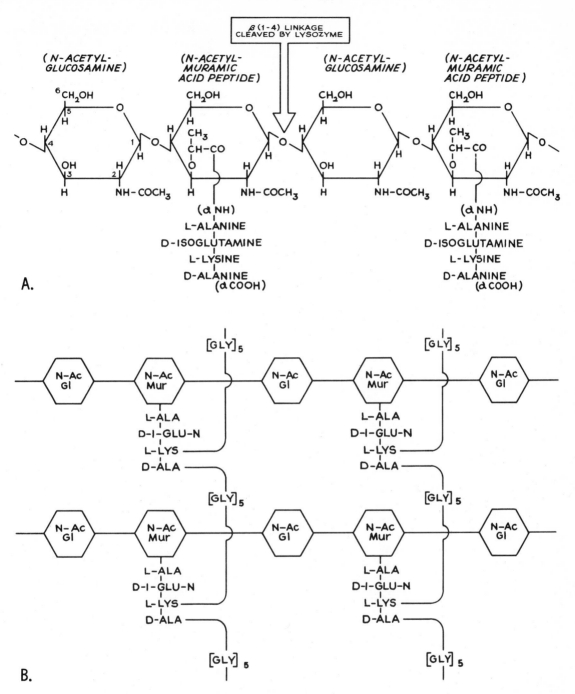

FIG 2–17. **A: A segment of the mucopeptide of** *Staphylococcus aureus.* The backbone of the polymer consists of alternating subunits of N-acetylglucosamine and N-acetylmuramic acid connected by $\beta(1-4)$ linkages. The muramic acid residues are linked to short peptides, the composition of which varies from one bacterial species to another. In some species the L-lysine residues are replaced by diaminopimelic acid, an amino acid which is found in nature only in procaryotic cell walls. Note the D-amino acids, which are also characteristic constituents of procaryotic cell walls. The peptide chains of the mucopeptide are cross-linked between parallel polysaccharide backbones, as shown in Fig 2–17B. **B: Schematic representation of the mucopeptide lattice which is formed by cross-linking.** Bridges composed of pentaglycine peptide chains connect the α-carboxyl of the terminal D-alanine residue of one chain with the ε-amino group of the L-lysine residue of the next chain.

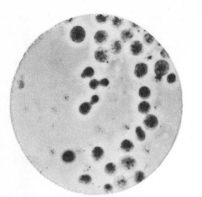

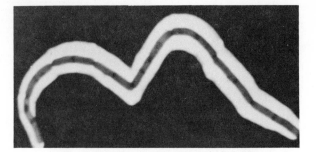

FIG 2–19. *Bacillus megaterium,* stained by a combination of positive and negative staining (1400 X). (See section on staining, below.) (Courtesy of H. Welshimer: J Bact 66:112–117, 1953.)

FIG 2–18. Phase contrast photomicrograph of protoplasts of *Bacillus megaterium* (2000 X). (Courtesy of K. McQuillen: Biochim Biophys Acta 18:458–461, 1955.)

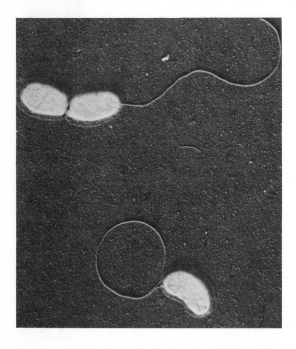

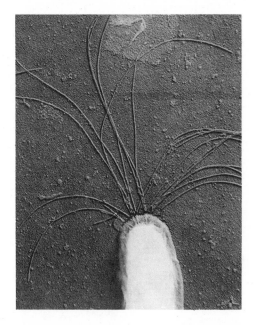

FIG 2–21. Electron micrograph of *Spirillum serpens,* showing lophotrichous flagellation (9000 X). (Courtesy of W. van Iterson: *Ibid.*)

FIG 2–20. *Vibrio metchnikovii,* a monotrichous bacterium (7500 X). (Courtesy of W. van Iterson: Biochim Biophys Acta 1:527–548, 1947.)

forms (see Chapter 23). An organism which is potentially gram-positive may appear so only under a particular set of environmental conditions and in a young culture.

The Gram staining procedure (see Chapter 24 for details) begins with the application of a basic dye, crystal violet. A solution of iodine is then applied; all bacteria will be stained blue at this point in the procedure. The cells are then treated with alcohol. "Gram-positive" cells retain the crystal violet-iodine complex, remaining blue; "gram-negative" cells are completely decolorized by alcohol. As a last step, a counterstain (such as the red dye safranin) is applied, so that the decolorized gram-negative cells will take on a contrasting color.

If gram-positive bacteria that have been gram-stained are treated with lysozyme to remove the cell wall, the protoplasts that are released are found to be stained. Such protoplasts, in contrast with whole cells, are readily decolorized by alcohol. These observations establish 2 facts: (1) The crystal violet-iodine complex is attached to the protoplast of a gram-stained bacterium, either inside or at the surface; and (2) the cell walls of gram-positive bacteria, but not of gram-

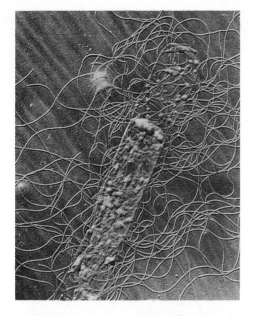

**FIG 2–22. Electron micrograph of *Proteus vulgaris,*
showing peritrichous flagellation (9000 X).** Note
basal granules. (Courtesy of Houwink, A., & W.
van Iterson: Biochim Biophys Acta 5:10–44,
1950.)

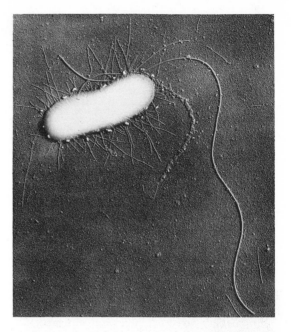

FIG 2–24. Surface appendages of bacteria. Electron
micrograph of a cell of *Escherichia coli* possessing
3 types of appendages: ordinary pili (short,
straight bristles); a sex pilus (longer, flexible, with
phage particles attached); and several flagella
(longest, thickest). Diameters: Ordinary pili: 7
nm; Sex pili: 8.5 nm; Flagella: 25 nm. (Courtesy
of Dr. Judith Carnahan & Dr. Charles Brinton.)

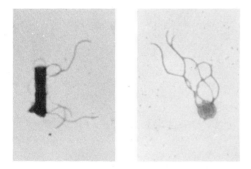

**FIG 2–23. *Bacillus megaterium* stained with flagella
stain (2000 X). Left:** Untreated cell. **Right:**
Protoplast freed from cell wall by treatment with
lysozyme and sucrose. (Courtesy of C. Weibull: J
Bact 66:688–695, 1953.)

negative bacteria, act as a barrier to the extraction of
the crystal violet-iodine complex by alcohol.

The Acid-Fast Stain

Acid-fast bacteria are those that retain carbolfuchsin (basic fuchsin dissolved in a phenol-
alcohol-water mixture) even when decolorized with
hydrochloric acid in alcohol. A smear of cells on a slide
is flooded with carbolfuchsin and heated on a steam
bath. Following this, the decolorization with acid-
alcohol is carried out, and finally a contrasting (blue or
green) counterstain is applied. Acid-fast bacteria

(Mycobacterium species and some of the related
actinomycetes) appear red; others take on the color of
the counterstain.

Negative Staining

This procedure involves staining the background
with an acidic dye, leaving the cells contrastingly colorless. The black dye nigrosin is commonly used. This
method is used for those cells or structures difficult to
stain directly.

The Flagella Stain

Flagella are too fine (0.013 μm in diameter) to be
visible in the light microscope. However, their presence
and arrangement can be demonstrated by treating the
cells with an unstable colloidal suspension of tannic
acid salts, causing a heavy precipitate to form on the
cell walls and flagella. In this manner the apparent
diameter of the flagella is increased to such an extent
that subsequent staining with basic fuchsin makes the
flagella visible in the light microscope. Fig 2–27 shows
cells stained by this method.

In some bacteria the flagella form into bundles
during movement, and such bundles may be thick
enough to be observed on living cells by darkfield or
phase contrast microscopy.

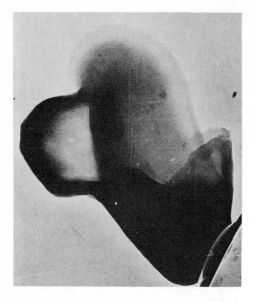

FIG 2–25. Electron micrograph of germinating spore of *Bacillus mycoides.* (Courtesy of Knaysi, G., Baker, R., & J. Hillier: J Bact 53:525–553, 1947.)

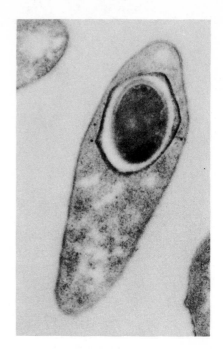

FIG 2–26. Thin section through a sporulating cell of a bacillus (33,000 ✕). Electron micrograph taken by Dr. C.L. Hannay. (From Stanier, R.Y., Doudoroff, M., & E.A. Adelberg: *The Microbial World,* 2nd ed. Copyright 1963. By permission of Prentice-Hall, Inc., Englewood Cliffs, N.J.)

The Capsule Stain

Capsules are usually demonstrated by the negative staining procedure or a modification of it (Fig 2–19). One such "capsule stain" (Welch method) involves treatment with hot crystal violet solution followed by a rinsing with copper sulfate solution. The latter is used to remove excess stain because the conventional washing with water would dissolve the capsule. The copper salt also gives color to the background, with the result that the cell and background appear dark blue and the capsule a much paler blue.

Staining the Cell Wall & the Cytoplasmic Membrane

Fig 2–13 shows the result of staining plasmolyzed cells with Victoria blue, which is specific for the cell wall and cell membrane. The Victoria blue dyes are water-soluble basic dyes belonging to the phenol-methane series; the reason for their specific reaction with the cell wall and membrane is not understood.

Staining of Nuclei

Nuclei are stainable with the Feulgen stain, which is specific for DNA.

The Spore Stain

Spores are most simply observed as intracellular refractile bodies in unstained cell suspensions or as colorless areas in cells stained by conventional methods. The spore wall is relatively impermeable, but dyes can be made to penetrate it by heating the preparation. The same impermeability then serves to prevent decolorization of the spore by a period of alcohol treatment sufficient to decolorize vegetative cells. The latter can finally be counterstained. Spores are commonly stained with malachite green or carbolfuchsin.

MORPHOLOGIC CHANGES DURING GROWTH

Cell Division

In general, bacteria reproduce by binary fission. Following elongation of the cell, a transverse cell membrane is formed, and subsequently a new cell wall. In bacteria, the new transverse membrane and wall grow inward from the outer layers (Fig 2–7). The nuclei, which have doubled in number preceding the division, are distributed equally to the 2 daughter cells.

Although bacteria lack a mitotic spindle, the transverse membrane is formed in such a way as to separate the 2 sister chromosomes formed by chromosomal replication. This is accomplished by the attachment of the chromosome to an invagination of the cell membrane, called a mesosome. The completion of a cycle of DNA replication apparently triggers active membrane synthesis between the sites of attachment of the 2 sister chromosomes, which are pushed apart

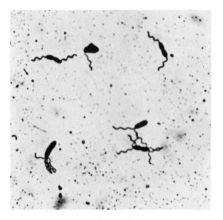

FIG 2–27. Flagella stain of Pseudomonas species. (Courtesy of E. Leifson: J Bact 62: 377–389, 1951.)

by the inward growth of the transverse membrane. The deposition of new cell wall material follows, resulting in the elongation and eventual doubling of the cell envelope.

One exception to this form of reproduction is the production of L-forms. In certain species of Proteus, Bacteroides, Escherichia, and Streptobacillus, normal cells may swell into large bodies which may then disintegrate into numerous particles about 0.2 μm in diameter. These particles can pass through bacteriologic filters, require a more complex medium than that which supports growth of the parent, are antigenically similar to the parent, and can revert to the parent bacterial form. In some species, the large bodies form spontaneously; in others, an inducing stimulus is required. The production of L-type growth by penicillin has revealed that L-forms are essentially naked protoplasts.

Cell Groupings

If the cells remain temporarily attached following division, certain characteristic groupings result. Depending on the plane of division and the number of divisions through which the cells remain attached, the following arrangement may occur in the coccal forms: chains (streptococci), pairs (diplococci), cubical bundles (sarcinae), or flat plates. Rods may form pairs or chains.

Following fission of some bacteria, characteristic postfission movements occur. For example, a "whipping" motion can bring the cells into parallel positions; repeated division and whipping results in the "palisade" arrangement characteristic of diphtheria bacilli.

Life Cycle Changes

As bacteria progress from the dormant to the actively growing state, certain changes usually take place. The cells tend to become larger, granules disappear, and the protoplasm stains more deeply with basic dyes. When growth slows down again, a gradual change in the reverse direction takes place. Finally, in very old cultures there appear morphologically unusual cells called involution forms. These include filaments, buds, and branched cells, many of which are nonviable.

● ● ●

General References

Books

Gunsalus, I.C., & R.Y. Stanier (editors): *The Bacteria.* Vol 1: *Structure.* Academic Press, 1960.

Murray, R.G.E.: Fine structure and taxonomy of bacteria. Pages 119–144 in: *Microbial Classification.* Cambridge Univ Press, 1962.

Pollock, M.R., & M.H. Richmond (editors): *Function and Structure in Microorganisms.* Cambridge Univ Press, 1965.

Salton, M.R.J.: *The Bacterial Cell Wall.* Elsevier, 1964.

Articles & Reviews

Cairns, J.: The chromosome of *Escherichia coli.* Cold Spring Harbor Symposium 28:43–46, 1963.

Doetsch, R.N., & G.J. Hageage: Motility in procaryotic organisms. Biol Rev 43:317–362, 1968.

Ryter, A.: Association of the nucleus and the membrane of bacteria: A morphological study. Bacteriol Rev 32:39–54, 1968.

Salton, M.R.J.: Structure and function of bacterial cell membranes. Ann Rev Microbiol 21:417–442, 1967.

Symposium on the fine structure and replication of bacteria and their parts. Bacteriol Rev 29:277–358, 1965.

3...
The Major Groups of Bacteria

PRINCIPLES OF CLASSIFICATION

Although it may be said of the higher organisms that no 2 individuals are exactly alike, it is nevertheless true that such individuals tend to form clusters of highly similar types. Furthermore, between any 2 clusters there is generally a sharp discontinuity. It is common practice to speak of each cluster as a **species.**

For hundreds of years, biologists have been naming and describing species of plants, animals, and microorganisms. Having at hand a large number of such names and accompanying descriptions, the next step was to compile this information in some orderly and systematic manner, ie, to classify it. In order to understand the problems and limitations of bacterial classification, it is necessary first to discuss 2 fundamental issues: the meaning of the term "species," and the types and purposes of classification.

"Species" Defined

A "species" is a stage in the evolution of a population of organisms. To understand this it is necessary to consider how species originate in higher plants and animals with obligatory sexual life-cycles.

A. Evolution in Higher Organisms: Imagine an island inhabited by a large, interbreeding population of a given species of plant. For the purposes of illustration, we will oversimplify and characterize the species as "broad-leaved plants." As generation follows generation, any mutant genes which arise will be thoroughly distributed throughout the population by interbreeding; in this way the population always remains homogeneous. The entire population may gradually change, as an adaptive response to a changing environment, but it cannot, as long as all individuals are free to interbreed at random, undergo divergent evolution into 2 or more different species. This can only occur if a segment of the population becomes isolated.

1. Geographic isolation—Isolation must at first be geographic, ie, 2 segments of an interbreeding population must become physically separated from each other. This can occur in many ways. For example, seeds may be transmitted by animals over a usually impassable mountain range, or seeds may be waterborne to a neighboring island. In any case, the result is that interbreeding between individuals on either side of the barrier is prevented. Within each segment, however, homogeneity is maintained by continued interbreed-

ing; 2 independent populations are thus established.

Each population continues to evolve. The probability is high, however, that evolution—owing either to different selective forces in their environments or to pure chance—will follow different courses in the 2 populations. We may thus picture the plants in the 2 populations as becoming more and more dissimilar. Up to a certain point the possibility remains that the 2 populations, upon removal of the geographic barrier, will mingle and finally "homogenize" as free interbreeding is once again established. But eventually, if they remain isolated, a point in their divergent evolution is reached where differences have accumulated to such an extent as to make interbreeding between the 2 populations impossible. They are then said to have become physiologically isolated.

2. Physiologic isolation—Two temporarily separated populations may become physiologically isolated in a variety of ways: For example, they may evolve different flowering seasons, or factors which cause hybrid progeny to be sterile. In any case, physiologic isolation represents a "point of no return"; removal of the geographic barrier now will permit intermingling but not interbreeding, with the result that the 2 populations are destined to remain different. Furthermore, the discontinuity will be a fairly large one, since many genetic differences will usually have accumulated before physiologic isolation occurs.

The point in evolution at which physiologic isolation occurs is thus a highly significant one and is therefore chosen as the point at which new species are said to have arisen. A "species" may thus be defined as follows: "A given stage of evolution at which actually or potentially interbreeding arrays of forms become segregated into two or more separate arrays which are physiologically incapable of interbreeding."*

Coming back to the oversimplified illustration, let us assume that the population of broad-leaved plants becomes split into two geographically isolated segments. On one side of the barrier, the population gradually evolves so as to possess short stems, serrated leaves, and a flowering season in the spring; whereas on the other side the population evolves long stems, smooth-edged leaves, and a fall flowering season. At this point, should the geographic barrier disappear (for

*Dobzhansky, T.: *Genetics and the Origin of Species.* Columbia, 1957.

example, by geologic change), the 2 types will spread and intermingle; but due to their different flowering seasons they will be physiologically isolated. A taxonomist visiting the island would then find 2 "species" of plants. He would probably classify them as follows:

Genus I: Broad-leaved plants.
    Species 1: Short stems, serrated leaves, spring-flowering.
    Species 2: Long stems, smooth-edged leaves, fall-flowering.

Note that what was originally a description of a species (possession of broad leaves) is now the description of a genus, illustrating that a "species" is really a stage in evolution.

3. Repetition of the process—All the individuals of "species 1" are freely interbreeding, as are the individuals of "species 2." Assume that a segment of the "species 1" population again becomes geographically isolated; further evolution will lead to physiologic isolation, and again new species will emerge. For example, in the cut-off segment of the "species 1" population, evolution may lead to the acquisition of the deciduous habit, while the other segment continues to retain its leaves all year. Let us assume also that the 2 types evolve different pollination systems. The taxonomist will probably then set up the following classification:

Family I: Broad-leaved plants.
    Genus I: Short stems, serrated leaves, spring-flowering.
        Species 1: Deciduous; wind-pollinated.
        Species 2: Nondeciduous; insect-pollinated.
    Genus II (one species): Long stems, smooth-edged leaves, fall-flowering.

Note that the original species has now become a family which includes 2 genera and 3 species. Thus, as the processes of geographic and physiologic isolation have repeated themselves over millions of years, organisms with obligate sexual life cycles have evolved along more and more divergent lines, until the present-day array of species has been reached.

B. Evolution in Bacteria: Unlike higher plants and animals, bacteria (and many other microorganisms) multiply almost entirely vegetatively. There is thus no mechanism by which discontinuous "species" can arise; instead, mutations accumulate so as to produce gradients of related types. As bacteria evolve to occupy their niches more and more efficiently, divergent lines of evolution will occur to the extent that the niches differ; groups of related ecologic types can thus often be recognized, but within each group there may be few real discontinuities. The term "species" thus has no real meaning when applied to bacteria; it cannot even be defined, as it can for sexually reproducing organisms. Bacterial taxonomists must be purely arbitrary in deciding to what extent 2 types must differ before being classed as different "species."

While it is thus unlikely that bacterial taxonomy can ever become the exact science that the taxonomies of higher organisms represent, nevertheless the recognition of natural ecologic groups is important and to a degree attainable. One great obstacle, however, is the exclusive use of pure cultures for the systematic study of bacteria. First of all, it is well known that this practice results in selection of mutations which adapt the organisms to growth in laboratory media; the cultures which are finally studied are thus artifacts, or "hot-house cultures," often quite different from the organism as it existed in nature. Second, the properties which are studied as the basis for classification are not necessarily significant in the organism's ecology; for example, the ability to liquefy gelatin is of questionable significance in describing an organism which in its natural environment is never called upon to hydrolyze proteins.

The only solution to this problem would be to study the properties of bacteria in "dirty" enrichment cultures, to the extent that this is possible. The enrichment culture (Table 6–2) represents the closest approach to the study of bacteria in their natural environment.

Types and Purposes of Classification

While many sorts of systematic compilations are conceivable, only 2 are generally used in taxonomy: keys, or "artificial classifications"; and phylogenetic (or "natural") classifications.

A. Keys: In a "key," descriptive properties are arranged in such a way that an organism on hand may be readily identified. Organisms which are grouped together in a "key" are not necessarily related in the phylogenetic sense; they are listed together because they share some easily recognizable property. It would be perfectly reasonable, for example, for a key to bacteria to include a group such as "bacteria forming red pigments," even though this would include such unrelated forms as *Serratia marcescens* and purple sulfur bacteria. The point is that such a grouping would be useful; the investigator having a red-pigmented culture to identify would immediately narrow his search to a relatively few types.

B. Phylogenetic Classification: A phylogenetic classification groups together types that are **related**, ie, those that share a common ancestor. Species which have arisen through divergent evolution from a common ancestor are grouped together in a single genus; genera with a common origin are grouped in a single family, etc. Recognition of phylogenetic relationships in higher organisms is greatly aided by the existence of fossil remnants of common ancestors and by the multitude of morphologic features which can be studied. Bacteria, on the other hand, have not been preserved as recognizable fossils and exhibit relatively few morphologic properties for study. Evolutionary trends are thus difficult to determine or even to guess at, and a phylogenetic classification of bacteria is certainly a long way from being realized.

Bergey's Manual of Determinative Bacteriology

There is no universally accepted natural classification of bacteria since there is no mechanism for the evolution of discrete bacterial species and we are almost totally ignorant of bacterial evolution. A few groups, such as the photosynthetic bacteria, have been thoroughly classified by studies with enrichment cultures, but we do not know how such major groups are related to each other. The few evolutionary lines which are discernible will be presented later in this chapter.

In spite of these objections, however, an attempt at a phylogenetic classification of bacteria has been published in the USA as *Bergey's Manual of Determinative Bacteriology.** First published in 1923, it has now reached its 7th edition. The 6th edition, in 1948, grouped the bacteria in 6 orders containing 36 families. The 7th edition has rearranged the genera into 10 orders and 47 families. In view of the divergent views that exist among authorities regarding bacterial classification, it is probable that the manual will undergo further major changes with each edition. We will therefore not follow Bergey's classification in this chapter but instead will describe the major groups of bacteria, using common names. We will also refer to the most important genera, about which there is good agreement among bacteriologists; and, in the case of the eubacteria, we will describe certain families about which there is also fairly good agreement.

Bergey's Manual does serve several useful purposes, however, if we ignore its attempt to represent a phylogeny. First, it represents an exhaustive compilation of names and descriptions; second, the latest edition includes a completely practical although artificial key to the genera, as an aid to identification of newly isolated types. The *Manual* has a companion volume, called *Index Bergeyana,* containing the literature index, the host and habitat index, and descriptions of organisms which the editors consider inadequately described or whose taxonomic positions are undertain.

A key to the genera of bacteria has also been published separately in Skerman, V.B.D.: *Guide to the Identification of the Genera of Bacteria.* Williams & Wilkins, 1959.

An informal classification is presented on the following pages and in Tables 3−1 and 3−2.†

Computer Taxonomy of Bacteria

Taxonomy by computer has been developed for groups of bacteria in which a large number of strains exist which can be described in terms of 100 or more clear-cut taxonomic properties (eg, presence or absence of certain enzymes, presence or absence of certain pig-

*Breed, Murray, & Smith, editors: *Bergey's Manual of Determinative Bacteriology,* 7th ed. Williams & Wilkins, 1957.

†Modified and reproduced, with permission, from Stanier, R.Y., Doudoroff, M., & E.A. Adelberg: *The Microbial World,* 2nd ed. Copyright 1963. By permission of Prentice-Hall, Inc, Englewood Cliffs, N.J.

ments, presence or absence of certain morphologic structures). Punch cards are prepared for each strain; the computer then compares the cards and prints out a list of the strains in such an order that each strain is followed in the list by the strain with which it shares the most characteristics. When this is done, the list often reveals several broad subgroups of strains, each subgroup characterized by a larger number of shared common characteristics. The median strain within each subgroup can then be arbitrarily considered as a type species.

DESCRIPTIONS OF THE MAJOR GROUPS OF BACTERIA

Three principal groups of bacteria can be recognized on the basis of the mechanism of movement and the character of the cell wall. The **eubacteria** have thick, rigid walls; motility, when present, is by means of flagella. The **spirochetes** have thin, flexible walls; motility is by contraction of an axial filament wound helically about the cell and anchored at both ends. The **gliding bacteria** move smoothly along solid surfaces by an unknown mechanism; no motility organelles have been detected. One group of gliding bacteria are colorless derivatives of blue-green algae and, like the blue-green algae, have thick, rigid walls. The other gliding bacteria, the myxobacteria, have thin, flexible walls.

A fourth group of bacteria, the **mycoplasmas**, are characterized by the absence of a cell wall. Similar forms, called L forms, can be induced in various eubacteria by removal of the cell wall. The surviving protoplasts, which closely resemble mycoplasmas, are capable of reverting to typical walled cells. It seems highly probable that mycoplasmas are similarly derived from eubacteria but have lost the ability to revert. The mycoplasmas were formerly called PPLO's (pleuropneumonia-like organisms). They are described in Chapter 20.

The Eubacteria

These organisms possess thick, rigid walls. Movement is accomplished by means of flagella, but motility is not an invariable property: Many eubacteria are immotile. Cell division always occurs by binary transverse fission. In addition to the simple unicellular types, several related types are set apart on the basis of special physiologic or morphologic properties; an outline of the eubacterial groups is presented below.

A. Unicellular, Nonphotosynthetic Eubacteria: This group contains nearly all of the well-known bacteria, including most of the pathogens. The important families and genera are characterized in Tables 3−1 and 3−2. The rickettsiae, which belong with the eubacteria, are described in Chapter 25.

A clear separation of 2 subgroups can be made on the basis of the Gram reaction, which appears to be a fundamental property of true phylogenetic signifi-

---

Outline of the Major Groups of Eubacteria

A. **Unicellular, nonphotosynthetic forms**
  1. Gram-negative forms (See Table 3—1.)
  2. Gram-positive forms (See Table 3—2.)
B. **Unicellular, photosynthetic forms**
  1. Family: Chlorobacteriaceae (green bacteria)
  2. Family: Thiorhodaceae (purple sulfur bacteria)
  3. Family: Athiorhodaceae (non-sulfur purple bacteria; brown bacteria)
C. **Stalked forms**
  1. Genus: Caulobacter
  2. Genus: Gallionella
D. **Filamentous forms (Caryophanon)**
E. **Sheathed forms (Sphaerotilus)**
F. **Mycelial forms (Actinomycetes)**
  1. Family: Mycobacteriaceae
  2. Family: Actinomycetaceae
  3. Family: Streptomycetaceae
  4. Family: Actinoplanaceae
G. **Budding forms**
  1. Genus: Hyphomicrobium (nonphotosynthetic)
  2. Genus: Rhodomicrobium (photosynthetic)

---

cance. The gram-positive and the gram-negative forms each appear to constitute closely related groups of bacteria.

Within the group of gram-positive eubacteria we have some evidence for a phylogenetic series. At the lower end of the series we would place the genus Lactobacillus, members of which carry out a fermentation of sugars to lactic acid (Figs 5—23 to 5—28). The next genus, Propionibacterium, is distinguishable on the basis of its fermentation, which yields propionic acid as the major product; and its morphology, which is intermediate between the more regular rod-shaped lactobacilli and the pleomorphic, club-shaped Corynebacterium. The latter group, standing third in the phylogenetic line, are weakly fermentative, relying primarily on a respiratory type of metabolism. They strongly resemble the lowest members of the actinomycetes, the mycobacteria, which form a rudimentary mycelium which fragments later into branching, club-shaped cells. The mycobacteria will be discussed below in the section on the mycelial bacteria, which stand at the upper end of our phylogenetic line.

B. Unicellular, Photosynthetic Eubacteria: The photosynthetic bacteria include all of the common eubacterial types: rods, cocci, and spheres. There is also a photosynthetic budding bacterium, Rhodomicrobium (Fig 3—12).

There are 3 clear-cut families of unicellular photosynthetic eubacteria, separated on the basis of their pigments and physiology. Fig 3—2 shows cells of purple sulfur bacteria which have accumulated droplets of sulfur as a result of photo-oxidation of H_2S.

From ecologic considerations it is clear that the photosynthetic bacteria form a natural phylogenetic group; their morphology indicates an affinity with the nonphotosynthetic eubacteria.

C. Unicellular Stalked Eubacteria: These are typical gram-negative eubacteria, except for their property of forming stalks. There are 2 principal genera, Caulobacter and Gallionella. Members of the genus Caulobacter are organotrophic bacteria, each cell of which is attached to the substrate by means of a fine stalk which is an extension of the cell. In dense cultures, the stalks may attach to each other, forming rosettes (Fig 3—3). When a cell divides, the daughter cell swims away by means of a polar flagellum, eventually secreting a new stalk and attaching itself to the substrate.

Cells of the genus Gallionella oxidize ferrous iron as a source of energy, forming ferric hydroxide which is excreted to form a ribbon-like stalk. When the cells divide, the new cells remain attached to the stalk, which thus becomes branched (Fig 3—4).

D. Filamentous Eubacteria: The loosely-connected chains of cells which form when rods or cocci adhere together following cell division are not true filaments. On the other hand, a few forms are known which form continuous filaments, subdivided into compartments by numerous cross-walls. The best known is Caryophanon (Fig 3—5), a relatively enormous bacterium reaching as much as 4 μm in width and 40 μm in length (an ordinary coccus is about 1 μm in diameter). Reproduction occurs by binary division of the entire filament, which is peritrichously flagellated. Carophyanon and related types occur in the intestinal tracts of cows and other animals.

E. Sheathed Eubacteria: The genus Sphaerotilus comprises types in which a loosely-connected chain of cells is held together as a permanent "filament" by a rigid sheath (Fig 3—6).

In an environment rich in iron, Sphaerotilus forms ferric hydroxide, which impregnates the sheath and gives it a yellow or brown color. It was formerly thought that the iron-depositing sheathed bacteria constituted a separate genus, Leptothrix, but it is now evident that "Leptothrix" is merely one growth form of Sphaerotilus.

F. Mycelial Eubacteria (the Actinomycetes): Although the higher actinomycetes form mycelia which resemble the structures of higher fungi, they are clearly related to the unicellular eubacteria through a continuous intergrading series of forms (see above). Furthermore, they share with all other bacteria the properties of procaryotic organisms. One group, the actinoplanes, produce, at one stage of their life-cycle, flagellated cells which are indistinguishable from simple unicellular eubacteria.

There are 4 families, which form an evolutionary series ranging from unicellularity (Mycobacteriaceae) to full mycelial habit (Streptomycetaceae and Actinomycetaceae).

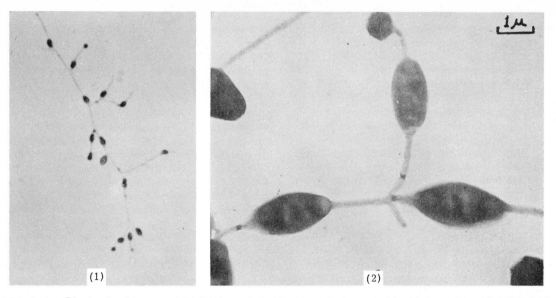

FIG 3-1. *Rhodomicrobium vannielii.* (1) Seven-day-old culture photographed in dilute gentian violet (1800 X); (2) electron micrograph showing constriction of filaments (10,000 X). (Courtesy of Duchow, E., & H. Douglas: J Bact 58:409–416, 1949.)

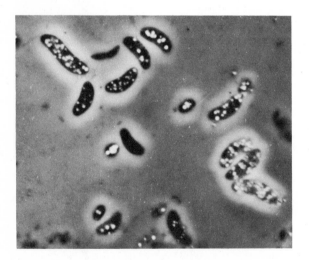

FIG 3-2. Cells of purple sulfur bacteria, containing sulfur droplets. Phase contrast (1400 X). (From Stanier, R.Y., Doudoroff, M., & E.A. Adelberg: *The Microbial World,* 2nd ed. Copyright 1963. By permission of Prentice-Hall, Inc., Englewood Cliffs, N.J.)

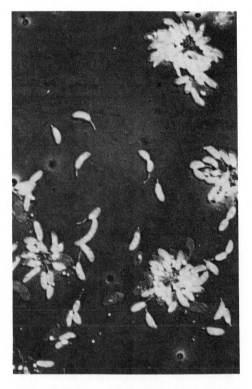

FIG 3-3. Caulobacter, single cells and rosettes (2500 X). (Courtesy of Houwink, A.E.: Antonie van Leeuwenhoek 21:59, 1955.)

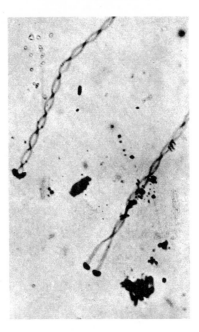

FIG 3–4. Stalked cells of Gallionella major, showing stages in cell division (1200 X). (From Cholodny, N.: Planta: Archiv für wissenschaftliche Botanik 8:252–268, 1929.)

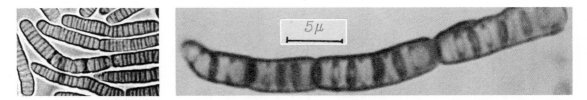

FIG 3–5. **Caryophanon: unstained filaments of** *Caryophanon latum.* **Left:** Live cells (the 2 refractile, biconcave segments are disintegrated cells). **Right:** Empty shells from old culture. Contents lysed, leaving outer walls and transverse cross-walls, many of the latter being incomplete "ring" structures. (Courtesy of Pringsheim, E., & C. Robinow: J Gen Microbiol 1:267–278, 1947.)

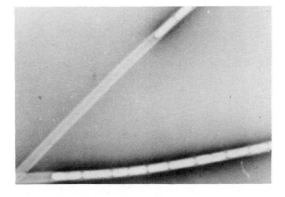

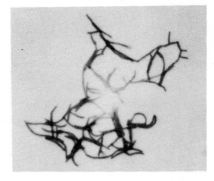

FIG 3–6. **Sheathed chains of** *Sphaerotilus natans* (1400 X). (Courtesy of Stokes, J.: J Bact 67:278–291, 1954.)

FIG 3–7. **Early growth, a species of Nocardia** (490 X). (Courtesy of E.J. Ordal: *The Biology of Bacteria,* 3rd ed. Heath, 1948.)

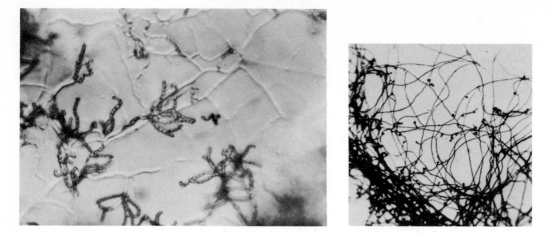

FIG 3–8. Streptomycetaceae. Left: Streptomyces, showing chains of aerial conidia (780 X). **Right:** Micromonospora, showing single conidia on short lateral branches. (From Stanier, R.Y., Doudoroff, M., & E.A. Adelberg: *The Microbial World,* 2nd ed. Copyright 1963. By permission of Prentice-Hall, Inc., Englewood Cliffs, N.J.)

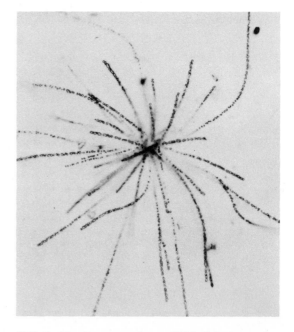

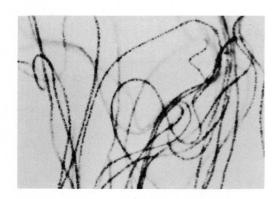

FIG 3–9. Filaments of Beggiatoa, containing sulfur granules (700 X). (From Stanier, R.Y., Doudoroff, M., & E.A. Adelberg: *The Microbial World,* 2nd ed. Copyright 1963. By permission of Prentice-Hall, Inc., Englewood Cliffs, N.J.)

FIG 3–10. A young colony of Thiothrix (a member of Beggiatoaceae) showing origin of filaments from a central holdfast. The inclusion bodies are refractile sulfur granules. Preparation not stained. (Courtesy of E. Ordal.)

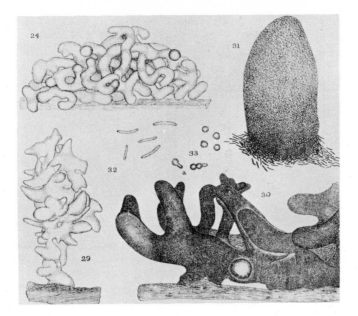

FIG 3–11. **Myxobacterial fruiting bodies (Thaxter).** Part of a drawing from the original article by Roland Thaxter in 1892, which first described myxobacteria. These drawings are still the best pictures available of myxobacterial fruiting bodies. **24:** Coalescent cysts of *Chondromyces serpens;* **29:** Fruiting body of *Myxococcus coralloides;* **30:** Highly magnified portion of fruiting body of *M coralloides;* **31:** Spore mass arising from mass of vegetative cells (*M coralloides*); **32:** Vegetative rods (*M coralloides*); **33:** Mature and developing microcysts (spores of *M coralloides*). (**Note:** Figures are drawn to different scales. Vegetative rods are approximately $4-7 \times 0.4$ μ; fruiting bodies [spore masses] attain sizes approaching several mm.)

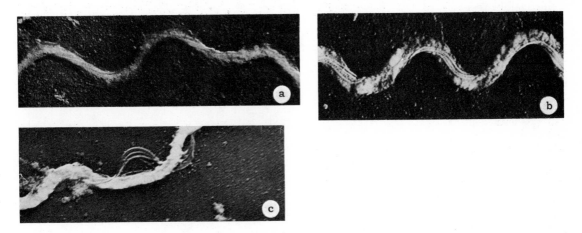

FIG 3–12. *Treponema pallidum.* **Electron micrographs showing intertwined fibrils or "axistyle." (a)** Without digestion. **(b)** After 20 minutes of tryptic digestion. **(c)** After 10 minutes of peptic digestion; several fine filaments have been freed, creating the appearance of external flagella. This artifact accounts for the earlier misconception concerning spirochete structure. (Courtesy of Swain, R.H.A.: J Path Bact 69:117–128, 1955.)

TABLE 3–1. Families and important genera of gram-negative eubacteria.*

Cell Shape	Motility	Other Distinguishing Properties	Family	Distinguishing Properties of the Genera	Genus
Cocci	Immotile		NEISSERIACEAE	Aerobic cocci	Neisseria
				Anaerobic cocci	Veillonella
Straight rods	Almost all immotile	Very small size; parasites and pathogens in animals.	PARVOBACTERIACEAE (BRUCELLACEAE*)	Require nutrients found in blood (hemin, NAD or NADP)	Hemophilus
				Nutritionally less exacting; grow on ordinary media. — Bipolar staining	Pasteurella
				Not bipolar staining	Brucella
	Motile with peritrichous flagella, and related immotile forms	Facultative anaerobes	ENTEROBACTERIACEAE	Mixed acid fermentation of sugars — Lactose-fermenting — Habitat: Intestinal tract of animals	Escherichia
				Habitat: Plant materials	Erwinia
				Lactose non-fermenting — Motile, produce gas from sugars — Urease positive	Proteus
				Urease negative	Salmonella
				Nonmotile, no gas from sugars	Shigella
				Butylene glycol fermentation of sugars — Red pigmented	Serratia
				Not pigmented — Large capsules	Klebsiella
				Capsules smaller or absent	Aerobacter
		Free-living nitrogen-fixers — Aerobes	AZOTOBACTERIACEAE	Free-living nitrogen fixers	Azotobacter
		Symbiotic nitrogen-fixers	RHIZOBIACEAE	Symbiotic nitrogen-fixers	Rhizobium
	Motile with polar flagella	Oxidize inorganic nitrogen compounds	NITROBACTERIACEAE	Oxidize NH_3 to NO_2^-	Nitrosomonas
				Oxidize NO_2^- to NO_3^-	Nitrobacter
		Oxidize inorganic sulfur compounds	THIOBACTERIACEAE	Oxidize inorganic sulfur compounds	Thiobacillus
		Oxidize organic compounds	PSEUDOMONADACEAE	Aerobic — Carry out complete oxidations	Pseudomonas
				Carry out blocked oxidations	Acetobacter
				Facultatively anaerobic — Luminescent marine forms	Photobacterium
				Nonluminescent — Alcoholic fermentation of sugars	Zymomonas
				Butylene-glycol fermentation of sugars	
Curved rods	Motile with polar flagella		SPIRILLACEAE	Comma-shaped — Aerobic	Vibrio
				Anaerobic	Desulfovibrio
				Spiral-shaped	Spirillum

*Nomenclature adopted in *Bergey's Manual*, 7th ed. Williams & Wilkins, 1957.

TABLE 3–2. Families and important genera of gram-positive eubacteria.*

Cell Shape	Motility	Other Distinguishing Properties	Family	Aerobes / Anaerobes	No spores / Endospores	Metabolism / fermentation	Morphology	Genus
Cocci	Nearly all immotile	Cells in cubical packets or in irregular masses	MICROCOCCACEAE	Aerobes	No spores		Cocci in cubical packets	Sarcina
					Endospores			Sporosarcina
				Anaerobes				Zymosarcina
						Aerobes (oxidative metabolism)	Cocci in irregular masses	Micrococcus
						Facultative anaerobes (fermentative)		Staphylococcus
		Cells in chains; lactic acid fermentation of sugars.	LACTOBACTERIACEAE (LACTOBACILLACEAE*) (Includes both cocci and rods.)			Homofermentative	Cocci in chains	Streptococcus
								Diplococcus
						Heterofermentative		Leuconostoc
		Lactic acid fermentation of sugars				Homofermentative	Straight rods	Lactobacillus
Straight rods	Nearly all immotile	Propionic acid fermentation of sugars	PROPIONIBACTERIACEAE					Propionibacterium
		Aerobic respiration; weakly fermentative.	CORYNEBACTERIACEAE					Corynebacterium
	Motile with peritrichous flagella, and related immotile forms	Endospores formed	BACILLACEAE			Aerobic spore formers		Bacillus

*Nomenclature adopted in *Bergey's Manual*, 7th ed. Williams & Wilkins, 1957.

1. Mycobacteriaceae—The only genus is Mycobacterium, pathogenic members of which are discussed in Chapter 17. Most mycobacteria are **acid-fast,** a staining property which they share with some members of Actinomycetaceae, the next higher group of actinomycetes. They tend to form a rudimentary mycelium during early stages of growth, but this breaks up into irregular, branching cells which resemble corynebacteria. They make a perfect transitional group, and the line between unicellular eubacteria and actinomycetes could just as easily have been drawn between the mycobacteria and the Actinomycetaceae as between the corynebacteria and mycobacteria.

2. Actinomycetaceae—The 2 genera, Actinomyces and Nocardia, form much more advanced mycelia, although these, too, tend to break up in older cultures to form irregularly shaped cells. A typical young mycelium of Nocardia is shown in Fig 3—7.

Actinomyces species are parasitic anaerobes; Nocardia species are aerobes. Many are acid-fast. The pathogenic forms are described in Chapter 22.

3. Streptomycetaceae—The 2 genera, Streptomyces and Micromonospora, remain fully mycelial throughout the life-cycle. Both reproduce by spores: Streptomyces by forming chains of conidia, Micromonospora by forming single spores at the ends of hyphae (Fig 3—8). In both cases the spores are formed in the aerial portion of the mycelium, so that they can become airborne. There are no pathogens; most of the useful antibiotics are produced by members of Streptomyces.

4. Actinoplanaceae—This family was set up to provide for the aquatic actinomycetes, Actinoplanes. Members of this genus form sporangia at the tips of hyphae; the sporangia rupture to liberate flagellated, rod-shaped cells which can initiate new mycelia.

G. Budding Eubacteria: These unique organisms, one photosynthetic and one nonphotosynthetic, reproduce in a manner unlike any other bacterium. The oval cells produce a fine thread at the end of which a bud appears. The bud enlarges to form a new oval cell, and cross-walls are laid down in the connecting threads. The cell at the tip of a stalk produces a flagellum, then breaks off and swims away to start a new organism. The photosynthetic form, Rhodomicrobium, is shown in Fig 3—1.

The Spirochetes

The spirochete cell is constructed in a unique fashion which makes its phylogenetic relationship to other bacteria obscure. The spiral cell is intertwined with a slimmer filament, which is composed of a single fibril in some species and of many fibrils in others. The filament is difficult to see unless loosened from the body of the spirochete by enzymatic digestion; too drastic treatment of the cell can break up the fibrils, so that the cell appears flagellated. Fig 3—12 illustrates these statements.

The axial filament lies between the cell membrane and cell wall. It is not a continuous structure but is composed of 2 overlapping sets of fibrils which are anchored at the 2 poles of the cell. Indeed, the cell of a spirochete is analogous to that of a polarly flagellated spirillum: The basic difference is that in a spirochete the polarly inserted fibrils lie inside the wall, whereas in a spirillum they extend through it.

The mechanism of spirochete motility is thus not comparable to that of the flagellated eubacteria. Contortions of the cell body are presumably involved, in which contraction of the axial filament may play a role.

There are 2 families, the Treponemataceae and the Spirochaetaceae. The former includes several pathogens (see Chapter 21): Treponema, Borrelia, and Leptospira. All are parasites, and all are relatively small (20 μm long or less). The Spirochaetaceae are mostly free-living, although one genus, Cristispira, inhabits the digestive tracts of molluscs. Members of this family are all large forms, 30—500 μm long.

The Gliding Bacteria

There are 2 assemblages of bacteria which, like many of the blue-green algae, move by a peculiar gliding motion without benefit of detectable organelles. In fact, one of the assemblages, the filamentous gliding bacteria, obviously consists of nonphotosynthetic descendants of blue-green algae. The other gliding group are the myxobacteria: unicellular rod-shaped bacteria which are highly flexible.

A. Filamentous Gliding Bacteria: In the blue-green algae are found certain pigmented filamentous forms which move by gliding action. Some of these have their exact counterparts in the colorless, chemosynthetic bacteria. Two of the best known "colorless blue-green algae," Beggiatoa and Thiothrix, obtain energy by oxidation of H_2S to sulfur, which is stored as intracellular granules (Figs 3—9 and 3—10).

Although Thiothrix filaments are attached to the substrate by holdfasts, the tips of the filaments liberate single cells ("gonidia") which move by gliding motion. Gonidia aggregate to form rosettes, from which new filaments grow out.

There also exist organotrophic filamentous gliding bacteria: Vitreoscilla resembles Beggiatoa morphologically, and Leucothrix resembles Thiothrix, but no sulfur granules are formed in the organotrophic species.

B. Myxobacteria: These are rod-shaped, unicellular gliding bacteria; on solid surfaces they swarm outward in a layer of secreted slime. Most species form microcysts: spherical or oval resting cells, formed by the rounding-up of individual rods.

With the exception of Cytophaga, the myxobacteria characteristically form fruiting bodies by aggregation of millions of cells (Fig 3—11). In the fruiting bodies the cells transform themselves into microcysts. (This cooperative action of independent cells to form a multicellular structure is observed also in the slime molds, a group related to the protozoa rather than to the bacteria.)

The cytophagas are cellulose-decomposing organisms. Myxobacteria which do not decompose cellulose are capable of killing and digesting various eubacteria and fungi, and are grown readily in the laboratory on killed suspensions of microorganisms.

•   •   •

General References

Books

Ainsworth, G.C., & P.H.A. Sneath (editors): *Microbial Classification.* Cambridge Univ Press, 1962.

Bergey's Manual of Determinative Bacteriology, 7th ed. Williams & Wilkins, 1957.

Skerman, B.V.D.: *A Guide to the Identification of the Genera of Bacteria,* 2nd ed. Williams & Wilkins, 1967.

Sokal, R.R., & P.H.A. Sneath: *Principles of Numerical Taxonomy.* Freeman, 1963.

Stanier, R.Y., Doudoroff, M., & E.A. Adelberg: *The Microbial World,* 3rd ed. Prentice-Hall, 1970.

Articles & Reviews

Marmur, J., Falkow, S., & M. Mandel: New approaches to bacterial taxonomy. Ann Rev Microbiol 17:329–372, 1963.

4...

Microbial Genetics

THE PHYSICAL BASIS OF HEREDITY

In formulating a general concept of the mechanism of inheritance, 2 basic biologic phenomena must be accounted for: **heredity**, or stability of type (eg, the progeny formed by the division of a unicellular organism are identical with the parent cell); and the rare occurrence of **heritable variations**. Genetic and cytologic analyses of plant and animal cells have established that the physical basis for both of these phenomena is the **gene** (the genetic determinant controlling the properties of organisms). The genes are located along the thread-like **chromosomes** in the cell nucleus. The chromosomes undergo duplication (replication) prior to cell division; when the cell divides, each cell receives an identical set of chromosomes and therefore an identical set of genes.

This duplication is usually an exact process, which accounts for heredity; any given gene, however, has a low probability of **mutation**, and mutation accounts for variation. Mutated genes are usually stable and are replicated in the new form in subsequent generations. A gene mutation thus causes a heritable change in one or more properties of the organism.

In eucaryotic and procaryotic cells (see Chapter 2), the chemical substance of the chromosome which is responsible for both gene replication and gene function is deoxyribonucleic acid (DNA). In viruses, it can be either DNA or RNA (ribonucleic acid). One of the basic problems of genetics is thus to explain gene replication and function in terms of nucleic acid structure. In the following sections this problem will be discussed with particular reference to the **procaryotic** chromosome of the bacterium, *Escherichia coli.* In general, however, the material to be presented applies equally to the **eucaryotic** microorganisms: protozoa, fungi, slime molds, and algae. The exceptions are as follows:

(1) Every eucaryotic cell contains several different chromosomes in its nucleus. Following chromosomal replication, nuclear division takes place by **mitosis,** such that each daughter nucleus receives a copy of each chromosome.

(2) Sexuality in eucaryotic organisms involves **cell fusion,** followed by the fusion of 2 haploid nuclei. (A haploid nucleus contains one set of chromosomes.) Nuclear fusion produces a diploid nucleus containing 2 identical sets of chromosomes.

(3) A diploid nucleus may undergo **meiosis,** in which a reductive division first produces 2 haploid nuclei and a mitotic division then produces 4 haploid nuclei. At the start of meiosis, the homologous chromosome of the diploid nucleus pair and exchange segments. This process of "crossing over," together with the random distribution of homologues to the daughter nuclei, is the basis of **genetic recombination** in eucaryotic organisms. All true plants, true animals, and higher protists exhibit classical mendelian inheritance as a result of the meiotic process.

(4) A eucaryotic microorganism may go through meiosis immediately after nuclear fusion, so that the organism remains haploid throughout most of its life cycle. In some eucaryotic organisms, however, meiosis may be postponed for many cell generations, so that the organism is diploid throughout a major part of its life cycle. Many fungi, for example, are capable of such alteration between haploid and diploid phases of growth.

THE PROCARYOTIC CHROMOSOME

Chromosome Structure

The electron micrograph in Fig 2–7 shows the bacterial nucleus to be a packed mass of DNA fibers when seen in cross section. When bacterial DNA is extracted and purified by ordinary chemical methods, a preparation is obtained having an average molecular weight of about 5×10^6. Recently, however, evidence has been accumulating that the bacterial nucleus consists of a single continuous DNA molecule with a molecular weight of about 5×10^9 which is sheared into several thousand fragments by the extraction procedure. Using gentler methods, Cairns has been able to extract the unbroken chromosome of *Escherichia coli* (Fig 4–1). Cairns's pictures show the bacterial chromosome to be a continuous DNA structure approximately 1 mm long. The structure of the DNA molecule is now well known through the work of Watson and Crick; it consists of a double helix made up of 2 complementary polynucleotide strands in each of which purine and pyrimidine bases are arranged along a backbone made of alternating deoxyribose and phosphate groups (Fig 4–2). The 2 strands are held together by hydrogen bonds between neighboring

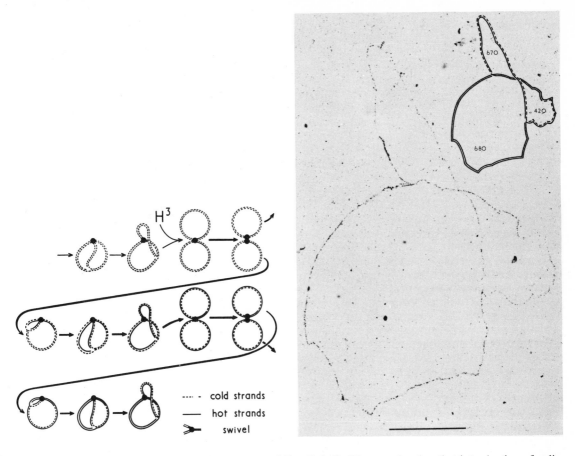

FIG 4–1. Replication of the circular chromosome of *E coli*. Left: Diagram showing that introduction of radioactive tritium (H³) toward the end of a replication cycle would lead, 2 cycles later, to a chromosome labeled as found experimentally. Replication begins at the "swivel" and proceeds counterclockwise along the 2 complementary strands of the DNA double helix. **Right:** Autoradiograph of a chromosome extracted from an Hfr cell of *E coli* 2 generations after addition of H³. Grain counts per unit length in the regions indicated by solid lines are double those in the regions indicated by dashed lines. The numbers in the inset are the lengths (in microns) between the 2 forks. (Courtesy of Cairns, J.: Cold Spring Harbor Symp Quant Biol 28:43, 1963.)

bases; the stereochemistry is such that hydrogen bonds can be formed only between adenine and thymine (A-T pair) and between guanine and cytosine (G-C pair). Thus, a sequence of bases along one strand such as G-C-C-A-C-T-C-A must be matched on the opposite strand by the complementary sequence C-G-G-T-G-A-G-T.

The chromosome of *E coli*, with a molecular weight of 3×10^9, contains about 5×10^6 base pairs. It has been shown both by genetic analysis and by Cairns's photographs to be a circular structure.

Chromosome Replication

In viruses, procaryotic cells, and eucaryotic cells, DNA has been shown to replicate according to the semi-conservative mechanism first proposed by Watson and Crick. The complementary strands separate, each then acting as a **template** on which is assembled a complementary strand by the enzymatic polymerization of nucleotide subunits. The sequence of bases in the new strand is rigidly dictated by the hydrogen bonding possibilities described above, ie, wherever the template carries adenine the new strand will acquire a thymine, etc. Replication thus leads to the formation of 2 new double helices, each identical with the original double helix.

The bacterial chromosome replicates sequentially along the entire structure, starting at a particular site called the **replicator**. There may be several replicators on the chromosome, with only one functioning during a particular cycle of replication. In order for chromosomal replication to keep in step with cell division, some type of regulatory system must exist. It has been postulated that a gene elsewhere on the chromosome produces a regulator substance, or "initiator." Replication would then start when a molecule of initiator combines with a replicator. Control of replication, according to this model, would involve activation

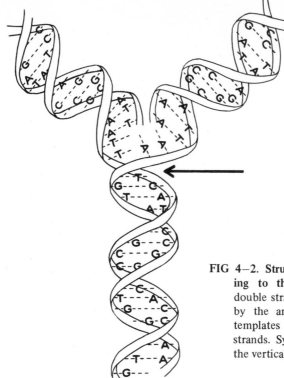

FIG 4–2. Structure and replication of DNA according to the Watson-Crick model. The vertical double strand is unwinding at the point indicated by the arrow, and the 2 arms have acted as templates for the synthesis of complementary strands. Synthesis is proceeding downward along the vertical double strand.

or inhibition of initiator formation or action (or both).

In a bacterial cell, several different genetic (DNA) structures may be present and replicating independently at the same time; eg, chromosome, sex factor (see p 41), and bacteriophage particles. The term **replicon** has been coined to describe an independent unit of replication.

Chromosome Function

The chromosome, consisting of about 1×10^7 nucleotide pairs, is subdivided into segments each of which determines the amino acid sequence, and hence the structure, of a discrete protein. These proteins, as enzymes and as components of membranes and other cell structures, determine all the properties of the organism. A segment of chromosomal DNA which determines the structure of a discrete protein is called a unit of genetic function or a **gene**. The mechanism by which the sequence of nucleotides in a gene determines the sequence of amino acids in a protein is as follows:

(1) An RNA polymerase forms a single polyribonucleotide strand, called "messenger RNA (mRNA)," using DNA as a template. The mRNA has a nucleotide sequence complementary to one of the strands in the DNA double helix.

(2) Amino acids are enzymatically activated and transferred to specific adaptor molecules of RNA, called "soluble RNA (sRNA)." Each adaptor molecule has at one end a triplet of bases complementary to a triplet of bases on mRNA, and at the other end its specific amino acid.

(3) mRNA and sRNA comes together on the surface of the ribosomes. As each sRNA finds its complementary nucleotide triplet on mRNA, the amino acid which it carries is put into peptide linkage with the amino acid of the preceding (neighboring) sRNA molecule. The polypeptide grows sequentially until the entire mRNA molecule has been translated into a corresponding sequence of amino acids. This concept is diagrammed in Fig 4–3.

Thus, the nucleotide sequence of the DNA gene represents a code which determines, through the mediation of mRNA, the structure of a specific protein. In many cases such proteins act as subunits which polymerize to form active enzymes; many high molecular weight enzymes are now known to be made up of identical subunits having molecular weights in the range of 10^4 to 10^5. The triplet code requires that a gene governing the formation of a protein of molecular weight 10^5 should contain on the order of 2000 nucleotide pairs; the chromosome of *E coli* has sufficient DNA for 5000 such genes.

MUTATION

Mutation at the Molecular Level

Any change in the nucleotide sequence of a gene which changes the structure—and hence the function—

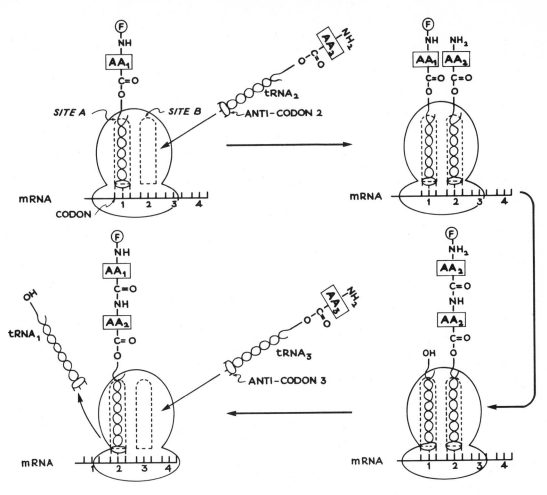

FIG 4–3. **Four stages in the lengthening of a polypeptide chain on the surface of a 70 S ribosome. Top left:** A tRNA molecule, bearing the anti-codon complementary to codon 1 at one and AA_1 at the other, binds to site A. AA_1 is attached to the tRNA through its carboxyl group; its amino nitrogen bears a formyl group (F). **Top right:** A tRNA molecule, bearing AA_2, binds to site B; its anti-codon is complementary to codon 2. **Bottom right:** An enzyme complex catalyses the transfer of AA_1 to the amino group of AA_2, forming a peptide bond. (Note that transfer in the opposite direction is blocked by the prior formulation of the amino group of AA_1). **Bottom left:** The ribosome moves to the right, so that sites A and B are now opposite codons 2 and 3; in the process, $tRNA_1$ is displaced and $tRNA_2$ moves to site A. Site B is again vacant, and is ready to accept $tRNA_3$ bearing AA_3. (When the polypeptide is completed and released, the formyl group is enzymatically removed.) (Redrawn and reproduced by permission of Stanier, R.Y., Doudoroff, M., & E.A. Adelberg: *The Microbial World,* 3rd ed. Copyright 1970. Prentice-Hall Inc., Englewood Cliffs, N.J.)

of a specific protein constitutes a mutation. The nucleotide sequence can conceivably change in either of 2 ways: by substitution of one base-pair for another as the result of an error during replication; or by breakages of the sugar-phosphate backbone of DNA with subsequent deletion or inversion of the segment between the breaks.

A. Sequence Changes Due to Base-Pair Substitution: Many mutations are capable of reversion, ie, the original base sequence can be restored. There is ample evidence that most revertible mutations involve only a single base-pair change, resulting from a replication error. The position of such "point mutations" can be accurately mapped within the structural gene by crossing 2 mutants and measuring the frequency with which they recombine to produce a nonmutant ("wild type") sequence. (See Recombination, below, and pertinent sections in Chapter 5.) When this is done, all point mutations are found to recombine with each other and to occupy positions along a one-dimensional genetic map.

1. Spontaneous mutation—As pointed out by Watson and Crick in their first paper on the structure of DNA, the most likely basis of spontaneous point

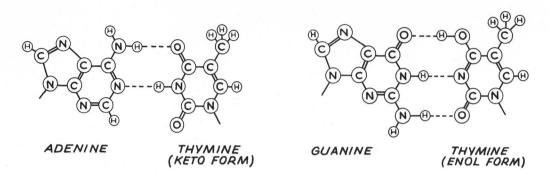

ADENINE   **THYMINE**   **GUANINE**   **THYMINE**
                   (KETO FORM)   **(ENOL FORM)**

FIG 4–4. Base pairing in DNA. Left: Thymine in its normal (keto) state forms 2 hydrogen bonds with adenine. **Right**: Thymine may exist in the enol state as the result of a rare tautomeric shift of electrons. In this state, thymine forms 3 hydrogen bonds with guanine. If the tautomeric shift occurred during replication, guanine would be incorporated into DNA in place of adenine, and a G-C pair would ultimately replace an A-T pair in the nucleotide sequence.

mutations is a rare tautomeric shift of electrons in a purine or pyrimidine base. For example, thymine normally exists in the keto state, in which state it forms a hydrogen bond with adenine. If, however, thymine exists in the rare enol state at the moment that it is acting as template during DNA replication, it will form a hydrogen bond with guanine instead (Fig 4–4). The new strand will then carry a guanine in place of adenine, and in all future replications a guanine and cytosine (G-C) pair will be formed where the original DNA carried an adenine and thymine (A-T) pair.

Any of the 4 bases is capable of tautomerization at a rate compatible with the observed rates of spontaneous mutation, and it is possible that many spontaneous mutations have occurred by this mechanism. The evidence comes from experiments in which spontaneous mutations have been reversed by mutagenic agents of the types discussed below.

2. Induced mutation—Several types of mutagenic agents apparently act by greatly increasing the rate of tautomerization of the bases, or by otherwise permitting hydrogen bond formation with a "wrong" base during replication. For example, 5-bromouracil is mutagenic because it is incorporated into DNA in place of thymine, and tautomerizes to the enol form more frequently than thymine. 2-Aminopurine acts similarly, being incorporated in place of adenine. It is capable of forming hydrogen bonds with cytosine in either of its tautomeric forms, and thus can cause G-C pairs to replace A-T pairs.

Certain mutagens act by chemically altering the bases in DNA in such a way as to promote a replication error. Nitrous acid, for example, deaminates adenine, guanine, or cytosine. The deaminated product of adenine (hypoxanthine) forms hydrogen bonds with cytosine instead of thymine, causing an A-T to be replaced by G-C at a later replication; the deaminated product of cytosine (uracil) forms hydrogen bonds with adenine instead of guanine, causing a G-C pair to be replaced by A-T at a later replication. (Deamination of guanine to xanthine does not change the hydrogen bonding possibilities.)

The most effective chemical mutagens known are certain alkylating agents, of which ethylmethane-sulfonate is a good example. These agents preferentially ethylate the 7 position of guanine and, to a lesser extent, of adenine. The ethylated base promotes base-pair substitution during subsequent replication; more frequently, however, the ethylated base is spontaneously hydrolyzed off of the DNA strand, leaving a "purine gap" at that position. At the next replication, a "wrong" base is often inserted opposite the gap, causing a heritable base-pair substitution.

The mutagen proflavine (and, in rare instances, ethylating agents) acts in a different way. Proflavine intercalates between the stacked base-pairs of DNA in such a way as to cause the **insertion** or **deletion** of a single base-pair during replication. This shifts the "reading frame" of the coded message from that point on, forming an entirely new set of triplets. For example, if a portion of the correct messages reads –/AGG/CTC/CAA/GCC/GAT/TCG/–, deletion of the fourth base changes the message to –AGG/TCC/AAG/CCG/ATT/CG–. This mechanism of mutation has been proved by showing that a second proflavine-induced mutation near the first one can reverse the effect of the first by restoring the reading frame. In the above hypothetical case, imagine that a second proflavine treatment causes insertion of a G between the seventh and eighth bases. The new sequence is now –AGG/TCC/AGA/GCC/GAT/TCG/–. Note that the final message differs from the wild type sequence only in the second and third triplets; if these code for amino acids that are not critical to the functioning of the protein produced by this gene, wild type activity will have been restored. Either of the proflavine-induced mutations alone, however, produces a reading frame shift leading to "missense triplets" throughout the remainder of the gene and thus to the mutant state.

A mutation which restores the function of a gene inactivated by a previous mutation is called a **suppressor mutation**. The above situation is an example of an **intragenic** suppressor mutation. Suppressor mutations can also occur at other places on the chromosome (**extragenic** suppressors); some of these may act by altering the adaptor (sRNA and activating enzyme system) to compensate for the original coding error.

Radiations (x-rays, ultraviolet light, etc) are commonly used to induce mutations. The mechanism of radiation-induced mutation is not well understood. It has recently been established, however, that ultraviolet light (UV) acts principally by causing covalent bond formation between neighboring thymine bases in DNA. Such "thymine dimers" apparently cause copying errors at replication, but the nature of these errors is not yet known. The second most frequent products of the action of UV on DNA are hydrated pyrimidines, in which a molecule of water has been added across the 4-5 double bond. Polynucleotides containing hydrated pyrimidines have been directly shown to cause copying errors in replication experiments in vitro.

B. Sequence Change Due to Breakage of Sugar-Phosphate Linkages: When a large number of spontaneous or induced mutations are studied, many are found which never revert. When a nonreverting mutation is mapped, it is usually found to overlap (fail to recombine with) a series of point-mutation sites. The mutation has thus affected a sequence of bases rather than a single base-pair, and can be accounted for on the theory that **deletion** of a segment of DNA has occurred. In at least one case (involving a mutant bacterial virus), the deletion hypothesis has been proved by showing that mutational sites on either side of the affected region have been brought closer together as the result of the mutation. It remains possible, however, that some "long span" mutations involve inversion (rather than deletion) of the segment lying between 2 breaks in the sugar-phosphate backbone of DNA.

Mutation at the Cellular Level

The set of genetic determinants carried by a cell is called its **genotype**. The observable properties of the cell are called its **phenotype**. A gene mutation can only be recognized if it brings about an observable phenotypic change; such changes may be described in terms of gross morphology or physiology, but in most cases it is now possible to define the phenotypic change in terms of the loss or gain of a particular protein or its function (eg, a specific enzyme or its activity). For convenience, we will discuss phenotypic change in terms of enzyme activity only.

A. Phenotypic Expression in Uninucleate Cells:

1. Gain mutations—When a mutation confers on the cell the ability to synthesize an active enzyme, there is no detectable lag between the time of mutation and the beginning of enzyme synthesis.

2. Loss mutations—Most cell proteins are stable. In *Escherichia coli,* for example, there is no protein turnover in actively growing cells, and a turnover of only about 5% per hour in resting cells. Thus, when a mutation causes the synthesis of an enzyme to stop, the cell remains enzymatically active. If the cell continues to grow, however, the amount of preexisting enzyme per cell is halved at each generation. After 6

generations, the progeny of the original mutant will each have less than 1% of the wild type enzyme level.

This **phenotypic lag** has certain practical consequences. For example, the sensitivity of bacteria to attack by viruses (bacteriophages, or "phages") depends upon the presence in the cell wall of specific receptor sites. The mutation to phage resistance reflects the loss of synthesis of phage receptor. If such mutations are induced, the phage resistance phenotype will not be detected until a sufficient number of generations has taken place to dilute out the original receptors. In other words, there is a **delay in phenotypic expression.**

B. Phenotypic Expression in Multinucleate Cells:

1. Gain mutations—Many microbial cells are multinucleate. *Escherichia coli,* for example, has an average of about 4 nuclei per cell during exponential growth. When a gain mutation occurs in a multinucleate cell, the mutant nucleus synthesizes the new active enzyme and phenotypic expression is immediate. A gain mutation is thus **dominant**; the active form ("allele") of the gene is expressed, and the inactive allele is not.

2. Loss mutations—When, in a multinucleate cell, a loss mutation occurs, only the mutant nucleus ceases to make active enzyme while the other nuclei continue. The loss mutation is thus **recessive**, and is not expressed in the original cell. After several generations, however, the mutant nucleus will have segregated into a separate cell (Fig 4–5), and this segregant cell will be genetically pure for the mutant state. Phenotypic expression of a loss mutation must thus await both phenotypic lag and nuclear segregation.

Mutation at the Population Level

A. Mutant Frequency and Mutation Rate:

1. Relation between frequency and rate—The proportion of mutants in a cell population is the **mutant frequency**. Frequencies ranging from 1×10^{-5} to 1×10^{-10} are commonly observed when individual phenotypes are considered. The frequency of mutants in a given culture reflects 3 independent parameters: (1) The probability that a cell will mutate during a given interval, such as a generation. This is the **mutation rate**. (2) The distribution in time of mutational events over the growth period of the culture. For example, exceptionally early mutations will produce extremely large **clones** of mutant progeny. (A clone constitutes the total progeny of a single cell.) (3) The growth rates of the mutant cells relative to the parental type.

2. Measurement of mutation rate—The mutation rate can be related to average mutant frequencies by a complex equation which takes into account all of the above parameters. However, there are methods which permit a **direct estimation** of the number of mutations which have occurred in a culture (as opposed to the number of mutant cells in the culture) and thus permit a simple estimation of the mutation rate.

The mutation rate is commonly expressed in units of "mutations per cell per generation"; in other words,

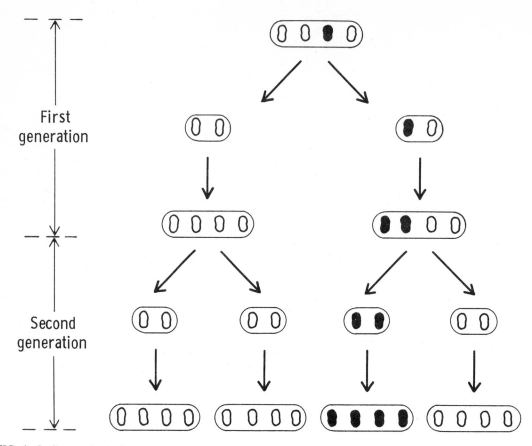

First
generation

Second
generation

FIG 4–5. Segregation of a mutant nucleus. The nucleus containing the mutation is shown in black. If the mutation occurs in a cell with 4 nuclei, 2 generations are required before a pure mutant cell is produced.

the probability that a mutation will occur during the event of a single cell doubling in size and dividing to become 2 cells. When one cell goes through 2 successive generations to become 4 cells, for example, 3 such "cell doubling events" occur (Fig 4–5). In general terms, when N_0 cells increase to form N_1 cells, the number of doubling events is equal to $N_1 - N_0$. The mutation rate (a) is thus expressed by the simple formula,

$$a = \frac{M}{N_1 - N_0}$$

where M = the number of mutations occurring during the growth of N_0 cells to form N_1 cells.

B. Selection:

1. Relative selection–Although any given type of mutant may be present in a culture at very low frequency (eg, 10^{-6}), small differences between the mutant and parent in either growth rate or death rate can lead to tremendous population shifts. For example, consider a culture containing 10^7 penicillin-sensitive (pen-s) cells and 10 penicillin-resistant (pen-r) cells. If the pen-s cells have a generation (doubling) time of 60 minutes and the pen-r cells a generation time of 50 minutes, then after 3 transfers of the cul-

ture, permitting 30 generations of the pen-s cells, the frequency of pen-r cells will have changed from 1×10^{-6} to 1×10^{-4}–a 100-fold increase. After 3 more such transfers, 1% of the culture will be penicillin-resistant.

2. Absolute selection–In medical or microbiologic practice, microbial populations are commonly subjected to absolute selection, either consciously or unconsciously. For example, growth of the above-described culture in the presence of penicillin will lead to the death of all pen-s cells, so that the final culture will be 100% pen-r after one transfer. Since most mutants occur in cultures at very low frequencies, absolute selection is generally employed for their detection. The usual practice is to plate the culture on an agar medium which will permit only the sought-for mutant type to form colonies.

INTERCELLULAR TRANSFER & GENETIC RECOMBINATION IN BACTERIA

The Formation of Bacterial Zygotes

In eucaryotic organisms, the diploid cell formed by the fusion of 2 haploid sexual cells (gametes) is

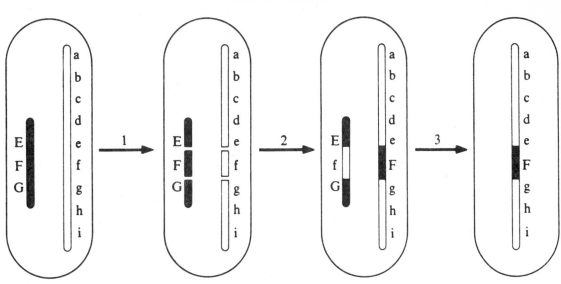

FIG 4–6. **The model of genetic recombination by breakage and reunion.** (From Stanier, R.Y., Doudoroff, M., & E.A. Adelberg: *The Microbial World,* 2nd ed. Copyright 1963. By permission of Prentice-Hall, Inc., Englewood Cliffs, N.J.)

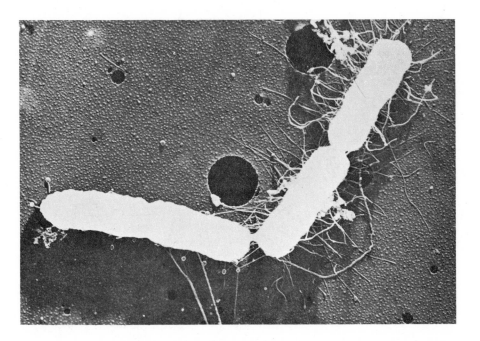

FIG 4–7. **Mating cells of** *Escherichia coli* **(23,000 ✕).** Before mixing the 2 types, the Hfr cells were labeled by being allowed to adsorb inactive phage particles; these are clearly seen attached to the cell at the bottom. The F⁻ partner is recognized by the protein threads, or fimbriae, extending from it. (Fimbriation is a genetically determined property, not related to mating type. The function of fimbriae is not known; they are not flagella.) The Hfr and F⁻ cells are attached by a conjugation bridge. (Courtesy of Anderson, Wollman, & Jacob: Ann Inst Pasteur 93:450–455, 1957.)

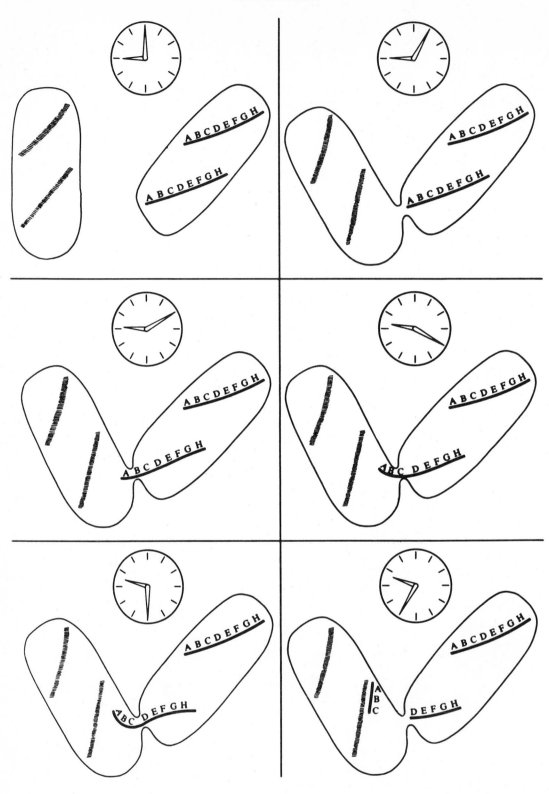

FIG 4–8. The oriented transfer of the chromosome in conjugation. Transfer starts 5 minutes after mixing. By 10 minutes, marker A has reached the recipient; by 20 minutes, marker B has reached the recipient, and so on. Rupture of the chromosome, a chance event, is shown in the diagram as interrupting the process after the entry of marker C. Mating cells separate spontaneously after varying lengths of time. A clone of recombinants is formed from the zygote. (From Stanier, R.Y., Doudoroff, M., & E.A. Adelberg: *The Microbial World,* 2nd ed. Copyright 1963. By permission of Prentice-Hall, Inc., Englewood Cliffs, N.J.)

called the **zygote**. Zygotes may also be formed in bacteria, but true cell fusion does not take place; instead, part of the genetic material of a donor cell is transferred to a recipient cell, and the recipient thus becomes diploid for only a part of its genetic complement. In the partial zygote, the genetic fragment from the donor is called the **exogenote** and the genetic complement of the recipient is called the **endogenote**. Exogenote and endogenote usually pair and exchange segments immediately after transfer. This recombinational step occurs by breakage and reunion of the paired genotes (Fig 4–6).

During succeeding nuclear and cell divisions, the **recombinant chromosome** is segregated into a single haploid cell. This cell can be experimentally detected by plating the partial zygotes on a selective medium on which only recombinants can grow.

The 3 processes by which recombination occurs in bacteria differ from each other primarily in the mechanism of the transfer process. These processes—transformation, conjugation, and transduction—are briefly summarized in the following sections.

Restriction & Modification

Bacterial cells of many species contain 2 enzymes with complementary functions. One enzyme **modifies** all the DNA in the cell; the methylation of bases at a few specific sites on the DNA is believed to be involved. The other enzyme degrades all DNA which is not so modified; this process is called **restriction**.

When a zygote is formed by the transfer of DNA between bacterial strains with different specificities of restriction and modification, the DNA which penetrates the recipient will be rapidly degraded in most of the cells. In a few cells, however (10^{-2} to 10^{-7} of the zygotes), the exogenote may escape restriction and recombination can take place.

For example, a conjugation between *E coli* strain B and *E coli* strain K12 yields recombinants at an extremely low frequency. From such crosses, however, a few recombinants have been isolated which are K12 strains carrying strain B's genes for modification and restriction. Such recombinants show high frequencies of recombination with *E coli* strain B.

Restriction and modification also affect the transfer of phages from one strain of bacterium to another (see p 105).

Transformation

In transformation, the recipient cell takes up soluble DNA released from the donor cell. In some cases, transforming DNA is released spontaneously; eg, it is found in the extracellular slime of certain Neisseria species. Usually, however, it is necessary to extract the DNA from donor cells by chemical procedures and to protect it from degradation by DNases.

Transformation occurs only in bacteria which are capable of taking up high molecular weight DNA from the medium. Originally discovered in the pneumococcus, it was subsequently carried out in Hemophilus and later in Bacillus, as well as in Neisseria. Transformable bacteria are capable of taking up DNA from any source, although they form genetic recombinants only if the donor is a closely related organism. This specificity presumably reflects the requirement of endogenote and exogenote to **pair** before exchanges can take place: pairing of DNA molecules demands close homology of nucleotide sequences.

Little is known about the mechanism of DNA uptake. The ability to take up DNA is called **competence**; the state of competence appears only at certain stages in the division cycle or in the culture, and only a fraction of the population is usually competent at any one time. Competent cells do not take up DNA molecules of molecular weight less than about 4 X 10^5; only double-stranded DNA is taken up.

After penetration, one strand of the donor DNA is integrated with recipient DNA and the other strand is degraded. The recombinant chromosome thus formed consists of double-stranded DNA of the recipient in which a short region of one of the 2 strands has been replaced by a strand of donor DNA.

Conjugation

In conjugation, a transient physical contact between donor and recipient cell is required in order for DNA to be transferred. A true fusion cell is not formed. Unlike transformation, in which only small fragments of DNA are taken up by the recipient, conjugation results in the transfer of long pieces of the donor's chromosome. Conjugation has so far been demonstrated only in a closely related group of enteric gram-negative bacteria—Escherichia, Shigella, and Salmonella—and in *Pseudomonas aeruginosa*. Any 2 members of the enteric genera can conjugate with each other. A pair of conjugating cells is shown in Fig 4–7.

A. Male and Female Mating Types: Male and female (donor and recipient) mating types are genetically determined in *E coli*. Maleness depends upon the presence in the cell of a small DNA element called the **sex factor** or F. Cells lacking F (F⁻) can act only as recipients, and can conjugate only with males. Cells possessing F (F⁺) can act as donors or as recipients, and can conjugate with either females or with males. F⁺ cells transmit F during conjugation at high frequency, although only about one in 10^4 F⁺ cells transfers chromosomal DNA. Thus, the female cell is converted to a male during the conjugation process.

The sex factor carries within its DNA the functional genes which determine the presence of sites on the cell surface for conjugation. The sex factor also acts to mobilize the donor cell's chromosome for transfer, as described below.

B. Hfr Males: Only a small minority of the cells in an F⁺ culture behave as donors of chromosomal DNA. The donor cells in the culture are "mutants," many of which are stable and can be isolated. Male "mutants" are termed **Hfr** (for "high frequency of recombination"); when mixed with an excess of F⁻ cells, every Hfr cell in the culture transfers chromosomal DNA to a female. The following facts have emerged from studies on Hfr mutants:

1. An Hfr mutant transmits its chromosome in an oriented manner, starting with a leading end (called "Origin") and continuing until spontaneous rupture of the chromosome occurs (Fig 4–8). The farther a gene is from Origin, the less chance it has of being transferred; in the rare conjugation which results in complete chromosome transfer, the process requires about 2 hours.

2. Each Hfr mutant has its own specific Origin and order of gene transfer. Analysis of a large number of Hfr mutants shows that the linkage group of the F^+ cell is circular; in each Hfr mutation the circle has broken in a different place, one of the broken ends becoming Origin. (See Fig 4–10.)

3. Hfr cells do not transmit free F particles; recombinants from Hfr F^- crosses are usually F^-. However, if a selection is made for recombinants receiving the last marker to be transferred by any Hfr, most of the recombinants are themselves male. This indicates that a sex factor particle (F) is attached at the distal end of the chromosome of the Hfr cell.

4. Hfr cells can revert (back-mutate) to F^+, in which case the sex factor becomes detached from the chromosome and is once more present as a population of intracellular, transmissible particles.

These facts indicate that the "mutation" $F^+ \rightarrow$ Hfr consists of the attachment of a sex factor particle to the chromosome, with 3 discernible consequences: (1) The chromosome becomes transferable; it appears to break at the point of sex factor attachment during conjugation. (2) The broken end at which F is attached is the last point to be transferred, the other end becoming Origin. (3) Attached F prevents further vegetative multiplication of F particles. They are diluted out by growth of the Hfr cells, so that an isolated Hfr culture possesses F only in the attached state.

The "breakage" of the chromosome actually reflects the fact that a cycle of chromosomal replication is initiated at that point. Replication creates a new "free end," which acts as the Origin for transfer.

C. The Transfer of Chromosomal Markers by Sex Factor: As stated above, Hfr cells sometimes revert to the F^+ state, F detaching from the chromosome and becoming once again autonomous. On rare occasion the sex factor is found to have attached to it a fragment of chromosomal DNA from the region adjacent to its former site of attachment. The new element, with its included chromosomal DNA, replicates autonomously and is transferred at very high frequency. (See Fig 4–10.)

For example, in the strain labeled "Hfr-2" in Fig 4–9, the sex factor is attached next to the galactose (gal) locus. From such an Hfr, an F^+ strain has been isolated in which the gal locus is now a part of the sex factor. If the F-gal$^+$ element is transferred to a gal$^-$ female, the resulting zygote produces a clone of cells each of which carries F-gal$^+$ and is a partial diploid for the gal region. Such diploids have been of major importance in studying the nature of regulatory genes, as described on p 46.

D. Autotransferable Genetic Elements: The sex factor (F) carries genes which govern the ability of the cell harboring it to mate and to transfer F itself; F is thus an autotransferable element. Chromosome transfer is a secondary consequence of the integration of F and chromosome; if this integration is prevented, only F is transferred.

A number of other autotransferable elements have been discovered in gram-negative bacteria. These include "resistance transfer factors" and certain "colicinogeny factors." The resistance transfer factors carry genes which respectively render the host bacterium resistant simultaneously to chloramphenicol, streptomycin, tetracyclines, and sulfonamides. The origin of resistance transfer factors is obscure, but they are efficiently transferred from one cell to another and are now widespread among gram-negative enteric bacteria. Some of them can act as sex factors, ie, they can cause chromosome transfer in the same manner as F.

Colicinogeny factors carry genes that cause the cell to liberate colicins: proteins which are toxic to noncolicinogenic strains of *E coli*. A single colicin molecule is sufficient to kill a sensitive cell. Only an occasional cell in a clone of colicinogenic bacteria liberates colicin; the cell is killed in the process. Colicin production can be induced by UV light in some instances, in a manner reminiscent of the induction of expression of prophage genes (see p 103).

Transduction by Bacteriophage

In transduction, a fragment of donor chromosome is carried to the recipient by a temperate bacteriophage which has been produced in the donor cell. (A temperate phage is one capable of becoming prophage; see Chapter 9.) As in transformation, only a small fragment of the donor's chromosome is transferred to the recipient. Transduction occurs in many bacterial genera. First discovered in Salmonella, it has since been shown to occur in the gram-negative organisms Escherichia, Shigella, Pseudomonas, Vibrio, and Proteus as well as in the gram-positive organisms Staphylococcus and Bacillus. Transduction may be generalized or restricted: in **generalized transduction**, the phage has a roughly equal chance of carrying any segment of the donor's chromosome; in **restricted transduction**, the transducing particles carry only those segments which are immediately adjacent to the site of prophage attachment.

A. Restricted Transduction: The mechanism of prophage attachment is shown in Fig 9–8, for phage λ (lambda). When λ is induced, λDNA is detached from the chromosome by the reversal of the steps shown in Fig 9–8; detachment is followed by phage replication, maturation, and host cell lysis. As a rare event (about 10^{-5} to 10^{-6} of the cells), the cross-over event occurs at a different position, generating a transducing particle in which part of the λ genome has been replaced by a segment of host chromosome (Fig 4–10). (The transducing particles, lacking certain essential phage genes, are defective; they cannot replicate or mature unless the cell is simultaneously infected with a normal phage

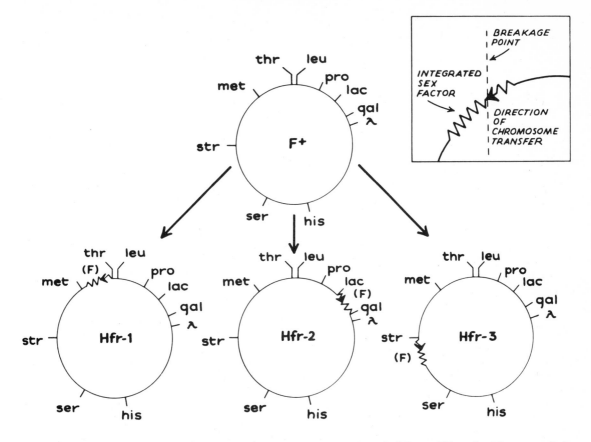

FIG 4–9. Integration of the sex factor and F⁺ chromosome to produce 3 different Hfr males. The upper circle represents the F⁺ chromosome; only a few of the known genetic loci, or "markers," are shown. The lower circles represent cases in which the sex factor (F) has integrated with the chromosome between met and thr, between lac and gal, and between str and ser, respectively. (The three-letter symbols represent genes governing biochemical activities of the cell, eg, "lac," the set of loci governing the utilization of β-galactosides; "his," the set of loci governing the biosynthesis of histidine, etc).

that supplies the missing phage gene products.) When the transducing particle is adsorbed by a recipient cell, it injects its DNA in the normal fashion; the recipient thus receives a segment of the donor's chromosome.

B. Generalized Transduction: Generalized transducing phages are capable of incorporating host DNA by the mechanism described above. The great majority of their transducing particles, however, contain only host DNA; it thus appears that phage heads can be assembled around condensed segments of host DNA as well as around condensed phage genomes. The mechanism by which this assembly takes place is not known. It is only known that the products of certain phage genes are essential for normal head assembly; presumably these "morphopoietic factors" complex with phage DNA and provide a matrix for assembly of the head subunits. Transducing phage particles may thus arise when morphopoietic factors complex with fragments of host DNA of the right size. As in restricted transduction, only about one particle in 10^5 or 10^6 is a transducing particle.

C. High-Frequency Transduction: In restricted transduction, the transducing particle contains part of a phage genome linked to a segment of host DNA. When this is injected into the recipient, the entire DNA structure becomes integrated into the bacterial chromosome. The transduced recipient then produces a clone of cells every one of which carries the defective prophage plus the extra segment of donor DNA. If these cells also carry a normal prophage (as a result of simultaneous infection of the original recipient by a normal particle and a transducing particle), then, on induction, a lysate is produced in which half of the particles are transducing particles. This is the phenomenon of "high-frequency transduction."

D. Abortive Transduction: In high-frequency transduction the transducing particle persists and replicates. In many low-frequency transductions, however, failure of the exogenote to be integrated may lead to persistence without replication. Thus, when the zygote divides, only one of the daughter cells receives the exogenote. In further cell generations, the exogenote is again transmitted without replicating, so that only one

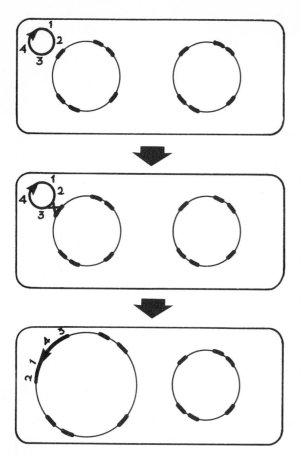

GENES OF STRUCTURE & GENES OF REGULATION

A gene which determines the structure of a particular protein (eg, an enzyme) is called a **structural gene.** The activity of a structural gene, in terms of production of messenger RNA for enzyme synthesis, is strictly regulated in the cell. It has been shown that many structural genes lie adjacent to specific sites concerned with the regulation of structural gene activity. Such a site is called an **operator.** Under certain conditions, the cell produces cytoplasmic substances called **repressors;** when an operator gene binds its specific repressor substance, the structural gene adjacent to it is prevented from producing mRNA and is thus inactivated. In many cases, a series of structural genes determining a series of coordinated enzymes (eg, the enzymes of a particular metabolic pathway) form a continuous segment of DNA under the control of a single adjacent operator gene. A gene sequence under the coordinated control of single operator is called an **operon.**

Each specific type of repressor molecule of the cell must, of course, be formed by its own structural gene. A gene concerned with the production of a repressor substance is called a **regulator gene.** Both operator genes and regulator genes can be detected when they occur in mutant form. For example, the operator can mutate to a state in which it is unable to bind repressor. The operon now functions under all conditions, and is said to be "derepressed."

Mutations of the regulator gene produce phenotypes similar to those produced by mutations of the corresponding operator gene. For example, a mutated regulator gene may fail to make repressor, giving rise to the derepressed phenotype (Fig 4–11). Regulator genes can be distinguished from operator genes, however, by the behavior of diploid cells carrying one normal gene and one mutated gene. In such diploids the derepressed state is **dominant** if the mutation has altered the operator gene but **recessive** if the mutation has inactivated the regulator gene.

The biochemical basis of enzyme regulation will be discussed in Chapter 5.

FIG 4–10. **The attachment of F to chromosome.** The sex factor (F) is shown as a smaller circle, not drawn to scale. The dark segments along the chromosome (larger circle) represent sites having base-pair homology with F DNA. The numbers represent regions of F DNA; the arrowhead represents the site at which the circle breaks at the time of conjugal transfer.

cell in the clone at any given time is a partial diploid. This situation is called "abortive transduction."

In abortive transduction, as in high-frequency transduction, the genes of the exogenote function normally. Thus, if a gal^+/gal^- cell is produced by an abortive transduction, the cell in which the non-replicating gal^+ gene resides will produce the galactose-fermenting enzyme. During further generations the clone of cells arising from each gal^- segregant will produce no more enzyme, and the enzyme will be diluted out by the cell division process. If a gal^+/gal^- abortive transductant is plated on a medium in which galactose is the sole source of carbon and energy, it will produce a minute colony (containing about 10^6 cells) after 4 days of growth as a result of the limited production of the galactose-fermenting enzyme. (A normal gal^+ cell would produce a very large colony, containing over 10^9 cells, in 2 days of growth.) The production of a minute colony as the result of abortive transduction is shown in Fig 4–12.

GENETICS OF DRUG RESISTANCE

Bacteria can become resistant to drugs by any one of 3 genetic mechanisms: mutation, recombination, or the acquisition of a plasmid carrying drug resistance genes.

Mutation to Drug Resistance

Mutations occurring in genes on the bacterial chromosome may confer drug resistance on the cell. Such mutations are of the ordinary kinds described on pp 36–40, occurring at rates of 10^{-5} to 10^{-9} per

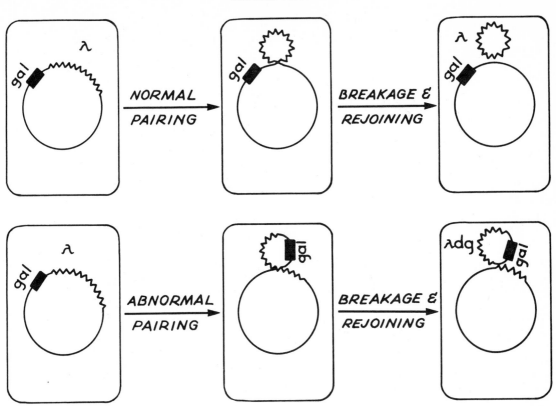

FIG 4–11. Upper Row: Detachment of λ prophage to form a normal λ vegetative DNA. **Lower Row**: Detachment of λ prophage to form λ dg DNA, which will mature as a transducing particle. ("λ dg" is an abbreviation for "lambda defective carrying gal genes.")

cell per generation. They are discussed further in Chapter 10.

Recombination

Once a mutation to drug resistance has arisen in a population of bacterial cells, it can be transferred to other cells by any of the 3 mechanisms described earlier in this chapter—transformation, transduction, or conjugation—depending on which mechanism the species in question is capable of performing. Recombination between 2 cells, each resistant to a different drug, can produce a cell resistant to both. The transfer of mutant chromosomal genes, including genes for drug resistance, occurs at a very low rate in nature, 10^{-5} per cell per generation being a rough average for the transfer of any particular chromosomal gene by transduction or by conjugation. The rate at which transformation occurs in nature is not known, but is probably much lower.

Acquisition of Episomes & Plasmids

A genetic element that exists in a bacterial cell in the autonomous state (ie, not attached to the bacterial chromosome) is called a **plasmid.** If the element is capable of alternating between the autonomous state and a state in which it is attached to the chromosome, it is called an **episome.** The sex factor, F, described earlier in this chapter, is a typical episome.

A. Gram-Negative Bacteria: Some episomes and plasmids of gram-negative bacteria are autotransferable by conjugation, as discussed on p 41. This is usually a very high frequency event, so that, shortly after such a plasmid-carrying cell is introduced into a population, every cell becomes infected with it. If the plasmid carries a gene for drug resistance, then the entire population of bacterial cells rapidly becomes drug resistant.

In 1959, during an outbreak of dysentery in Japan, cells of Shigella were isolated and found to be simultaneously resistant to streptomycin, chloramphenicol, tetracyclines, and sulfonamides. The Shigella cells were found to contain a hitherto unknown plasmid carrying 4 closely linked but different drug resistance genes. The plasmid was called **resistance transfer factor, or RTF**; since 1959, many different RTF's have been discovered in England and the USA as well as in Japan.

The origin of RTF's is completely obscure. Some of them behave as sex factors in that they bring about chromosome transfer; they appear to be related to the F factor of *E coli* and—like F—may have picked up genes from the chromosome. On the other hand, the mechanisms of resistance conferred by RTF genes are

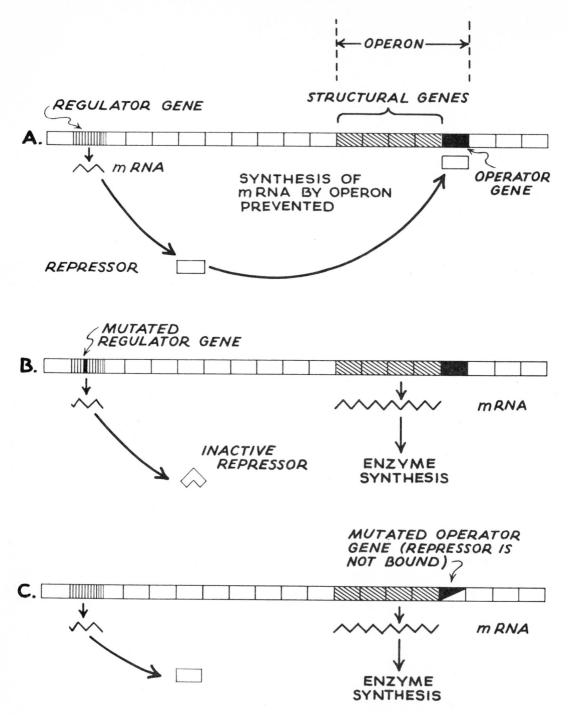

FIG 4–12. Genetic regulation of enzyme synthesis. The product of the regulator gene, the repressor, prevents the functioning of the operon which it controls by binding to the operator site. (Alternatively, the operator may govern a binding site for repressor on the mRNA, so that repressor prevents the reading of the message by the ribosomes.) Mutations at either the regulator gene or the operator gene can interfere with repression, thus permitting enzyme synthesis. (**Note:** Enzyme inducers are believed to act by inactivating repressors. In feedback repression of biosynthetic enzymes, however, the repressor is normally inactive and must be activated by the biosynthetic end product. See p 52.)

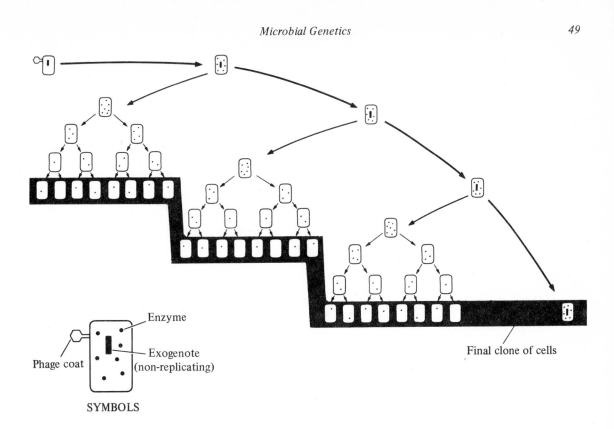

FIG 4–13. Abortive transduction. At each division only one of the daughter cells receives the active gene. The other cell goes through a few cell divisions, until the active gene product (eg, enzyme) is diluted out. Plating an abortive transductant produces a minute colony, in which only one cell is capable of further growth and division. (From Stanier, R.Y., Doudoroff, M., & E.A. Adelberg: *The Microbial World,* 2nd ed. Copyright 1963. By permission of Prentice-Hall, Inc., Englewood Cliffs, N.J.)

completely different from the mechanisms conferred by known chromosomal genes, so that it is not yet possible to establish the origin of the RTF drug resistance loci. Recombination does occur between different RTF's, producing new combinations of drug resistance genes.

B. Gram-Positive Bacteria: One group of gram-positive bacteria, the staphylococci, has become highly resistant to penicillin by virtue of an extracellular penicillinase. This character has never been observed to arise by chromosomal gene mutation; rather, it is determined by a locus carried by an autonomous plasmid, which also carries genes for resistance to

mercurous ion and to erythromycin. Other plasmids have been found in staphylococci which carry genes for resistance to a variety of antibiotics.

That the resistance genes are carried on plasmids is known from experiments showing that they are simultaneously lost at cell division at a rate of about 10^{-3} per cell per generation, and that they have a UV target size comparable to that of the phage which transduces them. They are not able to transfer from cell to cell by conjugation, but are transferred by phage transduction. The rate of transduction in some strains of Staphylococcus is extremely high (about 10^{-3} per phage particle), which presumably accounts for the maintenance of these plasmids in nature.

● ● ●

General References

Books

Adelberg, E. (editor): *Papers on Bacterial Genetics,* 2nd
  ed. Little, Brown, 1966.

Braun, W.: *Bacterial Genetics,* 2nd ed. Saunders, 1965.

Cold Spring Harbor Symposium on Quantitative Biology:
  Vol 31: *The Genetic Code.* Cold Spring Harbor,
  New York, 1966.

Gunsalus, I.C., & R.Y. Stanier (editors): *The Bacteria.* Vol
  5: *Heredity.* Academic Press, 1964.

Hartman, P., & S. Suskind: *Gene Action,* 2nd ed. Prentice-
  Hall, 1969.

Hayes, W.: *The Genetics of Bacteria and Their Viruses,*
  2nd ed. Blackwell, 1968.

Jacob, F., & E. Wollman: *Sexuality and the Genetics of
  Bacteria.* Academic Press, 1961.

Meselson, M.: The molecular basis of recombination. In:
  Heritage From Mendel. R. Brink (editor). Univ of
  Wisconsin Press, 1967.

Speyer, J.: The genetic code. In: *The Molecular Genetics.*
  Part 2. J.H. Taylor (editor). Academic Press, 1967.

Stent, G.: *Papers on Bacterial Viruses,* 2nd ed. Little,
  Brown, 1965.

Articles & Reviews

Orgel, L.: The chemical basis of mutation. Adv Enzymol
  27:289–346, 1965.

Microbial Metabolism

The principles of biochemistry are the same for microorganisms as for animals and plants. The student of medical microbiology is already familiar with the general principles of intermediary metabolism. The purpose of this chapter is to outline those principles briefly and then to discuss metabolic systems which are unique to microorganisms or which have been uniquely studied in microbial cells.

GENERAL PRINCIPLES
OF INTERMEDIARY METABOLISM

"Metabolism" is the totality of chemical reactions which occur in living cells. By means of these reactions energy is extracted from the environment and expended for biosynthesis and growth as well as for such secondary activities as motility, luminescence, and heat. Energy may be obtained from the environment in the form of light (**photosynthesis**) or by the oxidation of chemical substances (**chemosynthesis**). In both photosynthetic and chemosynthetic organisms, the pathways by means of which the acquired energy is used for cell synthesis are similar and are collectively known as **anabolism**; conversely, the energy-liberating pathways involved in the breakdown of chemical substances are grouped under the heading of **catabolism**. Since many cell materials (eg, carbohydrate and lipid inclusions) are constantly being broken down and replaced, certain catabolic pathways are common to both photo- and chemosynthetic organisms. These concepts are diagrammed in Fig 5—1.

Metabolic Reactions

When the equation for a chemical reaction is written, eg,

$$2H_2 + O_2 \rightleftharpoons 2H_2O$$

several points may be considered: (1) The direction (from left to right, or from right to left) in which the reaction will proceed; (2) the requirement for activation (failure in most cases to proceed spontaneously in the favorable direction); and (3) the case in living cells (how the above considerations apply to **metabolic** reactions).

A. Direction of the Reaction: Hydrogen and oxygen gases unite explosively (energy liberated) to form water; on the other hand, water breaks down to hydrogen and oxygen gases if electric current is passed through it (energy supplied). The above equation is thus incomplete, and should be written as follows:

$$2H_2 + O_2 \rightleftharpoons 2H_2O + \text{Energy (113 kcal)}$$

When hydrogen and oxygen react to produce water, the liberation of energy demonstrates that the chemical bonds in the gas molecules contained more energy than the bonds in the formed water molecules. If no energy is supplied from without, it is this relationship that determines the direction in which a reaction will proceed; ie, a reaction will proceed in the direction that results in the liberation of energy. Such reactions are called **exergonic**; the reverse reactions, requiring an input of energy (such as the electric current in the above example, or heat in the case of most laboratory reactions), are called **endergonic**.

B. Requirement for Activation: Since exergonic reactions proceed with no input of energy, why do not all such reactions proceed spontaneously? Cellulose, for example, can react with oxygen to produce water, CO_2, and a large amount of heat (as when wood or paper burns). Why did not the cellulose in contact with the atmosphere burn long ago? The answer lies in the requirement of reacting substances for activation: Before they can react, they must be raised to a critical energy level. The energy that must be put into the system for this purpose is called the "energy of activation." Once a few molecules have been activated, the exergonic reaction that follows releases sufficient heat energy to activate nearby molecules and the reaction will proceed spontaneously. Thus a match, for example, can supply the initial activation energy for an entire forest fire.

Although exergonic reactions are commonly initiated by supplying activation energy (usually in the form of heat), one other method is possible: **catalysis**. A catalyst is a substance that speeds up the rate of a reaction without itself being consumed in the process. Catalysts, by their action, make it possible to dispense with the requirement for activation energy. (Presumably they act by chemically binding the reactants temporarily, holding them in juxtaposition long enough for the reaction to take place.) In the above example, the reaction between hydrogen and oxygen is

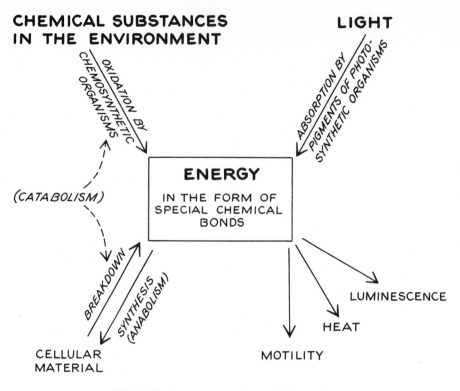

CHEMICAL SUBSTANCES IN THE ENVIRONMENT

LIGHT

OXIDATION BY CHEMOSYNTHETIC ORGANISMS

ABSORPTION BY PIGMENTS OF PHOTO-SYNTHETIC ORGANISMS

(CATABOLISM)

ENERGY
IN THE FORM OF SPECIAL CHEMICAL BONDS

BREAKDOWN

SYNTHESIS (ANABOLISM)

LUMINESCENCE

HEAT

CELLULAR MATERIAL

MOTILITY

FIG 5–1. Energy metabolism of living cells.

catalyzed by heated platinum surfaces. In industry, many exergonic reactions are catalyzed chemically in order to avoid the necessity for high activation energies.

C. The Case in Living Cells: Since living cells must operate at relatively low temperatures, 2 limitations are imposed upon their chemical activities: (1) Only exergonic reaction series can be used for either catabolism or anabolism. (2) Catalysis must be employed since there is no source of activation energy. The consequence of limiting metabolism to exergonic reaction series will be described in the section on the trapping and utilization of energy for synthesis. The properties of cell catalysts are discussed in the following paragraphs.

Enzymes

In order to carry out the chemical reactions necessary for life, cells produce a host of catalysts called "enzymes." Their properties are as follows:

A. Chemical Nature: All enzymes are proteins. In some (but not all) cases, enzyme action requires the participation also of nonprotein ions (activators) such as Mg^{++} or Mn^{++}. When a coenzyme is involved, the protein portion is called the **apoenzyme**; the combination of apo- and coenzyme is called the **holoenzyme**. The substance acted upon by the enzyme is called the **substrate** for that enzyme.

Enzymes retain their catalytic activity on extraction from the cell, and many hundreds have been studied in cell-free extracts. A large number of these have been isolated in crystalline form.

B. Specificity: Enzymes exhibit a high degree of specificity in most cases, catalyzing only one type of reaction efficiently. The proteolytic enzymes, for example, specifically attack the peptide bond. The enzyme is thus specific for a particular chemical configuration in each case; substrates that share this configuration may vary in the remainder of their structure to a limited extent and still be susceptible to attack by a given enzyme. The specificity of the enzyme resides in the apoenzyme moiety: One organic compound (such as pyridoxal phosphate) will serve as coenzyme for many different reactions.

C. Concentration: Any given enzyme exists in the cell at very low concentrations. High concentrations are not required because enzymes are true catalysts and are not consumed in the reactions in which they participate; furthermore, most enzymes have very high turnover numbers, which means that one molecule of enzyme can catalyze the successive reaction of thousands of substrate molecules per minute. Mineral activators and organic coenzymes are likewise used at very low concentrations; hence the low requirement for these substances in nutrition.

The concentration of most enzymes is actively regulated by the cell, primarily by repression of enzyme synthesis. The synthesis of many enzymes concerned with energy utilization is prevented by endogenously produced repressor substances; these repressors are inactivated by the substrates for the enzymes or by closely related compounds.

Other enzymes, called **constitutive enzymes**, are not inducible (the term "adaptive" has also been used) but are formed in the absence of their substrates. Even these, however, may be subject to regulation: The formation of many enzymes of the biosynthetic pathways is repressed by the end products of the pathways, and this provides the cell with a mechanism of negative feedback control. In other cases, the end product inhibits the activity, rather than the formation, of the biosynthetic enzymes. The mechanisms of repression, induction, and feedback inhibition are discussed below (see p 64).

D. Conditions Affecting Enzyme Function: Enzymatic activity is influenced by pH, so that each enzyme shows a characteristic pH optimum, with activity falling to zero about 2.0 pH units on either side of the optimum. Like all chemical reactions, enzymatic reactions increase in rate as temperature increases. However, proteins are generally unstable to heat: the higher the temperature, the greater the heat inactivation of the enzyme. The net effect of these 2 tendencies is to produce an activity curve with a temperature similar to that produced by pH changes. It is generally believed that the pH optima and temperature optima of the enzymes in a bacterial cell determine the optimal pH and temperature for that organism's growth. According to this concept, thermophilic bacteria that grow optimally at 60−70° C should contain enzymes that are relatively heat-stable; this has been found to be the case in the thermophils whose enzymes have been carefully studied.

Enzyme activity may also be affected by the presence of poisons or inhibitors. These are substances that combine chemically with a given enzyme, interfering with its attack on its normal substrate. Some inhibitors combine loosely with the enzyme and can be displaced by relatively large concentrations of the normal substrate. In this instance, the inhibitor competes with the normal substrate for an active site on the enzyme ("competitive inhibition"). In other instances ("noncompetitive inhibition"), the inhibitor cannot be displaced by any concentration of substrate (see p 84).

E. Allostery: Many enzymes are "allosteric"−ie, they possess special binding sites for inhibitors or activators. Small molecules that bind specifically to these sites can drastically alter enzyme activity without being structurally related to the substrate; such small molecules, called "effectors," play a major role in the regulation of enzyme activity in vivo. Allostery is discussed further on p 64.

F. Coenzyme Function: In the course of a catalyzed reaction, the coenzyme is itself changed chemically by action of the apoenzyme. It is thus a special kind of substrate, considered a catalyst because it is regenerated in its original form at the end of the reaction process. This property makes possible one of the most important coenzyme functions, the coupling of different biochemical reactions, by serving as a link between different apoenzymes (Fig 5−2). For examples, see the electron carrying coenzymes (p 55) and coenzyme A (p 59).

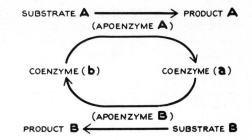

FIG 5−2. Coenzyme coupling. The coenzyme exists in 2 forms, (a) and (b). In the absence of coenzyme, neither substrate A nor substrate B can be acted on by the respective apoenzymes. In the presence of coenzyme, the 2 reactions proceed in coupled fashion, one molecule of substrate B reacting for each molecule of substrate A converted to product A. (Courtesy of Stanier, R.Y., Doudoroff, M., & E.A. Adelberg: *The Microbial World,* 2nd ed. Copyright 1963. By permission of Prentice-Hall, Inc., Englewood Cliffs, N.J.)

CATABOLIC REACTIONS INVOLVED IN CHEMOSYNTHESIS

Chemosynthesis is the process by which cells obtain energy from substances taken up from the environment. If the substance (energy source) that is oxidized is **inorganic,** the organism is a **lithotroph***; if the oxidation substrate is **organic,** the organism is an **organotroph*.**

Most bacteria are organotrophic. For these, catabolism of an exogenous substrate involves a complex series of enzymatic reactions including 4 phases: digestion, penetration, preparation for oxidation, and oxidation itself. Only oxidation liberates biologically utilizable energy, although all phases involve exergonic reactions. If the organic molecule oxidized in this way still retains some usable energy, it may undergo further series of preparatory and oxidative reactions until it has been completely oxidized to CO_2 and water.

Organic material in the environment is, of course, ultimately derived from plant, animal, and microbial cells. Aside from water, the bulk of protoplasm consists of proteins, carbohydrates, fats, and nucleic acids; these, then, are the principal categories of energy sources for the chemosynthetic organotrophs. In addition, living cells contain coenzymes, sterols, and many other types of organic molecules; all are subject to attack by the enzymes of one or many species of microorganisms.

*The terms lithotroph and organotroph, proposed at the Cold Spring Harbor Symposium on Quantitative Biology in 1945, have not come into general usage. They are extremely useful, however, in that they stress fundamental properties.

TABLE 5–1. Digestion of large molecules by exoenzymes.

Large Molecule	Structure	Bonds Hydrolyzed by Digestive Enzymes	Products of Digestion
Protein	Polypeptide	Peptide linkages	Oligopeptides and free amino acids
Carbohydrate	Polysaccharide	Glycosidic linkages	Oligo- and monosaccharides
Nucleic acid	Polynucleotide	Ester linkages between hydroxyl groups on pentoses and phosphate groups	Nucleosides and inorganic phosphate
Fat	Long-chain fatty acids esterified to the hydroxyl groups of glycerol	Ester linkages	Fatty acids and glycerol

Digestion

Many suitable organic energy sources are too large to penetrate the cell membrane and reach the site of oxidation. Such molecules must first be broken down by the cell into smaller fragments; this is accomplished by excreting into the medium enzymes that catalyze their hydrolysis (splitting by addition of water). Enzymes that function outside the cell in this manner are called **exoenzymes**, whereas those that act inside the cell are called **endoenzymes**. "Digestion," whether it occurs in the alimentary tract of higher animals or in the medium surrounding bacterial cells, may thus be defined as the exoenzyme-catalyzed hydrolysis of large molecules into fragments small enough to penetrate the cell.

Penetration

Small molecules, such as the products of digestion shown in Table 5–1, can penetrate the cell by one or more of the following 3 mechanisms:

A. Passive Diffusion: Uncharged molecules will diffuse slowly through the cell membrane until the internal and external concentrations are equal. At ordinary concentrations, such diffusion is much too slow to support metabolism and growth; cells therefore have evolved the mechanisms of facilitated diffusion and active transport.

B. Facilitated Diffusion: In certain cases, the cell membrane contains a system that catalyzes diffusion of a specific type of molecule. This system is enzyme-like in that it exhibits typical saturation kinetics and acts to accelerate attainment of equilibrium between internal and external substrate concentration.

C. Active Transport: In other cases, the cell membrane contains a system that acts as a "pump"; in steady state, the internal concentration of the substrate may exceed the external concentration by a factor of several hundred. Such systems require the expenditure of metabolic energy. All of the enzymatic components for active transport are embedded in the cell membrane, as shown by the fact that purified membranes of *E coli* will form closed vesicles and will actively transport amino acids and disaccharides into their interiors. In one case (alpha-glycosides), the mechanism of active transport involves phosphorylation of the substrate as it passes through the membrane; in other cases (eg, proline), the substrate is concentrated in its free form. The active transport system is inferred to be protein in nature, since its induced synthesis is blocked by chloramphenicol. In several cases, proteins have been isolated from the cell envelope that specifically bind transportable metabolites and seem to play an essential role in active transport.

Preparation for Oxidation

In some cases, the molecule that penetrates the cell membrane is a suitable substrate for an oxidative enzyme, eg, some bacteria possess an enzyme oxidizing

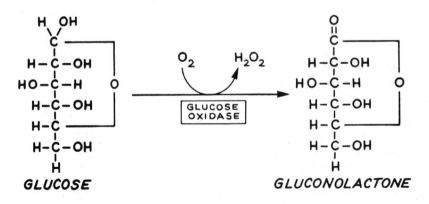

FIG 5–3. Oxidation of glucose to gluconolactone.

glucose directly to gluconolactone (as shown in Fig 5–3).

More frequently, however, preparation for oxidation is necessary; eg, in some bacteria no less than 5 successive reactions must be carried out in order to transform glucose into 3-phosphoglyceraldehyde, the substrate for which an oxidative enzyme exists. There are several types of exergonic reactions that are "preparative," such as nonoxidative removal of carboxyl or amino groups (decarboxylation and deamination), removal of a hydroxyl together with a hydrogen to form water (dehydration), and removal of a sulfhydryl together with a hydrogen to form hydrogen sulfide (desulfuration). The most important reaction, however, is the attachment of a phosphate group (phosphorylation), since the phosphate bond permits the trapping of energy (see p 57). The phosphate group can be enzymatically attached in one of several ways:

(1) It may be taken up as inorganic phosphate simultaneously with the oxidation itself:

3-Phosphoglyceraldehyde + Inorganic phosphate

$$\xrightarrow[\textit{Dehydrogenase}]{-2H} \text{1,3-Diphosphoglyceric acid}$$

(2) It may be transferred from one organic compound to another:

$$\text{Adenosine triphosphate + Glucose} \xrightarrow{\textit{Hexokinase}}$$
Glucose-6-phosphate + Adenosine diphosphate

(3) A large molecule may be split by phosphorylysis to yield 2 fragments, one of which is phosphorylated:

$$\text{Sucrose} \xrightarrow[\textit{Sucrose phosphorylase}]{+H_3PO_4} \text{Glucose-1-phosphate} + \beta\text{-D-Fructofuranose}$$

Oxidation

A. Mechanism: While the reactions described above are all exergonic, in general it is only by the oxidation of phosphorylated compounds that energy becomes trapped in a form suitable for later cell use (see p 57). Oxidation is defined as the removal of electrons from a substrate, with removal of accompanying hydrogen ions (if such exist). Most organic compounds lose hydrogen ions as a result of the removal of electrons; hydrogen ions are not involved in such cases as the oxidation of simple inorganic ions (eg, $Fe^{++} \longrightarrow Fe^{+++}$).

Electrons cannot remain free in solution and hence cannot be removed from a substrate unless a suitable compound is present to accept them. In so doing, the latter substance is said to have been reduced. In accepting electrons and thereby gaining negative charge, the electron acceptor also acts to

accept any hydrogen ions evolved by oxidation. In biology, the substance being oxidized is usually termed the hydrogen donor and the substance being reduced the hydrogen acceptor. It should be remembered, however, that it is the transfer of electrons that constitutes oxidation and reduction.

The final result of the transfer is the formation of an oxidized product, a reduced product, and the liberation (or trapping, in certain cases) of energy. The energy liberated or trapped represents the excess in the amount released by oxidation over that required for the reduction (Fig 5–4).

Some bacteria possess an enzyme called hydrogenase, which catalyzes the reduction of 2 hydrogen ions with 2 electrons to produce hydrogen gas:

$$2H^+ + 2\text{ electrons} \dashrightarrow H_2$$

Bacteria possessing hydrogenase always employ other reducing systems also.

B. Biologic Oxidations: Different types of biologic oxidation are classified according to the nature of the final hydrogen acceptor; examples of each type are presented in Table 5–3.

1. Respiration–The final hydrogen acceptor is molecular oxygen (O_2).

2. Anaerobic respiration–The final hydrogen acceptor is an inorganic compound other than oxygen (nitrate, sulfate, carbonate).

3. Fermentation–The final hydrogen acceptor is an organic compound.

In the foregoing discussion the term "final hydrogen acceptor" was used because electrons are usually transferred from the donor to the acceptor in a series of steps. Thus, the pair of electrons removed from the hydrogen donor may first be transferred to a coenzyme, which we will call "A." "A" thereby becomes reduced; we will designate the reduced form "AH_2." Another apoenzyme now catalyzes transfer of the electrons from "AH_2" to a second coenzyme, "B." "AH_2" is thus oxidized back to "A," and "B" has become reduced to "BH_2." This process may continue over several additional steps, as in the case of electron transfer from a hydrogen donor all the way to oxygen. This "bucket-brigade" system may be diagrammed as shown in Fig 5–5.

Known electron-carrying coenzymes include nicotinamide-adenine-dinucleotide (NAD)* and nicotinamide-adenine-dinucleotide-phosphate (NADP),* riboflavin phosphate and flavin-adenine-

*These terms have replaced the earlier terms "diphosphopyridine nucleotide (DPN) and triphosphopyridine nucleotide (TPN).

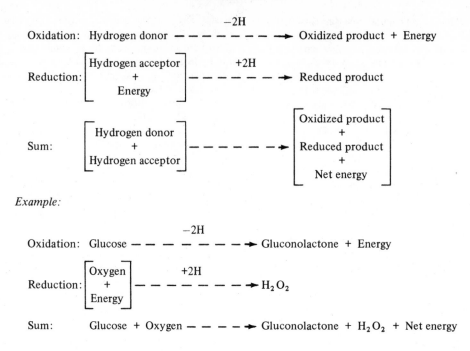

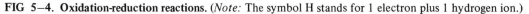

$$-2H$$
Oxidation: Glucose — — — — — — — ⟶ Gluconolactone + Energy

Reduction: $\begin{bmatrix} \text{Oxygen} \\ + \\ \text{Energy} \end{bmatrix}$ $\xrightarrow{+2H}$ — — — — ⟶ H_2O_2

Sum: Glucose + Oxygen — — — — ⟶ Gluconolactone + H_2O_2 + Net energy

FIG 5–4. Oxidation-reduction reactions. (*Note:* The symbol H stands for 1 electron plus 1 hydrogen ion.)

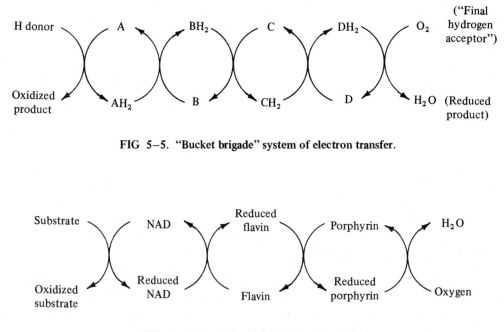

FIG 5–5. "Bucket brigade" system of electron transfer.

FIG 5–6. Example of electron transport chain.

dinucleotide (FAD), and various porphyrins. Different combinations of carriers are used depending on the substrate and on the enzymes present in the cell. In some aerobic oxidations, the complete series of carriers is required as shown in Fig 5–6.

The relative position of the carrier in the "bucket brigade" is determined by its oxidation-reduction potential (relative affinity for electrons).

Other aerobic oxidations employ only the flavin "FAD" as intermediate carrier; hydrogen peroxide is the final reduced product:

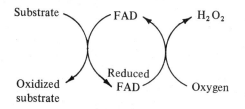

FIG 5–7. Coupling of substrate to oxygen by FAD.

In fermentations, NAD is usually the only intermediate carrier.

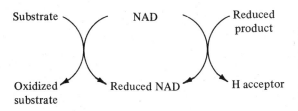

FIG 5–8. Electron transport in fermentation.

Other "bucket-brigade" arrangements undoubtedly exist. However, no matter what combinations of carriers are used they will always occupy the same relative position in the chain. The significance of the "bucket brigade" is discussed on p 59. Note that each coupled reaction shown in the diagrams requires a specific apoenzyme. (In the case of the porphyrin enzymes, the cytochromes, the porphyrin moiety is so tightly bound to the protein that it is not generally spoken of as a "coenzyme.")

STORAGE & UTILIZATION OF ENERGY

In the preceding discussions on metabolism, it has been pointed out that energy for cell synthesis is obtained primarily by oxidation. Since the cell cannot tolerate the temperatures that would be required in order to maintain heat-driven endergonic reactions, a mechanism has been evolved whereby the energy released by oxidation is trapped as chemical bond energy rather than appearing as heat. The newly formed bond can be transferred to another molecule for storage and can eventually be attached to one of the reactants in an anabolic step, raising its energy content to the level needed to make the synthetic reaction exergonic.

Trapping of Energy at Oxidation

In most cases the energy released by oxidation appears as heat:

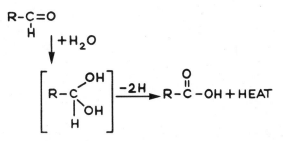

In the above example an aldehyde, such as 3-phosphoglyceraldehyde,

$$R = (H_2PO_3) - O - CH_2 - CH - \\ \qquad\qquad\qquad\qquad\quad OH$$

is hydrated and then oxidized to the homologous acid. About 8-9 kilocalories of heat are liberated per mol of reactant oxidized.

To prevent this waste of energy in the form of heat, an enzyme in the cell catalyzes the addition of a phosphate group instead of the molecule of water:

$$R-C=O \xrightarrow{+H_3PO_4} \quad$$

Now when oxidation occurs, less than 1 kcal/mol is liberated, and the bulk of the energy from the oxidation is retained in the bond between the phosphate group and the organic molecule:

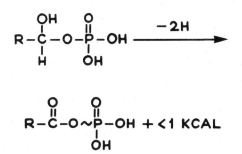

The energy-rich bond is indicated above by the symbol ∼; it can be demonstrated experimentally to contain the trapped energy: Hydrolysis of the new acid-phosphate to RCOOH and inorganic phosphage breaks this bond and releases the missing 8 kcal/mol as heat.

Storage of Energy-Rich Bonds

The newly formed bond is rich in energy because it joins a phosphate (an acid) to another acid, forming an anhydride; the anhydride linkage is characteristically energy-rich. If the phosphate group is now transferred to a different acid molecule, the new linkage will again be of the anhydride type and will therefore retain the high energy.

Certain nitrogenous compounds can also serve as acceptors, forming a different type of energy-rich linkage between a nitrogen atom and a phosphate group; in bacteria, however, energy-rich phosphate bonds are stored exclusively on the acidic molecule adenosine diphosphate (ADP) (Fig 5–9 and 5–10).

Thus energy is trapped by the formation of an energy-rich phosphate bond and stored when the phosphate group is transferred to ADP, forming ATP. The latter can donate energy-rich phosphate groups for the purpose of synthesis, as discussed in the following paragraphs.

The Use of Energy-Rich Bonds for Synthesis

As an example, consider the case of synthesis of the 6-carbon molecule citric acid from a 2-carbon building block (acetic acid) plus a 4-carbon building block (oxaloacetic acid). The condensation reaction is highly endergonic (Fig 5–11).

That reaction, in order to proceed as written, would require an energy input of several kilocalories per mol. In the living cell, this can be accomplished by the transfer of an energy-rich phosphate to one of the building-blocks from ATP:

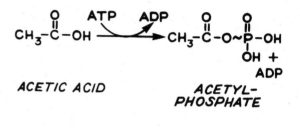

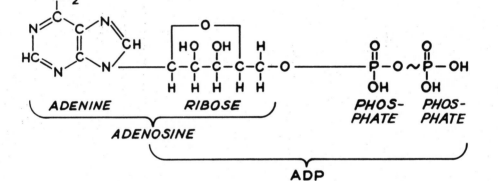

FIG 5–9. The structure of ADP.

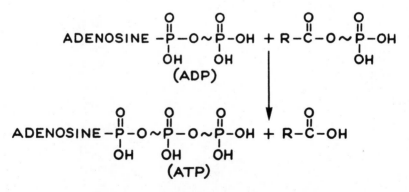

FIG 5–10. The formation of ATP from ADP.

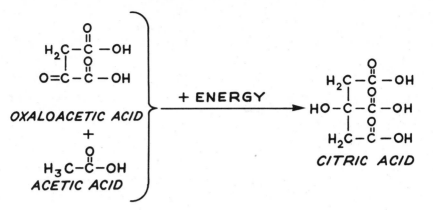

FIG 5–11. Endergonic synthesis of citric acid.

The energy content of the bonds in the building blocks is thereby raised by approximately 8 kcal/mol; the synthesis of citric acid thus becomes an exergonic reaction (since the bonds in the reactants now contain more energy than the bonds in the products):

$$ACETYL \sim PHOSPHATE$$
$$+$$
$$OXALOACETIC\ ACID$$
$$\downarrow$$
$$CITRIC\ ACID + H_3PO_4 + HEAT$$

Note that in the last 2 reactions above, inorganic phosphate and ADP are regenerated, becoming available again for use in trapping, storing, and transferring energy from further oxidations.

Trapping of Energy in Aerobic Oxidations

It has previously been stated that the transfer of electrons from an oxidation substrate to oxygen is accomplished via a "bucket brigade" of intermediary electron carriers (see p 56). We can now examine the significance of this mechanism in the light of our knowledge of energy-rich phosphate bond formation.

In any one-step electron transfer (oxidation-reduction), a maximum of one energy-rich phosphate bond can be generated, yielding a maximum of about 8 kilocalories of trapped energy per mol of substrate oxidized. However, the transfer of a pair of electrons from some substrates to oxygen involves a net liberation of about 58 kilocalories of heat energy per mol. Thus, if the entire transfer were allowed to go in one step, 8 kilocalories would be trapped and 50 kilocalories wasted as heat for each mol of substrate oxidized.

The "bucket-brigade" system avoids this waste by employing a series of consecutive oxidations, an energy-rich phosphate bond being generated at each step. Thus, as many as 4 energy-rich bonds can be formed for each molecule of substrate oxidized by

oxygen, yielding 32 kilocalories of trapped energy per mol of substrate and wasting very little as heat.

Other Energy-Rich Bonds

Energy-rich bonds can also be formed between acyl groups and the sulfur atoms of certain sulfhydryl compounds. Of the latter, the most important in metabolism is coenzyme A (Co A), which has the following structure (Fig 5–12).

In metabolism, those oxidations that result in the formation of organic acids frequently employ Co A instead of phosphate as the energy-trapping system (Fig 5–13).

Acetyl-Co A can now be used to donate acetate as a 2-carbon building block, since the acetate is held to the coenzyme by an energy-rich bond. In fact, Co A acts as intermediate acyl carrier in a wide variety or reactions, a few of which are shown in Fig 5–14. These are examples of the coupling function of coenzyme discussed on p 53.

THE ROLE OF METABOLISM IN BIOSYNTHESIS & GROWTH

Major Functions Served by Metabolism

The major function of any microbial cell is growth. Other functions, such as motility, luminescence, and synthesis of capsular substances, also exist but are often dispensable. Growth is defined as the orderly increase in mass or number of all components of the cell; cell multiplication is a common but not an essential consequence of growth. In some microorganisms, such as certain slime molds, growth is accompanied by repeated nuclear division but not by cell division. The result is the formation of a greatly enlarged, multinucleate cell or "coenocyte."

Since the major cell components (chromosomes, protein-synthesizing systems, enzymes, membranes, walls, flagella) are made up of macromolecules, the

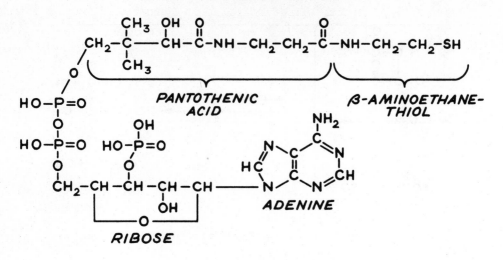

FIG 5–12. Structure of coenzyme A.

major function served by the metabolism of a microbial cell can be more precisely stated in terms of the **synthesis of macromolecules.** These macromolecules are assembled from their respective subunits: proteins from amino acids; nucleic acids from nucleotides; polysaccharides from simple sugars; and lipids from glycerol or other alcohols, fatty acids, and (in phospholipids) special subunits such as choline.

In every case, the condensation of subunits to form a macromolecule requires that the subunit be **activated**—ie, coupled by means of a suitable energy-rich bond to a substituent group such as phosphate (P), pyrophosphate (PP), adenosine monophosphate (AMP), or coenzyme A (Co A). The energy of the

activating group's linkage then provides the energy needed for the condensation, and the activating group is split off in the process. In general, the ultimate source of such activating groups is adenosine triphosphate (ATP).

The arrangement (sequence) of subunits in the ultimate macromolecule is determined in one of 2 ways. In nucleic acids and in proteins, it is **template-directed:** DNA serves as template for its own synthesis and for the synthesis of the various types of RNA; messenger RNA serves as template for the synthesis of proteins. In carbohydrate and lipids, on the other hand, the arrangement of subunits is determined entirely by enzyme specificities.

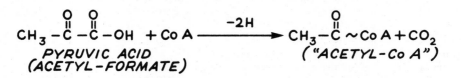

FIG 5–13. The formation of acetyl-Co A from pyruvic acid.

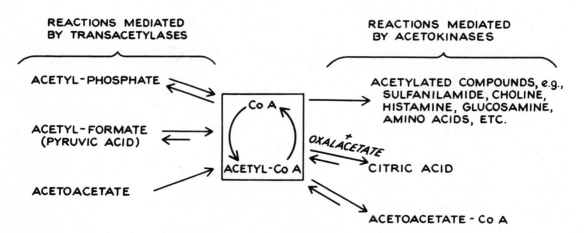

FIG 5–14. Coupling function of coenzymes.

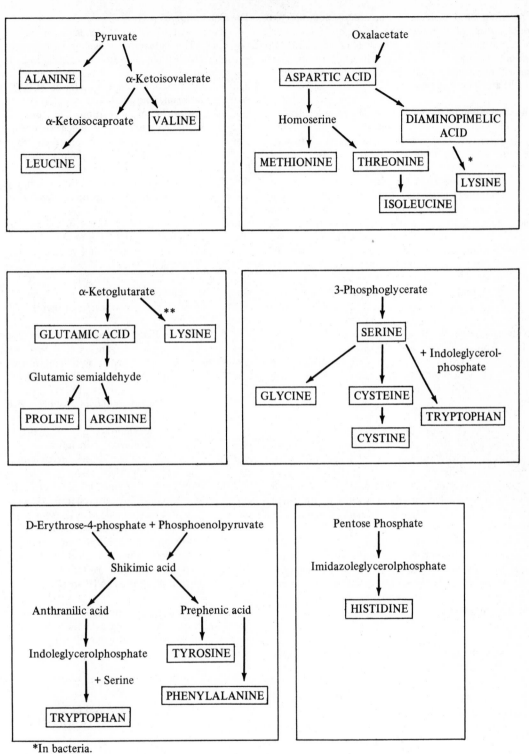

*In bacteria.
**In fungi.

FIG 5—15. Biosynthetic families of amino acids.

Given these systems for the orderly and directed condensation of subunits, the principal functions of metabolism are seen to be 2-fold: (1) to generate the subunits themselves from intermediates of metabolism, and (2) to generate ATP from adenosine diphosphate (ADP) and inorganic phosphate.

The Generation of the Subunits of Macromolecules

The subunits of macromolecules (amino acids, nucleotides, fatty acids, and simple sugars) are formed by biosynthetic pathways which originate from a relatively small number of metabolic intermediates. All of the aliphatic amino acids, for example, derive from just 4 intermediates: pyruvate, 3-phosphoglycerate, oxalacetate, and α-ketoglutarate. The aromatic ring of phenylalanine, tyrosine, and tryptophan derives from a condensation of D-erythrose-4-phosphate and p-enolpyruvate; and most of the carbon skeleton of histidine comes from pentose phosphate. These relationships are shown schematically in Fig 5–15.

The pyrimidine ring is formed by the addition of a carbamyl group to aspartic acid, followed by ring closure; the purine ring is built up by condensations involving glycine, formate, CO_2, and amido or amino groups from glutamine and aspartic acid. The fatty acids are all synthesized primarily from acetate as a building block, while the simple sugars are formed by a series of transformations starting with hexose phosphate.

All of these biosynthetic pathways are outlined in other sources. (See, for example, Harper, H.A.: *Review of Physiological Chemistry,* 12th ed. Lange, 1969.) They are essentially the same in all organisms which possess them. Different organisms lack one or another biosynthetic enzyme system, however, and in such cases the macromolecular subunits must be furnished by the environment. Man, for example, requires 8 amino acids in his diet.

The subunits, then, are either supplied by the environment or are derived through biosynthetic pathways from a number of **key intermediates** of metabolism. As shown in Table 5–2, these intermediates are in turn generated by relatively few metabolic pathways that are common to most organisms.

TABLE 5–2. Pathways of carbohydrate metabolism.

Pathway	Key Intermediates for Biosynthesis
Embden-Meyerhof pathway	Glucose-1-phosphate 3-Phosphoglyceraldehyde p-Enolpyruvate Pyruvate CO_2
Direct oxidative pathway	Pentosephosphates D-Erythrose-4-phosphate
Tricarboxylic acid (TCA) cycle	Acetyl-Co A Oxalacetate α-Ketoglutarate CO_2

The Generation of ATP

There are 3 general mechanisms for the generation of ATP: substrate phosphorylation, oxidative phosphorylation, and photophosphorylation. In all cases, bond energy from a metabolic intermediate or light energy is used to create a molecule of ATP from ADP and inorganic phosphate (Pi).

A. Substrate Phosphorylation: This term is used to describe the 2 steps in the Embden-Meyerhof pathway at which an energy-rich phosphate bond is created: (1) The oxidation of 3-phosphoglyceraldehyde by nicotinamide-adenine-dinucleotide (NAD) in the presence of Pi produces 1,3-diphosphoglyceric acid, and the new phosphate group is then transferred to ADP. (2) The dehydration of 2-phosphoglyceric acid redistributes the bond energy of the molecule so that the phosphate bond of the product, p-enolpyruvate, is energy-rich and transferable to ADP also.

An analogous process occurs when α-ketoglutarate is oxidized to succinic acid in the TCA cycle. One of the intermediates in this process is succinyl-Co A; the energy of the Co A bond can then be used to form ATP from ADP plus Pi.

B. Oxidative Phosphorylation: In respiration, a pair of electrons is passed from reduced NAD to oxygen through a series of catalytic intermediates— principally the flavoproteins and cytochromes. At 3 of the steps involved in this process, the transfer of electrons is coupled, in an unknown manner, with the phosphorylation of ADP.

C. Photophosphorylation: In photosynthesis by plants, algae, and bacteria, a quantum of light is absorbed by chlorophyll and causes the ejection of an electron. The electron is then passed to a coenzyme, and the chlorophyll is reduced by an electron from a cytochrome molecule. The latter step is coupled with the generation of one molecule of ATP from ADP + Pi. The cytochrome is in turn reduced, in one of 2 ways.

1. In cyclic photophosphorylation, common to all photosynthetic organisms, the electron taken from chlorophyll by a coenzyme is transferred to cytochrome, generating another ATP in the process (Fig 5–16).

2. In noncyclic photophosphorylation by green plants and algae, cytochrome is reduced by H_2O. The net effect is the reduction of NADP coupled with the oxidation of H_2O to gaseous O_2 (Fig 5–17).

SPECIALIZED ASPECTS OF MICROBIAL METABOLISM

The Regulation of Enzyme Formation & Activity

The regulation of enzymes is not peculiar to microorganisms; indeed, the enzymes of higher organisms must be even more exquisitely regulated. Nevertheless, most of our present information on this subject comes from experiments with microorganisms.

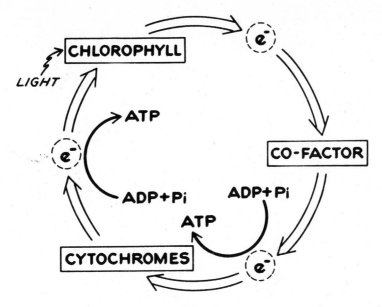

FIG 5–16. Cyclic photophosphorylation.

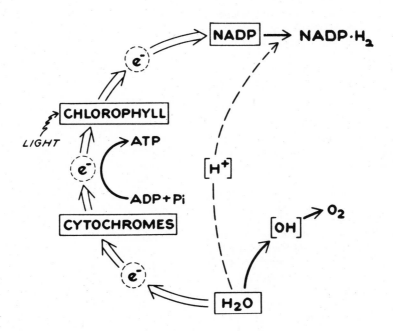

FIG 5–17. Noncyclic photophosphorylation in green plants and algae.

A. Feedback Inhibition of Biosynthetic Enzyme Activity: The subunits of the macromolecules must be synthesized in regulated amounts if, for reasons of cell economy, excesses of any are to be avoided. (This argument is not teleologic but teleonomic—a term used to describe the origin of useful properties in biologic systems through natural selection.) The first level at which regulation acts is the inhibition of enzyme activity: The first enzyme in each biosynthetic pathway (following any branch points leading to other products) is highly sensitive to inhibition by the end product of the pathway. For example, the first enzyme in isoleucine biosynthesis is L-threonine deaminase, which catalyzes the deamination of L-threonine to a-ketobutyric acid. This enzyme is strongly and specifically inhibited by L-isoleucine; other compounds, including many which are much closer analogues of threonine, have no effect. The evolutionary advantage of this system is obvious: As soon as the cell has obtained enough isoleucine for protein synthesis, further synthesis of isoleucine is shut off and carbon ceases to flow into this pathway to be wasted.

B. Enzymes as Allosteric Proteins: The inhibition of threonine deaminase by isoleucine is not competitive; furthermore, several types of treatment (eg, mild heat) will change the enzyme so that it is no longer sensitive to inhibition while retaining full catalytic activity. Such observations on a variety of enzymes subject to specific inhibition by compounds structurally unrelated to the substrates show that the catalytic site and binding site for the inhibitor are completely separate. Enzymes which have, in addition to their catalytic site, one or more binding sites for either inhibitors or activators are called **allosteric proteins.**

The evolutionary advantage of allostery is also obvious, since natural selection can thus produce organisms in which an enzyme activity is regulated by any desirable molecule—eg, a hormone. Indeed, the enzyme glutamic dehydrogenase is an allosteric protein whose activity is inhibited by certain steroids as well as by several other small molecules.

C. Repression of Enzyme Synthesis: In Chapter 4 we saw that structural genes are controlled by specific **repressors;** the existence of repressors provides for 2 kinds of regulation of enzyme synthesis:

1. Feedback repression— The repressors of the genes producing biosynthetic enzymes are normally inactive. They are activated, however, by the biosynthetic end product in each case. For example, the structural genes producing the 9 enzymes of histidine biosynthesis form one operon under the control of a single repressor. This repressor is activated by histidine; therefore, if the cell produces more histidine than is needed for protein synthesis, the enzymes for histidine synthesis are no longer produced. All biosynthetic enzymes seem to be under such regulation, so that the cell never synthesizes a biosynthetic enzyme that it does not need.

2. Enzyme induction—The repressors of the genes producing the enzymes of catabolic pathways, such as the enzymes that catalyze the breakdown of carbo-

hydrates, are normally active. They are inactivated, however, by **inducers.** For example, the breakdown of β-galactosides such as lactose requires the presence of the enzyme β-galactosidase. The formation of this enzyme is normally repressed; if a β-galactoside is present in the medium, however, it inactivates the repressor and thereby induces formation of the necessary enzyme. Once again, the cell is spared making any enzyme that it does not need.

3. The nature of repressor—The repressor of the gene for β-galactosidase (and the other genes of the "lac" operon) has been isolated and characterized as a protein. Indirect evidence suggests that repressors in general are proteins. Such evidence comes from observations on **suppressor mutations** (see p 38). In *Escherichia coli,* for example, an extragenic suppressor mutation is known that restores the activity of alkaline phosphatase, a protein lost by a previous mutation of the structural gene. The same suppressor restores the activity of a repressor lost by a previous mutation of a regulator gene.

Repressors being proteins, their response to specific activators and inactivators can readily be explained by assuming them to be allosteric.

Many of the enzymes of catabolic pathways are subject to a regulation process called **catabolite repression.** If the cell is provided with a rapidly metabolizable energy source, such as glucose, the resulting increase in the intracellular concentration of ATP leads to the repression of enzymes which degrade alternative sources of energy. β-Galactosidase synthesis, for example, is repressed in cells which are actively catabolizing glucose.

The manner in which an increase in ATP concentration leads to the repression of specific enzymes is not yet fully understood, but it has been found that such repression may be overcome by the addition of 3',5'-cyclic AMP. Cyclic AMP is normally present in bacterial cells, and it may be that it serves as an **activator** of the synthesis of many catabolic enzymes. It has been suggested that the accumulation of ATP leads to a decrease in the intracellular concentration of cyclic AMP; if so, this might account for the failure of many catabolic enzymes to be synthesized when the ATP concentration is high.

How cyclic AMP activates enzyme synthesis is not known. It does not act on the operator locus, since both operator-constitutive mutants and regulator-constitutive mutants are still subject to catabolite repression. Rather, cyclic AMP may be necessary for the correct binding of RNA polymerase to the DNA template.

Unique Pathways for the Generation of Key Intermediates

Table 5–2 lists the principal pathways, common to all groups of organisms, by which the key intermediates for biosynthesis are formed. In certain microorganisms these have been supplemented by several unique pathways, including the following:

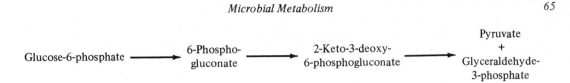

FIG 5–18. Entner-Doudoroff pathway.

A. The Entner-Doudoroff Pathway: In addition to the Embden-Meyerhof and the direct oxidative pathways, many microorganisms break down hexose via the Entner-Doudoroff pathway, first discovered in the bacterium *Pseudomonas saccharophilia.*

B. The Glyoxylate Cycle: A special problem of biosynthesis arises in the case of microorganisms that are furnished acetate as the sole source of carbon for growth under aerobic conditions. Since, under aerobic conditions, acetate is completely oxidized to CO_2 in the TCA cycle, this pathway cannot provide a net synthesis of C_4 compounds necessary for many biosynthetic pathways. Instead, acetate is metabolized by the set of reactions shown in Fig 5–19.

Note that with each turn of the cycle, 2 molecules of acetate (activated as acetyl-Co A) are converted to one molecule of succinate. Note also that several enzymes of this pathway are also those of the TCA cycle; indeed, the glyoxylate cycle and the TCA cycle go on simultaneously when acetate is the sole carbon source. Under these conditions, the 2 unique enzymes of the glyoxylate cycle (isocitritase and malate synthetase) are induced.

C. Other Pathways Unique to Microorganisms: A number of microorganisms found in the soil have evolved specialized pathways for producing their biosynthetic substrates. Since they do not occur in human pathogens, they will be mentioned here only in passing:

1. Nitrogen fixation—Certain bacteria are capable of fixing atmospheric nitrogen (N_2), converting it to NH_3 inside the cell. This microbiologic process is an essential part of the overall nitrogen cycle in nature, compensating for the loss of nitrogen from the soil by another microbial activity called "denitrification." (In denitrification, which occurs under anaerobic conditions, certain bacteria utilize nitrate [NO_3^-] in place of oxygen as the terminal electron acceptor for the respiratory [cytochrome] enzyme chain. In so doing, they reduce the nitrate to N_2, which is lost from the soil.)

The principal nitrogen-fixing bacteria are the symbiotic forms in the genus Rhizobium and free-living forms in the genera Azotobacter and Clostridium, as well as certain blue-green algae. The symbiotic forms inhabit the root tissues of leguminous plants (peas, beans, alfalfa, clover, etc), causing formation of root nodules. In the nodule, true hemoglobin is formed, which is apparently essential to the fixation process. Neither the bacteria alone nor the plant tissues alone form hemoglobin or fix nitrogen.

2. The synthesis of carbohydrates from CO_2—A special mechanism is found in organisms that use CO_2 as the sole source of carbon for the production of

intermediates. This occurs in photosynthetic organisms and in "lithotrophic" bacteria which obtain their energy by the oxidation of inorganic substances (see p 53). In such organisms, CO_2 is converted to carbohydrate according to the general scheme shown in Fig 5–20. Note the requirement for 12 molecules of $NADPH_2$ for each molecule of hexose produced. These are furnished by noncyclic photophosphorylation, as in Fig 5–17, or (in the case of lithotrophic bacteria) by the oxidation of reduced inorganic substances from the environment.

The key step in this cycle is the fixation of CO_2 by ribulose diphosphate to form 3-phosphoglyceric acid (Fig 5–21).

The conversion of 3-phosphoglyceric acid to hexose and ribulose diphosphate via 3-phosphoglyceraldehyde is a complex process involving 12 separate enzymatic reactions. (For details, see Elsden, S.R.: Photosynthetic and lithotrophic carbon dioxide fixation. In: *The Bacteria*. Vol 3: *Biosynthesis*. Gunsalus, I.C., & R.Y. Stanier [editors]. Academic Press, 1962.)

Unique Biosynthetic Pathways: Synthesis of Cell Wall Mucopeptide

For most subunits of macromolecules, as well as for the macromolecules themselves, the biosynthetic pathways are universal. The pathway for purine synthesis, for example, is identical in bacteria, fungi, plants, and animals. There is one class of macromolecule which is unique to bacteria, however, and for this substance—the mucopeptide of the cell wall—a unique pathway exists.

The structure of the mucopeptide is shown in Fig 4–17; the pathway by which it is synthesized is shown in simplified form in Fig 5–22. The major precursors of the mucopeptide are UDP-linked acetylglucosamine (UDP-AcGLN) and UDP-linked muramic acid pentapeptide (UDP-MA-pentapeptide). The pentapeptide, in the case of *Staphylococcus aureus,* is the tetrapeptide shown in Fig 4–17 plus one additional (terminal) D-alanine residue.

The synthesis of mucopeptide begins with the stepwise synthesis in the cytoplasm of UDP-MA-pentapeptide. Acetyl-glucosamine is first attached to UDP and then converted to UDP-muramic acid by condensation with *p*-enolpyruvate and reduction. The amino acids of the pentapeptide are sequentially added, each addition catalyzed by a different enzyme and each involving the split of ATP to ADP + Pi.

The UDP-MA-pentapeptide is attached to a lipid of the cell membrane, and receives a molecule of AcGLN from UDP. The pentaglycine derivative is next

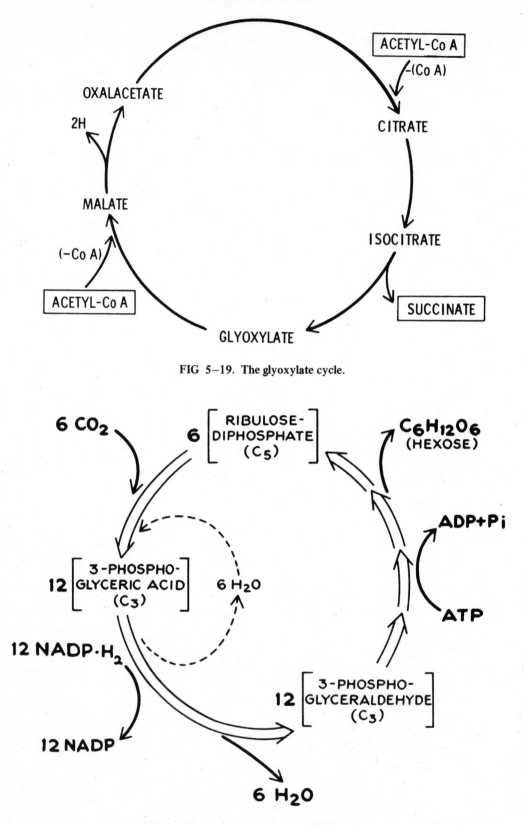

FIG 5–19. The glyoxylate cycle.

FIG 5–20. Path of carbon in photosynthesis.

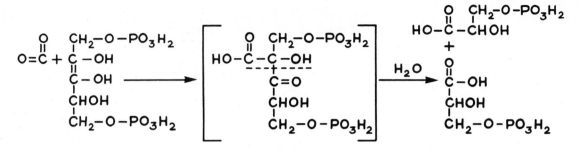

FIG 5−21. Synthesis of 3-phosphoglyceric acid.

formed in a series of reactions, using glycyl-tRNA as the donor; the completed disaccharide is then transferred to the growing end of a glycopeptide polymer in the cell wall. Finally, cross-linking is accomplished by a transpeptidation reaction, in which the free amino group of a pentaglycine residue displaces the terminal D-alanine residue of a neighboring pentapeptide.

This biosynthetic pathway is of particular importance in medicine, as it provides a basis for the selective antibacterial action of several chemotherapeutic agents. Unlike their host cells, bacteria are not isotonic with the body fluids. Their contents are under high osmotic pressure, and their viability depends on the integrity of the mucopeptide lattice in the cell wall being maintained throughout the growth cycle. Any compound that inhibits any step in the biosynthesis of the mucopeptide causes the wall of the growing bacterial cell to be weakened and the cell to lyse. The sites of action of several antibiotics are shown in Fig 5−22.

Unique Pathways Involved in ATP Generation

A. Fermentations: Fermentation can be defined as a class of biologic oxidation-reduction reactions in which both the electron donor and the electron acceptor are organic compounds. From the study of mammalian biochemistry, the student will already be familiar with the lactic acid fermentation ("glycolysis") of muscle tissue, which provides an anaerobic mechanism for the generation of ATP. In this fermentation the $NADH_2$ formed during the oxidation of triose phosphate in the Embden-Meyerhof pathway is reoxidized by pyruvic acid, forming lactic acid as the reduced product.

Many microorganisms, including all of the pathogenic forms, are capable of living under anaerobic conditions, generating their ATP through fermentation. Seven different types of fermentation have been discovered; they differ from each other principally in the pathways which they utilize for the reoxidation of $NADH_2$ formed during the breakdown of carbohydrates. The 7 types are summarized in Figs 5−23 to 5−29.

B. Other Unique Pathways in ATP Generation: In all nonphotosynthetic forms of metabolism, energy is obtained by **oxidation-reduction systems,** coupled with the formation of energy-rich bonds in ATP or in Co A-linked products. Any oxidation-reduction system

can be characterized in terms of 2 half-reactions: the oxidation half-reaction (H donor → oxidized product) and the reduction half-reaction (H acceptor → reduced product). In these notations, H stands for one electron plus one hydrogen ion. For example, mammalian tissues are generaly aerobic, and the 2 half-reactions are as follows:

$$\text{Oxidation: Organic compound} \xrightarrow{-4H} CO_2 + H_2O$$

$$\text{Reduction: } O_2 \xrightarrow{+4H} 2H_2O$$

In glycolysis, however, which is anaerobic, the 2 half-reactions are:

$$\text{Oxidation: Organic compound} \xrightarrow{-2H} \text{Pyruvate}$$

$$\text{Reduction: Pyruvate} \xrightarrow{+2H} \text{Lactic acid}$$

Biologic oxidation-reduction reactions in which the H acceptor is O_2 are called "aerobic respiration." When the H acceptor (as well as the H donor) are organic compounds, the process is called "fermentation."

The parasitic microorganisms, by virtue of their organic environment, all generate ATP either by aerobic respiration of organic substrates found in the host or by the fermentations outlined above. Many soil organisms exist, however, which can use **inorganic substances** as H donor or H acceptor (or both).

1. Inorganic H acceptors—The term **anaerobic respiration** is used to describe metabolism in which inorganic substances other than O_2 are used as H acceptors. These are **sulfate,** which is reduced to H_2S by bacteria of the genus Desulfovibrio; **nitrate,** which is reduced to N_2 by many so-called "denitrifying bacteria"; and **carbonate,** which is reduced to methane by several genera of "methane bacteria."

The sulfate and carbonate reducing organisms are obligate anaerobes that rely exclusively on these H acceptors for their metabolism. The denitrifying bacteria are facultative aerobes, and only use nitrate when O_2 is not available. The reduction of nitrate and of sulfate has been shown to involve electron transport over special cytochrome systems.

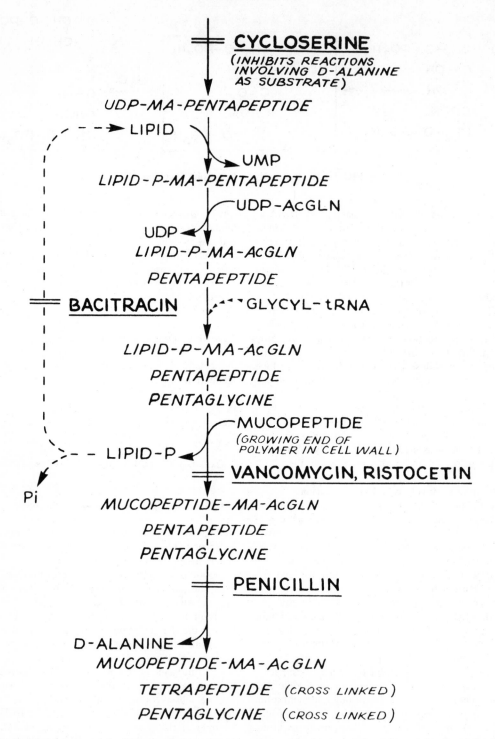

FIG 5—22. The biosynthesis of cell wall mucopeptide, showing the sites of action of 5 antibiotics which inhibit cell wall synthesis.

TABLE 5–3. Oxidation-reduction systems used by nonphotosynthetic microorganisms.

H DONOR	H ACCEPTOR				Organic Compounds (Fermentation)
	Oxygen (Aerobic Respiration)		Inorganic Substances NO_3^-, $SO_4^=$, $CO_3^=$ (Anaerobic Respiration)		
	Organism	Oxidative Half-Reaction	Organism	Oxidation-Reduction	
Inorganic substances (lithotrophy)	Beggiatoa, Thiobacillus	$H_2S \rightarrow S$ $S \rightarrow SO_4^=$	Some "hydrogen bacteria"	$H_2 \rightarrow H_2O$ $NO_3^- \rightarrow N_2$	(NONE)
	Nitrosomonas	$NH_3 \rightarrow NO_2^-$	Some species of Desulfovibrio	$H_2 \rightarrow H_2O$ $SO_4^= \rightarrow H_2S$	
	Nitrobacter	$NO_2^- \rightarrow NO_3^-$			
	Sphaerotilus, Leptothrix	$Fe^{++} \rightarrow Fe^{+++}$	Some "methane bacteria"	$H_2 \rightarrow H_2O$ $CO_3^= \rightarrow CH_4$	
	Hydrogenomonas	$H_2 \rightarrow H_2O$	*Clostridium aceticum*	$4H_2 + 2CO_2 \rightarrow$ $CH_3COOH + 2H_2O$	
	Carboxydomonas	$CO \rightarrow CO_2$	*Thiobacillus denitrificans*	$S \rightarrow SO_4^=$ $NO_3^- \rightarrow N_2$	
Organic substances (organotrophy)	For every naturally-occurring organic compound, a microorganism exists which can use it as H donor for aerobic respiration.		A variety of organic compounds may serve as H donors.		See Table 5–4 and Figs 5–23 to 5–29.
			Organism	Reductive Half-Reaction	
			Denitrifying bacteria	$NO_3^- \rightarrow N_2$	
			Nitrate-reducing bacteria	$NO_3^- \rightarrow NH_3$	
			Desulfovibrio	$SO_4^= \rightarrow H_2S$	
			Methane bacteria	$CO_3^= \rightarrow CH_4$	

TABLE 5–4. Microbial fermentations.

Fermentation	Organisms	Products
Ethyl alcohol (Fig 5–23)	Some fungi (notably some yeasts)	Ethyl alcohol, CO_2.
Lactic acid (homofermentation) (Fig 5–24)	Streptococcus Some species of Lactobacillus	Lactic acid (accounting for at least 90% of the energy source carbon).
Lactic acid (heterofermentation) (Fig 5–25)	Leuconostoc Some species of Lactobacillus	Lactic acid (between 25% and 90% of the energy source carbon), acetic acid, ethyl alcohol, glycerol, CO_2.
Propionic acid (Fig 5–26)	*Clostridium propionicum* Propionibacterium *Corynebacterium diphtheriae* Some species of: Neisseria Veillonella Micromonospora	Propionic acid, acetic acid, succinic acid, CO_2.
Butyl alcohol-butyric acid (Fig 5–27)	Butyribacterium *Zymosarcina maxima* Some species of: Clostridium Neisseria	Butyl alcohol, butyric acid, acetone, isopropanol, acetic acid, ethyl alcohol, H_2, CO_2.
Mixed acid (Fig 5–28)	Escherichia Salmonella Shigella Proteus	Lactic acid, acetic acid, formic acid, succinic acid, H_2, CO_2, ethyl alcohol. (Total acids = 159 mols.*)
Butylene glycol (Fig 5–29)	Aerobacter Aeromonas *Bacillus polymyxa*	Ethyl alcohol, acetoin, 2,3-butylene gylcol, H_2, CO_2, lactic acid, acetic acid, formic acid. (Total acids = 21 mols.*)

*Per 100 mols of glucose fermented.

2. Inorganic H donors—The use of inorganic H donors has been called lithotrophy. (The more common term autotrophy has the more restricted meaning of growth in the total absence of organic compounds, even as growth factors.) Soil organisms are known that can obtain energy by oxidizing H_2S or S (Beggiatoa, Thiobacillus); NH_3 (Mitrosomonas); NO_2^- (Nitrobacter); ferrous iron (Sphaerotilus, Gallionella); hydrogen gas (Hydrogenomonas); and carbon monoxide (Carboxydomonas). All of these are aerobes, using O_2 as the final H acceptor.

Some bacteria can couple the oxidation of an inorganic H donor with the reduction of an inorganic H acceptor. For example, *Thiobacillus denitrificans* can use the following oxidation-reduction system (involving electron transport over a cytochrome chain):

Oxidation: $S \rightarrow SO_4^=$

Reduction: $NO_3^- \rightarrow N_2$

All of the lithotrophs must produce all of their organic intermediates from CO_2 by the cycle discussed on p 65.

3. Unique H donors in noncyclic photophosphorylation—Fig 5–17 shows the mechanism by which green plants and algae use the energy of light to drive electrons from H_2O to such acceptors as NADP. The photosynthetic bacteria use a similar system, except that H_2O is not the ultimate H donor. The green bacteria (Chlorobacteriaceae) and purple sulfur bacteria (Thiorhodaceae) use H_2S or S as H donor in noncyclic photophosphorylation; the nonsulfur purple bacteria

(Athiorhodaceae) use organic compounds. In each case an oxidized product appears, eg, sulfate from H_2S or S. Oxygen is never produced in bacterial photosynthesis since H_2O cannot serve as H donor.

C. Summary of Metabolic Systems for ATP Generation: All nonphotosynthetic organisms generate ATP from ADP plus Pi at the expense of energy obtained by oxidation-reduction reactions. The various oxidation-reduction reactions used by microorganisms are summarized in Table 5–3.

Photosynthetic organisms generate ATP both by cyclic and by noncyclic photophosphorylation. In the former, an electron ejected from chlorphyll by light is passed over a series of electron acceptors and back to chlorophyll, ATP being generated by coupled reactions at 2 steps. In noncyclic photophosphorylation, the oxidized chlorophyll is reduced by exogenous H donors: H_2O in green plants and algae, and H_2S, S, or organic compounds in photosynthetic bacteria. ATP is generated in this process also. The photophosphorylation processes are diagrammed in Figs 5–16 and 5–17.

THE REOXIDATION OF NADH$_2$ IN FERMENTATIONS

In Figs 5–24 to 5–29, the symbol $-2H$ represents the transfer of 2 electrons plus 2 hydrogen ions to NAD, forming $NADH_2$. The symbol $+2H$ represents the transfer of 2 electrons plus 2 hydrogen ions from $NADH_2$ to the H acceptor shown.

Products that accumulate are shown in bold type.

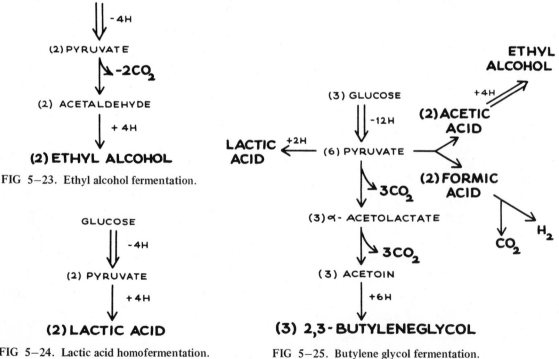

FIG 5–23. Ethyl alcohol fermentation.

FIG 5–24. Lactic acid homofermentation.

FIG 5–25. Butylene glycol fermentation.

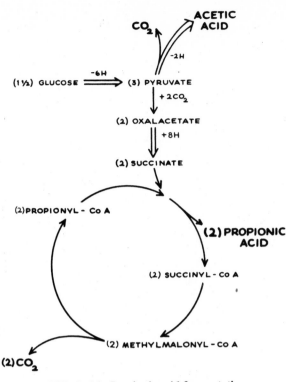

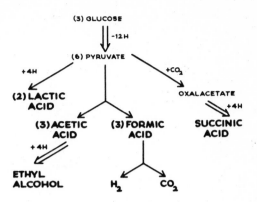

FIG 5–27. Mixed acid fermentation.

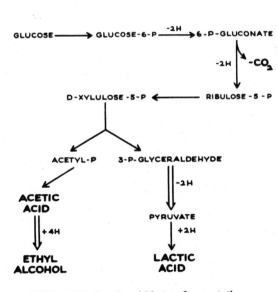

FIG 5–26. Propionic acid fermentation.

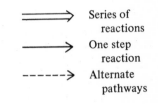

⟹ Series of reactions

⟶ One step reaction

------> Alternate pathways

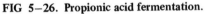

FIG 5–28. Lactic acid heterofermentation.

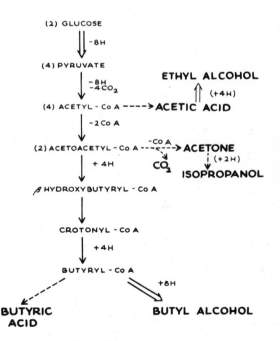

FIG 5–29. Butyl alcohol-butyric acid fermentation.

•   •   •

General References

Books

Barker, H.A.: *Bacterial Fermentations.* Wiley, 1957.

Cohen, G.N.: *Biosynthesis of Small Molecules.* Harper, 1967.

Cold Spring Harbor Symposia on Quantitative Biology: Vol 26: *Cellular Regulatory Mechanisms.* Vol 28: *Synthesis and Structure of Macromolecules.* Vol 33: *Replication of DNA in Microorganisms.* Cold Spring Harbor, New York, 1961, 1963, 1968.

Doelle, H.W.: *Bacterial Metabolism.* Academic Press, 1969.

Gunsalus, I.C., & R.Y. Stanier (editors): *The Bacteria.* Vol 2: *Metabolism.* Vol 3: *Biosynthesis.* Academic Press, 1961, 1962.

Hartman, P., & S. Suskind: *Gene Action,* 2nd ed. Prentice-Hall, 1969.

Haynes, R., & P. Hanawalt (editors): *The Molecular Basis of Life–An Introduction to Molecular Biology: Readings from Scientific American.* Freeman, 1968.

Kornberg, A.: *Enzymatic Synthesis of DNA.* Wiley, 1962.

Maaløe, O., & N. Kjeldgaard: *Control of Macromolecular Synthesis.* Benjamin, 1965.

Mandelstam, J., & K. McQuillen (editors): *The Biochemistry of Bacterial Growth.* Wiley, 1968.

Sokatch, J.R.: *Bacterial Physiology and Metabolism.* Academic Press, 1969.

Watson, J.D.: *Molecular Biology of the Gene.* Benjamin, 1965.

Articles & Reviews

Cohen, G.N., & J. Monod: Bacterial permeases. Bacteriol Rev 21:169–194, 1957.

Horecker, B.L.: Biosynthesis of bacterial polysaccharides. Ann Rev Microbiol 20:253–290, 1966.

Kornberg, A.: Active center of DNA polymerase. Science 163:1410–1418, 1969.

Monod, J., Changeux, J., & F. Jacob: Allosteric proteins and cellular control systems. J Molec Biol 6:306–329, 1963.

6...

Cultivation of Microorganisms

Cultivation is the process of propagating organisms by providing the proper environmental conditions: nutrients, pH, temperature, and aeration. Other factors which must be controlled include the salt concentration and osmotic pressure of the medium and such special factors as light for photosynthetic organisms.

NUTRITION

The provision of nutrients for the growth of an organism is called nutrition. In the following discussion, the nutrients are classified according to their role in metabolism.

Hydrogen Donors

All chemosynthetic organisms require an energy source in the form of H donors (ie, oxidizable substrates). In addition, photosynthetic organisms require H donors in order to carry on photosynthesis. Types of compounds which can serve as H donors are discussed in Chapter 5.

Hydrogen Acceptors

H acceptors are required in energy-yielding oxidation-reduction reactions. For aerobes, gaseous oxygen (O_2) is required. Anaerobes require either inorganic compounds (sulfate, nitrate, carbonate) or organic compounds. In the latter case (called "fermentation"), either the carbon source or a fragment derived from it by catabolism usually serves; in a few instances, however, there is a requirement for a unique H acceptor which must be present in the medium.

Carbon Source

All organisms require a source of carbon for synthesis of the numerous organic compounds which comprise protoplasm. For photosynthetic and lithotrophic organisms, CO_2 is the sole source. Other organisms use the organic energy source as carbon source also; in addition, they require small amounts of CO_2. In most cases, sufficient CO_2 is produced in catabolism to satisfy this requirement; however, growth frequently cannot be initiated unless CO_2 is present in the environment.

Nitrogen Source

Many cell constituents, principally the proteins, contain nitrogen; in bacteria, nitrogen accounts for approximately 10% of the cellular dry weight.

The form in which nitrogen is required depends on the organism's enzymatic reducing abilities; although in protoplasm nitrogen is organically combined ($R-NH_2$), a given microbial species may obtain it from the environment in one or more of the forms shown in Table 6–1.

TABLE 6–1. Sources of nitrogen in microbial nutrition.

Compound	Valence of N
NO_3^-	+5
NO_2^-	+3
N_2	0
NH_3	−3
$R - NH_2$	−3

When the nitrogen source is $R-NH_2$ (R = organic radical), the organism uses it by deamination to NH_3, which is then incorporated into nitrogenous compounds, or by direct transfer of the amino group to suitable acceptors (transamination), or both:

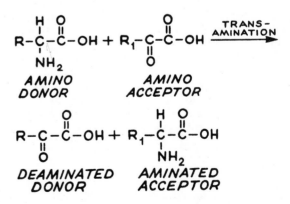

Most microorganisms can use NH_3 as the sole nitrogen source. The principal reaction by which NH_3 is introduced into organic molecules is the reaction catalyzed by glutamic dehydrogenase:

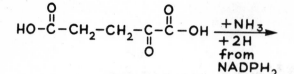

α-KETOGLUTARIC ACID

$$HO-\overset{\overset{O}{\|}}{C}-CH_2-CH_2-\overset{\overset{H}{|}}{\underset{\underset{NH_2}{|}}{C}}-\overset{\overset{O}{\|}}{C}-OH + H_2O$$

GLUTAMIC ACID

Distribution of the nitrogen into other compounds can then be affected by transamination between glutamic acid and various keto acids and by modification of the new amino acids thus formed.

A limited number of microorganisms can fix atmospheric nitrogen (N_2) by converting it to NH_3 in the cell. The intermediate steps in this process are not known. Some bacteria can use nitrate as nitrogen source, reducing it to the level of NH_3 in the cell.

Minerals

In addition to carbon and nitrogen, living cells require a number of other minerals for growth:

A. Sulfur: Like nitrogen, sulfur is a component of many organic cell substances; the bulk of it occurs as sulfhydryl (–SH) groups in proteins. Some organisms require organic sulfur (R–SH) or H_2S, but most species can reduce sulfate ($SO_4^=$) to the organic form.

B. Phosphorus: Phosphate ($PO_4^\equiv$) is required as a component of ATP, of nucleic acids, and of such coenzymes as NAD, NADP, and flavins. Phosphate is always taken into the cell as free inorganic phosphate.

C. Enzyme Activators: Numerous minerals are needed as enzyme activators. Magnesium ion (Mg^{++}) and ferrous ion are also found in porphyrins: magnesium in the chlorophyll molecule and iron as a part of the coenzymes of the cytochromes and peroxidases. In formulating a medium for the cultivation of most microorganisms, it is necessary to provide sources of potassium, magnesium, calcium, and iron, usually as their ions (K^+, Mg^{++}, Ca^{++}, and Fe^{++}). Many other minerals are required, but are adequately provided as contaminants of tap water and of other medium ingredients.

Growth Factors

A growth factor is an organic compound which a cell must contain in order to grow but which it is unable to synthesize. Many microorganisms, when provided with the nutrients listed above, are able to synthesize all of the organic constituents of their complex protoplasm, including amino acids (the subunits of protein), vitamins (for coenzymes), purines and pyrimidines (components of nucleic acid), fatty acids (components of fats and lipids), and various other compounds.

Each of these essential compounds is synthesized by a discrete sequence of enzymatic reactions; each enzyme is produced under the control of a specific gene. When an organism undergoes a gene mutation resulting in failure of one of these enzymes to function, the chain is broken and the end product is no longer produced. The organism must then obtain that compound from the environment; in other words, that compound has become a growth factor for the affected organism.

Different microbial species vary widely in their growth factor requirements. The compounds involved are found in and are essential to all organisms; the differences in requirement reflect differences in synthetic abilities. Some species require no growth factors, while others (like some of the lactobacilli) have lost, by mutation, the ability to synthesize as many as 30–40 essential compounds and hence require them in the medium. This type of mutation can be readily induced in the laboratory.

ENVIRONMENTAL FACTORS AFFECTING GROWTH

A suitable growth medium must contain all the nutrients required by the organism to be cultivated, and such factors as pH, temperature, and aeration must be carefully controlled. A liquid medium is used; the medium can be gelled for special purposes by adding agar or silica gel. Agar, a polysaccharide extract of a marine alga, is uniquely suitable for microbial cultivation because it is resistant to microbial action and because it dissolves at 100° C but does not gel until cooled below 45° C; cells can be suspended in the medium at 45° C, and the medium quickly cooled to a gel without harming them.

Nutrients

On the previous pages the function of each type of nutrient is described and a list of suitable substances presented. In general, the following must be provided: (1) Hydrogen donors and acceptors: about 2 gm/liter. (2) Carbon source: about 1 gm/liter. (3) Nitrogen source: about 1 gm/liter. (4) Minerals: sulfur and phosphorus, about 50 mg/liter of each; trace elements, 0.1–1 mg/liter of each. (5) Growth factors: amino acids, purines, pyrimidines, about 50 mg/liter of each; vitamins, 0.1–1 mg/liter of each.

For studies of microbial metabolism it is usually necessary to prepare a completely synthetic medium in which the characteristics and concentration of every ingredient are exactly known. Otherwise it is much cheaper and simpler to use natural materials such as yeast extract, protein digest, or similar substances.

Most free-living microbes will grow well on yeast extract; parasitic forms may require special substances found only in blood or in extracts of animal tissues.

For many organisms, a single compound (such as an amino acid) may serve as energy source, carbon source, and nitrogen source; others require a separate compound for each. If natural materials for non-synthetic media are deficient in any particular nutrient, they must be supplemented.

Hydrogen Ion Concentration (pH)

Most organisms have a fairly narrow optimal pH range. The optimal pH must be empirically determined for each species. Most organisms grow best at a pH of 6.0–8.0, although some forms have optima as low as pH 2.0 (*Thiobacillus thioxidans*) and others have optima of pH 8.5 (*Alcaligenes faecalis*).

Temperature

Psychrophilic forms grow best at low temperatures (15–20° C); mesophilic forms grow best at 30–37°C; and thermophilic forms grow best at 50–60° C. Most organisms are mesophilic; 30° C is optimal for the free-living forms and 37° C for the animal parasites.

Aeration

The role of oxygen as hydrogen acceptor is discussed in Chapter 5. Many organisms are obligate aerobes, specifically requiring oxygen as hydrogen acceptor; some are facultative, able to live aerobically or anaerobically; and others are obligate anaerobes, requiring a substance other than oxygen as hydrogen acceptor and being sensitive to oxygen inhibition. The organisms in the latter group lack catalase, and thus are killed by the H_2O_2 which they form by the flavin-catalysed reduction of O_2.

The supply of air to cultures of aerobes is a major technical problem. Vessels are usually shaken mechanically to introduce oxygen into the medium, or air is forced through the medium by pressure or suction. The diffusion of oxygen often becomes the limiting factor in growing aerobic bacteria; when a cell concentration of $4-5 \times 10^9$ per ml is reached, the rate of diffusion of oxygen to the cells sharply limits the rate of further growth.

Obligate anaerobes, on the other hand, present the problem of oxygen exclusion. Many methods are available for this: Reducing agents such as sodium thioglycollate can be added to liquid cultures; tubes of agar can be sealed with a layer of petrolatum and paraffin; or the culture vessel can be placed in a container from which the oxygen is removed by evacuation or by chemical means.

Other Factors

To a lesser extent, such factors as osmotic pressure and salt concentration may have to be controlled. For most organisms the properties of ordinary media are satisfactory; but for marine forms and organisms adapted to growth in strong sugar solutions, for example, these factors must be considered. Organisms requiring high salt concentrations are called *halophilic;* those requiring high osmotic pressures are called *osmophilic.*

CULTIVATION METHODS

Two problems will be considered: the choice of a suitable medium, and the isolation of a bacterial organism in pure culture.

The Medium

The technic used and the type of medium selected depend upon the nature of the investigation. In general, 3 situations may be encountered: (1) One may need to raise a crop of cells of a particular species which is on hand; (2) one may need to determine the numbers and types of organisms present in a given material; or (3) one may wish to isolate a particular type of microorganism from a natural source.

A. Growing Cells of a Given Species: Microorganisms observed microscopically to be growing in a natural environment may prove exceedingly difficult to grow in pure culture in an artificial medium. Certain parasitic forms, for example, have never been cultivated outside the host. In general, however, a suitable medium can be devised by carefully reproducing the conditions found in the organism's natural environment. The pH, temperature, and aeration are simple to duplicate; the nutrients present the major problem. The contribution made by the living environment is important and difficult to analyze; a parasite may require an extract of the host tissue, and a free-living form may require a substance excreted by a microorganism with which it is associated in nature. Considerable experimentation may be necessary in order to determine the requirements of the organism, and success depends upon providing a suitable source of each category of nutrient listed at the beginning of this chapter. The cultivation of obligate parasites, such as rickettsiae, is a special problem and is discussed in Chapter 28.

B. Microbiologic Examination of Natural Materials: A given natural material may contain many different micro-environments, each providing a niche for a different species. Plating a sample of the materials under one set of conditions will allow a selected group of forms to produce colonies but will cause many other types to be overlooked. For this reason it is customary to plate out samples of the material using as many different media and conditions of incubation as is practicable. Six to 8 different culture conditions is not an unreasonable number if most of the forms present are to be discovered.

Since every type of organism present must have a chance to grow, solid media are used and crowding of colonies is avoided. Otherwise, competition will prevent some types from forming colonies.

C. Isolation of a Particular Type of Microorganism: A small sample of soil, if handled properly, will yield a different type of organism for every micro-environment present. For fertile soil (moist, aerated, rich in minerals and organic matter) this means that hundreds or even thousands of types can be isolated. This is done by selecting for the desired type. One gm of soil, for example, is inoculated into a flask of liquid medium which has been made up for the purpose of favoring one type of organism, eg, aerobic nitrogen fixers (Azotobacter). In this case the medium contains no combined nitrogen and is incubated aerobically. If cells of Azotobacter are present in the soil, they will grow well in this medium; forms unable to fix nitrogen will grow only to the extent that the soil has introduced contaminating fixed nitrogen into the medium. When the culture is fully grown, therefore, the percentage of Azotobacter in the total population will have increased greatly; the method is thus called "enrichment culture." Transfer of a sample of this culture to fresh medium will result in further enrichment of Azotobacter; after several serial transfers, the culture can be plated out on a solidified enrichment medium and colonies of Azotobacter isolated.

Liquid medium is used to permit competition and hence optimal selection, even when the desired type is represented in the soil as only a few cells in a population of millions. Advantage can be taken of "natural enrichment." For example, in looking for kerosene oxidizers, oil-laden soil is chosen as the inoculum since such soil is already an enrichment environment for such forms.

Enrichment culture, then, is a procedure whereby the medium is prepared so as to duplicate the natural environment ("niche") of the desired microorganisms, thereby selecting for it. An important principle involved in such selection is the following: The organism selected for will be the type whose nutritional requirements are barely satisfied. Azotobacter, for example, grows best in a medium containing organic nitrogen, but its minimum requirement is the presence of N_2; hence it is selected for in a medium containing N_2 as the sole nitrogen source. If organic nitrogen is added to the medium, the conditions no longer select for Azotobacter but rather for a form for which organic nitrogen is the minimum requirement.

When searching for a particular type of organism in a natural material, it is advantageous to plate the organisms obtained on a differential medium if available. A differential medium is one which will cause the colonies of a particular type of organism to have a distinctive appearance. For example, colonies of *Escherichia coli* have a characteristic iridescent sheen on agar containing the dyes eosin and methylene blue (EMB agar). EMB agar containing a high concentration of one sugar will also cause organisms which ferment that sugar to form reddish colonies. Differential media are used for such purposes as recognizing the presence of enteric bacteria in water or milk and the presence of certain pathogens in clinical specimens from patients.

Table 6–2 presents some examples of enrichment culture conditions and the types of bacteria which they will select.

Isolation of Microorganisms in Pure Culture

In order to study the properties of a given organism, it is necessary to handle it in pure culture free of all other types of organisms. To do this, a single cell

TABLE 6–2. Some enrichment cultures.

Constituents of all media: $MgSO_4$, K_2HPO_4, $FeCl_3$, $CaCl_2$, $CaCO_3$, trace elements.

Nitrogen Source	Carbon Source	Atmosphere	Illumination	Predominant Organism Initially Enriched
N_2	CO_2	Aerobic or anaerobic	Dark	None
			Light	Blue-green algae
	Alcohol, fatty acids, etc	Anaerobic	Dark	None
		Air	Dark	Azotobacter
	Glucose	Anaerobic	Dark	*Clostridium pasteurianum*
		Air	Dark	Azotobacter
$NaNO_3$	CO_2	Aerobic or anaerobic	Dark	None
			Light	Green and blue-green algae
	Alcohol, fatty acids, etc	Anaerobic	Dark	Denitrifiers
		Air	Dark	Aerobes
	Glucose	Anaerobic	Dark	Fermenters
		Air	Dark	Aerobes
NH_4Cl	CO_2	Anaerobic	Dark	None
		Aerobic	Dark	Nitrosomonas
		Aerobic or anaerobic	Light	Green and blue-green algae
	Alcohol, fatty acids, etc	Anaerobic	Dark	Sulfate or carbonate reducers
		Aerobic	Dark	Aerobes
	Glucose	Anaerobic	Dark	Fermenters
		Aerobic	Dark	Aerobes

must be isolated from all other cells and cultivated in such a manner that its collective progeny also remain isolated. Several methods are available:

A. Plating: Unlike cells in a liquid medium, cells in or on a gelled medium are immobilized. Therefore, if few enough cells are placed in or on a gelled medium, each cell will grow into an isolated colony. In the pour-plate method, a suspension of cells is mixed with melted agar at 45° C and poured into a Petri dish. When the agar solidifies, the cells are immobilized in the agar and grow into colonies. If the cell suspension was sufficiently dilute, the colonies will be well separated, so that each has a high probability of being derived from a single cell. To make certain of this, however, it is necessary to pick a colony of the desired type, suspend it in water, and replate. Repeating this procedure several times ensures that a pure culture will be obtained.

Alternatively, the original suspension can be streaked on an agar plate with a wire loop. As the streaking continues, fewer and fewer cells are left on the loop, and finally the loop may deposit single cells on the agar. The plate is incubated and any well-isolated colony is then removed, resuspended in water, and again streaked on agar. If a suspension is streaked (and not just a bit of growth from a colony or slant), this method is just as reliable and much faster than the pour-plate method.

B. Dilution: A much less reliable method is that of extinction dilution. The suspension is serially diluted and samples of each dilution are plated. If only a few samples of a particular dilution exhibit growth, it is presumed that some of these cultures started from single cells. This method is not used unless plating is for some reason impossible. An undesirable feature of this method is that it can only be used to isolate the predominant type of organism in a mixed population.

● ● ●

General References

Luria, S.E.: The bacterial protoplasm: Composition and organization. Page 1 in: *The Bacteria.* Vol 1: *Structure.* Gunsalus, I.C., & R.Y. Stanier (editors). Academic Press, 1960.

Meynell, G.G., & E. Meynell: *Theory and Practice in Experimental Bacteriology.* Cambridge Univ Press, 1965.

Schlegel, H.G. (editor): *Anreicherungskultur und Mutantenauslese. [Enrichment Culture and Mutant Selection.]* Fischer (Stuttgart), 1965. [The only systematic description of enrichment methods. Many of the articles are in English.]

7...

The Growth & Death of Microorganisms

DEFINITION & MEASUREMENT OF GROWTH

The Meaning of Growth

Growth is the orderly increase in all of the components of an organism. Thus, the increase in size which results when a cell takes up water or deposits lipid is not true growth. Cell multiplication is a consequence of growth; in unicellular organisms, multiplication leads to an increase in the number of individuals making up a population or a culture.

The Measurement of Growth

Microbial growth can be measured in terms of cell concentration (the number of cells per unit volume of culture) or of cell density (dry weight of cells per unit volume of culture). These 2 parameters are not always equivalent because the average dry weight of the cell varies at different stages in the history of the culture. Nor are they of equal significance: In studies on microbial biochemistry or nutrition, cell density is the significant quantity; in studies on microbial inactivation, cell concentration is the significant quantity.

A. **Cell Concentration**: The viable cell count (Table 8–1) is usually considered the measure of cell concentration. However, the general practice is to measure the light absorption or light scattering of a culture by photoelectric means and to relate viable counts to optical measurements in the form of a standard curve. By means of the standard curve, all further optical readings can be converted to cell concentration. However, it is essential that a separate standard curve be determined for each stage in the growth of the culture so that differences in average cell size can be taken into account.

B. **Cell Density**: Since it is technically difficult to perform a large number of dry weight measurements, and since such measurements are accurate only with relatively large amounts of cells, various indirect methods are used. These include photoelectric measurements, nitrogen determination, and centrifugation in special vessels. In each case it is necessary to construct a standard curve equating the measurement values with known dry weights.

EXPONENTIAL GROWTH

The Growth Constant

Since the 2 new cells produced by the growth and division of a single cell are each capable of growing at the same rate as the parent cell, the number of cells in a culture increases with time as a geometric progression—ie, exponentially.

The rate of growth of a culture at a given moment is directly proportionate to the number of cells present at that moment. This relationship is given by the following equation:

$$\frac{dN}{dt} = kN \qquad \dots (1)$$

Integration of the above expression gives:

$$N = N_0 e^{kt} \qquad \dots (2)$$

where N_0 is the number of cells at time zero and N is the number of cells at any later time, t.

In equation (2) above, k is the growth constant. Solving the equation for k gives:

$$k = \frac{\ln(N/N_0)}{t} \qquad \dots (3)$$

Thus, k represents the rate at which the natural logarithm of cell number increases with time, and can be determined graphically as shown in Fig 7–1.

The Generation

In practice it is customary to express the growth rate of a microbial culture in terms of generations per hour. For organisms which reproduce by binary fission, a generation is defined as a doubling of cell number. Thus, the number of cells (N) increases with generations (g) as follows:

g	N
0	1
1	2
2	4
3	8
4	16
5	32

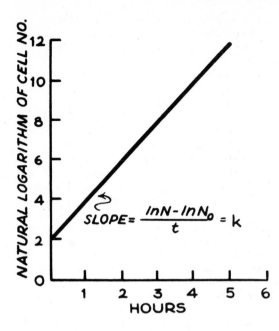

FIG 7–1. The rate at which the natural logarithm of cell number increases with time.

This relationship can be expressed as follows:

$$N = N_0 2^g \qquad \ldots (4)$$

Combining equations (2) and (4), we find

$$N_0 e^{kt} = N_0 2^g \qquad \ldots (5)$$

Equation (5) can be rearranged to give:

$$\frac{g}{t} = \frac{k}{\ln 2} \qquad \ldots (6)$$

Equation (6) thus relates g/t (generations per hour) with k, the growth constant.

The number of generations per hour is usually determined by plotting cell number against time on a semi-logarithmic scale and reading off directly the time required for the number to double. For example, if such a plot shows the doubling time ("generation time") to be 40 minutes, the growth rate of the culture is said to be 1.5 generations per hour.

Alternatively, the generation time can be calculated directly from equation (4), which can be solved for g (the number of generations) as follows:

$$g = \frac{\log N - \log N_0}{\log 2} \qquad \ldots (7)$$

Thus, for example, if an inoculum of 10^3 cells grows exponentially to 1×10^9 cells,

$$g = \frac{\log(10^9) - \log(10^3)}{\log 2} = \frac{9 - 3}{0.3} = 20 \text{ generations}$$

If, for example, this growth required 13.3 hours, the growth rate was 20/13.3, or 1.5 generations per hour.

THE GROWTH CURVE

If a liquid medium is inoculated with microbial cells taken from a culture which has previously been grown to saturation and the number of viable cells per ml determined periodically and plotted, a curve of the type shown in Fig 7–2 is usually obtained. The curve may be discussed in terms of 6 phases, represented by the letters A–F.

The Lag Phase

The lag phase represents a period during which the cells, depleted of metabolites and enzymes as the result of the unfavorable conditions which obtained at the end of their previous culture history, adapt to their new environment. Enzymes and intermediates are formed and accumulate until they are present in concentrations which permit growth to resume.

If the cells are taken from an entirely different medium, it often happens that they are genetically incapable of growth in the new medium. In such cases, the lag represents the period necessary for a few mutants in the inoculum to multiply sufficiently for a net increase in cell number to be apparent.

The Exponential Phase

During the exponential phase, the mathematics of which has already been discussed, the cells are in steady state. New cell material is being synthesized at a constant rate, but the new material is itself catalytic and the mass increases in an exponential manner. This continues until one of 2 things happens: Either one or more nutrients in the medium becomes exhausted, or toxic metabolic products accumulate and inhibit growth. For aerobic organisms, the nutrient which

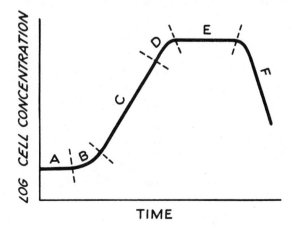

FIG 7–2. Cell concentration curve.

TABLE 7–1.

Section of Curve	Phase	Growth Rate
A	Lag	Zero
B	Acceleration	Increasing
C	Exponential	Constant
D	Retardation	Decreasing
E	Maximum stationary	Zero
F	Decline	Negative (death)

becomes limiting is usually oxygen: When the cell concentration exceeds about 1×10^7/ml (in the case of bacteria), the growth rate will decrease unless oxygen is forced into the medium by agitation or by bubbling in air. When the cell concentration reaches $4-5 \times 10^9$/ml, the rate of oxygen diffusion cannot meet the demand even in an aerated medium, and growth is progressively slowed.

The Maximum Stationary Phase

Eventually, the exhaustion of nutrients or the accumulation of toxic products causes growth to cease completely. In most cases, however, cell turnover takes place in the stationary phase: There is a slow loss of cells through death, which is just balanced by the formation of new cells through growth and division. When this occurs, the total cell count slowly increases although the viable count stays constant.

The Phase of Decline (the Death Phase)

After a period of time in stationary phase, which varies with the organism and with the culture conditions, the death rate increases until it reaches a steady level. The mathematics of steady-state death are discussed below. Frequently, after the majority of cells have died, the death rate decreases drastically, so that a small number of survivors may persist for months or even years in the culture. This persistence may in some cases reflect cell turnover, a few cells growing at the expense of nutrients released from cells which die and lyse.

THE MAINTENANCE OF CELLS IN EXPONENTIAL PHASE

Cells can be maintained in exponential phase by transferring them repeatedly into fresh medium of identical composition while they are still growing exponentially. Two devices have been invented for carrying out this process automatically: the chemostat and the turbidostat.

The Chemostat

This device consists of a culture vessel equipped with an overflow siphon and a mechanism for dripping in fresh medium from a reservoir at a regulated rate. The medium in the culture vessel is stirred by a stream of sterile air; each drop of fresh medium that enters causes a drop of culture to siphon out.

The medium is prepared so that one nutrient limits growth yield. The vessel is inoculated, and the cells grow until the limiting nutrient is exhausted; fresh medium from the reservoir is then allowed to flow in, at such a rate that the cells use up the limiting nutrient as fast as it is supplied. Under these conditions, the cell concentration remains constant and the growth rate is directly proportional to the flow rate of the medium.

The chemostat thus provides a steady-state culture of exponentially-growing cells, and permits the growth rate to be regulated. It has the disadvantage, however, that the cells are always in a state of semi-starvation for one nutrient, and must be grown at less than maximal rate if good regulation is to be achieved. These disadvantages are not present in the turbidostat.

The Turbidostat

This device resembles the chemostat except that the flow of medium is controlled by a photoelectric mechanism which measures the turbidity of the culture. When the turbidity exceeds the chosen level, fresh medium is allowed to flow in. Thus, the cells can grow at maximum rate at a constant cell concentration. The growth rate can be controlled in the turbidostat only by varying the nature of the medium or the culture conditions (eg, temperature).

SYNCHRONOUS GROWTH

In ordinary cultures the cells are growing nonsynchronously: At any moment, cells are present in every possible stage of the division cycle. In order to study the sequence of events that takes place in a single cell during the division cycle, the culture must be synchronized.

Synchrony has been achieved for a variety of microorganisms by several technics. Some yeast strains, for example, go through one or 2 synchronous divisions when diluted from a stationary phase culture into fresh medium. In most cases, however, it is necessary to bring the cells into synchrony by a more involved process. Pneumococci, for example, will divide synchronously after several alternating periods of incubation at high and low temperature. *Escherichia coli* has been synchronized by 2 different methods: In one, a thymine-requiring mutant is starved for thymine until viability begins to drop. Replacing thymine in the culture then causes the surviving cells to undergo several synchronous divisions. In the other method, a heavy cell suspension is forced through a filter paper pile. The cells which emerge first are often found to be a selected population which undergoes synchronous growth after a lag period.

In all cases, synchrony only persists for 1–4 cycles. After that time the cells become more and more out of phase until their division times become completely random.

GROWTH PARAMETERS

Physiologic studies may be carried out by introducing controlled variations in individual environmental factors and then quantitatively determining the effect of such variations on bacterial growth. To be most useful, experiments of this type should involve determination of meaningful growth parameters. Growth parameters which may be determined include total growth and exponential growth rate.

Total Growth

A culture eventually stops growing when one of 3 things occurs: (1) when one or more nutrients are exhausted; (2) when toxic products accumulate; or (3) when an unfavorable ion equilibrium develops (eg, unfavorable pH).

If total growth (G) is limited by exhaustion of a nutrient, then

$$G = KC \qquad \dots (8)$$

where K is a constant and C is the initial concentration of the limiting nutrient. Such an equation implies a straight line relationship between C and G.

Exponential Growth Rates

If some nutrient is initially present at a sufficiently low concentration, metabolic intermediates will be formed at a limited rate and the overall growth rate will be a function of the concentration of the limiting nutrient. Experiments show that a hyperbolic curve results, in accordance with the following general equation:

$$R = R_K \frac{C}{C_1 + C} \qquad \dots (9)$$

where R = Growth rate
    R_K = Maximum rate reached with increasing concentration of nutrient
    C = Concentration of the limiting nutrient
    C_1 = Value of C at which R = ½ R_K

Total growth is a useful parameter in many microbial assays; for example, in the assay of a vitamin or a carbon source in some natural material. For most physiologic studies, however, growth rate is the most meaningful parameter. One method, for example, is to compare concentrations of nutrients or inhibitors which give half-maximal growth rates.

DEFINITION & MEASUREMENT OF DEATH

The Meaning of Death

For a microbial cell, death means the irreversible loss of the ability to reproduce (grow and divide). The empiric test of death is the culture of cells on solid media: A cell is considered dead if it fails to give rise to a colony on any medium. Obviously, then, the reliability of the test depends upon choice of medium and conditions: A culture in which 99% of the cells appear "dead" in terms of ability to form colonies on one medium may prove to be 100% viable if tested on another medium.

The conditions of incubation in the first hour following treatment are also critical in the determination of "killing." For example, if bacterial cells are irradiated with ultraviolet light and plated immediately on any medium, it may appear that 99.99% of the cells have been killed. If such irradiated cells are first incubated in a suitable buffer for 20 minutes, however, plating will indicate only 10% killing. In other words, irradiation determines that a cell will "die" if plated immediately, but will live if allowed to repair irradiation damage before plating.

A microbial cell that is not physically disrupted is thus "dead" only in terms of the conditions used to test viability.

The Measurement of Death

When dealing with microorganisms, one does not customarily measure the death of an individual cell but the death of a population. This is a statistical problem: Under any condition which may lead to cell death, the probability of a given cell's dying is constant per unit

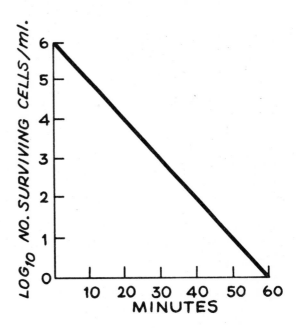

FIG 7–3. Death curve of microorganisms.

time. For example, if a condition is employed which causes 90% of the cells to die in the first 10 minutes, the probability of any one cell dying in a 10-minute interval is 0.9. Thus, it may be expected that 90% of the surviving cells will die in each succeeding 10-minute interval, and a death curve similar to that shown in Fig 7–3 will be obtained.

The number of cells dying in each time interval is thus a function of the number of survivors present, so that death of a population proceeds as an exponential process according to the general formula:

$$S = S_0 e^{-kt} \qquad \ldots (10)$$

where S_0 is the number of survivors at time zero, and S is the number of survivors at any later time, t. As in the case of exponential growth, $-k$ represents the rate of exponential death when the fraction $ln\ (S/S_0)$ is plotted against time.

Sterilization

In practice, we speak of "sterilization" as the process of killing all of the organisms in a preparation. From the above considerations, however, we see that no set of conditions is guaranteed to sterilize a preparation. Consider Fig 7–3, for example. At 60 minutes, there is one organism (10^0) left per ml. At 70 minutes there would be 10^{-1}, at 80 minutes 10^{-2}, etc. By 10^{-2} organisms per ml we mean that in a total volume of 100 ml, one organism would survive. How long, then, does it take to "sterilize" the culture? All we can say is that after any given time of treatment, the probability of having any surviving organisms in 1 ml is that given by the curve. After 2 hours, in the above example, the probability is 1×10^{-6}. This would be considered a safe sterilization time in most situations, but a thousand-liter lot might still contain one viable organism.

Note that such calculations depend upon the curve's remaining unchanged in slope over the entire time range. Unfortunately, it is very common for the curve to bend upward after a certain period, as a result of the population being heterogeneous with respect to sensitivity to the inactivation agent. Extrapolations are thus dangerous, and can lead to such errors as those which were encountered in early preparations of sterile poliovaccine.

The Effect of Drug Concentration

When antimicrobial substances (drugs) are used to inactivate microbial cells, it is commonly observed that the concentration of drug employed is related to the time required to kill a given fraction of the population, as shown in the following expression:

$$C^n t = K \qquad \ldots (11)$$

where C is the drug concentration, t is the time required to kill a given fraction of the cells, and n and K are constants.

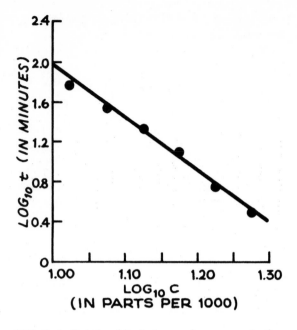

FIG 7–4. Relationship between drug concentration and time required to kill a given fraction of a cell population.

This expression says that, for example, if $n = 5$ (as it is for phenol), then doubling the concentration of the drug will reduce the time required to achieve the same extent of inactivation 32-fold. That the effectiveness of a drug varies with the fifth power of the concentration suggests that 5 molecules of the drug are required to inactivate a cell, although there is no direct chemical evidence for this conclusion.

In order to determine the value of n for any drug, inactivation curves are obtained for each of several concentrations, and the time required at each concentration to inactivate a fixed fraction of the population is determined. For example, let the first concentration used be C_1 and the time required to inactivate 99% of the cells be t_1. Similarly, let C_2 and t_2 be the second concentration and time required to inactivate 99% of the cells. From equation (11), we see that

$$C_1{}^n t_1 = C_2{}^n t_2 \qquad \ldots (12)$$

Solving for n gives:

$$n = \frac{\log t_2 - \log t_1}{\log C_1 - \log C_2}$$

Thus, n can be determined by measuring the slope of the line which results when log t is plotted against log C (Fig 7–4). If n is experimentally determined in this manner, K can be determined by substituting observed values for C, t, and n in equation (11).

ANTIMICROBIAL AGENTS

Definitions

The following terms are commonly employed in connection with antimicrobial agents and their uses.

A. Bacteriostatic: Having the property of inhibiting bacterial multiplication; multiplication resumes upon removal of the agent.

B. Bactericidal: Having the property of killing bacteria. Bactericidal action differs from bacteriostasis only in being irreversible; ie, the "killed" organism can no longer reproduce, even after being removed from contact with the agent. In some cases the agent causes lysis (dissolving) of the cells; in other cases the cells remain intact and may even continue to be metabolically active.

C. Sterile: Free of life of every kind. Sterilization may be accomplished by filtration (in the case of liquids or air) or by treatment with microbicidal agents. Since the criterion of death for microorganisms is the inability to reproduce, sterile material may contain intact, metabolizing microbial cells.

D. Disinfectant: Having the property of killing infectious organisms.

E. Septic: Characterized by the presence of pathogenic microbes in living tissue.

F. Aseptic: Characterized by absence of pathogenic microbes.

Possible Modes of Action

Antibacterial agents may affect cells in a variety of ways, many of which are poorly understood. Some broad generalizations can be made, however. At high concentrations many agents are so destructive that, among other things, the cell proteins precipitate from the colloidal state ("coagulate"). Under certain conditions, some agents may specifically disrupt the cell membrane. Many of the cell's essential enzymes possess sulfhydryl (−SH) groups and can only function if these remain free and reduced; hence agents which oxidize or combine with sulfhydryl groups are strongly inhibitory. Finally, many agents may act by interfering with one or a few specific enzymatic reactions (chemical antagonism).

A. Protein Coagulation: The proteins of the cell, most or all of which are enzymatic, exist in the finely dispersed colloidal state. If the properties of the proteins are drastically altered by an antibacterial agent, they will coagulate and become nonfunctional. The changes that take place when egg white is heated or when milk sours are good examples of coagulation, but little is known about the chemical changes preceding and accompanying the visible change.

B. Disruption of Cell Membrane or Wall: The cell membrane acts as a selective barrier, allowing some solutes to pass through and excluding others. Indeed, some compounds are actively transported through the membrane, becoming concentrated within the cell. The mechanisms involved in these actions are obscure at the present time, but it seems certain that an undisturbed, intact membrane is required. For this reason, substances which concentrate at the cell surface may alter the physical and chemical properties of the membrane, preventing its normal function and therefore killing or inhibiting the cell.

The cell wall acts as a corseting structure, protecting the cell against osmotic lysis. Thus, agents which destroy the wall (eg, lysozyme) or prevent its normal synthesis (eg, penicillin) bring about lysis of the cell.

C. Removal of Free Sulfhydryl Groups: Enzyme proteins containing cysteine have side-chains terminating in sulfhydryl groups. In addition to these, at least one key enzyme (coenzyme A, required for acyl group transfer) contains a free sulfhydryl group. Such enzymes and coenzymes cannot function unless the sulfhydryl groups remain free and reduced. Oxidizing agents thus interfere with metabolism by tying neighboring sulfhydryls in disulfide linkages:

$$R-SH + HS-R \xrightarrow{-2H} R-S-S-R$$

Many metals such as mercuric ion likewise interfere by combining with sulfhydryls:

$$\begin{matrix} R-SH \\ R-SH \end{matrix} + \begin{matrix} Cl \\ | \\ Hg \\ | \\ Cl \end{matrix} \longrightarrow \begin{matrix} R-S \\ R-S \end{matrix}\!\!\searrow\!\!\nearrow Hg + 2HCl$$

There are many sulfhydryl enzymes in the cell; therefore, oxidizing agents and heavy metals do widespread damage. The exact reason for the requirement of free sulfhydryl groups is not certain, although in many cases (eg, coenzyme A) they probably represent the normal site of substrate attachment.

D. Chemical Antagonism: The interference by a chemical agent with the normal reaction between a specific enzyme and its substrate is known as "chemical antagonism." The antagonist acts by combining with some part of the holoenzyme (either the protein apoenzyme, the mineral activator, or the coenzyme), thereby preventing attachment of the normal substrate. ("Substrate" is here used in the broad sense to include cases in which the inhibitor combines with the apoenzyme, thereby preventing attachment to it of coenzyme.)

An antagonist combines with an enzyme because of its chemical affinity for an essential site on that enzyme. Enzymes perform their catalytic function by virtue of their affinity for their natural substrates; hence any compound structurally resembling a substrate in essential aspects may also have an affinity for the enzyme. If this affinity is great enough, the "analogue" will displace the normal substrate from the enzyme and prevent the proper reaction from taking place.

Many holoenzymes include a mineral ion either as a bridge between enzyme and coenzyme or between enzyme and substrate. Chemicals which combine readily with these minerals will again prevent attachment of coenzyme or substrate; for example, carbon monoxide and cyanide ($-C\equiv N$) combine with the iron atom in the porphyrin enzymes and prevent their function in respiration.

Chemical antagonists can be conveniently discussed under 2 headings: antagonists of energy-yielding processes, and antagonists of biosynthetic processes. The former include poisons of respiratory enzymes (carbon monoxide, cyanide) and of oxidative phosphorylation (dinitrophenol); the latter include analogues of the building-blocks of proteins (amino acids) and of nucleic acids (nucleotides). In some cases the analogue simply prevents incorporation of the normal metabolite (eg, 5-methyltryptophan prevents incorporation of tryptophan into protein), and in other cases the analogue replaces the normal metabolite in the macromolecule, causing it to be nonfunctional. The incorporation of p-fluorophenylalanine in place of phenylalanine in proteins is an example of the latter type of antagonism.

Reversal of Antibacterial Action

In the section on definitions, the point was made that bacteriostatic action is, by definition, reversible. Reversal can be brought about in several ways:

A. Removal of Agent: When cells which are inhibited by the presence of a bacteriostatic agent are removed by centrifugation, washed thoroughly in the centrifuge, and resuspended in fresh growth medium, they will resume normal multiplication.

B. Reversal by Substrate: When a chemical antagonist of the analogue type forms a dissociating complex with the enzyme, it is possible to displace it by adding a high concentration of the normal substrate. Such cases are termed "competitive inhibition." The ratio of inhibitor concentration to concentration of substrate reversing the inhibition is called the **antibacterial index**; it is usually very high (100–10,000), indicating a much greater affinity of enzyme for its normal substrate.

C. Inactivation of Agent: Agents can often be inactivated by adding to the medium a substance which combines with it, preventing its combination with cellular constituents. For example, mercuric ion can be inactivated by addition to the medium of sulfhydryl compounds such as thioglycollic acid.

D. Protection Against Lysis: Osmotic lysis can be prevented by making the medium isotonic for naked bacterial protoplasts. Concentrations of 10–20% sucrose are required. Under such conditions penicillin-induced protoplasts remain viable and grow into normal cells on removal of the penicillin.

Resistance to Antibacterial Agents

The ability of bacteria to become resistant to antibacterial agents is an important factor in their control. The mechanisms by which resistance is acquired are discussed on p 109.

Physical Agents

A. Heat: Application of heat is the simplest means of sterilizing materials, providing the material is itself resistant to heat damage. A temperature of 100° C will kill all but spore forms of bacteria within 2–3 minutes; a temperature of 120° C for 15 minutes is required to kill spores. Steam is generally used, both because bacteria are more quickly killed when moist and because steam provides a means for distributing heat to all parts of the sterilizing vessel. Steam must be kept at a pressure of 15 lb/square inch above atmospheric pressure to obtain a temperature of 120° C; autoclaves or pressure cookers are used for this purpose. For sterilizing materials which must remain dry, circulating hot air electric ovens are available; since heat is less effective on dry material, it is customary to apply a temperature of 160° C for 1 hour.

Under the conditions described above (ie, excessive temperatures applied for long periods of time), heat undoubtedly acts by coagulating cell proteins and breaking down all vital cell structures. The mode of action of heat when applied so as to barely kill the more sensitive cells in a population is purely a matter of conjecture at the present time. However, it has been found that a significant fraction of a heat-killed suspension of bacteria can be revived by incubation in a buffered solution of certain common metabolites such as citric acid or pyruvic acid. This suggests that, at threshold levels, heat acts by producing a reversible impairment of only one or a few key metabolic reactions.

B. Radiation: Ultraviolet light is commonly used as a sterilizing agent. Its action is due in part to the production of peroxides ($R-O-O-R$) in the medium, which in turn act as oxidizing agents. Some of the more penetrating radiations, such as x-rays, ionize (and hence inactivate) the cell constituents through which they pass. However, some of the effect of x-ray irradiation can be traced again to peroxide formation, since cells can be partially protected by the exclusion of oxygen during irradiation.

Much of the killing action of radiation, however, is due to a direct effect on the nucleic acids of the cell. The major effect of ultraviolet absorption by DNA is the production of cross-links between neighboring pyrimidine residues (production of pyrimidine dimers).

Bacteria contain 2 enzymatic systems for the repair of DNA which contains pyrimidine dimers. One system, called *photoreactivation*, consists of an enzyme which cleaves the pyrimidine dimers. This enzyme is activated by visible light; hence, cells which have been "killed" by ultraviolet light can be reactivated by exposure to intense light of wavelength 400 μm. The second system is called the *dark repair* system. It requires the action of 4 enzymes operating in succession: (1) a specific endonuclease which makes single-strand cuts on either side of the dimer, excising it from the DNA; (2) a 3′ exonuclease, which widens the gap in the DNA strand by sequential digestion; (3) DNA polymerase, which fills in the gap by lengthening the 3′ end using the opposite strand as template;

and (4) polynucleotide ligase, which rejoins the free ends.

The relative resistance of different bacterial strains to radiation and other agents which directly damage DNA is due to the relative effectiveness of their repair enzyme systems.

Chemical Agents

Because antibacterial agents must be safe for the host organism under the conditions employed (selective toxicity), the number of commonly used antibacterial agents is much lower than the number of cell poisons and inhibitors available. Thus cyanide, arsenic, and other poisons are not included below because of the limitations on their practical usefulness.

A. Alcohols: Compounds with the structure $R-CH_2OH$ (where R means "alkyl group") are toxic to cells at relatively high concentrations. Ethyl alcohol (CH_3CH_2OH) and isopropyl alcohol ($[CH_3]_2CHOH$) are commonly used. At the concentrations generally employed (70% aqueous solutions) they act as protein coagulants; however, as in the case of heat, their mode of action at marginal concentrations is not known. Revival of "killed" cells by incubation with certain metabolites has been observed with alcohol-treated suspensions also.

B. Phenol: Phenol and many phenolic compounds are strong antibacterial agents. At the high concentrations generally employed (1—2% aqueous solutions) they coagulate proteins; this is not due to their acidity, however, since they are extremely weak acids. At low concentrations phenol acts by a different mechanism, since at these concentrations its action is reversed by a component of yeast extract.

C. Heavy Metal Ions: Mercury, copper, and silver salts are all protein coagulants at high concentrations but are too injurious to human tissues to be used in this manner. They are commonly used at very low concentrations, under which conditions they act by combining with sulfhydryl groups. Mercury can be made safer for external use by combining it with organic compounds (eg, Mercurochrome, Merthiolate). Except when used on clean skin surfaces these organic mercurials are of doubtful practical value, since they are readily inactivated by extraneous organic matter.

D. Oxidizing Agents: Strong oxidizing agents inactivate cells by oxidizing free sulfhydryl groups. Useful agents include hydrogen peroxide, iodine, hypochlorite, chlorine, and compounds slowly liberating chlorine (chloride of lime).

E. Detergents: Compounds which have the property of concentrating at interfaces are called "surface-active agents" or "detergents." The interface between the lipid-containing membrane of a bacterial cell and the surrounding aqueous medium attracts a particular class of surface-active compounds, namely, those possessing both a fat-soluble group and a water-soluble group. Long-chain hydrocarbons are very fat-soluble, while charged ions are very water-soluble; a compound possessing both structures will thus concentrate at the surface of the bacterial cell:

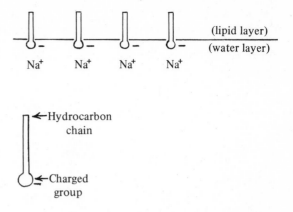

Two general types of such surface-active agents or detergents are known: anionic and cationic.

1. Anionic detergents—Detergents in which the long-chain hydrocarbon has a negative charge are called "anionic." These include soaps (sodium salts of long-chain carboxylic acids); synthetic products resembling soaps except that the carboxyl group is replaced by a sulfonic acid group; and bile salts, in which the fat-soluble portion has a steroid structure. Some examples are shown in Figs 7—6, 7—7, and 7—8.

The synthetic detergents have advantages in solubility and cost over the natural soaps (obtained by saponification of animal fat). Bile salts are notable in that they completely dissolve pneumococcus cells, thus providing an aid in identification.

2. Cationic detergents—The fat-soluble moiety can be made to have a positive charge by combining it with a quaternary (valence = +5) nitrogen atom (Fig 7—5).

Since the detergents concentrate at the cell membrane, and since the latter is a delicate, essential cell component, the inference is drawn that detergents act by disrupting the normal function of the cell membrane. Support for this view comes from experiments showing that cells exposed to detergents "leak" soluble nitrogen and phosphorus compounds into the medium.

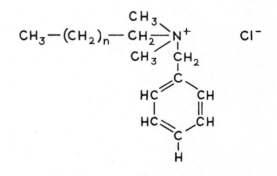

FIG 7—5. **Alkyl-dimethyl-benzyl-ammonium chloride (Roccal).**

$$CH_3\,CH_2\,CH_2\,CH_2\,CH_2\,CH_2\,CH_2\,CH_2\,CH_2\,CH_2\,CH_2\,CH_2\,CH_2\,CH_2\,CH_2\,C\overset{\overset{\displaystyle O}{\|}}{{-}}O^-Na^+$$

FIG 7–6. Sodium salt of palmitic acid (a soap).

$$CH_3\,CH_2\,CH_2\,CH_2\,CH_2\,CH_2\,CH_2\,CH_2\,CH_2\,CH_2\,CH_2\,CH_2-O-\overset{\overset{\displaystyle O}{\|}}{\underset{\underset{\displaystyle O}{\|}}{S}}-O^-Na^+$$

FIG 7–7. Sodium lauryl sulfate (a synthetic anionic detergent, Duponol WA).

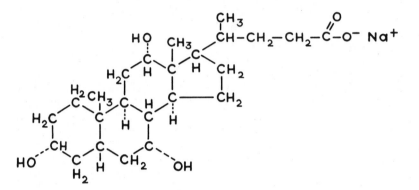

FIG 7–8. Sodium salt of cholic acid (a bile salt).

Chemtherapeutic Agents

To be a useful chemotherapeutic agent, a compound must be either bacteriostatic or bactericidal in vivo (action not reversed by substances in host tissues or fluids), and at the same time remain noninjurious to the host. These requirements for in vivo effectiveness and selective toxicity narrow the list of important chemotherapeutic agents to a very few compounds, principally the sulfonamides, the antibiotics, and the antituberculosis agents.

The natures and modes of action of these drugs are discussed in Chapter 10.

• • •

General References

Books

Gunsalus, I.C., & R.Y. Stanier (editors): *The Bacteria.* Vol 4: *Physiology of Growth.* Academic Press, 1962.

Mandelstam, J., & K. McQuillen (editors): *The Biochemistry of Bacterial Growth.* Wiley, 1968.

Articles & Reviews

Novick, A.: Growth of bacteria. Ann Rev Microbiol 9:97–110, 1955.

Scherbaum, O.H.: Synchronous division of microorganisms. Ann Rev Microbiol 14:283–310, 1960.

Senez, J.C.: Some considerations on the energetics of bacterial growth. Bacteriol Rev 26:95–107, 1962.

8...

The Microbiology of Special Environments

WATER

Methods of Study

A. **Quantitative Analysis:** Bacteria cannot be counted by direct microscopic examination unless there are at least 100 million (10^8) cells per ml. Natural bodies of water, however, rarely contain more than 10^5 cells per ml. The method employed is therefore the plate count: A measured volume of water is serially diluted (see below), following which 1 ml from each dilution tube is plated in nutrient agar and the resulting colonies counted. Since only those cells which are able to form colonies are counted, the method is also known as the "viable count."

A typical example of serial dilution would be the following: One ml of the water sample is aseptically transferred by pipet to 9 ml of sterile water. The mixture is thoroughly shaken, yielding a 1:10 dilution. (For obvious reasons, this is also known as the "10^{-1}" dilution.) The process is repeated serially until a dilution is reached which contains between 30–300 colony-forming cells per ml, at which point several 1 ml samples are plated in a nutrient medium. Since the original sample may have contained up to one million (10^6) viable bacteria, it is necessary to dilute all the way to 10^{-5}, plate 1 ml samples from each dilution tube, and then count the colonies only on those plates containing 30–300 colonies. The reasons for these numerical limits are that below 30 the percent counting error becomes too large, whereas over 300 the plate becomes too crowded to permit each cell to form a visible colony. For example, assume the above procedure has been carried out with the results shown in Table 8–1. The 10^{-3} dilution has a suitable number of colonies, the others being either too high or too low for accuracy. The original water sample is calculated to

TABLE 8–1. Example of a viable count.

Dilution	Plate Count*
Undiluted	} Too crowded
10^{-1}	} to count
10^{-2}	510
10^{-3}	72
10^{-4}	6
10^{-5}	1

*Each count is the average of 3 replicate plates.

have contained 72,000 (72×10^3) viable cells per ml.

B. **Qualitative Analysis:** The methods of plating and enrichment culture (see Chapter 6) are used to obtain a picture of the aquatic bacterial population. While such methods are satisfactory for general biologic studies, they are inadequate for the purpose of sanitary water analysis; this involves the detection of intestinal bacteria in water, since their presence indicates sewage pollution and the consequent danger of the spread of enteric diseases (see Chapter 18). Since any enteric bacteria would be greatly outnumbered by other types present in the water samples, a selective technic is necessary in order to detect them. A widely used procedure for sanitary water analysis is as follows: A large measured volume of water is filtered through a sterilized membrane of a type which retains bacteria on its surface while permitting the rapid passage of smaller particles and water. The membrane is then transferred to the surface of an Endo agar plate. (Endo's medium is a selective, differential medium for coliform bacteria.) Upon incubation, coliform bacteria give rise to typical colonies on the surface of the membrane. The advantages of this method are speed (the complete test takes less than 24 hours) and quantitation, the number of coliform cells being determined for a given volume of water.

Control of Bacteria in Water

Bacteria are controlled in water only in connection with sanitation measures. Two problems are encountered: the sanitation of drinking water and the purification of sewage.

A. **Sanitation of Drinking Water:** Since drinking water supplies may at any time become contaminated with sewage and cause an epidemic of enteric disease, water supplies for large cities are usually filtered and chlorinated. The presence of only 2 parts per million of chlorine will rid the water of the most dangerous contaminant, the typhoid organism. Before chlorination, however, the majority of the bacteria are removed by filtration through beds of sand. In "slow sand filters" removal of bacteria is actually accomplished by their adsorption on the gelatinous film of slime-forming microbes which build up in the sand layers. In "rapid sand filters" chemicals are first added to coagulate organic matter and bacteria; after the precipitate is settled out or is removed mechanically, a rapid filtration through clean sand completes the purification.

B. **Sewage Purification:** In modern cities, domestic sewage is pumped through a disposal plant which accomplishes the following general objectives:

1. **Screening**—Bulky, nondecomposable material is screened and removed (bottles, paper, boxes, gravel, etc).

2. **Sludge formation**—The screened sewage is allowed to settle in large tanks. The sediment, containing much of the organic matter and microorganisms, is called **sludge**. It is drained off at the bottom of the tank and separated from the supernatant, which still contains large amounts of putrescible organic matter. The sludge and supernatant are then treated separately as described below.

The amount of organic matter in the supernatant can be greatly reduced if, instead of simply allowing sludge to form by settling, an activated sludge is caused to form by aeration of the sewage. As air is forced through the sewage, a floc or precipitate is formed, the particles of which teem with actively oxidizing microbes. After a period of time, during which the organic matter is oxidized to a very great extent, the sludge is allowed to settle. The supernatant and part of the sludge are removed for treatment as described below, and part of the sludge is returned to the tank to activate fresh sewage.

3. **Sludge digestion**—The sludge obtained by either process described above consists of organic matter rich in bacteria and other microbes. It is then pumped to anaerobic tanks where fermentation is allowed to go on for weeks or months. Much of the organic matter is converted to gases (CO_2, CH_4, NH_3, H_2, and H_2S). The methane content of the gas may be as high as 75%, and the collected gas may consequently be burned with the production of useful heat. When fermentation is complete, the sludge is removed and disposed of in one of several ways: It may be dried and discarded, or dried and sold as fertilizer (nitrogen may have to be added), or it may be pumped into a large body of water.

4. **Disposal of supernatant**—The supernatant, after chlorination, may be pumped into a large body of water. When none is nearby, however, the supernatant must be treated to remove remaining putrescible material as well as enteric bacteria. This is accomplished by aerating and filtering the fluid: It is sprayed over a bed of sand or broken stone, which then filters it as in the process described earlier for drinking water purification. The aeration is necessary to ensure formation of an oxidizing microbial film on the filter-bed particles.

In some cases, the untreated supernatant is used directly for subsurface irrigation of crop land. Some authorities feel, however, that this introduces the danger of spreading enteric disease.

MILK

Methods of Study

A. **Quantitative Analysis:** Bacteria in milk are counted either directly under the microscope or by plate count. The direct procedure has been rigidly standardized and is known as the "Breed count." The plate count method employs a medium containing skimmed milk in addition to other ingredients, ensuring maximal development of colonies of milk-inhabiting organisms.

Most procedures connected with the bacteriologic analysis of milk have been devised as tests of the safety of the product for human consumption. In addition to the counting procedures, a rough index of bacterial activity in milk is provided by the reductase test. Bacteria contain many enzymes which reduce various substrates. Various dyes are available which are susceptible to bacterial reduction ("reductase activity") and change color when reduced. These dyes thus serve as indicators; in a typical test, a standard amount of a dye such as methylene blue is added to a measured volume of milk, and the time necessary for it to change from blue to colorless is determined. Grade A raw milk which is to be pasteurized, for example, should show a reduction time under standard conditions of 6 hours or more.

B. **Qualitative Analysis:** The types of organisms present in milk are determined by the procedures described above for water bacteriology. Milk, like water, is subject to fecal contamination and is thus also analyzed for the presence of coliform organisms.

Nature of the Environment & of the Bacterial Population

A. **The Environment:** Milk constitutes an ideal bacterial habitat, consisting of emulsified fat droplets and dissolved, physiologic concentrations of salts, sugars, and proteins in water. Milk also contains enzymes originating in the animal. Sugar is present in the form of lactose, a disaccharide in which glucose is linked to one of its stereoisomers, galactose. The pH of fresh milk is about 6.8, which is within the optimal range for most bacteria. As normally handled (in filled containers), milk tends to be anaerobic.

B. **The Bacterial Population:** Because bacteria invade milk usually as dust-borne contaminants, almost any type may be present. Milk constitutes a typical enrichment culture medium, however, and so only the most suited types will predominate. The first organism to flourish in milk is usually *Streptococcus lactis,* which ferments the lactose principally to lactic acid. As the pH drops, other species, such as *Lactobacillus casei* and *L acidophilus,* may replace *S lactis* as the predominant type. If the milk is kept at body temperature, *Aerobacter aerogenes* and *Escherichia coli* may be favored.

Other organisms which may develop in milk under special conditions include anaerobic sporeformers (clostridia), *Streptococcus faecalis* and related enterococci, *Pseudomonas aeruginosa* (producing blue pigment), and lactose-fermenting yeasts.

Ecology

A. Effect of the Environment on Bacteria: As discussed above, the environmental factors which most affect the bacterial population are the degree of anaerobiosis, the temperature, the presence of lactose as the principal sugar, and the pH (which drops as fermentation ensues). The selective effect of these factors has been described above.

B. Effect of Bacteria on Milk:

1. Souring—Milk, whether raw or pasteurized (see below), will sour on standing, mainly as a result of the production of lactic acid by *S lactis* or by the lactobacilli. Many dairy products are purposely allowed to sour in this way, as in the manufacture of "buttermilk," butter, sour cream, yoghurt, and cheese. When *E coli* or *A aerogenes* propagate, mixed acid or butylene glycol fermentations take place; these produce less acidity than lactic acid bacteria but cause the production of gas and unpleasant flavors.

2. "Abnormal fermentations"—All changes due to microbial activity other than souring are referred to as "abnormal fermentations," although many of the processes involved are not fermentative. Included are gas formation by yeasts or bacteria; "ropiness," due to gum secretion by bacteria; "sweet curdling," due to secretion by bacteria of the protein coagulating enzyme rennin; and various color productions due to pigment-forming bacteria.

Control of Bacteria in Milk

It has not yet proved economically feasible to sterilize milk completely except by drastic heating, and this destroys the flavor of fresh milk. (Heat sterilization is used in the production of canned evaporated milk.) However, because contaminated milk is a method of transmission of many diseases, rigid control is necessary.

A. Diseases Transmitted by Milk: Two general classes of disease may be transmitted by milk: those which are transmitted from the animal, the causative microbe being able to infect both animals and men; and those transmitted from other contaminating sources, which are ultimately derived from infected persons.

1. Transmission from the animal—Tuberculosis and undulant fever are the most important of these diseases. Both are transmissible from animal to animal or from animal to man. The route from the animal's tissues to the milk is not known for certain, but it is possible that Brucella organisms, which cause undulant fever, may be secreted directly from the blood stream into the udder. Some authorities also list streptococcal infections in this category, since the streptococci pathogenic for man (Lancefield group A) can be transmitted to cows from infected dairy workers, causing udder infections. One rickettsial disease, Q fever, is also transmitted in milk (probably from the animal).

2. Transmission from infected persons—Milk which is not handled under scrupulously clean conditions may at any time become contaminated by dust or droplets bearing pathogenic microorganisms. Still more likely is direct infection from diseased milk-handlers and dairy workers. The diseases most commonly transmitted by contaminated milk are typhoid fever, dysentery, tuberculosis, and streptococcal infections.

B. Control of Pathogenic Bacteria in Milk: Since many diseases transmitted by milk are the result of milk contamination, an obvious control measure is to insist on sanitary procedures in milk production and bottling. Communities which enforce the provisions of their own Medical Milk Commission with regard to "Certified Raw Milk" or of the USPHS with regard to "Grade A Raw Milk" supervise the production of milk under sanitary conditions. However, even the most sanitary handling procedures cannot prevent the transmission of tuberculosis or undulant fever from infected animals, and the only safe milk is therefore that which has been pasteurized. In the USA, it is becoming the practice to check all dairy cattle by the tuberculin test; an agglutinin test is used to detect infection with Brucella.

Pasteurization may be carried out by maintaining the milk at 62° C (143° F) for 30 minutes and then rapidly cooling it; this will kill all pathogenic bacteria which may be present, although many harmless forms (eg, *S lactis*) survive. Alternatively, pasteurization can be accomplished by heating an extremely thin layer of milk for 3—5 seconds at 74° C. Pasteurization is the only procedure which renders milk absolutely safe without destroying its flavor and palatability.

C. Safety Standards: A very sensitive, practical method used to determine whether milk has been properly pasteurized is known as the phosphatase test, which consists of quantitatively determining the activity of the enzyme phosphatase in a sample of the milk. Because this enzyme is more resistant than any pathogenic bacterium to pasteurization, its destruction indicates that the milk is safe. Phosphatase activity indicates improper pasteurization or adulteration with raw milk.

A satisfactory phosphatase test, however, does not guarantee that the milk has not become contaminated by handlers after pasteurization. To determine this, milk is analyzed for the presence of coliform organisms by the procedures described in the section on water bacteriology above. Even a negative coliform test does not eliminate the possibility that diphtheria or streptococcal organisms may have been introduced. The best protection against this danger is the insistence on sanitary procedures of dairies and medical examination of milk handlers.

FOODS

Methods of Study

The plate count and enrichment culture methods are also used for the examination of foods. Solid food samples must be ground and suspended in liquid for dilution and plating; care must be taken to avoid introducing bacteria from other sources during preparation of the sample. Coliform analysis is carried out on food samples as well as on water and milk to determine whether fecal contamination has occurred.

Nature of the Environment & of the Bacterial Population

A. Meat: The interior of intact meat is usually sterile or nearly so unless taken from an infected animal. The surface, however, becomes contaminated from dust or from handling immediately upon dismemberment of the animal. Any organotrophic bacterium may be found, including those from soil, dung, or human handlers.

B. Ground Meat: The grinding process introduces the surface contaminants into the interior of the meat and may also warm the meat enough to encourage considerable bacterial multiplication. The interior of the meat is somewhat anaerobic, and fermentative organisms are enriched for. The number of bacteria in ground meat is so high that a count of 10 million per gram is considered a safe maximum. (Since such counts are made on aerobic plates, the many obligate anaerobes present are not included in this figure.)

C. Fish: The general picture is similar to that for unground meat, but the bacterial population will include many marine halophilic and psychrophilic forms. The "phosphorescence" of spoiling fish is due to the growth of luminescent marine bacteria (such as Achromobacter) on the surface.

D. Shellfish: These become contaminated during handling, but they also bear organisms acquired from their marine environment. Shellfish gathered near a sewage outlet will contain numbers of sewage bacteria, including both pathogenic enterobacteria and viruses. Outbreaks of infectious hepatitis have been traced to oysters contaminated with the viral agent of this disease. Oysters are often "planted" near sewage outlets because they fatten rapidly on sewage. In recent years it has become mandatory that such oysters be transported to fresh water and left there long enough so that they will cleanse themselves of sewage organisms before they are marketed.

E. Fruits and Vegetables: Most vegetables have a considerable surface contamination of soil organisms. Fruits acquire a surface flora through dust contamination and handling. Fruits and vegetables with tough skins are fairly proof to penetration by bacteria unless bruised; soft fruits and vegetables will spoil much more readily. Acid fruits offer a selective environment for yeasts and molds; otherwise, a typical array of soil microorganisms is found.

F. Eggs: Bacteria may be incorporated into eggs from infected ovaries or oviducts; otherwise the interiors of eggs are usually sterile. The surface becomes contaminated immediately after laying, but penetration of the egg by bacteria is normally prevented by a dry, mucilaginous coating on the surface. This coating is easily removed, however, by washing or overhandling, in which case the interior of the egg becomes contaminated. Bacteria on eggs comes from soil and from the feces of the birds. A mixed flora is common, but fermenters predominate inside the egg. Egg products, like ground meat, show the result of mixing surface contaminants throughout the material; counts are similar to those of ground meat.

G. Bread: The flour from which bread is made contains polysaccharide carbohydrates and protein; fats are added in the form of "shortening." Hydrolysis of the polysaccharides by the yeast or bacteria added to make the bread rise, and partial hydrolysis of the protein by enzymes in the flour, yields a mixture which is ideal for bacterial growth. Baking kills most microorganisms, but spores of bacilli, clostridia, and of fungi persist and will germinate to produce a new flora unless preservatives are added.

Ecology

A. Effect of Environment on Bacterial Population: When organisms begin to grow in food products, selection will determine the predominant type (eg, fermentative organisms are selected for in the anerobic interior of ground meat). Variables which most affect bacterial growth are moisture, factors permitting penetration (bruising of fruits, washing of eggs, etc), and autolysis ("self-dissolving"); as cells die, enzymes are released which dissolve cell walls and protoplasts to a variable extent depending upon the tissue and the environmental conditions. The "ripening" or "tenderizing" of meat, for example, is a result of autolysis. Autolysis results in digestion of polysaccharides, proteins, and fats, rendering the product much more susceptible to bacterial growth.

B. Effect of Bacteria on Food: The interest in food bacteriology is focused on spoilage and disease transmission. Since pathogens affect the consumer rather than the food, only spoilage need be considered here. Disease transmission is discussed below.

Spoilage is the result of microbial growth in or on food. The metabolic activity associated with growth causes both a breakdown of the food substance and the release of the products of fermentation, digestion, and other processes. Spoilage may be defined as the process by which food is rendered unfit for human consumption. Only rarely does this involve actual poisoning of the food ("food poisoning" is restricted to infection by enteric pathogens contaminating food, or ingestion of food containing exotoxins produced by staphylococci or Clostridium botulinum).

Spoilage usually involves alterations in flavor, odor, and color, the production of sliminess, etc—in other words, esthetics. Many types of spoiled food can be eaten with safety; there is no reason, for example, to throw away moldy bread, bacon, or other foods if the taste and odor have not become unpleasant. Other types of spoiled food might, if eaten, cause a mild indigestion. The one danger is that spoiled food may have supported growth of *Clostridium botulinum,* which produces a deadly toxin. This organism requires anaerobic conditions such as are found in the interior of ground meat or various food mixtures.

Unpleasant odors and tastes are produced by "putrefactive" organisms, ie, those which digest proteins and produce H_2S, sulfhydryl compounds, or amines. These compounds, while not poisonous in the concentrations involved, have vile smells. Molds produce a "musty" odor and taste, and some bacteria produce great quantities of slime (as in "ropy bread"). Eggs have a high sulfur content, and their spoilage results in H_2S production, rendering them completely unpalatable. Canned oysters may become covered with a layer of red yeast, in which case they are considered "spoiled" although unchanged in odor, taste, and safety.

Control of Bacteria in Food

A. Prevention of Spoilage: For some foods, such as meats, much can be accomplished along the lines of preventing contamination through the use of sanitary procedures. Some foods, however, already have a rich surface flora from their natural environment (fruits, vegetables, etc), and contamination during handling plays a relatively minor role. In the case of meat, fruit, eggs, and vegetables, it is important to prevent penetration of the food by bacteria (see above). Most effort, however, is directed toward preservative measures; the following measures are used either singly or in combination.

1. Irradiation—Meat packers often keep refrigerated meat under constant ultraviolet irradiation to cut down on surface spoilage.

2. Low temperature—Bacterial activity is markedly slowed at refrigeration temperatures and virtually negligible at temperatures below freezing. Refrigeration and freezing are well-known methods of food preservation and need no further discussion here.

3. Drying—Foods which are kept completely dry will stay preserved indefinitely, since moisture is essential to microbial activity. Examples of dried foods are hay, raisins, "cured" meat, powdered eggs, and powdered milk. All of these contain dormant microorganisms and will spoil if exposed to humidity.

4. Heat—A temperature of 120° C (248° F) for 15 minutes is necessary to kill heat-resistant bacterial spores. Such conditions are obtainable with steam at a pressure of 15 lb per square inch above atmospheric pressure. Industrial autoclaves and home pressure cookers are used for heat-sterilization of canned foods.

5. Salt—Most bacteria are unable to grow at high salt concentrations. Meat and fish are often "salt-cured" by immersion in brine or by rubbing salt into the surface.

6. Sugar—High sugar concentrations produce osmotic pressures which are too high for most bacteria.

Many fruits are packed in syrup, and meat is sometimes rubbed with sugar instead of, or mixed with, salt ("sugar-cured" ham).

7. Smoking—Smoke contains volatile bactericidal substances which are gradually absorbed by the meat or fish being smoked. The smoking process is slow, however, and the food is often salt-treated first to prevent spoilage early in the process.

8. Chemical preservatives—Only a few chemicals are useful preservatives at concentrations harmless to humans. Calcium propionate is used to prevent growth of molds in bread; sodium benzoate is used in cider and some vegetable products; sulfite is used to preserve some fruits.

9. Acids—Many foods which are soured for the purpose of flavor are thereby preserved, since few bacteria can tolerate the pH values produced by the lactic acid or acetic acid bacteria. Examples are buttermilk, pickles, sauerkraut, and vinegar.

B. Prevention of Disease Transmission: Since few of the preservative measures listed above are bactericidal, it is essential that pathogenic organisms be prevented from contaminating food. The infectious diseases transmissible by food are typhoid fever, Salmonella infection, dysentery, and streptococcal infection; the diseases due to bacterial toxins in food are botulism and staphylococcal food poisoning. Botulism is caused by the toxin of the obligate anaerobe *Clostridium botulinum;* it is usually found in improperly sterilized canned foods. Since the canning industry now observes rigid standards of sterilization, most cases of botulism arise from home-canned foods. Correct pressure-cooking technics can eliminate most incidents of botulism; food suspected of contamination with botulinus toxin can be rendered completely safe by boiling for 10–20 minutes.

Staphylococci grow particularly well in cream foods and produce a potent exotoxin. This can usually be prevented by careful refrigeration and sanitary measures to prevent their introduction into foods.

Typhoid fever, Salmonella infections, and dysentery are enteric diseases transmitted by fecal contamination of food. They are preventable only by rigid sanitation control and medical examination of food handlers. Salmonella infection may also be acquired by the ingestion of meat or eggs from infected animals.

AIR

The air does not constitute a bacterial habitat; bacteria exist in the air only as accidental contaminants. However, many pathogens are transmitted through the air on dust particles or on the dry residues of saliva droplets, and control measures are attempted for this reason.

Types of Infectious Particles

Pathogenic microorganisms occur in the air associated with 2 types of particles: the residues of evaporated exhalation droplets (**droplet nuclei**), and the much larger **dust particles**. These 2 types of particles are very different with respect to their source, their settling behavior, their significance in disease, and the methods which must be used to assess them and to control them. Some of these differences are summarized in Table 8–2.

Viability of Air-Borne Organisms

Both dust-borne and droplet-nuclei-borne organisms lose viability in air, and the kinetics of survival are similar to those shown in Fig 8–1. Usually the curve changes slope sharply, revealing the presence of a more resistant fraction, even in experiments dealing with a single type of organism. The presence of 2 populations with different death rates probably reflects differences in the microenvironments of the particles rather than genetic differences in the organisms. The death rates are markedly affected by the humidity and temperature of the air, and there are great differences in death rates among different species of organisms. In general, organisms which are normally air-borne (eg, *M tuberculosis*) are more resistant to inactivation than organisms which are normally water-borne (eg, *E coli*).

Epidemiology of Droplet-Nuclei-Borne Infections

In propagated epidemics, succeeding crops of cases, or "generations," occur as a result of the incubation period which intervenes between successive cases. At each generation, the relationship between the number of new cases (C), the number of infectors (I), and the number of susceptibles (S) is given by the equation

$$C = KIS \qquad \ldots . (1)$$

where K is a constant representing the effective contact rate.

For droplet-nuclei-borne infections, K is related to the volume of air (s) breathed by a susceptible, the number of infectious doses (i) liberated by an infector, and the volume of air (V) which passes through the space in which contact occurs, all measured over the same interval of time, by the equation

$$K = si/V \qquad \ldots . (2)$$

For an epidemic to occur, C/I must exceed 1; the greater the ratio C/I, the more severe the epidemic. Since equation [1] can be rearranged as

$$C/I = KS \qquad \ldots . (3)$$

it is seen that the severity of an epidemic is directly proportionate to K, the effective contact rate, and to S, the number of susceptibles.

These simple equations have been used to make some illuminating calculations. For example, in a measles epidemic occurring in a school where contact took place only in a well-defined classroom area, K was estimated by equation [1] to be 0.1. Since both s and V were known, i could be calculated from equation [2]; it was found to be 270. Thus each infector liberated enough measles virus to infect 270 persons. This

TABLE 8–2. Characteristics of and control measures for air-borne infections.

	Droplet Nuclei	Dust Particles
Source of particles in air	Evaporation of droplets expelled from the respiratory tract by sneezing, coughing, and talking (in decreasing order of effectiveness).	Movements which cause the shedding of particles from skin and clothing; air turbulence sufficient to redistribute previously settled dust.
Settling behavior	Remain suspended indefinitely as a result of minor air turbulence (average settling velocity in still air, 0.04 feet/minute).	Settle rapidly to the ground (average settling velocity, 1.5 feet/minute). Redistributed by major air turbulence.
Organisms per particle	Rarely more than one.	Usually many.
Access to susceptible tissues and significance in disease	Deposited in lungs; probably responsible for most pulmonary infections.	Deposited on external surfaces and in upper respiratory tract.
Epidemiologic characteristics	Propagated epidemics (disease transmitted serially from person to person).	Epidemics associated with specific places as reservoirs of infection.
Control measures	Ventilation; ultraviolet irradiation of the air; evaporation of glycols.	Prevention of accumulation of infectious material (eg, by sterilization of clothing and bedding); prevention of dispersal (eg, by oiling of floors and bedding, and by proper design of ventilation system).

represented about 1 infectious dose per 3000 cubic feet of air, which was the volume breathed by 10 children during the time interval used for the calculation. Thus, under such conditions, one child in 10 could be expected to be infected. (Since, however, the distribution of particles in air is random, there is about one chance in 3 under such conditions that no child would be infected. Chance thus may play a significant part in deciding whether an epidemic will occur.)

Control of Epidemics of Air-Borne Infections

Some control measures for dust-borne infections are indicated in Table 8–2. The accumulation of infectious organisms on fabrics can be minimized by a bactericidal rinse at the end of the laundering process, or by heat sterilization when feasible. The dispersal of dust can be minimized by the oiling or other wetting of blankets and floors; however, the design of the ventilation system often limits what can be accomplished by such measures.

The control measures for droplet-nuclei-borne infections include the following:

A. Sanitary Ventilation: If equations [2] and [3] above are combined, it is found that

$$C/I = si/V_S \qquad \ldots . (4)$$

where V_S is the volume of air per susceptible. Thus, the severity of an epidemic as well as its probability of being initiated (which are proportionate to C/I) are inversely proportionate to V_S. In order to achieve a value of C/I less than 1, the corresponding V_S may require **1 air change per minute** under ordinary circumstances of room size and occupancy. This is more than 5 times that supplied by ordinary air-conditioning installations.

B. Ultraviolet Irradiation: The use of ultraviolet light can accomplish the equivalent of 1 air change per minute by the killing of air-borne organisms. This can be done either by installing high-intensity ultraviolet lamps in the air supply ducts, or by irradiating the air in the upper levels of the room by indirect lamps. The latter method requires good mixing of upper and lower air, but this condition does obtain in many situations. Ultraviolet barriers or "curtains" can also be set up at room entrances so that personnel can pass through quickly and avoid radiation injury.

C. Chemical Disinfection: Propylene glycol and some related compounds are effective germicides in the vapor phase. They presumably act by condensing on droplet nuclei and dehydrating the nuclei-borne organisms. This method is only successful within a narrow range of relative humidities, and is therefore not always reliable.

D. Evaluation: Control measures against dust-borne and droplet-nuclei-borne infections must be separately evaluated by methods which assay only the appropriate particles. The best criterion of success is the lowering of the incidence of disease; in practice, however, it is almost impossible to design valid controls for comparison. For this reason, there are very

few data which permit a valid evaluation of the efficacies of the methods listed above.

When the data indicate that a control measure has failed, it can mean that the transmission route which is being controlled is not significant in the spread of the disease being studied, or the exposure to the disease is taking place outside of the controlled area.

SOIL

The earth is covered with green plants which rapidly convert nitrate, sulfate, and CO_2 into organic matter. The plants die—or are eaten by animals which in turn die—and so return the elements to the soil in organic form. The nitrogen and sulfur are then present principally as the amino ($-NH_2$) and sulfhydryl ($-SH$) groups of proteins; the carbon is present principally in the form of the reduced "carbon skeletons" of carbohydrates, proteins, fats, and nucleic acids.

Without a mechanism for the "mineralization" of these elements, the surface of the earth would long ago have been depleted of the nitrate, sulfate, and CO_2 needed for plant growth, and life on the earth would have ceased. But, as we have seen in the previous sections on metabolism, such a mechanism does exist, in the form of microbial metabolic activities. Thus nitrogen, sulfur, and carbon are constantly undergoing cycles of transformations, from the oxidized, inorganic state to the reduced, organic state and back again. These cycles, and hence all life on the earth, are completely dependent on microbial action, as illustrated in the following paragraphs.

One other major element, phosphorus (as phosphate), is converted to organic form during plant growth, being incorporated chiefly into nucleic acids. On return to the soil, nucleic acids are hydrolyzed by microbial enzymes, again liberating free phosphate. No oxidation or reduction is involved.

The Nitrogen Cycle (See Fig 8–1.)

A. Decomposition: The proteins of organic matter are digested by many microorganisms to free amino acids, from which ammonia (NH_3) is then liberated by deamination. Urea, the principal form in which higher animals excrete nitrogen, is hydrolyzed to NH_3 and CO_2 by various urea-decomposing bacteria.

B. Oxidation of Ammonia: Soil rich in ammonia from decomposing organic matter is abundantly occupied by cells of Nitrosomonas, which obtain their energy for growth by oxidizing NH_3 to nitrite (NO_2^-). As nitrite is formed, the Nitrobacter cells which are present multiply and convert the nitrite to nitrate (NO_3^-).

C. Nitrate Reduction and Denitrification: Nitrate serves as the final hydrogen acceptor for various anaerobic bacteria, being reduced by some to NH_3 and by others to gaseous N_2. In the former case no nitrogen is lost from the soil, since the ammonia usually

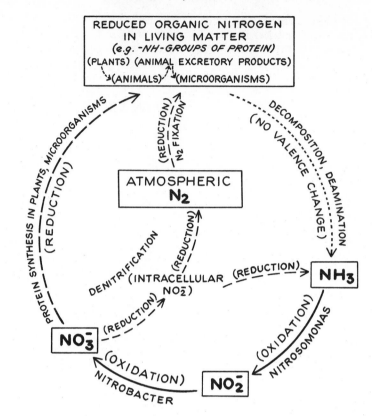

FIG 8–1. The nitrogen cycle.

stays in solution as ammonia ion (NH_4^+); N_2 escapes, however, and the latter process is hence termed "denitrification."

D. Conversion of Nitrate to Organic Nitrogen: Green plants, as well as many microorganisms, convert nitrate to organic nitrogen and reduce it once again to amino groups, thus completing the cycle.

E. Nitrogen Fixation: One other important source of nitrogen is the atmosphere. Atmospheric nitrogen is reduced to organic nitrogen by nitrogen-fixing bacteria and certain algae, balancing the losses due to denitrification. This process, although a reduction, is not a mechanism for anerobic respiration but rather a means of obtaining nitrogen. Many nitrogen fixers, in fact, are aerobes. Two types of fixation are distinguished: symbiotic and nonsymbiotic (see p 65).

The Sulfur Cycle (See Fig 8–2.)

A. Decomposition: Following digestion, the sulfur-containing amino acids are broken down by many microorganisms and in the process H_2S is released.

B. Oxidation of H_2S to Free Sulfur: H_2S spontaneously oxidizes to S in the presence of oxygen; in addition, it is oxidized as an energy source by certain chemolithotrophs and as a hydrogen donor by some photosynthetic bacteria.

C. Oxidation of S to $SO_4^=$: Certain chemolithotrophs and photosynthetic bacteria oxidize sulfur to sulfate.

D. Conversion of Sulfate to Organic Sulfur: This process is analogous to the conversion of nitrate to organic nitrogen in the nitrogen cycle.

E. Sulfate Reduction: Desulfovibrio uses $SO_4^=$ as the final hydrogen acceptor in anaerobic respiration.

The Carbon Cycle (See Fig 8–3.)

The valence changes of carbon are frequently associated with valence changes of oxygen; hence the inclusion of an "oxygen cycle." Since anaerobic respiration of organic matter may involve electron transfer from carbon to sulfate or nitrate, the sulfur and nitrogen cycles are also "geared" to the carbon cycle. By "gearing" we mean that the organic carbon oxidation is coupled with a reduction of nitrate or sulfate by electron transfer.

A. Green Plant Photosynthesis and Aerobic Oxidation: For each molecule of CO_2 reduced in photosynthesis, one molecule of O_2 is produced from H_2O. This process just balances the reduction of O_2 to H_2O in aerobic oxidations, so that the oxygen content of the atmosphere remains remarkably constant at about 20%.

B. Other CO_2 Reductions: A relatively small amount of CO_2 is reduced to organic carbon by processes which do not result in the formation of oxygen. These include chemolithotrophic reduction, bacterial photosynthesis, carbonate reduction in anaerobic respiration, and CO_2 fixations in chemoorganotrophic nutrition.

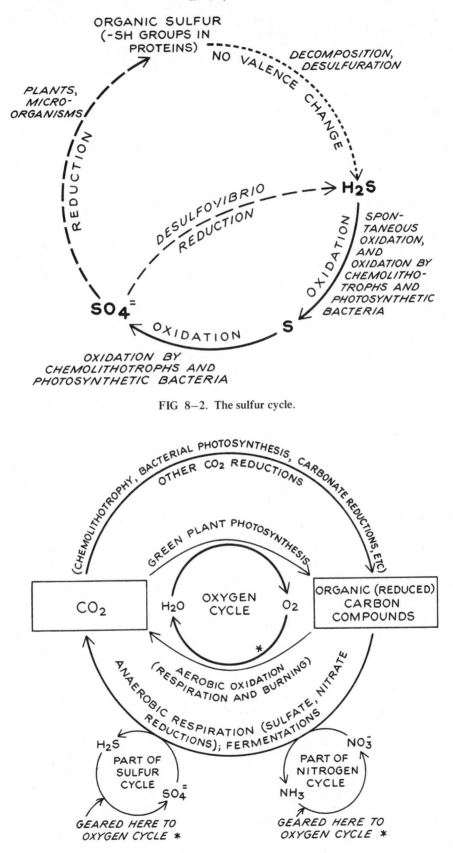

FIG 8–2. The sulfur cycle.

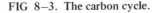

FIG 8–3. The carbon cycle.

   C. Anaerobic Respiration: Anaerobic organotrophs oxidize carbon compounds to CO_2 with nitrate, sulfate, or organic molecules as electron acceptors. When nitrate or sulfate is reduced, their respective cycles are affected; reoxidation of the nitrogen and sulfur is usually accomplished aerobically, causing a half-turn of the oxygen cycle.

●   ●   ●

General References

Frazier, W.C.: *Food Microbiology,* 2nd ed. McGraw-Hill, 1967.
Gregory, P.H., & J.L. Monteith (editors): *Airborne Microbes.* Cambridge Univ Press, 1967.

Riley, R., & F. O'Grady: *Airborne Infection.* Macmillan, 1961.
Stanier, R.Y., Doudoroff, M., & E.A. Adelberg: *The Microbial World,* 3rd ed. Prentice-Hall, 1970.

9 . . .

Bacteriophage

Bacteria are host to a special group of viruses called bacteriophage, or "phage." Although any given phage is highly host-specific, it is probable that every known type of bacterium serves as host to one or more phages. Phages have not been successfully used in therapy. They are important, however, because they furnish ideal materials for studying host-parasite relationships and virus multiplication. Information gained from studies on phage may in the future help solve many problems in the control of animal and plant viruses.

LIFE CYCLES OF PHAGE & HOST

Fig 9–1 summarizes our concepts of phage-host life cycles. The remainder of this chapter is devoted to a detailed account of these cycles and to the experimental evidence for their existence.

Fig 9–1 shows the following:

(1) Life cycle of uninfected bacterium: An uninfected bacterium may reproduce by binary fission, showing no involvement with phage.

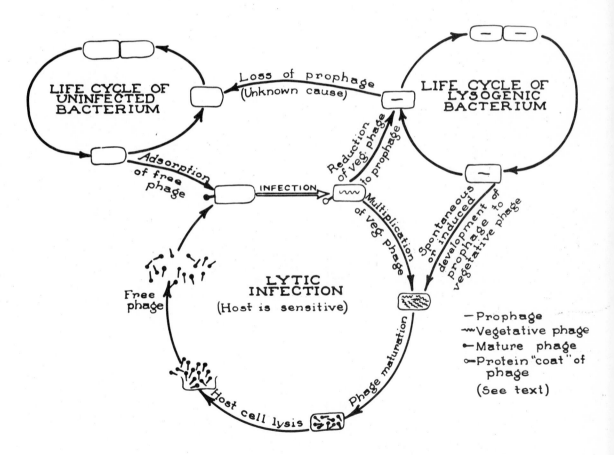

FIG 9–1. Phage-host life cycles.

(2) Adsorption of free phage: When an uninfected bacterium is exposed to free phage, infection will take place if the cell is sensitive. Bacteria may also be genetically resistant to phage infection; such cells lack the necessary receptors on their surface. (Contrast this with "immunity" due to the presence of prophage. See p 103.)

When infection takes place, the phage is adsorbed onto the cell surface and the nucleic acid of the phage penetrates the cell. In this state, the phage nucleic acid is called "vegetative phage."

(3) Lytic infection: The injected vegetative phage material may be reproduced, forming many replicas. These mature by acquisition of protein coats, following which the host cell lyses and free phage is liberated.

(4) Reduction of vegetative phage to prophage: Many phages, termed "temperate," are capable of reduction to prophage as an alternative to producing a lytic infection. The prophage attaches to the bacterial chromosome, with which it reproduces in harmony. The bacterium is now lysogenic (see pp 102–105); after an indeterminate number of cell divisions, one of its progeny may lyse and liberate infective phage.

(5) Loss of prophage: Occasionally a lysogenic bacterium may lose its prophage, remaining viable as an uninfected cell. The cause of this spontaneous loss is unknown.

METHODS OF STUDY

Assay

Since phage (like all viruses) multiplies only within living cells, and since their size precludes direct observation except with the electron microscope, it is necessary to follow their activities by indirect means. For this purpose, advantage is taken of the fact that one phage particle introduced into a crowded layer of dividing bacteria on a nutrient agar plate will produce a more or less clear zone of lysis in the opaque film of bacterial growth. This zone of lysis is called a "plaque"; it results from the fact that the initially infected host cell bursts (lyses) and liberates dozens of new phage particles, which then infect neighboring cells. This process is repeated cyclically until bacterial growth on the plate ceases as a result of exhaustion of nutrients and accumulation of toxic products. When handled properly, each phage particle produces one plaque; any material containing phage can thus be titrated by making suitable dilutions and plating measured samples with an excess of sensitive bacteria. The plaque count is analogous to the colony count for bacterial titration.

Isolation & Purification

In order to study the physical and chemical properties of phage, it is necessary to prepare a large batch of purified virus as free as possible of host cell material. For this purpose, a liquid culture of the host bac-

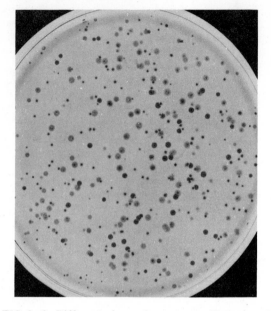

FIG 9–2. Different phage plaque types. (Courtesy of G.S. Stent.)

terium is inoculated with phage and incubated until the culture is completely lysed. The now clear culture fluid, or lysate, contains in suspension only viral particles and bacterial debris. These are easily separated from each other by differential centrifugation. The centrifuged pellet of phage material can be resuspended and washed in the centrifuge as often as needed and may then be used for chemical and physical analysis or for electron microscopy.

PROPERTIES OF PHAGE

One group of phages has been studied more extensively than any other: certain phages which attack *Escherichia coli* strain B (coliphages). Of the numerous coliphages, 7 have been selected for intensive study. Unless otherwise noted, the information given below applies to this group, which has been numbered T1 through T7.

Morphology

A typical phage particle consists of a "head" and a "tail." The head represents a tightly packed core of nucleic acid, surrounded by a protein coat or capsid. The protein capsid of the head is made up of identical subunits, packed to form a prismatic structure, usually hexagonal in cross-section. The smallest known phage has a head diameter of 25 nm; others range from 55 X 40 nm up to 100 X 70 nm.

The phage tail varies tremendously in its complexity from one phage to another. The most complex tail is found in phage T2 and in a number of other coli and typhoid phages. In these phages, the tail consists of at least 3 parts: a hollow core, ranging from 6–10 nm in width; a contractile sheath, ranging from 15–25 nm in width; and a terminal base-plate, hexagonal in shape, to which may be attached prongs, tail fibers, or both. Electron micrographs of phage preparations embedded in electron-dense material such as phosphotungstate show the phages to exist in 2 states: in one, the head contrasts highly with the medium, the sheath is expanded, and the base-plate appears to have a series of prongs. In the second state, the head is of low contrast, the sheath is contracted, and the base-plate is now revealed to have 6 fibers attached to it. The former state presumably represents active phage, containing nucleic acid; the latter state presumably represents phage which has ejected its nucleic acid (eg, into a host cell). These 2 states are diagrammed in Fig 9–3.

A number of other tail morphologies have been reported. In some of these, sheaths are visible but the contracted state has not been observed; and in one case no sheath can be seen. The phages also vary with respect to the terminal structure of the tail: Some have base-plates, some have "knobs," and some appear to lack specific terminal structures.

The phage tail is the adsorption organ for those phages which possess them. Some phages lack tails altogether; in the RNA phages, for example, the capsid is a simple icosahedron.

Although most phages have the head-and-tail structure described above, some **filamentous phages** have been discovered which possess a very different morphology. One of these, called "fd," has been characterized in some detail. It is a rod-shaped structure measuring 6 nm in diameter and 800 nm in length. It contains DNA and protein, which are complexed in a manner which is not completely understood. The DNA may be intertwined with the protein, rather than forming a core, and there is evidence that the entire phage structure penetrates the host cell. Liberation of this phage is also unique in that the phage filaments are extruded through the cell wall without cell lysis occurring.

Chemistry

Phage particles contain only protein and one kind of nucleic acid. Most phages contain only DNA; however, a group of phages which specifically attack male strains of *E coli* contain only RNA. The nucleic acid makes up about 50% of the dry weight, and (in the T-even phages) consists of a single molecule with a molecular weight of 1.3×10^8. In phages T2, T4, and T6, a unique base (hydroxymethylcytosine) is present, to which are attached short chains of glucose units. This pyrimidine has never been found in the nucleic acid of the bacterial host.

The proteins which make up the head membrane, the core, the sheath, and the tail fibers are distinct from each other; in each case, the structure appears to be made of repeating subunits.

PHAGE REPRODUCTION

Adsorption

The kinetics of phage adsorption have been thoroughly analyzed, and the process has been shown to be a first-order reaction; the rate of adsorption is proportionate to the concentration both of the phage and of the bacterium. Under optimal conditions, the observed rates are compatible with the assumption that almost every collision between phage and host cell results in adsorption. If the bacteria are mixed with an excess of phage, adsorption will continue until as many as 300 particles are adsorbed per cell. For the T-phages, this represents a coating of most or all of the cell surface.

Before the phage can be adsorbed onto the host cell, the phage surface must be modified by attachment of positively charged cations (the nature and number of cations varying from one phage to another) and, in some cases, of the amino acid, tryptophan. Each phage is quite specific with regard to the cofactors required for adsorption.

The bacterial surface, ie, the cell wall, is complex and heterogeneous. In gram-negative bacteria, there

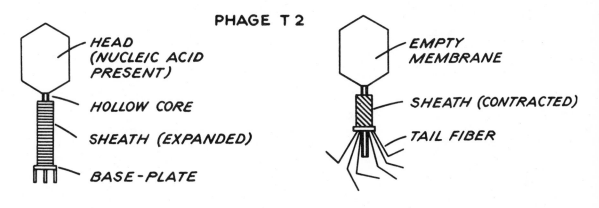

FIG 9–3. Diagrams of phage T2 based on electron micrographic observation. (*Note:* In some micrographs, the base-plate is found attached at the end of the core after contraction of the sheath.)

appear to be 3 distinct layers: an inner layer composed of mucopeptide (see Chapter 2) and 2 outer layers of lipoprotein and lipopolysaccharide. Different bacterial strains are highly specific with regard to the phages which they will adsorb. For example, a strain able to adsorb phages T2, T4, and T6 can give rise to mutants unable to combine with one or another of these viruses. This specificity has been found to reside in the cell wall; when cell walls are isolated and purified, they exhibit the same adsorption patterns as the cells from which they are prepared. The factors in the cell wall responsible for adsorption appear to be discrete, localized "receptors"; the receptors for phages T3, T4, and T7 reside in the lipopolysaccharide layer, whereas the receptors for phages T2 and T6 reside in the lipoprotein layer. Ability to adsorb phage is obviously a factor in the determination of bacterial sensitivity to infection.

Intracellular Development of Phage

Some phages always lyse their host cells shortly after infection, generally in a matter of minutes and usually before the host cell can divide again. (See "lytic infection" cycle in Fig 9–1.) Once such a phage injects its contents into the host cell, ensuing events can be only indirectly ascertained. The most informative data have come from experiments with isotopically labeled phage and labeled metabolites, and from experiments involving premature lysis of infected cells by artificial means.

The process of intracellular development is probably as follows:

(1) Experiments in which the phage nucleic acid was labeled with ^{32}P and the phage protein with ^{35}S have shown that the nucleic acid enters the host cell, whereas the protein coat of the invading virus remains outside. The protein can be removed by mechanical agitation after infection without interfering with reproduction of the phage within. (The exceptions are the filamentous DNA phages, in which the entire phage particle appears to penetrate the host cell.)

(2) For several minutes following infection (eclipse period), active phage is not detectable by artificially induced premature lysis (eg, by sonic oscillation). However, chemical analysis and isotopic tracer studies show that during this period the host cell stops synthesizing bacterial DNA and shifts to production of viral DNA. This involves not only a new arrangement of nucleic acid "building blocks" (purines, pyrimidines, deoxyribose, phosphate) but also, at least in the case of T2, T4, and T6, production of a new type of pyrimidine, hydroxymethylcytosine. The invading phage thus directs the synthesis of new enzymes in the host.

(3) Immediately after penetration of the host cell by phage DNA, a number of new proteins ("early proteins") are synthesized. These include certain enzymes necessary for the synthesis of phage DNA: a new DNA polymerase, new kinases for the formation of nucleoside triphosphates, and a new thymidylate synthetase. The T-even phages (T2, T4, T6), which incorporate hydroxymethylcytosine instead of cytosine into their DNA, also cause the appearance of a series of enzymes needed for the synthesis of hydroxymethylcytosine, as well as an enzyme that destroys the deoxycytidine-triphosphate of the host. Later on in the eclipse period, "late proteins" appear, which include the subunits of the phage head and tail as well as a lysozyme which degrades the mucopeptide layer of the host cell wall. All of these enzymes and phage proteins are synthesized by the host cell using the genetic information provided by the phage DNA.

(4) During the eclipse period, up to several hundred new vegetative phages are produced; as fast as they are formed, they undergo random exchanges of genetic material (see below). The newly formed phage DNA is built with building block compounds which come partly from the medium and partly from degraded host DNA.

(5) Maturation consists of irreversible combination of phage nucleic acid with a protein coat. The mature particle is a morphologically typical infectious virus and no longer reproduces in the cell in which it was formed. If the cells are artificially lysed late in the eclipse period, immature phage particles are found in which the DNA and protein are not yet irreversibly attached, so that the DNA is easily removed.

Lysis & Liberation of New Phage

Phage synthesis continues until the cell disintegrates, liberating infectious phage. The cell bursts as a result of osmotic pressure after the cell wall has been weakened by the phage lysozyme. (The exceptions are the filamentous DNA phages, in which the mature virus particles are extruded through the cell wall without killing the host.)

PHAGE GENETICS

Phage particles exhibit the same 2 fundamental genetic properties that are characteristic of organized cells: general stability of type and a low rate of heritable variation (see Chapter 4).

Phage Mutation

All phage properties are controlled by phage genes and are subject to change through gene mutation. The mechanisms of gene mutation described in Chapter 4 apply equally well to phages; indeed, most of our knowledge concerning the chemical basis of mutation comes from studies on phage genetics.

A phage particle such as T2, which contains 1.3×10^8 daltons of DNA, has sufficient DNA to code for about 100 different proteins of molecular weight 100,000, assuming the triplet code to be correct.

Phage Recombination

If a bacterium simultaneously adsorbs 2 related but slightly different phage particles, both can infect

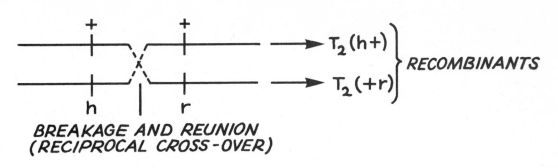

FIG 9—4. Recombination between phage genomes by breakage and reciprocal reunion.

and reproduce; on lysis, the cell releases both types. When this occurs, many of the progeny are observed to be recombinants. For example, one can prepare a double mutant of T2 which differs from wild-type in the type of plaque it forms (large plaques, due to rapid lysis of the host) and in its host range (ability to lyse *E coli* B/2, a mutant strain resistant to lysis by T2). The mutant is designated T2hr ("h" for "host range"; "r" for "rapid lysis"). The wild-type is designated T2++. When a cell of *E coli* B is simultaneously infected with both types and allowed to lyse, the following 4 types of progeny are found:

Parental Types	Recombinant Types
T2++	T2+r
T2hr	T2h+

The "r" mutation occurs very frequently; when a large number of "r" mutants of independent origin were isolated and crossed with each other 2 at a time, it was found that most of them were nonallelic and produced wild-type recombinants. Recombination between phage genomes occurs by the breakage and rejoining of DNA molecules (Fig 9—4).

The closer together 2 markers lie on the same strand, the lower will be the probability of a "crossover" between them. The different pairs of r mutants were found to give widely different recombination frequencies, and these data permitted construction of a linkage map of phage T2, part of which is diagrammed in Fig 9—5.

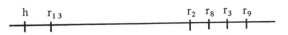
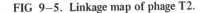

FIG 9—5. Linkage map of phage T2.

Proof of linkage was obtained by showing that map distances were additive: eg, the distance between h and r_2 equaled the sum of the distance h-r_{13} and r_{13}-r_2.

Simultaneous infection of a cell by 3 parental phage types can yield 3-way recombinants, ie, a single progeny may have genes from all 3 parents. Evidence so far obtained supports the concept that "mating" of vegetative phage takes place in pairs but that it is repeated many times between different particles before maturation. When a particle matures, it is removed from the "mating pool."

Genetic Fine Structure

Phage T2 forms plaques when plated on *E coli* strain K12; r mutants, however, do not. This discovery made possible the detection of extremely low frequencies of recombination between different r mutants: a culture of *E coli* B is infected with the 2 r mutants, and the lysate plated on K12. Since 10^8 phage particles can easily be plated, and since only wild-type recombinants can form plaques, a recombination frequency lower than 10^{-6} can be accurately measured.

In a great many such crosses, the lowest frequency observed has been 10^{-4}, or 0.01%. The total genetic map of T2 is estimated to be about 800 crossover units long (1 unit = the distance separating 2 markers which give 1% recombinant progeny). The minimum recombinational unit is thus 0.01/800, or 1.2×10^{-5} of the total map. It has also been estimated that the total DNA of the phage genome contains about 4×10^5 nucleotide pairs, in terms of the Watson-Crick structure (Fig 4—2). If these estimates are correct, a mutation need involve a segment of DNA only 1 or 2 nucleotide pairs in length, and recombination can separate 2 mutant loci which are only 1 or 2 nucleotide pairs apart.

The Genetic Map of Phage T4 (See Fig 9—6.)

Two special classes of phage mutants have greatly extended our knowledge of the phage chromosome: temperature sensitive (ts) mutants and a certain group of host-range mutants. The latter, which have been given the scientifically meaningless name of "amber" (am) mutants, are unable to grow on *E coli* strain B (the normal host of T4) but are able to grow on certain strains of *E coli* strain K12. The ts mutants are able to form plaques on *E coli* B at 25° C but not at 42° C, in contrast with wild-type T4, which forms plaques at both temperatures.

By infecting bacterial cells with ts and am mutants and examining the infected cells and their lysates by serology, electron microscopy, and bio-

chemical tests, it has been shown that a variety of
different classes are represented: Some mutations have
affected DNA replication, some the head protein, some
the tail fibers, and so on. Recombination tests have
allowed the mapping of the ts and am mutations in
relation to the classical markers such as the r loci and
the h loci; the results are shown in Fig 9–6. As in *E
coli,* the genetic map is circular.

LYSOGENY

Earlier in this chapter it was mentioned that some
phages ("temperate phages") fail to lyse the cells they
infect, and then appear to reproduce synchronously
with the host for many generations. Their presence can
be demonstrated, however, because every so often one

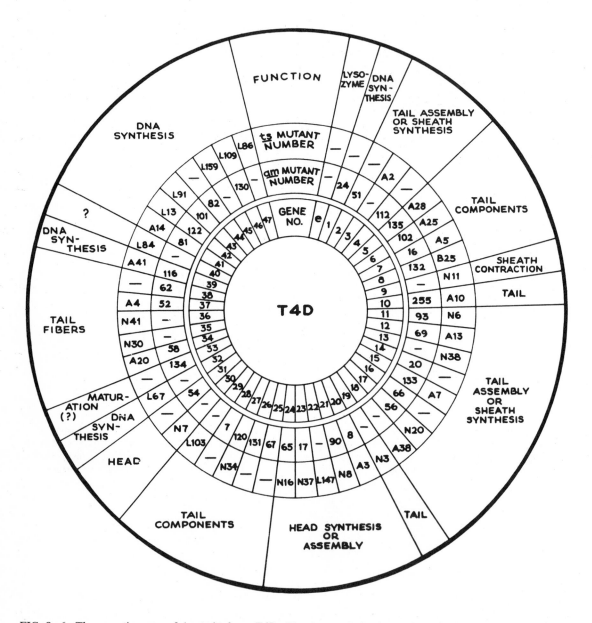

FIG 9–6. The genetic map of bacteriophage T4D. The inner circle shows the division of the map into 48
functional units. Each unit has been shown to be functionally distinct from the others by complementation
test. The size shown for each unit is arbitrary. The next 2 circles show the location of the am and ts
mutations which have been used to reconstruct the map. The outer circle describes the functions controlled
by each unit, as determined by studies on the defects exhibited by the various mutants. (After Epstein &
others: Cold Spring Harbor Symp Quant Biol 28:375, 1963.)

of the progeny of the infected bacterium will lyse and liberate infectious phage. To detect this event it is necessary to use a sensitive indicator strain of bacterium, ie, one that is lysed by the phage. The bacteria which liberate the phage are called "lysogenic"; when a few lysogenic bacteria are plated with an excess of sensitive bacteria, each lysogenic bacterium grows into a colony in which are liberated a few phage particles. These particles immediately infect neighboring sensitive cells, with the result that plaques appear in the film of bacterial growth; in the center of each plaque is a colony of the lysogenic bacterium.

A culture of lysogenic bacteria can also be centrifuged, removing the cells and leaving the temperate phage particles in the supernatant. Their number can be measured by plating suitable dilutions of the supernatant on a sensitive bacterial indicator strain and counting typical plaques.

The release of infectious phage in a culture of lysogenic bacteria is restricted to a very few cells of any given generation. For example, in one bacterial type about 1 in 200 lyse and liberate phage during each generation; in another type it may be 1 in 50,000. The remainder of the cells, however, retain the potentiality to produce active phage and transmit this potentiality to their offspring for an indefinite number of generations.

That lysogenic bacteria bear internal, latent phage was first proved by experiments with a lysogenic spore-former, *Bacillus megaterium.* Heating a culture to a temperature far in excess of that required to destroy free phage permitted the survival of spores which, on germination, yielded lysogenic vegetative cells. Most striking proof of the nature of lysogeny has come from experiments in which single cells, free of infectious phage, were isolated by micromanipulation and grown into lysogenic cultures. In further experiments, single cells were isolated and observed for long periods of time. Only an occasional cell lysed, and only when this occurred was free phage detected.

With the rare exceptions mentioned, lysogenic bacteria contain no detectable phage, either as morphologic, serologic, or infectious entities. However, the fact that they carry the potentiality to produce, generations later, phage with a predetermined set of characteristics means that each cell must contain one or more specific noninfectious structures endowed with genetic continuity. This structure is termed "prophage."

Prophage

Prophage has the following properties: (1) From studies on the life cycle of virulent phage, genetic continuity is known to imply persistence of phage nucleic acid; serologic studies fail to detect the presence of phage protein. (2) Since all the cells in the clone are lysogenic, prophage must be reproduced regularly along with the host. This is accomplished by integration of the prophage DNA into the bacterial chromosome.

The Nature of Prophage Integration

Two entirely different mechanisms of prophage formation are found in different phages. In one mechanism, discovered in phage P1, the phage chromosome circularizes and enters a state of "quiescent" replication which is synchronous with that of the host; no phage proteins are formed. The prophage in the "P1 type" of system is not integrated with the chromosome; it is probably attached to the cell membrane, as are other autonomous replicons in the cell.

In the other system, discovered in phage λ, the prophage is integrated with the host chromosome. The chromosomes of *E coli* and of phage λ are circular; the length of the phage chromosome is about 1/50 that of the bacterial chromosome. A short region of the phage chromosome carries a sequence of nucleotide pairs which is homologous with a sequence in the bacterial chromosome close to the "gal" locus discussed above. When λ infects a cell of *E coli,* pairing of the 2 circular chromosomes occurs in the region of homology. Recombination then takes place by breakage and reciprocal rejoining, with the result that the 2 circles are integrated (Fig 9–7). The enzymes which catalyze the breakage and rejoining (recombination) steps are specified by phage genes. Phage mutants defective in this system are unable to lysogenize the cell.

Further Properties of the Lysogenic System

A. Immunity: Lysogenic bacteria are immune to infection by phage of the type already carried in the cell as prophage. When nonlysogenic cells are exposed to temperate phage, many permit phage multiplication and are lysed, while other cells are lysogenized. Once a cell carries prophage, however, neither it nor its progeny can be lysed by homologous phage. Adsorption takes place, but the adsorbed phage simply persists without reproducing and is quickly "diluted out" by continued cell division.

The immune state is exactly correlated with the presence of prophage. The moment prophage is transformed into vegetative phage and begins to reproduce, immunity is lost. It has been shown that attached prophage causes the appearance in the cytoplasm of a repressor substance which inhibits multiplication of vegetative phage. Repressor also blocks the detachment of prophage (which otherwise would occur by the reversal of the integration process described above) as well as the expression of phage genes (eg, formation of phage proteins). The establishment of the lysogenic state is thus dependent on the production and action of repressor. The λ repressor has been isolated and characterized as a protein which specifically binds to λ DNA.

The immunity of a lysogenic cell to homologous phage is clearly different from the phenomenon of "resistance" to virulent phage, which is exhibited by certain bacteria. In the latter case, resistance is caused by failure to adsorb the phage.

B. Induction: "Vegetative phage" is defined as rapidly reproducing phage on its way to mature infective phage, whereas "prophage" reproduces synchro-

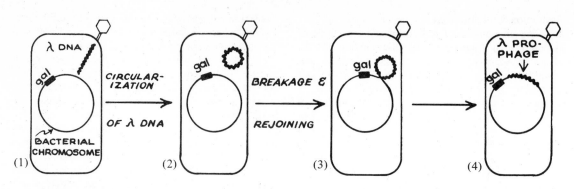

FIG 9—7. The integration of prophage and host chromosome. (1) The phage DNA is injected into the host. **(2)** The ends of the phage DNA are covalently joined to form a circular element. **(3)** Pairing occurs between a sequence of bases adjacent to the gal locus and a homologous sequence on the phage DNA. **(4)** Breakage and reciprocal rejoining ("crossing over") within the region of pairing integrates the 2 circular DNA structures. The integrated phage DNA is called prophage. The length of λ DNA has been exaggerated for diagrammatic purposes. It is actually 1—2% of the chromosomal length.

nously with the host cell. On rare occasions prophage "spontaneously" develops into vegetative (and later into mature) phage. This accounts for the sporadic cell lysis and liberation of infectious particles in a lysogenic culture. However, the prophage of practically every cell of certain lysogenic cultures can be induced by various treatments to form and liberate infectious phage. For example, ultraviolet light will induce phage formation and liberation by most of the cells in a lysogenic culture at a dose which would kill very few nonlysogenic bacteria.

The susceptibility of prophage to induction depends on the genetic constitution of the prophage and on the physiologic state of the host prior to the induction treatment. The state of the host can be experimentally modified by controlling conditions of cultivation.

In some cases, infection of a lysogenic bacterium with a virulent phage will induce development of the prophage present; when the cells lyse, the liberated phage particles include genetic recombinants of the virulent and prophage "parents."

Induction requires the inactivation or destruction of repressor molecules present in the cell. Phage mutants have been obtained which produce thermolabile repressors: These phages can be induced simply by raising the temperature to 44° C. Inducing agents such as UV, on the other hand, appear to cause the accumulation in the cell of an inducer which inactivates the phage repressor; the nature of this inducer is still unknown.

C. Mutation to Virulence: When temperate phage is mixed with nonlysogenic bacteria, some of the cells reproduce the phage and are lysed, while others are lysogenized.

The outcome of the infection of any given cell appears to be determined by a race between phage replication and the formation of repressor: If the former proceeds far enough before repressor appears, the cell will lyse; if repressor is formed early, the cell will survive and become lysogenic.

Temperature phage can mutate to the virulent state. Virulent mutants can then be used in multiple infection experiments with temperate phage and recombinants obtained, showing that virulence is genetically determined like other properties of phage.

Two types of virulent mutants have been found. In one type, the mutation has made the phage resistant to the repressor, so that it can multiply even in lysogenic cells which are otherwise immune; in the other type, the phage has lost the ability to produce repressor. Virulent mutants of temperate phages are quite different from the naturally virulent phages such as T2. The latter cause the appearance of enzymes which degrade host DNA and stop the synthesis of ribosomal RNA, whereas the former do not interfere with the normal metabolism of the host.

D. Effect on Genotype of Host: When a lysogenic phage, grown on host "A," infects and lysogenizes host "B" of a different genotype, some of the cells of host "B" may acquire one or more closely linked genes from host "A." For example, if the phage is grown in a lactose-nonfermenting host, about 1 in every million cells infected becomes lactose-fermenting. The transferred property is heritable. This phenomenon, called "transduction," is described in more detail in Chapter 4.

In other instances, phage genes may themselves determine new host properties. For example, cells of *Corynebacterium diphtheriae* become toxigenic when lysogenized by a certain phage, with 100% efficiency. In Salmonella, phage infection confers a new antigenic surface structure on the host cell. The acquisition of new cell properties as the result of phage infection is called "phage conversion." Phage conversion differs from transduction in that the genes controlling the new properties are found only in the phage genome, and are never found in the chromosome of the host bacterium.

Restriction & Modification

The phenomena of restriction and modification, as described in Chapter 4, were discovered as a result of their effects on phage multiplication. It was observed that if phage λ is grown in *E coli* strain K12, only about 1 in 10^4 particles can multiply in strain B. The few that succeed, however, liberate progeny which infect B with an efficiency of 1.0, but infect strain K12 with an efficiency of 10^{-4}.

It was shown that the DNA of particles formed in K12 is modified by a K12 enzyme so as to be immune to degradation in K12. In strain B, however, the DNA of such particles is rapidly degraded by the restricting enzyme of the host. The few particles which escape restriction are modified by the specific modification enzyme of strain B; the progeny formed are now susceptible to degradation in K12, but not in B.

Certain temperate phages carry genes which govern the formation of new modification and restriction enzymes in the host. Thus, *E coli* cells carrying P1 prophage will degrade all DNA not modified in a P1-containing cell.

It seems likely that a given restricting enzyme recognizes a particular site on DNA and causes hydrolysis at that site unless the site has already been protected by the homologous modifying enzyme. Restriction appears to be a mechanism by which a cell protects itself against invasion by foreign DNA.

•   •   •

General References

Books

Hayes, W.: *The Genetics of Bacteria and Their Viruses,* 2nd ed. Blackwell, 1968.

Stent, G.: *The Molecular Biology of Bacterial Viruses.* Freeman, 1963.

Stent, G. (editor): *Papers on Bacterial Viruses,* 2nd ed. Little, Brown, 1965.

Articles & Reviews

Horne, R.W., & P. Wildy: Symmetry in virus structure. Virology 15:348–373, 1961.

Lwoff, A.: The concept of virus. J Gen Microbiol 17:239–253, 1957.

Lwoff, A., Horne, R., & P. Tournier: A system of viruses. Cold Spring Harbor Symposium 27:51–55, 1962.

10 . . .

Antimicrobial Chemotherapy

Although various chemicals have been used for the treatment of infectious diseases since the 17th century (eg, quinine for malaria and emetine for amebiasis), chemotherapy as a science begins with Paul Ehrlich. He was the first to formulate the principles of selective toxicity and to recognize the specific chemical relationships between parasites and drugs, the development of drug-fastness in parasites, and the role of combined therapy in combating this development. Ehrlich's experiments in the first decade of the twentieth century led to the arsphenamines, the first major triumph of planned chemotherapy.

The current era of rapid development in antimicrobial chemotherapy began in 1935, with the discovery of the sulfonamides by Domagk. In 1940, Chain and Florey demonstrated that penicillin, which had been observed in 1929 by Fleming, could be made into an effective chemotherapeutic substance. During the past 25 years, chemotherapeutic research has largely centered around antimicrobial substances of microbial origin called antibiotics. The isolation, concentration, purification, and mass production of penicillin was followed by the development of streptomycin, tetracyclines, chloramphenicol, and many other agents. Although these substances were all originally isolated from filtrates of media in which their respective molds, or streptomyces, had grown, several have subsequently been synthesized. In recent years chemical modification of molecules by biosynthesis has been a prominent method of new drug development. Brief summaries of antimicrobial agents commonly employed in medical treatment are presented at the end of this section.

SELECTIVE TOXICITY

The fundamental principle of chemotherapy is the principle of selective toxicity, which may be stated as follows: In order to be useful for systemic treatment of infectious disease, a substance must be harmful to parasites but relatively innocuous to host cells. This is the main difference between useful systemic antimicrobial drugs and disinfectants, which are highly active against the parasite in vitro but are not sufficiently well tolerated by the host to permit systemic administration. "Selective toxicity" must be based on certain

unique features of structure or of function of the parasite which set it apart from the host cell. A few known features of this sort are discussed below. In many other instances, the precise reason for the selective toxicity of useful antimicrobial drugs is not presently understood. For each antimicrobial drug found safe for therapeutic use, hundreds have been discarded because they proved toxic not only to the parasite but also to the host.

MECHANISM OF ACTION OF ANTIMICROBIAL DRUGS

It was once believed that most types of antibacterial effects could be explained by competitive antagonism. An enzyme usually catalyzes a single reaction. The substrate attaches to the enzyme's active center where it is activated, metabolized, and released. A competitor is a chemical compound similar to (but not identical with) the substrate which can combine with the enzyme's active center but cannot be metabolized and released. It remains attached to the active center and prevents combination of the active center with the true substrate.

However, it is now apparent that competitive antagonism is rare among antimicrobial drugs and that most effective antimicrobial substances act by interfering with the synthesis, assembly, or function of the macromolecular components of microbial cells. A brief summary of the probable mechanisms of action of certain antimicrobial drugs is given below.

Inhibition of Growth by Means of Analogues of Essential Metabolites (Competitive Antagonism) (*Example:* Sulfonamides.)

For many microorganisms, para-aminobenzoic acid (PABA) is an essential metabolite in the synthesis of folic acid, which serves as an important step in the eventual synthesis of purines. The specific mode of action of PABA probably involves an ATP-dependent condensation of a pteridine with PABA to yield dihydropteroic acid, which is subsequently converted to folic acid. Sulfonamides are structural analogues of PABA.

Sulfonamides can enter into the reaction in place of PABA and compete for the active center of the

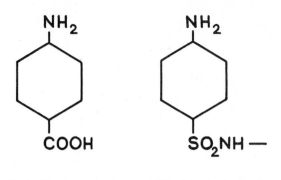

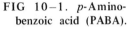

FIG 10−1. *p*-Amino-
benzoic acid (PABA).

FIG 10−2. Basic ring
structure of sulfon-
amides.

enzyme. As a result, nonfunctional analogues of folic acid are formed, preventing further growth of the bacterial cell.

This is the outstanding example of competitive antagonism among antimicrobial drugs. For a given sulfonamide and a given microorganism, the ratio of the inhibitory concentration of a sulfonamide in the presence of different concentrations of PABA is almost constant. This S/PABA ratio is an index of sulfonamide activity and varies greatly with different drugs, eg, it might be 2000 for sulfanilamide and 27 for sulfathiazole.

Animal cells cannot synthesize folic acid and depend on an exogenous source. Some bacteria likewise do not synthesize folic acid, but require it for growth. These bacteria, like animal cells, are not inhibited by sulfonamides. Many other bacteria cannot use the form of folic acid that occurs in most tissues but synthesize folic acid by the reaction described above, and consequently are susceptible to sulfonamide action. The inhibiting action of sulfonamides on bacterial growth can be counteracted by an excess of PABA in the environment.

Tubercle bacilli are not inhibited markedly by sulfonamides, but their growth is inhibited by aminosalicylic acid (para-aminosalicylic acid, PAS). Conversely, most sulfonamide susceptible bacteria are resistant to PAS. This suggests that the enzyme catalytic site for PABA differs in different types of organisms.

A later step in folic acid metabolism, the conversion of dihydro- to tetrahydrofolate, can be inhibited by trimethoprim. Sulfonamides plus trimethoprim can thus produce sequential blocking which results in marked enhancement of activity (eg, in urinary tract infections, malaria).

Inhibition of Cell Wall Synthesis
(*Example:* Penicillins.)

In contrast to animal cells, bacteria possess a rigid outer layer, the cell wall. It maintains the shape of microorganisms and "corsets" the bacterial cell, which has a high internal osmotic pressure. Removal of the cell wall (eg, by lysozyme) or inhibition of its formation may lead to lysis of the cell. In a hypertonic

environment (eg, 20% sucrose), cell wall inhibition leads to formation of spherical bacterial "protoplasts" limited only by the fragile cytoplasmic membrane. If such protoplasts are placed in an environment of ordinary tonicity, they may explode.

The cell wall contains a chemically distinct complex polymer "mucopeptide" consisting of polysaccharides and a highly cross-linked polypeptide ("peptidoglycan"). The polysaccharides regularly contain an amino sugar, acetylmuramic acid, which is found only in bacteria. (See Chapter 2.)

Penicillins are selective inhibitors of bacterial cell wall synthesis. It has been proposed that penicillin may be a structural analogue of acyl-D-alanyl-D-alanine and may inhibit the terminal cross-linking of linear glycopeptides, thus interfering with the complex mucopeptide synthesis. Under the influence of low concentrations of penicillin, the formation of dividing cross walls is inhibited, and bizarre, enormous forms develop from bacteria. With higher concentrations of penicillin, cell wall formation is completely blocked and cells may lyse or, if the medium is hypertonic, change to protoplasts. In penicillin-inhibited cells, nucleotides accumulate which are cell wall precursors. However, the synthesis of proteins and nucleic acids continues unabated.

All penicillins and all cephalosporins act through selective inhibition of cell wall synthesis. The difference in susceptibility of gram-positive and gram-negative bacteria to penicillins may depend on the chemical differences in cell wall composition which determine penetration or binding of the drugs.

Several other drugs likewise inhibit bacterial cell wall synthesis, but this may not be their principal or sole mode of action. Among them are bacitracin, vancomycin, novobiocin, and cycloserine. D-cycloserine, a structural analogue of the amino acid D-alanine, blocks cell wall synthesis by interfering with alanine incorporation into the peptide portion of the polymer.

Inhibition of Cell Membrane Function
(*Example:* Polymyxins.)

The cytoplasm of all living cells is bounded by the cytoplasmic membrane, which serves as a selective permeability barrier and thus controls the internal composition of the cell. If the functional integrity of the cytoplasmic membrane is disrupted, purine and pyrimidine nucleotides and proteins escape from the cell and cell damage or death ensues. The cytoplasmic membrane of certain bacteria and fungi can be more readily disrupted by certain agents than the membranes of animal cells. Consequently, selective chemotherapeutic activity is possible.

The outstanding examples of this mechanism are the polymyxins acting on gram-negative bacteria and the polyene antibiotics acting on fungi. However, polymyxins are inactive against fungi and polyenes are inactive against bacteria. This is because sterols are present in the fungal cell membrane and absent in the bacterial cell membrane. Polyenes must interact with a sterol in the fungal cell membrane prior to exerting their effect.

Bacterial cell membranes do not contain that sterol, and consequently are resistant to polyene action—a good example of cell individuality and of selective toxicity.

Inhibition of Protein Synthesis (*Examples: Chloramphenicol, Aminoglycosides*)

It is established that chloramphenicol, tetracyclines, streptomycins, and erythromycins can inhibit protein synthesis in bacteria. Puromycin is an effective inhibitor of protein synthesis in animal and other cells. The concepts of protein synthesis are undergoing rapid change, and the precise mechanism of action is not established for any one drug.

Chloramphenicol does not interfere with cell wall or nucleic acid synthesis. It acts on the 50 S unit of bacterial ribosomes and interferes markedly with the attachment of amino acids to nascent peptide chains. In animal cells with stably attached mRNA, chloramphenicol does not significantly inhibit protein synthesis. However, it inhibits new antibody synthesis, which requires attachment of new mRNA. Chloramphenicol is bacteriostatic for many bacteria, and its action is readily reversible.

Tetracyclines inhibit protein synthesis in bacteria by blocking the binding of charged amino-acyl transfer RNA (tRNA) to the 30 S unit of ribosomes. Macrolides (erythromycin group) and lincomycin also inhibit protein synthesis but their mode of action is not yet established.

Streptomycin can effectively inhibit protein synthesis in bacteria. Streptomycin binds to a protein of the 30 S unit of ribosomes and causes a misreading of the mRNA message. This results in the synthesis of nonfunctional proteins.

Streptomycin resistance is associated with an altered structure of ribosomal protein which otherwise serves as binding site for streptomycin. In streptomycin dependent bacteria, the misreading of the mRNA message is a requirement for growth.

Other aminoglycosides (kanamycin, neomycin, and gentamicin) act similarly to streptomycin.

Inhibition of Nucleic Acid Synthesis

Drugs such as the actinomycins are effective inhibitors of DNA synthesis. Actually they form complexes with DNA by binding to the deoxyguanosine residues. The DNA-actinomycin complex inhibits the DNA-dependent RNA polymerase and blocks mRNA formation. Actinomycin also inhibits DNA virus replication.

Mitomycin effectively depolymerizes DNA. Both actinomycins and mitomycin inhibit bacterial as well as animal cells and are not sufficiently selective to be employed in antibacterial chemotherapy.

The halogenated pyrimidines (eg, 5-iodo-2-deoxyuridine, idoxuridine, IDU) can block the synthesis of functionally intact DNA and thus interfere with the replication of infective DNA viruses. IDU can interfere with the incorporation of thymidine into viral DNA, and IDU itself is incorporated into DNA to form nonfunctional DNA. The systemic administration of IDU is rarely feasible because of its severe toxicity, but local application to DNA virus-producing cells (especially in herpes simplex keratitis) can result in significant suppression of viral replication in vivo.

Nalidixic acid, used mostly as a urinary antiseptic, is a potent inhibitor of DNA synthesis, but it is not known whether its antibacterial action depends on this effect.

DRUG RESISTANCE

Mutation & Adaptation

Drug-resistant organisms arise in a bacterial population by mutation or other genetic mechanisms, rarely by nongenetic adaptation.

A. Genetic Mechanisms of Drug Resistance: Most large bacterial populations contain mutants which are less susceptible to a given drug than the remainder of the population. Such mutations on the bacterial chromosome arise independently of exposure to the drug. The drug only serves to select the mutants from the susceptible organisms.

"Resistance patterns" vary with each drug and with different organisms. First step mutants to penicillins, tetracyclines, chloramphenicol, and other drugs tend to be of low and uniform resistance. Second step mutants (ie, those descended from a population of first step mutants) are uniformly of only slightly higher resistance. On the other hand, first step mutants to streptomycin may be of low or of very high resistance, including some which are completely unaffected by levels of streptomycin attainable in tissues.

Once a drug resistant mutant has arisen in a bacterial population, the mutation can be transferred to other cells by the mechanisms of transformation, transduction, or conjugation, depending on the type of mechanism which is applicable to the particular bacteria. The transfer of chromosomal genes by any of these mechanisms probably occurs at low rates in nature. Recombination between 2 cells, each resistant to a different drug, can produce a cell resistant to both drugs.

Drug resistance can also be transferred genetically through the transfer of episomes or plasmids. Outstanding examples are the resistance transfer factor (RTF) capable of transmitting multiple drug resistance among gram-negative bacteria by conjugation, and the plasmids controlling penicillinase production transmitted between staphylococci by bacteriophage transduction. These are described in more detail in the chapters on microbial genetics and bacteriophage.

B. Nongenetic Mechanisms of Drug Resistance: It has been postulated that drugs can act as a direct and necessary stimulus to the development of resistance of the entire exposed microbial population. Such "adaptation" probably contributes only rarely, if ever, to the development of significant drug resistance. However, environmental conditions can account for drug resistance independent of genotype. For example, metabolically inactive microorganisms can readily survive drug action. Such phenotypically resistant "persisters" may be important in chronic infection and failure of drug therapy.

Mechanisms of Drug Resistance

Among the many possible explanations of the mechanisms of drug resistance, the following appear attractive but are only in part supported by evidence: (1) Increased destruction of the drug, eg, production of penicillin destroying enzymes, penicillinases, by many penicillin resistant organisms. (2) Decreased permeability of the organism to the drug. (3) Increased formation of the metabolite with which the drug competes for an enzyme, eg, increased PABA synthesis in some sulfonamide resistant strains. (4) Increased synthesis of the inhibited enzyme. (5) Development of an alternate metabolic pathway, bypassing the inhibited reaction. (6) An altered enzyme which is still able to perform its metabolic function but is no longer affected by the drug. (7) An altered structure of ribosomal protein, eg, in streptomycin resistance.

When microbial variants are resistant to a certain drug and are selected out from the population by that drug, they may also be resistant to another drug to which they have not been exposed. This is known as cross-resistance. Such relationships exist principally between agents that are closely related chemically, eg, all tetracyclines; erythromycins-carbomycin-spiramycin-oleandomycins; streptomycin-dihydrostreptomycin; neomycin-kanamycin-paromomycin; polymyxin-colistin.

The emergence of drug resistance in infections may be minimized in the following ways: (1) by maintaining sufficiently high levels of the drug in the tissues to inhibit both the original population and first step mutants (of the "penicillin type"; see above); (2) by simultaneous administration of 2 drugs which do not give cross-resistance, each of which delays the emergence of mutants resistant to the other drug (eg, streptomycin and isoniazid in the treatment of tuberculosis); and (3) avoiding exposure of microorganisms to a particularly valuable drug by restricting its use, especially in hospitals.

Clinical Implications of Drug Resistance

In 1936, when sulfonamides were first employed for the treatment of gonorrhea, practically all strains of gonococci were susceptible and most cases were cured by these drugs. Six years later the majority of strains were resistant and most cases failed to respond to sulfonamide therapy. Until 1962, meningococci were regularly susceptible to sulfonamides. Subsequently, sulfonamide resistant group B meningococci appeared in and spread widely in some military populations. Sulfonamides have lost most of their usefulness in the prevention and treatment of meningococcal infections in military populations, and some spread to

civilians has occurred. A similar increase in resistance has taken place with staphylococci. In 1944 the vast majority of strains of staphylococci isolated from hospitalized patients or members of hospital staffs were found to be sensitive to penicillin. By 1948, 65−85% of staphylococci in hospitals were resistant to penicillin. This change has been attributed to the fact that large-scale use of penicillin in hospitals has resulted in elimination of penicillin sensitive staphylococci and their replacement by resistant variants (usually producing penicillinase). The widespread use of tetracyclines also resulted in elimination of tetracycline sensitive organisms and their replacement by tetracycline resistant ones. Thus, a majority of "hospital staphylococci" are both penicillin resistant and tetracycline resistant. These strains present both a clinical problem in the individual patient and an epidemiologic one with respect to the entire hospital population and the community. Tetracycline resistant strains of pneumococci and group A streptococci have appeared and, most recently, methicillin resistant staphylococci have been noted.

A similar situation has developed with respect to gram-negative enteric organisms, especially in hospitals. The excessive use of drugs leads to suppression of drug-susceptible microorganisms and favors the survival of drug resistant ones. This "selection pressure" of drugs in the hospital environment gradually brings about prevalence of drug resistant microbial species, eg, aerobacter, proteus, pseudomonas, and serratia.

To a limited extent, drug resistant mutants have arisen in tuberculosis. Streptomycin resistant and isoniazid resistant mutants may complicate the treatment of individual patients in whom they arise and may be transmitted to contacts, giving rise to primary drug resistant infections.

In closed environments, eg, hospitals or military establishments, the intensive exchange of drug resistant organisms between persons and their spread by fomites greatly contribute to the problem. The possibility also exists that certain drug resistant organisms may exhibit enhanced virulence or ability to disseminate.

DRUG DEPENDENCE

Certain organisms not only are resistant to a drug but even require it for growth. This has been best demonstrated for streptomycin, but it may apply to other antimicrobial drugs as well. When streptomycin dependent meningococci are injected into mice, progressive fatal disease results only if the animals are treated simultaneously with streptomycin. In the absence of streptomycin the microorganisms cannot proliferate and the animals remain well. This phenomenon probably plays no role in human infection and its treatment.

ANTIMICROBIAL ACTIVITY IN VITRO

Antimicrobial activity is measured in vitro in order to determine (1) the potency of an antibacterial agent in solution, (2) its concentration in body fluids or tissues, and (3) the sensitivity of a given microorganism to known concentrations of the drug.

A. Measurement of Antimicrobial Activity: Determination of these quantities may be undertaken by one of 2 principal methods: dilution or diffusion.

Using an appropriate standard test organism and a known sample of drug for comparison, these methods can be employed to estimate either the potency of antibiotic in the sample or the "sensitivity" of the microorganism.

1. Dilution tests—These are carried out by incorporating antimicrobial substances in graded amounts into liquid or solid bacteriologic media. The media are subsequently inoculated with test bacteria and incubated. The end point is taken as that amount of antimicrobial substance required to inhibit the growth of, or to kill, the test bacteria.

2. Diffusion method—A filter paper disk, a porous cup, or a bottomless cylinder containing measured quantities of drug is placed on a solid medium which has been heavily seeded with the test organisms. After incubation the diameter of the clear zone of inhibition surrounding the deposit of drug is taken as a measure of the inhibitory power of the drug against the particular test organism. Obviously this method is subject to many physical and chemical factors in addition to the simple interaction of drug and organisms (eg, nature of medium, diffusibility and molecular size of drug, stability of drug). Nevertheless, standardization of conditions permits quantitative assay of drug potency or sensitivity of the organism.

When determining bacterial sensitivity by the diffusion method, most laboratories use disks of antibiotic-impregnated filter paper. A concentration gradient of antibiotic is produced in the medium by diffusion from the disk. As the diffusion is a continuous process, the concentration gradient is never stable for long; but some stabilization can be achieved by allowing diffusion to start before bacterial growth begins. The greatest difficulties arise from the varying growth rates of different microorganisms and must be corrected by varying the density of the inoculum.

Since it is not feasible to state directly the antibiotic concentration in the medium at any given distance from the diffusion center, interpretation of the results of diffusion tests must be based on comparisons between dilution and diffusion methods. Such comparisons have been made, and, under the sponsorship of WHO, international reference standards are being established. Linear regression lines can express the relationship between log of minimum inhibitory concentration in dilution tests and diameter of inhibition zones in diffusion tests.

Use of a single disk for each antibiotic with careful standardization of the test conditions permits the evaluation of "susceptibility" for a microorganism by comparing the size of the inhibition zone against a standard of the same drug.

It is fundamentally wrong to regard inhibition around a disk containing a certain amount of antibiotic as implying sensitivity to the same concentration of the antibiotic per ml of medium.

B. Factors Affecting Antimicrobial Activity: Among the many factors which affect antimicrobial activity in vitro the following must be considered because they significantly influence the results of tests.

1. pH of environment—Some drugs are more active at acid pH (eg, nitrofurantoin); others at alkaline pH (eg, streptomycin, sulfonamides).

2. Components of medium—Salts may strikingly inhibit streptomycin. PABA in tissue extracts antagonizes sulfonamides. Serum proteins bind penicillins in varying degrees, ranging from 40% for methicillin to 96% for oxacillin.

3. Stability of drug—At incubator temperature, several antimicrobial agents lose their activity. Chlortetracycline is inactivated rapidly and penicillins more slowly, whereas streptomycin, chloramphenicol, and polymyxin B are quite stable for long periods.

4. Size of inoculum—In general, the larger the bacterial inoculum, the lower the apparent "sensitivity" of the organism. Large bacterial populations are less promptly and completely inhibited than small ones. In addition, the likelihood of the emergence of a resistant mutant is much greater in large populations.

5. Length of incubation—In many instances, microorganisms are not killed but only inhibited upon short exposure to antimicrobial agents. The longer incubation continues, the greater the chance for resistant mutants to emerge or for the least susceptible members of the microbial population to begin multiplying as the drug deteriorates.

6. Metabolic activity of microorganisms—In general, actively and rapidly growing organisms are more susceptible to drug action than those in the resting phase. "Persisters" are metabolically inactive organisms which survive long exposure to a drug but whose offspring are fully susceptible to the same drug. A specialized form of "persisters" might be L forms of bacteria. Under treatment with drugs which inhibit cell wall formation, protoplasts may be formed in certain tissues of suitable osmotic properties. These protoplasts could persist in tissues while the drug (eg, penicillin) was administered and might later revert to intact bacterial forms, giving rise to relapse of disease.

ANTIMICROBIAL ACTIVITY IN VIVO

The problem of the activity of antimicrobial agents in vivo is much more complex than in vitro. It

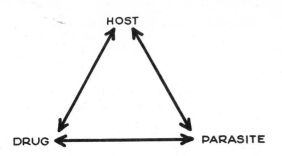

FIG 10—3. Interrelationships of host, drug, and parasite.

involves not only drug and parasite but also a third factor, the host. The interrelationships of host, drug, and parasite are diagrammed below. Drug-parasite and host-parasite relationships are discussed in the following paragraphs. Host-drug relationships (absorption, excretion, distribution, metabolism, and toxicity) are dealt with mainly in pharmacology texts.

DRUG-PARASITE RELATIONSHIPS

Several important interactions between drug and parasite have been discussed in the preceding pages. The following are additional important in vivo factors.

Environment

The environment in the test tube is constant for all members of a microbial population. In the host, however, varying environmental influences are brought to bear on microorganisms located in different tissues and in different parts of the body. Therefore, the response of the microbial population is much less uniform within the host than in the test tube.

A. State of Metabolic Activity: In the test tube the state of metabolic activity is relatively uniform for the majority of microorganisms. In the body it is diverse; undoubtedly, many organisms are at a low level of biosynthetic activity and are thus relatively insusceptible to drug action. These "dormant" microorganisms or "persisters" often survive exposure to high concentrations of drugs and subsequently may produce a clinical relapse of the infection. Alternatively, "persisters" may be bacterial L forms insusceptible to drugs which inhibit cell wall formation.

B. Distribution of Agent: In the test tube all microorganisms are equally exposed to the drug. In the body the antimicrobial agent is unequally distributed in tissues and fluids. Often the lesion induced by the microorganism tends to protect it from the drug. The walls of abscesses, for example, are avascular and may delay passage of the drug. Fibrin deposits may also impede the free diffusion of the drug; necrotic tissue or pus may adsorb the drug and thus prevent its contact with bacteria.

C. Location of Organisms: In the test tube the microorganisms come into direct contact with the drug. In the body they may often be located within tissue cells. Drugs enter tissue cells at different rates. Some (eg, oxytetracycline) reach about the same concentration inside monocytes as in the extracellular fluid. With others (eg, streptomycin) the intracellular concentration is only a small fraction (perhaps 5—10%) of the extracellular concentration.

D. Interfering Substances: In the test tube drug activity may be impaired by becoming bound to protein, by interacting with salts, and in similar ways. The biochemical environment of microorganisms in the body is much more complex and results in significant interference with drug action. The drug may be bound by blood and tissue proteins or lipids; it may also react with nucleic acids in pus and may be physically adsorbed onto exudates, cells, and necrotic debris. In necrotic tissue the pH may be highly acid and thus unfavorable for drug action (eg, streptomycin).

Concentration

In the test tube microorganisms are exposed to an essentially constant concentration of drug. In the body this is not so.

A. Absorption: The absorption of drugs from the intestinal tract (if taken by mouth) or from tissues (if injected) is irregular. There is also a continuous excretion, as well as the inactivation of the drug. Consequently the available levels of drug in the body fluctuate continuously, and the microorganisms are exposed to varying concentrations of the antimicrobial agent.

B. Distribution: The distribution of drugs varies greatly with different tissues. In some body cavities (eg, the pleura or the dural sac), many drugs penetrate poorly; drug concentrations following systemic administration are therefore inadequate for effective treatment. In such situations the drug must be administered locally (eg, injection of drugs into the pleural space in empyema). On surface wounds or mucous membranes local (topical) application of poorly-absorbed drugs permits highly effective local concentrations without toxic side-effects.

C. Variability of Concentration: The critical consideration in antimicrobial therapy is the necessity of maintaining an effective concentration of the drug in contact with microorganisms at their site of proliferation or establishment in the tissues for a sufficient length of time to cause eradication of infecting organism. Because the drug is administered intermittently and is absorbed and excreted irregularly, the levels constantly fluctuate at the site of infection. In order to maintain sufficient drug concentrations for a sufficient time, the time-dose relationship has to be considered. The larger each individual drug dose, the longer the permissible interval between doses. The smaller the individual dose, the shorter the interval which will ensure adequate drug levels. A good general rule in antimicrobial therapy is as follows: Give a sufficiently large amount of an effective drug as early as possible, and continue treatment long enough to ensure eradication of infection; but give an antimicrobial drug only when it is indicated by rational selection.

HOST-PARASITE RELATIONSHIPS

Host-parasite relationships may be altered by antimicrobial drugs in several ways.

Alteration of Tissue Response
The inflammatory response of the tissues to infections may be altered if the drug suppresses the multiplication of microorganisms but does not eliminate them from the body, and an acute process may in this way be transformed into a chronic one. Conversely, the suppression of inflammatory reactions in tissues by the corticosteroids may reduce the effectiveness of antimicrobial agents. The administration of antineoplastic chemotherapeutic agents depresses inflammatory reactions and immune responses and consequently leads to enhanced susceptibility to infection and diminished response to antimicrobial drugs.

Alteration of Immune Response
If an infection is modified by an antimicrobial drug, the immune response of the host may also be altered. Two examples will suffice to illustrate this phenomenon.

(1) In untreated salmonella infection, recovery is associated with the development of immunity, so that relapses are uncommon. When this disease is treated for a short time with chloramphenicol, recovery is greatly accelerated but a relapse is likely to occur when the drug has suppressed the microorganisms so that the normal immune mechanism is not adequately stimulated. When the drug is withdrawn, the organisms resume multiplication and illness returns. This sequence may repeat itself several times.

(2) Infection with beta-hemolytic group A streptococci is followed frequently by the development of antistreptococcal antibodies and occasionally by the development of rheumatic fever. If the infective process can be interrupted early and completely with antimicrobial drugs, the development of antibodies and rheumatic fever can be prevented (presumably by rapid elimination of the antigen). Drugs and doses which rapidly eradicate the infecting streptococci (eg, penicillin) are more effective in preventing rheumatic fever than those that merely suppress the microorganisms temporarily (eg, tetracycline).

Alteration of Microbial Flora
Antimicrobial drugs affect not only the infecting microorganisms but also susceptible members of the normal microbial flora of the body. An imbalance is thus created which in itself may lead to disease. A few examples will serve:

(1) In hospitalized patients who receive tetracyclines or penicillin the normal microbial flora is sup-pressed. This creates a partial void which is filled by the organisms most prevalent in the environment, particularly drug resistant "hospital" staphylococci, pseudomonas, etc. Such superinfecting organisms subsequently may produce serious drug resistant infections.

(2) In women taking tetracycline antibiotics by mouth, the normal vaginal flora may be suppressed, permitting marked overgrowth of candida. This leads to unpleasant local inflammation and itching which is difficult to control.

(3) In the presence of urinary tract obstruction, the tendency to bladder infection is great. When such urinary tract infection due to a sensitive microorganism (eg, *Escherichia coli*) is treated with an appropriate chemotherapeutic drug, the organism may be eradicated. However, very often a "superinfection" due to drug resistant proteus, pseudomonas, or aerobacter species occurs as soon as the drug sensitive microorganisms are suppressed. A similar process accounts for respiratory tract superinfections in patients being treated for chronic bronchitis or bronchiectasis.

(4) In persons receiving antimicrobial drugs by mouth, the normal intestinal flora may be suppressed. Drug resistant staphylococci may establish themselves in the bowel in great numbers and may cause serious enterocolitis.

CLINICAL USE OF ANTIBIOTICS

Dangers of Indiscriminate Use
(1) Widespread sensitization of the population, with resulting hypersensitivity, anaphylaxis, rashes, fever, blood disorders, cholestatic hepatitis, and perhaps connective tissue diseases.

(2) Changes in the normal flora of the body, with disease resulting from "superinfection" due to overgrowth of drug resistant organisms.

(3) Masking serious infection without eradicating it. For example, the clinical manifestations of an abscess may be suppressed while the infectious process continues.

(4) Direct drug toxicity, particularly with prolonged use of certain agents. Important examples are aplastic anemia due to inappropriate use of chloramphenicol; renal damage due to aminoglycoside antibiotics; auditory nerve damage due to kanamycin.

(5) Development of drug resistance in microbial populations, chiefly through the elimination of drug sensitive microorganisms from antibiotic-saturated environments (eg, hospitals) and their replacement by drug resistant microorganisms.

Selection of Antibiotics
The rational selection of antimicrobial drugs depends upon the following:

A. Diagnosis: A specific etiologic diagnosis must be formulated. This can often be done on the basis of a clinical impression. Thus in typical streptococcal sore throat, gonorrhea, or lobar pneumonia, the relationship between clinical picture and etiologic agent is sufficiently constant to permit selection of the antibiotic of choice on the basis of clinical impression alone. Even in these cases, however, as a safeguard against diagnostic error, it is preferable to obtain a representative specimen for bacteriologic study before giving antimicrobial drugs.

In most infections the relationship between etiologic agent and clinical picture is not constant. It is therefore important to obtain proper specimens for bacteriologic identification of the etiologic agent. As soon as such specimens have been secured, chemotherapy can be started on the basis of the "best guess." Once the etiologic agent has been identified by laboratory procedures, chemotherapy can be modified as necessary.

When the etiologic agent of a clinical infection is known, the drug of choice can often be selected on the basis of current clinical experience. At other times, laboratory tests for antibiotic sensitivity (see below) are necessary to determine the drug of choice.

B. Sensitivity Tests: Laboratory tests for antibiotic sensitivity are indicated in the following circumstances: (1) When the microorganism recovered is of a type which is often resistant to antimicrobial drugs (eg, staphylococci, enterococci, proteus, coliform organisms). (2) When an infectious process is likely to be fatal unless treated specifically (eg, meningitis, septicemia). (3) In certain infections where eradication of the infectious organisms requires the use of drugs which are rapidly bactericidal, not merely bacteriostatic (eg, bacterial endocarditis, acute osteomyelitis). The laboratory aspects of antibiotic sensitivity testing are discussed in Chapter 24.

C. Serum Assay of Bactericidal Activity: This test determines directly whether adequate amounts of the correct drugs are being administered to the patient from whom an etiologic organism has been isolated. Serum is obtained during therapy, diluted, inoculated with the previously isolated organism, and incubated. Subcultures at intervals must indicate bactericidal activity in significant serum dilutions (depending upon inoculum size, usually at least 1:10) to suggest adequate therapy.

COMBINED ANTIBIOTIC ACTION

Indications

Combinations of antimicrobial agents may rationally be used (1) in mixed infections; (2) to prevent or delay the emergence of resistant mutants; (3) to achieve additive or synergistic effects against a homogeneous population of resistant organisms; or (4) for emergency treatment of serious infections before laboratory studies are completed (eg, suspected gram-negative bacterial sepsis).

Mechanisms

When 2 antimicrobial agents act simultaneously on a homogeneous microbial population the effect may be one of the following: (1) Indifference, ie, the combined action is no greater than that of the more effective agent when used alone. (2) Addition, ie, the combined action is equivalent to the sum of the actions of each drug when used alone. (3) Synergism, ie, the combined action is significantly greater than the sum of both effects. (4) Antagonism, ie, the combined action is less than that of the more effective agent when used alone.

All these effects may be observed both in vitro (particularly in terms of bactericidal rate) and in vivo. Antagonism is sharply limited by time-dose relationships and is therefore a rare event in clinical antimicrobial therapy. Indifference and simple addition are most common with drug combinations. Synergism is the most desirable form of combined drug action in the treatment of infections, but it is rare.

The effects which can be achieved with combinations of antimicrobial drugs vary with different combinations and are specific for each strain of microorganism. Thus no combination is uniformly synergistic. Combined effects cannot be predicted from the behavior of the microorganism toward single drugs.

Combined therapy should not be used indiscriminately; every effort should be made to employ the single antibiotic of choice. In resistant infections detailed laboratory study can at times define synergistic drug combinations which may be essential to eradicate the microorganisms.

CHEMOPROPHYLAXIS

Anti-infective chemoprophylaxis implies the administration of drugs to prevent the establishment of pathogenic microorganisms in the body. The term may also include the administration of drugs soon after exposure to pathogens but before the development of symptoms and disease.

It is not possible to remove—or prevent the establishment of—all possible microorganisms with one or even with several antimicrobial drugs. **The useful effect of chemoprophylaxis is limited to the action of a specific drug against a specific microorganism.** Any effort to prevent the establishment of any or all microorganisms only selects the most drug resistant ones as the cause of subsequent infection. In all forms of chemoprophylaxis, the risk of a possible infection in a given individual must be weighed against the toxicity, cost, efficacy, and inconvenience of the proposed chemoprophylaxis.

Antibacterial chemoprophylaxis is an accepted clinical procedure for the prevention of group A streptococcus, gonococcus, syphilis, and plague infections. Prophylactic drugs have also been used against rickettsial and poxvirus infections. The prevention of bac-

Table 10–1. Practical chemical disinfectants.

Table tops, instruments, and other inanimate objects	Lysol phenolic disinfectant, 5%; $HgCl_2$, 1:1000; quaternary ammonium compounds (eg, Zephiran or Roccal).
Skin	Soap and water; soaps containing hexachlorophene 2–3%; surface-active agents (anionic detergents); weak (2%) tincture of iodine; PVP-bound iodine (eg, Betadine); 70% ethyl alcohol; or isopropyl alcohol.
Air	Aerosols in finely dispersed droplets, particularly propylene or diethylene glycols. Ultraviolet light.

Gases may be used for disinfection (eg, HCOH, SO_2, Cl_2) but are generally objectionable. Gaseous ethylene oxide is useful as a sterilizing agent for instruments and materials which tolerate heat poorly.

terial endocarditis, of postcoital cystitis, and of exacerbations in chronic bronchitis in persons at high risk at a particular time has also been recommended.

The reduction of lower bowel flora prior to elective bowel surgery has found wide application, but its efficacy as "chemoprophylaxis" is not proved. Specific bactericidal drugs aimed at the most dangerous pathogens likely to complicate cardiac surgical procedures may be helpful at times. In the large majority of elective surgical procedures, however, there is no evidence that "chemoprophylactic drugs" affect the incidence or severity of postoperative infections in any way.

ANTIMICROBIAL DRUGS FOR LOCAL (TOPICAL) APPLICATION

The following agents are occasionally applied to infected surface tissues (skin, mucous membranes, superficial wounds, burns); they may be used alone or in conjunction with systemic chemotherapy.

Dyes

Gentian violet; acridine dyes (acriflavines), 2–3% in aqueous solution or jelly.

Nitrofurans

Nitrofurazone (Furacin), 0.2% in solution or jelly.

Heavy Metal Compounds

Ammoniated mercury, 2–5% in ointment base; silver nitrate, 0.5% solution for wet compresses or 0.5% cream for burns.

Antimicrobial Drugs

Tyrothricin in concentrations of 0.5 mg/ml (cannot be administered systemically because it is hemolytic). Tyrothricin consists of 2 substances: tyrocidin and gramicidin, both polypeptides, active against gram-positive organisms.

Nystatin (Mycostatin) and amphotericin B (Fungizone) are effective for the local suppression of candida. Bacitracin, neomycin, and polymyxin B are used topically in high concentrations because they are poorly absorbed from wounds or mucous membranes. They can also be given systemically with suitable precautions.

Sulfamylon hydrochloride as a 10% emulsion can be applied to burns to control infection.

ANTIMICROBIAL DRUGS FOR SYSTEMIC ADMINISTRATION

PENICILLINS

The penicillins are derived from molds of the genus Penicillium (eg, *P notatum*) and obtained by extraction of submerged cultures grown in special media. The most widely used natural penicillin at present is penicillin G. From fermentation brews of penicillium, 6-aminopenicillanic acid has been isolated on a large scale. This made it possible to synthesize an almost unlimited variety of penicillin-like compounds by coupling the free amino group of the penicillanic acid to free carboxyl groups of different radicals.

All penicillins share the same basic structure. A thiazolidine ring (a) is attached to a beta-lactam ring (b) which carries a free amino group (c). The acidic radicals attached to the amino group can be split off by bacterial and other amidases. The structural integrity of the 6-aminopenicillanic acid nucleus is essential to the biologic activity of the compounds. If the beta-lactam ring is enzymatically cleaved by beta-lactamases (penicillinases), the resulting product, penicilloic acid, is devoid of antibacterial activity. However, it carries an antigenic determinant of the penicillins and acts as a sensitizing hapten when attached to serum proteins.

The different radicals (R) attached to the aminopenicillanic acid determine the essential pharmacologic properties of the resulting drugs. The clinically important penicillins of 1970 fall into 3 main groups. (1) Highest activity against gram-positive bacteria, inactivated by penicillinases (eg, penicillin G, penicillin V, benzathine penicillin); (2) somewhat lower activity against gram-positive bacteria but resistant to penicillinases (eg, methicillin, nafcillin, oxacillin, dicloxacillin); (3) broad spectrum activity against both gram-negative and gram-positive bacteria, inactivated by penicillinase (eg, ampicillin, carbenicillin). Some representatives are shown in Figs 10–4 to 10–10. Most penicillins are dispensed as sodium or potassium salts of the free acid. Potassium penicillin G contains about 1.7 mEq of K^+ per million units (2.8 mEq/gm). Procaine salts and benzathine salts of penicillin provide repository forms for intramuscular injection. In dry form, penicillins are stable, but solutions rapidly lose their activity and must be prepared fresh for administration.

Antimicrobial Activity

All penicillins have the same mode of action: They inhibit the synthesis of bacterial cell walls by blocking the terminal cross-linking of linear glucopeptides into the complex peptidoglycan. Since active cell wall synthesis is a requirement for susceptibility to penicillins, metabolically inactive cells, or L forms, are unaffected. Most penicillins are much more active against gram-positive than gram-negative bacteria, probably because of differences in cell wall composition.

Penicillin G and penicillin V are often measured in units (1 million units = 0.6 gm), but the semisynthetic penicillins are measured in grams. Whereas 0.002–1 µg/ml of penicillin G is lethal for a majority of susceptible gram-positive organisms, 10–100 times more is required to kill gram-negative (except neisseriae). The activity of penicillins also varies with their protein binding, which ranges from 40% to more than 95% for different drugs.

Resistance

Certain organisms (eg, many pathogenic staphylococci, coliforms, pseudomonas) produce beta-lactamases (penicillinases), which inactivate some penicillins. Penicillinase-producing staphylococci are susceptible to methicillin, oxacillin, dicloxacillin, nafcillin, and the cephalosporins.

Certain organisms (eg, coliforms) produce an enzyme, amidase, which splits off the R side chain from 6-aminopenicillanic acid and inactivates the drug.

Certain bacteria are genetically resistant to penicillins but do not destroy the drug. Their resistance must reside in the nature of the mucopeptide structure and synthesis. Such mutants arise infrequently in susceptible populations, and the resistance is of small magnitude.

Among penicillinase-producing staphylococci, mutants arise infrequently which are insusceptible to the penicillinase resistant penicillins (eg, methicillin) and cephalosporins.

Metabolically inactive cells, or L forms, are not susceptible to penicillin, but the offspring of these "persisters" are fully susceptible.

Absorption, Distribution, & Excretion

After intramuscular or intravenous administration, absorption of most penicillins is rapid and complete. After oral administration, only 1/20–1/3 of the dose is absorbed, depending on acid stability, binding to foods, presence of buffers, etc. After absorption, penicillins are widely distributed in tissues and body fluids. Protein binding is 40–60% for penicillin G, ampicillin, and methicillin; 90% for nafcillin; and 95% or more for oxacillin and dicloxacillin. For most rapidly absorbed penicillins, a parenteral dose of 3–6 gm/24 hours yields serum levels of approximately 1–6 µg/ml.

Special dosage forms have been designed for delayed absorption to yield drug levels for long periods. After a single IM dose of benzathine penicillin, 1.5 gm (2.4 million units), serum levels of 0.03 unit/ml are maintained for 10 days and levels of 0.005 unit/ml for 3 weeks. Procaine penicillin given intramuscularly yields levels for 24 hours.

In many tissues, penicillin concentrations are similar to those in serum. Lower levels occur in joints, eyes, and CNS. However, in meningitis, penetration is enhanced and levels of 0.2 µg/ml occur in the CSF with a daily parenteral dose of 12 gm.

Most of the absorbed penicillin is rapidly excreted by the kidneys. About 10% of renal excretion is by glomerular filtration and 90% by tubular secretion. The latter can be partially blocked by probenecid (Benemid) to achieve higher systemic levels. In the newborn and in persons with renal failure penicillin excretion is reduced, and systemic levels remain elevated longer.

Clinical Uses

Penicillins are the most widely used antibiotics, particularly in the following areas:

Penicillin G is the drug of choice in infections caused by streptococci, pneumococci, meningococci, nonpenicillinase-producing staphylococci, gonococci, spirochetes, clostridia, aerobic gram-positive rods, and bacteroides. Most of these infections respond to daily doses of penicillin G, 0.4–4 gm. Intermittent intramuscular injection is the usual method of administration. Much larger amounts (6–120 gm daily) can be given by intravenous infusion in serious infections. Oral administration of buffered penicillin G or penicillin V is indicated in minor infections in daily doses of 1–4 gm. Oral administration is subject to so many variables that it should not be relied upon in seriously ill patients.

Penicillin G is inhibitory for enterococci (*Streptococcus faecalis*); but for bactericidal effects (eg, in enterococcal endocarditis), kanamycin or streptomycin must be added. Penicillin G in ordinary doses is excreted in sufficiently high concentrations into the urine to inhibit some gram-negative organisms in urinary tract infections, particularly *Proteus mirabilis*. However, this treatment fails in the presence of large numbers of beta-lactamase-producing bacteria.

Benzathine penicillin G is a salt of very low solubility given intramuscularly for low but prolonged drug levels. A single injection of 2.4 million units (1.5 gm) is satisfactory treatment for group A streptococcal pharyngitis. The same injection once every 3–4 weeks is satisfactory prophylaxis against group A streptococcal reinfection in rheumatics.

Infection with beta-lactamase-producing staphylococci is the only indication for the use of the lactam-

TABLE 10–2. Drug selections, 1969–70.

Suspected or Proved Etiologic Agent	Drug(s) of First Choice	Alternative Drug(s)
Gram-negative cocci		
Gonococcus	Penicillin[1]	Erythromycin[2], cephalosporin[3],
Meningococcus		tetracycline[4]
Other neisseriae		
Gram-positive cocci		
Pneumococcus	Penicillin[1]	Cephalosporin, erythromycin,
Staphylococcus, nonpenicillinase-producing		lincomycin
Streptococcus viridans		
Streptococcus, hemolytic		
Staphylococcus, penicillinase-producing	Penicillinase-resistant penicillin[5]	Cephalosporin, vancomycin, erythromycin, lincomycin
Streptococcus faecalis (enterococcus)	Penicillin plus streptomycin	Penicillin plus kanamycin, ampicillin plus streptomycin
Gram-negative rods		
Aerobacter (Enterobacter)	Kanamycin	Tetracycline, gentamicin, chloramphenicol
Bacteroides	Tetracycline	Penicillin
Brucella	Tetracycline plus streptomycin	Streptomycin plus sulfonamide[6]
Escherichia		
E coli sepsis	Kanamycin	Cephalothin, ampicillin
E coli urinary tract infection (first attack)	Sulfonamide[7]	Ampicillin
Hemophilus (meningitis, respiratory infections)	Ampicillin	Chloramphenicol
Klebsiella	Cephalosporin plus ampicillin	Tetracycline plus streptomycin
Mima-Herellea	Kanamycin	Tetracycline, gentamicin
Pasteurella (plague, tularemia)	Streptomycin plus tetracycline	Sulfonamide[6]
Proteus		
P mirabilis	Penicillin, ampicillin	Kanamycin, gentamicin
P vulgaris and other species	Kanamycin	Chloramphenicol, gentamicin
Pseudomonas		
Ps aeruginosa	Polymyxin	Gentamicin
Ps pseudomallei (melioidosis)	Chloramphenicol	
Ps mallei (glanders)	Streptomycin plus tetracycline	
Salmonella	Chloramphenicol, ampicillin	Cephalosporins
Serratia	Gentamicin	Kanamycin
Shigella	Ampicillin	Tetracycline
Vibrio (cholera)	Tetracycline	Chloramphenicol
Gram-positive rods		
Actinomyces	Penicillin[1]	Tetracycline, sulfonamide
Bacillus (eg, anthrax)	Penicillin[1]	Erythromycin
Clostridium (eg, gas gangrene, tetanus)	Penicillin[1]	Tetracycline, erythromycin
Corynebacterium	Penicillin[1]	Erythromycin, cephalosporin
Nocardia	Sulfonamide[6]	Tetracycline
Acid-fast rods		
Actinomyces	Penicillin[1]	Tetracycline, sulfonamide
Mycobacterium tuberculosis	INH plus PAS plus streptomycin	Other antituberculosis drugs
Myco leprae	Dapsone or sulfetrone	Other sulfones
Nocardia	Sulfonamide[6]	Tetracycline, cycloserine
Spirochetes		
Borrelia (relapsing fever)	Tetracycline	Penicillin
Leptospira	Penicillin	Tetracycline
Treponema (syphilis, yaws)	Penicillin	Erythromycin, tetracycline
Mycoplasma	Tetracycline	Erythromycin
Psittacosis-lymphogranuloma-trachoma agents	Tetracycline, sulfonamide[6]	Erythromycin, chloramphenicol
Rickettsiae	Tetracycline	Chloramphenicol

[1] Penicillin G is preferred for parenteral injection; penicillin G (buffered) or penicillin V for oral administration. Only highly sensitive microorganisms should be treated with oral penicillin.
[2] Erythromycin estolate and triacetyloleandomycin are the preferred oral forms.
[3] Cephalothin and cephaloridine are the best accepted cephalosporins.
[4] All tetracyclines have the same activity against microorganisms and all have comparable therapeutic activity and toxicity. Dosage is determined by the rates of absorption and excretion of different preparations.
[5] Parenteral methicillin, nafcillin, or oxacillin. Oral dicloxacillin or other isoxazolylpenicillin.
[6] Trisulfapyrimidines have the advantage of greater solubility in urine over sulfadiazine for oral administration; sodium sulfadiazine is suitable for intravenous injection in severely ill persons.
[7] For previously untreated urinary tract infection, a highly soluble sulfonamide such as sulfisoxazole or trisulfapyrimidines is the first choice.

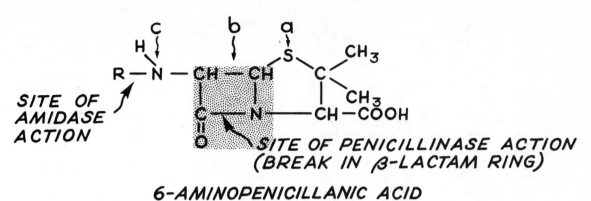

SITE OF AMIDASE ACTION

SITE OF PENICILLINASE ACTION (BREAK IN β-LACTAM RING)

6-AMINOPENICILLANIC ACID

FIG 10—4. 6-Aminopenicillanic acid.

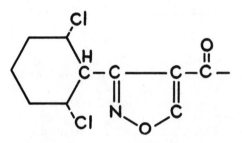

FIG 10—5. **Penicillin G.** Destroyed by penicillinase; active against gram-positive bacteria; acid-labile. Little protein-bound (50%).

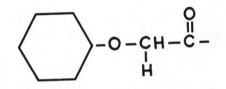

FIG 10—6 **Penicillin V.** Similar to penicillin G but relatively stable to acid.

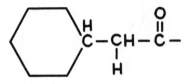

FIG 10—7. **Oxacillin, cloxacillin (1 Cl in structure), dicloxacillin (2 Cl in structure).** Not destroyed by penicillinase; active against gram-positive bacteria; relatively acid-stable; strongly (96%) protein-bound; can be given by mouth.

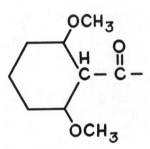

FIG 10—8. **Methicillin.** Not destroyed by penicillinase; active against gram-positive bacteria; acid-labile. Cannot be given by mouth. Little protein-bound (40%).

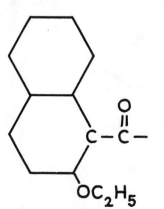

FIG 10—9. **Nafcillin.** Similar to dicloxacillin but less strongly protein bound (90%). Not destroyed by penicillinase, active against gram-positive bacteria. Relatively acid stable.

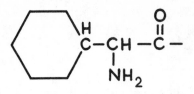

FIG 10–10. **Ampicillin.** Destroyed by penicillinase; acid-stable; active against gram-negative as well as gram-positive organisms. Little protein-bound (50%).

ase resistant penicillins, eg, methicillin, nafcillin, or oxacillin (8–16 gm IV for adults, 50–100 mg/kg/day IV for children); oxacillin, cloxacillin, dicloxacillin, or nafcillin, 2–6 gm/day by mouth, can be given for milder staphylococcal infections.

Ampicillin, 3–6 gm/day, can be given orally for treatment of some urinary tract infections with coliforms. In larger doses, ampicillin suppresses salmonella infections. For bacterial meningitis in small children, ampicillin, 150 mg/kg/day IV, is the present choice. Carbenicillin resembles ampicillin but is somewhat more active against pseudomonas; however, resistance emerges rapidly.

Side-Effects

Penicillins possess less direct toxicity than any of the other antimicrobial drugs. Most serious side-effects are due to hypersensitivity.

A. Toxicity: Very high doses (more than 30 gm/day IV) may produce CNS concentrations which are irritating. In patients with renal failure, smaller doses may produce CNS irritation. With such doses, direct cation toxicity (K^+) may also occur. Lactamase resistant penicillins rarely cause granulopenia and nephritis.

B. Allergy: All penicillins are cross-sensitizing and cross-reacting. Any material (including milk, cosmetics) containing penicillin may induce sensitization. The responsible antigens occur in degradation products, eg, penicilloic acid, bound to host protein. Skin tests with penicilloyl-polylysine, with alkaline hydrolysis products, and with undegraded penicillin identify some hypersensitive persons. Among positive reactors to skin tests the incidence of subsequent allergic reactions is

Table 10–3. **Some blood levels of antibiotics.**

Drug	Route	Daily Dose (gm)	Expected Average Concentration/ ml Blood
Penicillin G	IM	0.6 (1 million units)	0.3–1 unit
	Oral	0.6 (1 million units)	0.03–0.2 unit
Methicillin, nafcillin	IV	6–12	3–12 μg
Cloxacillin dicloxacillin	Oral	3–6	1–5 μg
Ampicillin	Oral	3–6	2–8 μg (10–30 μg in urine)
Cephalothin	IV	8–12	5–20 μg
Cephaloridine	IM	4	10–25 μg
Tetracycline	Oral	2	10–20 μg
Chloramphenicol	Oral	2	15–25 μg
Erythromycin	Oral	2	2–5 μg
Kanamycin	IM	1	1–5 μg
Streptomycin	IM	2	10–20 μg
Gentamicin	IM	0.15 (2–3 mg/kg)	3–5 μg
Polymyxin B	IV	0.15 (2.5 mg/kg)	1–2 μg
Colistin	IM	0.3 (3–5 mg/kg)	1–3 μg

high. Antibodies to penicillin are not correlated with allergic reactions, except rare hemolytic anemia. While a history of a penicillin reaction in the past is not reliable, the drug must be administered with caution to such persons.

Allergic reactions may occur as typical anaphylactic shock, typical serum sickness-type reactions (urticaria, joint swelling, angioneurotic edema, pruritus, respiratory embarrassment within 7–12 days of penicillin dosage), and a variety of skin rashes, fever, renal abnormalities, eosinophilia, vasculitis, etc. The incidence of hypersensitivity to penicillin is negligible in children, but may be 5–10% among adults in the USA. Corticosteroids can sometimes suppress allergic manifestations to penicillins.

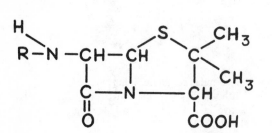

FIG 10–11. **6-Aminopenicillanic acid.**

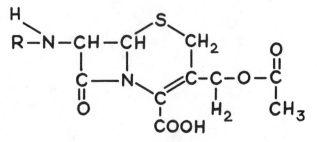

FIG 10–12. **7-Aminocephalosporanic acid.**

CEPHALOSPORINS

In 1945, Brotzu isolated a cephalosporium mold which yielded several antibiotics, called cephalosporins, which resembled penicillins but resisted the action of penicillinase and were active against both gram-positive and gram-negative bacteria. The nucleus of the cephalosporins, 7-aminocephalosporanic acid, bears a close resemblance to the nucleus of penicillin, 6-aminopenicillanic acid (Figs 10–11 and 10–12).

Although the intrinsic activity of the natural cephalosporins is low, modification of the nucleus by attachment of various R groups has yielded several compounds of high therapeutic activity and low toxicity. The cephalosporins have molecular weights of about 420; they are freely soluble in water and relatively stable. Cephalothin and cephaloridine must be injected parenterally since they are not well absorbed from the gastrointestinal tract. Serum levels of 5–15 μg/ml are reached with cephalothin, 8–10 gm/day IV, and 10–20 μg/ml with cephaloridine, 4 gm/day IM. The drugs are distributed widely in tissues and can penetrate into the CNS in the presence of meningitis. Cephalexin or cephaloglycin is sufficiently well absorbed from the gut to be excreted in significant amounts into the urine, so that urinary tract infections can be treated. Fusidic acid and helvolic acid are closely related to cephalosporins and have been used as antistaphylococcal drugs.

Activity

The cephalosporins are active in concentrations of 10 μg/ml or less against gram-positive organisms, including penicillinase-producing staphylococci, and against many gram-negative bacteria. Typically, aerobacter are resistant, whereas klebsiellae are susceptible. The antistaphylococcal activity of the cephalosporins is comparable to that of penicillinase resistant penicillins. Most enterococci, pseudomonas, proteus, and some strains of coliforms are resistant to 10 μg/ml but may be inhibited by the levels reached in urine (300–500 μg/ml). The cephalosporins are bactericidal because they interfere with cell wall synthesis (like penicillins) and are moderately resistant to penicillinase. A cephalosporinase can be produced by some bacteria.

Side-Effects

A. Allergy: The sensitizing potential of the cephalosporins is not yet established. Because of the chemical difference in drug nucleus structure, the antigenicity of the cephalosporins differs somewhat from that of the penicillins. Some individuals hypersensitive to the penicillins can tolerate the cephalosporins. However, anaphylaxis can occur with the cephalosporins, and there is increasing evidence of cross-antigenicity and cross-reactions between penicillins and cephalosporins. Ten to 30% of persons hypersensitive to penicillin also react to cephalosporins.

B. Toxicity: Pain on injection, thrombophlebitis, rashes, and granulocytopenia. There is occasional renal toxicity, particularly with cephaloridine.

THE TETRACYCLINE DRUGS

The tetracyclines have the basic structure shown below. The following radicals occur in the different chemical forms:

	R	R$_1$	R$_2$
Tetracycline	–H	–CH$_3$	–H
Chlortetracycline	–Cl	–CH$_3$	–H
Oxytetracycline	–H	–CH$_3$	–OH
Demethylchlortetracycline	–Cl	–H	–H
Methacycline	–H	–CH$_2$	–OH
Doxycycline	–H	–CH$_3$	–OH

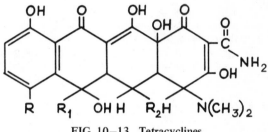

FIG 10–13. Tetracyclines.

The tetracyclines are available as hydrochlorides. They have virtually identical antimicrobial properties and give complete cross-resistance. However, they differ in physical and pharmacologic characteristics. Chlortetracycline is much less stable than the others. All tetracyclines are readily absorbed from the intestinal tract and distributed widely in tissues; they penetrate poorly, however, into the CSF. They can also be administered intramuscularly or intravenously. They are excreted into bile, stool, and urine at varying rates. With ordinary doses (1–2 gm daily by mouth), blood levels reach 3–10 μg/ml. Demethylchlortetracycline, methacycline, and doxycycline are excreted more slowly; similar blood levels are achieved by daily doses of 0.6–1.2 gm.

Activity

Tetracyclines inhibit protein synthesis by inhibiting the binding of amino-acyl tRNA to the 30 S units of bacterial ribosomes.

The tetracyclines are principally bacteriostatic and rickettsiostatic agents. They inhibit the growth of susceptible gram-positive and gram-negative bacteria (inhibited by 0.1–10 μg/ml), rickettsiae, chlamydiae, and *Mycoplasma pneumoniae* (Eaton agent). They have no suppressive effect against fungi or viruses and may even stimulate the growth of some yeasts. They temporarily suppress parts of the normal bowel flora.

Their therapeutic effectiveness is limited by the occurrence of "superinfections": While one microorganism is suppressed, another is permitted to multiply freely and produce pathogenic effects. This has occurred particularly with tetracycline resistant pseudomonas, proteus, staphylococci, and yeasts.

The tetracyclines are sometimes employed in combination with streptomycin in the treatment of brucellosis and pasteurella infections.

Side-Effects

The tetracyclines produce varying degrees of gastrointestinal upset (nausea, vomiting, diarrhea), skin rashes, mucous membrane lesions, and fever in many patients, particularly when administration is prolonged and dosage high. It is not definitely known what part is played by allergy and what part by direct toxicity. Replacement of bacterial flora (see above) occurs commonly. Overgrowth of yeasts on anal and vaginal mucous membranes during tetracycline administration is troublesome. Overgrowth of staphylococci in the intestines during tetracycline therapy may lead to enterocolitis.

Tetracyclines are deposited in bony structures and teeth, particularly during fetal life. Discoloration and fluorescence of the teeth occurs in newborns if tetracyclines are taken for prolonged periods by pregnant women. In pregnancy, hepatic damage may occur. Outdated tetracycline can produce renal damage.

Bacteriologic Examination

Because of its instability in vitro, chlortetracycline often appears less active than the other members of the group. Antimicrobial efficacy of the tetracyclines is virtually identical, so that only one stable tetracycline need be included in antibiotic sensitivity tests. Cross-resistance of microorganisms to tetracyclines is virtually complete; an organism resistant to one of the drugs may be assumed to be resistant to the others also.

CHLORAMPHENICOL

Chloramphenicol is a substance produced originally from cultures of *Streptomyces venezuelae* but now manufactured synthetically.

Crystalline chloramphenicol is a stable compound which is rapidly absorbed from the gastrointestinal

tract, widely distributed into tissues and body fluids, including the CSF, and penetrates well into cells. Most of the drug is inactivated in the liver by conjugation with glucuronide or by reduction to inactive arylamines. Excretion is mainly in the urine, 90% in inactive form. Although chloramphenicol is usually administered orally (2 gm daily gives blood levels up to 20 μg/ml), the succinate can be injected intramuscularly or intravenously.

Activity

Chloramphenicol interferes markedly with protein synthesis in microorganisms by blocking the attachment of amino acids to the nascent peptide chain on the 50 S unit of ribosomes. Chloramphenicol is principally bacteriostatic, and its spectrum is similar to that of the tetracyclines. Dosage and blood levels are also similar to those of the tetracyclines. Chloramphenicol is a drug of choice against salmonella infections.

Side-Effects

Chloramphenicol infrequently causes gastrointestinal upsets. However, prolonged administration of more than 3 gm daily to adults regularly results in abnormalities of early forms of red blood cells, elevation of serum iron, and anemia. These changes are reversible upon discontinuance of the drug. Very rare individuals exhibit an apparent idiosyncrasy to chloramphenicol and develop severe or even fatal depression of bone marrow function. The mechanism of this aplastic anemia is not understood, but it is distinct from the dose-related reversible effect described above. For these reasons the use of chloramphenicol is generally restricted to salmonella infections and those other infections where it is clearly the most effective drug by laboratory test.

In premature and newborn infants, chloramphenicol can induce collapse ("gray syndrome") because the normal mechanism of detoxification (glucuronide conjugation in the liver) is not yet developed.

Bacteriologic Examination

Chloramphenicol is very stable and diffuses well in agar media. For these reasons, it tends to give larger zones of growth inhibition by the "disk test" than the tetracyclines, even when tube dilution tests show identical effectiveness.

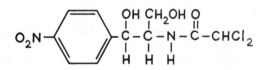

FIG 10–14. Chloramphenicol.

ERYTHROMYCINS
(Macrolides)

Erythromycin is obtained from *Streptomyces erythreus* and has the chemical formula $C_3H_{6\ 7-6\ 9}NO_{13}$. Drugs related to erythromycin are spiramycin, oleandomycin, and others. These drugs give partial or complete cross-resistance but are less effective than erythromycin.

The erythromycins inhibit gram-positive organisms. They are less effective than penicillin in most penicillin sensitive infections but are useful alternate drugs in cases of penicillin allergy. Erythromycin estolate and triacetyloleandomycin are the most readily absorbed forms and yield the highest levels. The base and the stearate are less well absorbed. The oral dose of either drug is 2 gm daily. A special form (erythromycin glucoheptonate) is given IV in a dose of 0.5 gm every 8–12 hours.

Most erythromycin-sensitive microbial strains produce significant numbers of erythromycin resistant mutants. In clinical infections, these mutants emerge and become dominant if the infection is not controlled within a few days. The rapidity of emergence of these mutants may be diminished by the simultaneous use of another drug exhibiting no cross-resistance.

Undesirable side-effects are drug fever, mild gastrointestinal upsets, and cholestatic hepatitis as a hypersensitivity reaction.

Because of the great frequency of resistant mutants, the "disk test" may suggest sensitivity and the tube dilution test resistance of large microbial populations.

LINCOMYCIN

Lincomycin is derived from *Streptomyces lincolnensis.* It resembles the erythromycins in antibacterial activity. It is acid-stable and can be given by mouth (30–60 mg/kg/day, or 2–3 gm/day) or by injection (10–20 mg/kg/day). Gastrointestinal absorption is greatly impaired by food. Serum levels reach 2–10 μg/ml. The drug is distributed widely in tissues. Diarrhea is a frequent side-effect. Lincomycin may be used as a substitute for penicillin in infections with pneumococci, group A streptococci (but not enterococci), and staphylococci in persons allergic to penicillins. Successful treatment of bone infections has been claimed.

VANCOMYCIN

Vancomycin is an amphoteric material produced by *Streptomyces orientalis,* dispensed as the hydrochloride. It has a high molecular weight (3300) and is poorly absorbed from the intestine.

Vancomycin is active mainly against gram-positive cocci, including drug resistant staphylococci, and is markedly bactericidal. Drug resistant strains do not emerge rapidly. The dosage is 0.5 gm every 6–12 hours IV for serious systemic staphylococcal or enterococcal infections; orally for staphylococcal enterocolitis.

Undesirable side-effects are thrombophlebitis, skin rashes, nerve deafness, and kidney damage.

BACITRACIN

Bacitracin is a polypeptide obtained from a strain of *Bacillus subtilis.* It is stable, and poorly absorbed from the intestinal tract or from wounds. Its best use is for topical application to skin, wounds, burns, or mucous membranes.

Bacitracin is mainly bactericidal for gram-positive bacteria, including penicillin resistant organisms. For topical use, concentrations of 500–2000 units/ml of solution are used. In combination with polymyxin B or neomycin, bacitracin is useful for the suppression of mixed bacterial flora in surface lesions. It has no place in systemic therapy.

Bacitracin is toxic for the kidney, causing proteinuria, hematuria, and nitrogen retention. For this reason, systemic administration is undesirable. Bacitracin is said not to induce hypersensitivity readily.

NOVOBIOCIN

Novobiocin is an acidic material produced by *Streptomyces niveus,* dispensed as the sodium or calcium salt. It is readily absorbed from the intestinal tract, distributed widely, and excreted in the urine. While high levels of the drug appear in blood and body fluids, much of it is bound to proteins and not available for antimicrobial action. Novobiocin is predominantly bacteriostatic.

Novobiocin is active against gram-positive cocci, including penicillin resistant staphylococci, and some strains of proteus and other gram-negative bacilli. Resistant variants occur in most bacterial strains and emerge very promptly. Novobiocin has been used in combination with a second antimicrobial drug in serious staphylococcal infections. The dosage is 0.5 gm every 6–8 hours orally. A special form may be given intravenously.

Frequent undesirable side-effects include fever, skin rashes, nausea, vomiting, eosinophilia, granulocytopenia, jaundice, and impaired renal function. At present there is no clear-cut indication for the use of this drug.

POLYMYXINS

Polymyxin B and polymyxin E (colistin) are 2 of a group of basic polypeptides derived from *Bacillus polymyxa.* The other members of the group (A, C, and D) are too toxic for use. These drugs are poorly absorbed from the intestinal tract. They are readily absorbed after intramuscular and intravenous injection but are not widely distributed in tissues and body fluids. Unless locally introduced, they do not reach the spinal fluid or pleural space. Colistin is dispensed as a methanesulfonate complex, and produces less intense local and systemic side-effects than polymyxin B sulfate.

Activity

The polymyxins are strongly bactericidal against gram-negative bacilli, including pseudomonas organisms that are resistant to other antibiotics. Polymyxins coat the bacterial cell membrane and destroy its osmotic function as a selective permeability barrier.

Polymyxin B sulfate can be injected IM or IV (2.5 mg/kg/day) in serious gram-negative infections, including pseudomonas sepsis. It can be given intrathecally (up to 5 mg/day) for pseudomonas meningitis. Colistin methane-sulfonate (3–5 mg/kg/day) IM for urinary tract infections is better tolerated than polymyxin B sulfate and equally effective, but it cannot be injected by other routes.

Side-Effects

The polymyxins are unpleasantly, though harmlessly, toxic for the CNS, causing drowsiness, abnormal sensations, and ataxia. Pain at the site of intramuscular injection necessitates simultaneous administration of a local anesthetic. Local pain of the sulfates may be avoided by intravenous administration. In doses exceeding 2.5 mg/kg/day, damage to the kidney may occur, particularly if renal function is impaired.

Bacteriologic Examination

The polymyxins are large molecules and diffuse poorly through agar. Consequently, inhibition zones in "disk tests" are always very small, even when the organism is highly sensitive by the tube dilution test. Organisms highly sensitive in vitro (inhibited by 0.1–1 μg/ml) may not respond in vivo if parenchymatous organs are involved in the infection. In susceptible strains of bacteria, resistance to polymyxin develops infrequently.

NEOMYCIN & KANAMYCIN

Neomycin sulfate is a group of complex substances isolated from *Streptomyces fradiae.* They are stable, poorly absorbed from the intestinal tract, readily absorbed and distributed after intramuscular injection, and slowly excreted in the urine. Their best use is for topical application to skin, wounds, or mucous membranes. Kanamycin is a close relative of neomycin and has similar activity and less toxicity, but complete cross-resistance. Paromomycin is also closely related and gives complete cross-resistance. All 3 drugs are aminoglycosides, and probably inhibit protein synthesis by the same mechanism as streptomycin.

Activity

Neomycin and kanamycin are bactericidal for gram-negative bacilli, including some strains of proteus and serratia, but ineffective against pseudomonas. There is some activity against *M tuberculosis* and against gram-positive cocci except enterococci. IM doses of 1–2 gm daily are administered in serious infections due to gram-negative organisms which are resistant to other drugs. Oral doses of 4–6 gm daily are used for reduction of intestinal flora preoperatively but are ineffective in most bacterial diarrheas except that caused by enteropathogenic *E coli.* Neomycin is also used for topical application to skin or wounds.

Side-Effects

Neomycin and kanamycin may cause some renal damage. They may also cause nerve deafness without warning signs, and are therefore limited in use. Intramuscular administration is usually limited to 1–2 weeks. Intraperitoneal administration of 3–5 gm has induced respiratory paralysis, which can be overcome by neostigmine.

GENTAMICIN

Gentamicin is an aminoglycoside complex which resembles kanamycin. Solutions of the sulfate are stable for weeks. The activity of the drug is enhanced at alkaline pH.

In concentrations of 0.5–5 μg/ml, gentamicin is bactericidal for many gram-positive and gram-negative bacteria, including many strains of proteus, serratia, and pseudomonas. Antibacterial activity is due to inhibition of protein synthesis probably associated with misreading of the mRNA message on the 30 S unit of the ribosome, similar to other aminoglycosides.

After IM injection of 2–3 mg/kg/day, serum levels reach 3–5 μg/ml and the drug is widely distributed. Gentamicin is indicated in serious infections caused by gram-negative bacteria insusceptible to other drugs.

Gentamicin is nephrotoxic and ototoxic, particularly in impaired renal function, which predisposes to cumulation and toxic effects. Gentamicin sulfate, 0.1%, has been used topically in creams or solutions for infected burns or skin lesions.

STREPTOMYCINS

Streptomycin is an aminoglycoside derived from *Streptomyces griseus.* It is available as the sulfate of the base, and is quite stable. It is bactericidal against both gram-positive and gram-negative bacteria and mycobacteria. Dihydrostreptomycin is similar to streptomycin in antibacterial properties but is not used clinically because of its ototoxicity.

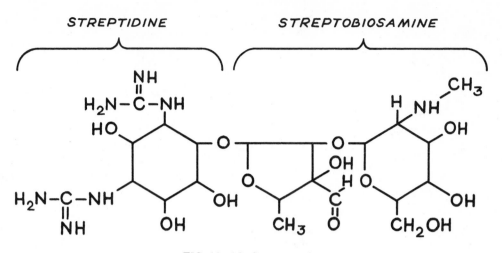

FIG 10—15. Streptomycin.

After intramuscular injection, streptomycin is rapidly absorbed and distributed in tissues and body fluids; it is excreted through the kidneys. It diffuses poorly into the synovial spaces or into the CSF. Only 1/20 of the extracellular concentration reaches the interior of cells. After oral administration, it is poorly absorbed from the gastrointestinal tract; most of it is excreted in the feces. Streptomycin diffuses poorly into the CNS.

Activity

Like other aminoglycosides, streptomycin inhibits protein synthesis. It attaches to a protein of the 30 S unit of the bacterial ribosome and causes a misreading of the mRNA message. In streptomycin resistant cells, this protein is altered or missing.

The streptomycins are predominantly bactericidal against susceptible microorganisms (inhibited in vitro by 0.1—20 μg/ml). The therapeutic effectiveness of streptomycin is limited by its toxicity and by the rapid emergence of resistant mutants. In tuberculosis, 1 gm is injected IM twice weekly (or daily), and other drugs (INH, PAS) are used with streptomycin to inhibit the emergence of resistant mutants.

In nontuberculous infections, streptomycin is not used alone. It may be given (1—2 gm/day IM) with penicillin in enterococcal endocarditis to enhance bactericidal action, and in pasteurella infection it is given with tetracyclines.

Resistance

All microbial strains produce streptomycin resistant mutants with relatively great frequency. Characteristically, mutants of both low and high resistance emerge at the same time; this is in contrast to the stepwise pattern of penicillin resistance. In tuberculosis, combinations with isoniazid or aminosalicylic acid (PAS) are most commonly employed. In this fashion, the period of useful streptomycin treatment is significantly prolonged.

Side-Effects

A. Allergy: Fever, skin rashes, and other allergic manifestations may result from hypersensitivity to streptomycin. This occurs most frequently upon prolonged contact with the drug, especially in those patients receiving a protracted course of treatment (particularly for tuberculosis) or in medical personnel preparing and handling the drug (eg, nurses preparing solutions should wear gloves). Patients sensitive to streptomycin may tolerate dihydrostreptomycin, and vice versa.

B. Toxicity: Streptomycin is markedly toxic for the vestibular portion of the eighth cranial nerve, causing tinnitus, vertigo, and ataxia, which are often irreversible. Dihydrostreptomycin has less vestibular toxicity but is more toxic for the auditory portion of the eighth nerve, causing deafness. Both drugs have some toxic effects on the kidney.

Bacteriologic Examination

Streptomycin is inactivated by semicarbazide. When sensitivity determinations are carried out in liquid media, a single resistant organism in the inoculum may grow out rapidly, although the bulk of the population is streptomycin sensitive. Conversely, testing on solid media may fail to reveal the presence of resistant mutants in the population unless a very large inoculum is employed.

AMINOSALICYLIC ACID
(Para-aminosalicylic Acid, PAS)

Aminosalicylic acid and its salts have weak antimycobacterial properties; PAS is used in the treatment of tuberculosis together with other more potent agents (eg, streptomycin or isoniazid) to delay the emergence of resistant variants. The drug is administered orally in an average dose of 8—14 gm daily. It is readily

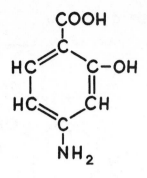

FIG 10–16. PAS.

absorbed but tends to produce anorexia and gastro-intestinal upsets. Its mode of action is based on competition with PABA (similar to the action of sulfonamides). It is being replaced by other antituberculosis drugs, eg, ethambutol.

ISONIAZID
(Isonicotinic Acid Hydrazide, INH)

Isoniazid has little effect on most bacteria but is strikingly active against mycobacteria, especially *M tuberculosis*. Most tubercle bacilli are inhibited by 0.1–1 μg/ml of isoniazid in vitro, but large populations of tubercle bacilli usually contain some isoniazid resis-

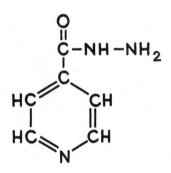

FIG 10–17. Isoniazid.

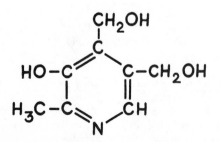

FIG 10–18. Pyridoxine.

tant organisms. For this reason, the drug is best employed in combination with other antimyco-bacterial agents (especially streptomycin or amino-salicylic acid) to reduce the emergence of resistant tubercle bacilli. Isoniazid has been shown to exert competitive antagonism against pyridoxine-catalyzed reactions in *E coli*. Isoniazid and pyridoxine are structural analogues. (See Chapter 5 for discussion of competitive inhibition.) Patients receiving isoniazid excrete pyridoxine in excess amounts, which results in peripheral neuritis. This can be prevented by the administration of pyridoxine, 0.3–0.5 gm daily, which does not interfere with the antituberculosis action of isoniazid.

Isoniazid is rapidly and completely absorbed from the gastrointestinal tract and is rapidly excreted in the urine. In the ordinary systemic dose of 4–6 mg/kg/day, toxic manifestations are negligible and blood levels reach an average of 0.5 μg/ml. Isoniazid freely diffuses into tissue fluids, including the CSF. In tuberculous meningitis, 8–10 mg/kg/day are given for many weeks.

AMPHOTERICIN B
(Fungizone)

Amphotericin B is a complex antibiotic polyene produced by a Streptomyces species which has negligible antibacterial properties but strongly inhibits the growth of several pathogenic fungi in vitro and in vivo. The microcrystals of the drug are dispensed with sodium deoxycholate and a buffer to be dissolved in dextrose solution. It is injected intravenously in daily doses of 50–100 mg, and can be given intrathecally up to 1 mg every other day in meningitis. Amphotericin B appears to be the most effective agent available for the treatment of disseminated coccidioidomycosis, blastomycosis, histoplasmosis, cryptococcosis, and candidiasis. It frequently produces marked toxic effects, including fever, chills, nausea and vomiting, renal failure, and anemia.

GRISEOFULVIN
(Grifulvin, Fulvicin)

Griseofulvin is an antibiotic obtained from certain Penicillium species. It has no effect on bacteria or fungi producing systemic mycoses but suppresses dermatophytes, particularly *Microsporum audouini* and *Trichophyton rubrum*. Oral daily doses of 0.2–1 gm are given for weeks or months. Toxic effects include headache, drowsiness, skin rashes, and gastrointestinal disturbances.

CYCLOSERINE

Cycloserine (D-4-amino-3-isoxazolidone, molecular weight 102) is an antibiotic active against many types of microorganisms, including coliforms, proteus, and tubercle bacilli. It acts by inhibiting the incorporation of D-alanine into mucopeptide of bacterial cell walls. It is occasionally used in urinary tract infections (15–20 mg/kg/day orally), but often causes neurotoxic side-effects or shock.

THE NITROFURANS

The nitrofurans are synthetic nitrofuraldehyde compounds which are strongly bactericidal in vitro for many gram-positive and gram-negative bacteria. Most nitrofurans are very insoluble in water. Some compounds (eg, nitrofuraldehyde semicarbazone, Furacin) are effective topical antibacterial agents used in surgical dressings and virtually not absorbed. Others (eg, Furoxone) can be taken orally to suppress organisms of bacterial diarrhea in the intestines, but are not significantly absorbed.

Nitrofurantoin (Furadantin) is absorbed after oral administration and excreted in the urine. With daily doses of 400–600 mg, urine concentrations reach 100–200 μg/ml, sufficient to inhibit most organisms commonly encountered in urinary tract infections. Activity is limited to the urine. In the blood stream, no antibacterial effect occurs because the drug is bound to blood proteins. Thus, nitrofurantoin has no effect on systemic infections but is a good urinary antiseptic (see below). Sodium nitrofurantoin can be given intravenously but likewise acts only in the urine.

Gastrointestinal intolerance is the commonest side-effect of orally administered nitrofurantoin, but occasionally hemolytic anemia, skin rashes, hepatitis, and other effects have been observed.

SULFONAMIDES

The sulfonamides are a large group of compounds with the basic formula shown in Fig 10–2. By substituting various R-radicals, a series of compounds is obtained with somewhat varying physical, pharmacologic, and antibacterial properties. The basic mechanism of action of all of these compounds appears to be competitive inhibition of para-aminobenzoic acid (PABA) utilization.

The sulfonamides are bacteriostatic for some gram-negative and gram-positive bacteria, chlamydiae, nocardia, and some protozoa. Several special sulfones (eg, diaminodiphenylsulfone, DDS) are employed in the treatment of leprosy.

The "soluble" sulfonamides (eg, trisulfapyrimidines, sulfisoxazole) are readily absorbed from the intestinal tract after oral administration in dosages of 4–8 gm daily and are distributed in all tissues and body fluids (required blood levels: 8–12 mg/100 ml). The sodium salts of sulfonamides may be injected intravenously or subcutaneously. Most sulfonamides are excreted rapidly in the urine. Some (eg, sulfamethoxypyridazine, sulfadimethoxine) are excreted very slowly and give high tissue and low urine levels. At present, sulfonamides are particularly useful in the treatment of trachoma, toxoplasmosis, and first attacks of urinary tract infections due to coliform bacteria. By contrast, many meningococci, shigellae, group A streptococci, and recurrent urinary tract infections are now resistant.

The "insoluble" sulfonamides (eg, succinylsulfathiazole, phthalylsulfathiazole) are poorly absorbed from the intestinal tract and exert their action largely by inhibiting the microbial population within the lumen of the tract. To prepare the bowel for surgery, 8–15 gm orally are given daily for 4–7 days.

Resistance

Microorganisms which produce an excess of PABA or those which do not use PABA but require preformed folic acid for growth are resistant to sulfonamides.

Side-Effects

The soluble sulfonamides may produce unpleasant and sometimes serious side-effects which fall into 2 categories:

A. Allergic Reactions: Many individuals develop hypersensitivity to sulfonamides after initial contact with these drugs and, on reexposure, may develop fever, hives, skin rashes, and chronic vascular diseases such as periarteritis nodosa.

B. Direct Toxic Effects: There may be fever, skin rashes, gastrointestinal disturbances, depression of the bone marrow leading to anemia or agranulocytosis, hemolytic anemia, and toxic effects on the liver and kidney. Some of the toxic action on the kidney can be prevented by keeping the urine alkaline and the water intake adequate; by using mixtures of sulfonamides such as trisulfapyrimidines (which are relatively more soluble than a single drug); or by employing sulfisoxazole, which is highly soluble in urine.

Bacteriologic Examinations

When culturing specimens from persons receiving sulfonamides, it is necessary to incorporate PABA (5 mg/100 ml) into the medium in order to overcome sulfonamide inhibition.

URINARY ANTISEPTICS

These are drugs with antibacterial effects limited to the urine. They fail to produce significant levels in tissues and thus have no effect on systemic infections. However, they effectively lower bacterial counts in the urine and thus greatly diminish the symptoms of lower urinary tract infection. They are used primarily for the suppression of bacteria in the urine of patients with chronic urinary tract infection.

The most prominent urinary antiseptics are methenamine mandelate (Mandelamine), nitrofurantoin, and nalidixic acid. The active compounds are liberated in the urine only and have no systemic effect. Therefore, it is meaningless to perform and report sensitivity tests with these substances in any systemic infections. Other materials, such as amino acids (methionine) or hippuric acid (cranberry juice), may be ingested in large doses to provide an acid, bacteriostatic urine. Nalidixic acid is effective in the urine, but microbial resistance tends to emerge rapidly.

ANTIVIRAL DRUGS

The rickettsiae and chlamydiae (agents of the psittacosis-LGV-trachoma group) resemble bacteria in structure and mode of replication and can be inhibited by certain antibacterial drugs. The tetracyclines are the drugs of choice for all of these agents, whereas the sulfonamides suppress some chlamydiae (eg, trachoma), but actually stimulate rickettsial growth.

True viruses, because of their distinct method of replication and structure, are not affected by the common antibacterial drugs. However, viral multiplication may be interrupted by a variety of chemicals at various stages. In addition to specific antibody globulins which block penetration of extracellular virus into the cell, several chemicals have found limited application in the treatment of viral infections. The following substances are currently used in the management of clinical viral disease.

Amantadine Hydrochloride

This tricyclic symmetric amine inhibits the penetration into susceptible cells of certain myxoviruses, especially influenza A, but not influenza B. A daily oral dose of 200 mg of amantadine hydrochloride for 3 days before and 7 days after influenza A virus infection reduces the incidence and severity of symptoms. The most marked side-effects are insomnia, dizziness, and ataxia.

Several dihydroxyisoquinolines also inhibit the penetration of myxoviruses into susceptible cells, and can prevent disease due to influenza A and B viruses.

Idoxuridine (5-Iodo-2-deoxyuridine)

This halogenated pyrimidine can inhibit the replication of DNA viruses by becoming incorporated into viral DNA in place of thymidine. Topical application to herpetic keratitis can result in marked improvement. The topically applied drug remains localized in the avascular cornea and inhibits herpesvirus replication. For the treatment of herpetic keratitis, 1 drop of 0.1% solution is instilled into the conjunctival sac every 2 hours around the clock. Ointments containing 0.5% idoxuridine can be applied less frequently.

Some toxic effects on corneal epithelium occur after prolonged use. While idoxuridine is too severely cytotoxic for use in most generalized virus infections, it has been employed in herpetic encephalitis (from 40 mg/kg/day IV to 6 gm/day IV).

Cytosine arabinoside (arabinofuranosylcytosine hydrochloride) also inhibits replication of DNA viruses. It has been used topically in herpetic keratitis, but it is more toxic than idoxuridine.

Methisazone (N-Methyl-isatin-betathiosemicarbazone)

This drug can block replication of poxviruses, probably by inhibiting the formation of a structural protein. If administered to contacts of smallpox cases within 1–2 days after exposure, 2–4 gm orally/day for 3–4 days (100 mg/kg/day for children) gives striking protection against smallpox.

Generalized or progressive vaccinia in immunologically deficient individuals can also be treated with methisazone.

The principal side-effect is vomiting.

•   •   •

General References

Braun, P.: Hepatotoxicity of erythromycin. J Infect Dis 119:300–306, 1969.

Garrod, L.P., & F. O'Grady: *Antibiotics and Chemotherapy,* 2nd ed. Livingstone, 1968.

Gingell, J.C., & P.M. Waterworth: Dose of gentamicin in patients with normal renal function and renal impairment. Brit MJ 2:19–22, 1968.

Jawetz, E.: Polymyxins, colistin, bacitracin, ristocetin, and vancomycin. P Clin North America 15:85–94, 1968.

Jawetz, E., & others: A laboratory test for bacterial sensitivity to combinations of antibiotics. Am J Clin Path 25:1016–1031, 1955.

Kaye, D., & others: Comparison of parenteral ampicillin and parenteral chloramphenicol in the treatment of typhoid fever. Ann New York Acad Sc 145:423–428, 1967.

Kirby, W., & R.J. Bulger: The new penicillins and cephalosporins. Ann Rev Med 15:393–412, 1964.

Kunin, C.M.: A guide to use of antibiotics in patients with renal disease. Ann Int Med 67:151–158, 1967.

Kunin, C.M., & M. Finland: Clinical pharmacology of the tetracycline antibiotics. Clin Pharmacol Therap 2:51–69, 1961.

McCracken, G.H., Jr., & H.G. Eichenwald: Antimicrobial therapy in infancy and childhood: 1966. P Clin North America 13:231–250, 1966.

Sabath, L.D.: Drug resistance of bacteria. New England J Med 280:91–94, 1969.

Weinstein, L.: Common sense (clinical judgment) in the diagnosis and antibiotic therapy of etiologically undefined infections. P Clin North America 15:141–156, 1968.

Weinstein, L., & A.C. Dalton: Host determinants of response to antimicrobial agents. New England J Med 279:467–473, 1968.

11 . . .

Host-Parasite Relationships

A parasite is an organism which resides on or within another living organism in order to find the environment and nutrients it requires for growth and reproduction. This does not imply that a parasite must harm its host. On the contrary, the most successful parasites achieve a balance with the host which ensures the survival, growth, and propagation of both parasite and host. Thus a majority of host-parasite interactions do not result in disease: The infection remains latent or subclinical.

The relationship between parasite and host is determined both by those characteristics of the parasite which favor establishment of the parasite and damage to the host and by the various host mechanisms which oppose these processes. Among the parasite's attributes are infectivity, invasiveness, pathogenicity, and toxigenicity. These are described below. If the parasite injures the host to a sufficient degree, disturbances will result in the host which manifest themselves as disease.

INFECTION

Infection is the process whereby the parasite enters into a relationship with the host. Its essential component steps in man and animals are the following:

(1) **Entrance of the parasite into the host**—The most frequent portals of entry are the respiratory tract (mouth and nose), the gastrointestinal tract, and breaks in the superficial mucous membranes and skin. Some parasites can penetrate intact mucous membrane and skin; still others are passively introduced by arthropods through these layers directly into the lymphatic channels or the blood stream.

(2) **Establishment and multiplication of the parasite within the host**—From the portal of entry the parasite may spread directly through the tissues or may proceed via the lymphatic channels to the blood stream, which distributes it widely and permits it to reach tissues particularly suitable for its multiplication. The biochemical environment of the tissues ultimately determines the susceptibility or resistance of a certain host to a given parasite.

Although the process of infection is of paramount interest to medicine, there are 2 other requirements for the perpetuation of a parasitic species: a satisfactory portal of exit of the parasite from the host and an effective mechanism for transmission to new hosts.

ATTRIBUTES OF MICROORGANISMS WHICH ENABLE THEM TO CAUSE DISEASE

There is no sharp semantic distinction between the terms "pathogenicity" and "virulence." **Pathogenicity** denotes the ability of microorganisms to cause disease or to result in the production of progressive lesions. **Virulence** introduces the concept of degree, ie, virulent organisms exhibit pathogenicity when introduced into the host in very small numbers. These properties may be subdivided into **toxigenicity** (ability to produce toxic substances) and **invasiveness** (ability to enter host tissues, multiply there, and spread). Different pathogenic microorganisms possess these attributes in varying degrees. Toxigenicity and invasiveness may be under separate genetic control.

The measurement of virulence in terms of the number of microorganisms necessary to kill a given host when administered by a certain route (usually expressed as LD_{50}, ie, the number of organisms which must be administered to kill 50% of the animals) largely reflects the invasive properties of the organism being tested.

A few representative substances known to play a role in the production of disease by microorganisms are mentioned below.

Toxins

Toxins are usually subdivided into exotoxins and endotoxins. Exotoxins are specific injurious substances secreted into the environment by certain gram-positive (and, rarely, gram-negative) bacteria. They are antigenic and are rapidly destroyed by heat ($60°$ C). Toxins of diphtheria, tetanus, and botulism have been highly purified; they are protein molecules having molecular weights between 10,000 and 100,000. Exotoxins are converted into nonpoisonous toxoids by heat, formalin, or prolonged storage.

Endotoxins are injurious substances which are intimately associated with the cell wall of most gram-negative bacteria and are liberated into the environment upon autolysis. They are relatively heat stable lipopolysaccharides which possess a large number of pathophysiologic effects. Among other effects, they may produce fever and irreversible shock.

Pathogenesis of Some Diseases Caused by Toxin-Producing Bacteria

(1) In botulism, a fatal type of food poisoning, *Clostridium botulinum* produces a potent toxin (lethal dose for man about 1 μg) in canned or anaerobically stored food. This toxin is ingested, absorbed from the intestinal tract, and reaches the CNS; the microorganism, however, never reaches the tissues at all.

(2) In tetanus, spores of *Clostridium tetani* are introduced into contaminated wounds. They germinate in the anaerobic environment of injured tissue and produce the toxin, which is absorbed and reaches the spinal cord. Thus tetanus organisms manufacture the toxin in the body but are themselves noninvasive.

(3) In diphtheria, *Corynebacterium diphtheriae* usually remains limited to the upper respiratory tract. The toxin is produced there, absorbed, and exerts its effects on many organs.

(4) In gas gangrene, *Clostridium perfringens* is introduced into a contaminated wound. Under the anaerobic conditions of injured tissue several toxins are produced which aid the active spread of the bacilli in tissue. Among these toxins the most important (alpha) is a lecithinase, an enzyme able to hydrolyze lecithin, an important constituent of cell walls. In this way hemolysis and injury to many tissue cells ensue.

Extracellular Enzymes

Certain bacteria produce substances that are not directly toxic but which do play an important role in the infectious process.

A. Collagenase: *Clostridium perfringens,* in addition to a lecithinase, also produces proteolytic enzymes (collagenase) capable of disintegrating collagen. This promotes the spread of bacilli in tissues.

B. Coagulase: Many pathogenic staphylococci produce a substance (coagulase) which, in conjunction with certain serum factors, coagulates plasma. Coagulase contributes to the formation of fibrin walls around staphylococcal lesions, which protect the organisms from the defenses of the body and aid in their persistence. Coagulase also causes a deposit of fibrin on the surface of individual staphylococci, which may protect them from phagocytosis or from destruction within phagocytic cells.

C. Hyaluronidases (enzymes hydrolyzing hyaluronic acid, a constituent of the ground substance of connective tissue) are produced by many microorganisms (eg, staphylococci, clostridia, streptococci, pneumococci) and aid in their spread through tissues.

D. Streptokinase (Fibrinolysin): Many hemolytic streptococci produce a substance (streptokinase) which activates a proteolytic enzyme of the plasma (plasminogen → plasmin). This enzyme (also called fibrinolysin) is then able to dissolve coagulated plasma and probably aids in the spread of streptococci through tissues.

E. Hemolysins and Leukocidins: Many microorganisms produce substances which dissolve red blood cells (hemolysins) and probably also tissue cells and leukocytes (leukocidins). Streptolysin O, for example, is produced by group A hemolytic streptococci and is lethal for mice in addition to being hemolytic for a variety of red cells. This substance is readily oxidized and thereby inactivated, but it is reactivated by reducing agents. It is antigenic. The same streptococci also produce oxygen-stable streptolysin S, which is nonantigenic. Clostridia produce a variety of hemolysins, among them the lecithinase previously mentioned. Hemolysins are also produced by staphylococci, pneumococci, and many gram-negative rods.

Factors in the Invasiveness of Microorganisms

A continuous scale of invasiveness could be drawn up for microorganisms. One end of this scale would be occupied by toxin producers like tetanus or diphtheria; the other, by highly invasive organisms like anthrax or plague, with staphylococci and streptococci in between. The toxin producers are pathogenic principally because of elaboration of poisonous chemical substances without much tissue invasion. Plague or anthrax bacilli produce disease and death because they are able to invade tissues rapidly and multiply extensively, with the production of several toxic materials. Pneumococci or meningococci also spread widely throughout the body. The invasiveness of such organisms may be aided by enzymes favoring spread, such as hyaluronidase or streptokinase, but invasiveness is not clearly related to toxic properties. A part of the invasiveness of microorganisms may be attributed to certain surface components which protect the bacteria from phagocytosis and destruction. Such surface substances may be polysaccharide capsules (eg, pneumococci, *Klebsiella pneumoniae, Hemophilus influenzae*), hyaluronic acid capsules and surface "M" proteins (beta-hemolytic streptococci), or a surface polypeptide (anthrax bacilli). Certain microorganisms may be invasive and "virulent" because they survive within phagocytic cells and are resistant to enzymatic attack. While these various factors contribute to the observed invasiveness of microorganisms, it must be concluded that this behavior is an expression of inherent biochemical properties not yet understood. On the other hand, invasiveness as such is by no means synonymous with disease production. Some organisms, eg, viruses, may be widely distributed in the body without causing illness.

How can one prove that a given microorganism really causes a disease? Traditionally, the etiologic relationship between a microorganism and a disease is established by fulfilling "Koch's postulates": (1) The microorganism must regularly be isolated from cases of the illness. (2) It must be grown in pure culture in vitro. (3) When such a pure culture is inoculated into susceptible animal species, the typical disease must result. (4) From such experimentally induced disease the microorganism must again be isolated.

While these postulates were adequate to prove the etiology of some bacterial diseases, they had to be modified extensively for other infections, particularly for virus diseases, which are highly species-specific for man.

ATTRIBUTES OF THE HOST WHICH DETERMINE RESISTANCE TO MICROORGANISMS

The various factors that operate to prevent infection of a host can be arranged in 2 groups: nonspecific factors, operating against a variety of parasites; and specific factors, directed only against a certain parasite.

SOME MECHANISMS OF NONSPECIFIC HOST RESISTANCE

Physiologic Barriers at the Portal of Entry

A. The Skin: Few microorganisms are capable of penetrating the intact skin, but many can enter sweat or sebaceous glands and hair follicles and establish themselves there. Sweat and sebaceous secretions, by virtue of their acid pH and possibly chemical substances (especially fatty acids), have antimicrobial properties which tend to eliminate pathogenic organisms. Lysozyme, an enzyme which dissolves some bacterial cell walls, and perhaps other enzymes are also present on the skin.

Skin resistance may vary with age. In childhood, susceptibility is high to ringworm infection. After puberty, resistance to such fungi increases markedly with the increased content of saturated fatty acids in sebaceous secretions.

B. Mucous Membranes: A film of mucus covers the surface and is constantly being driven by ciliated cells toward the natural orifices. Bacteria tend to stick to this film. Mucus and tears likewise contain lysozyme and other substances with antimicrobial properties. When organisms enter the mucous membrane, they tend to be taken up by phagocytes and to be transported into regional lymphatic channels which carry them to lymph nodes. These act as barriers toward further spread and are capable of disposing of large numbers of bacteria. The mucociliary apparatus for removal of bacteria in the respiratory tract is aided by pulmonary macrophages. This entire defense system can be suppressed by ethyl alcohol, cigarette smoke, hypoxia, and other influences. Additional special protective mechanisms include, in the respiratory tract, the hairs at the nares and the cough reflex; in the gastrointestinal tract, the saliva, stomach acidity, and numerous proteolytic enzymes. In the vagina the acid pH is maintained by lactobacilli.

It must be remembered that most mucous membranes of the body carry a constant normal microbial flora which itself opposes the establishment of pathogenic microorganisms and has important physiologic functions. (See Bacterial Interference.)

Phagocytosis

Microorganisms (and other particles) which enter the lymphatics, lung, bone marrow, or blood stream are engulfed by any of a variety of phagocytic cells. Among them are polymorphonuclear leukocytes, wandering macrophages, and fixed macrophages of the reticuloendothelial system (below). Many microorganisms elaborate chemotactic factors which attract phagocytic cells. Phagocytosis can occur in the absence of serum antibodies, particularly if aided by the architecture of tissue. Thus phagocytic cells are inefficient in large, smooth, open spaces like pleura, pericardium, or joint, but may be more effective in ingesting microorganisms which are trapped in small tissue spaces (eg, alveoli) or on rough surfaces. Such "surface phagocytosis" occurs early in the infectious process before antibodies are available.

Phagocytosis is made more efficient by the presence of antibodies (opsonins) which coat the bacterial surface and facilitate the uptake of bacteria by the phagocyte. The Fc fragment of immunoglobulins largely determines the opsonic activity of an antibody. Hyperosmolality of the environment inhibits phagocytosis (eg, in the renal medulla).

The ingestion of foreign particles, eg, microorganisms, has the following effects on the phagocytic cell: (1) O_2 consumption increases; (2) glycolysis increases; (3) lysosomes rupture and their hydrolytic enzymes are discharged into the cytoplasm—this is called "degranulation" of phagocytes; (4) RNA turnover increases, but there is no increased synthesis of protein; (5) synthesis of lecithin increases.

Phagocytes may kill the ingested microorganisms, or may permit their prolonged survival and even intracellular multiplication. One or the other outcome of phagocytosis is determined partly by the nature of the microorganism and partly by the conditioning of the phagocytic cell. Polymorphonuclear leukocytes contain at least 2 kinds of granules: (1) lysosomes, which are bags of hydrolases; and (2) basic proteins with antibacterial properties. Macrophages in blood have few lysosomal granules until they become "activated." This "activation" results from interaction with immunologically active lymphoid cells as a consequence of bacterial infection. "Activated" macrophages have many lysosomes, and are active in phagocytosis and intracellular killing of a variety of bacteria—not only the ones which induced the initial "activation." Clearly this is part of active cellular immunity (see below).

The functional mechanism of intracellular killing of microorganisms in phagocytes is uncertain. Oxidative mechanisms seem importantly involved. Myeloperoxidase (one of many lysosomal enzymes) appears to be important in intracellular killing of some bacteria and candida, which produce hydrogen peroxide. In certain congenital defects phagocytic cells may specifically lack enzymes which normally kill ingested bacteria. Thus, patients suffering from "granulomatous disease" usually die of overwhelming bacterial infection. Their phagocytes ingest bacteria normally but there is an abnormally low increase in O_2 consumption, there are metabolic defects in aerobic glycolysis, and phagocytized bacteria are not killed. The metabolic basis of other defects in phagocyte function remains to be demonstrated.

Corticosteroids stabilize many membrane structures. They probably also increase the stability of lysosomal membranes. This may contribute to the diminished ability of phagocytes to eradicate bacterial and fungal infection in persons receiving high doses of corticosteroids.

Reticuloendothelial (RE) System

This refers to a functional concept of fixed phagocytic cells in lymphoid tissue, liver, spleen, bone marrow, lung, and other tissues which are efficient in uptake and removal of particulate matter from lymph and blood streams. It includes cells lining blood (Kupffer cells of liver) and lymph sinuses and histiocytes of tissues (macrophages). This system of fixed phagocytic cells is the principal means of clearing particles, including bacteria, from blood and lymph. Phagocytosis by RE cells is greatly enhanced by opsonins.

Biochemical Tissue Constituents

Certain animal tissues are resistant to specific bacteria (eg, *Bacillus anthracis*) because of their content of polypeptides, which have antibacterial properties. Such biochemical constituents may determine tissue resistance to infection. Beta lysin of serum can kill some gram-positive bacteria. The nutritional status of the host plays an important role in susceptibility or resistance to a given infection. (Dubos, R.J.: J Exp Med 108:69, 1968.)

The role of interferon in resistance to virus infections is discussed in Chapter 27.

Many normal tissues have a high inherent ability to inhibit proliferation of microorganisms. This resistance is severely impaired by trauma, foreign bodies, disturbances in fluid and electrolyte balance, and by depression of the inflammatory response (x-ray radiation, corticosteroids, antineoplastic drugs, lymphomas).

Inflammatory Response

Any injury to tissue, such as that following the establishment and multiplication of microorganisms, calls forth an inflammatory response. This begins with dilatation of local arterioles and capillaries, from which plasma escapes. Edema fluid accumulates in the area of injury, and fibrin forms a network and occludes the lymphatic channels, tending to limit the spread of organisms. Polymorphonuclear leukocytes in the capillaries stick to the walls, then migrate out of the capillaries toward the irritant. This migration is probably stimulated by substances in the inflammatory exudate (chemotaxis). The phagocytes engulf the microorganisms, and intracellular digestion begins. Soon the pH of the inflamed area becomes more acid, and the cellular proteases tend to induce lysis of the leukocytes. Large mononuclear macrophages arrive on the site and, in turn, engulf leukocytic debris as well as microorganisms and pave the way for resolution of the local inflammatory process.

Different stages in this inflammatory sequence may predominate with different microorganisms as the inciting cause of the inflammation. The early edema fluid may actually promote bacterial growth. The degree of local fixation depends on the nature of the organism: Staphylococci tend to limit their spread through extensive lymphatic thrombi, fibrin walls, etc, precipitated by coagulase, while hemolytic streptococci, through the activity of streptokinase (fibrinolysin) and hyaluronidase, tend to spread rapidly through the tissue. Phagocytosis and intracellular residence is destructive to some bacteria (some pyogenic cocci), whereas for others (eg, tubercle bacilli) it serves as a means of transport and protection and even of multiplication.

Fever

Fever in itself may be a host mechanism of defense. It is certainly the most frequently observed systemic manifestation of the inflammatory response and a cardinal symptom of infectious diseases. Possible mechanisms of fever production must therefore be discussed.

The ultimate regulators of body temperature are the thermoregulatory centers in the brain. They are subject to physical and chemical stimuli. Direct mechanical injury or the application of chemical substances to these centers results in fever. Neither of these obvious forms of stimulation is present in the many types of fever which are associated with infection, neoplasia, hypersensitivity, and other processes which cause inflammation.

Among the substances known to induce fever upon injection into normal mammals are the endotoxins of gram-negative bacteria and sterile leukocytic exudates and extracts. The febrile response to these 2 types of substances is distinct:

(1) Endotoxins (lipopolysaccharides of gram-negative bacteria) are heat-stable. After intravenous injection there is a relatively long latent period (30–60 minutes) until fever appears. During that time marked leukopenia develops. Repeated injection of endotoxin makes the recipient **tolerant**; he becomes **unresponsive to endotoxins** and develops little fever or leukopenia.

(2) Leukocytic extracts are heat-labile. They can induce fever within a few minutes after injection (short latent period). They do not produce leukopenia. Repeated injections of leukocytic extracts do not induce tolerance: Recipients remain responsive to endotoxin. Leukocytic extracts produce fever in endotoxin-tolerant recipients.

After the administration of endotoxin to animals or man, elements of both A and B can be observed in

Injected pyrogen (exogenous)	→	Injury of leukocytes, monomyctes, and perhaps other cells	→	Release of endogenous pyrogen	→	Stimulation of thermoregulatory centers of brain	→ Fever

sequence. Some time after the injection of endotoxin a pyrogen can be demonstrated in the serum which behaves like leukocytic extract. That substance, called **endogenous pyrogen**, appears to have been released from leukocytes under the influence of endotoxin and appears to act directly on the thermoregulatory center of the brain. Thus the overall sequence of events shown above has been postulated for endotoxin-induced fever and other similar responses. (Wood, B.W.: New England J Med 258:1023, 1958.)

This type of fever is a function of available leukocytes. Experimental removal of leukocytes abolishes the febrile response. The chemical nature of leukocytic (endogenous) pyrogen appears to be a lipid-protein complex with a molecular weight of 14,000, non-dialyzable, stable at acid pH, resistant to ribonucleases inactivated by trypsin, pepsin, or heat (90° C for 30 min).

It is possible that many pyrogens act by this pathway. However, endotoxins or similar chemicals can at times enter the CNS and produce fever by direct stimulation of thermoregulatory centers.

Some Causes of Persistent Fever of Unknown Origin (FUO)

If the usual diagnostic procedures (including thorough bacteriologic and serologic studies) fail to reveal the diagnosis, consider early biopsy or exploratory laparotomy.

(1) **Infections (bacterial, fungal, parasitic; rarely viral)**: Especially tuberculosis, liver and biliary tract disease, bacterial endocarditis, abdominal abscess, urinary tract disease.

(2) **Neoplasms**: Consider especially those involving the kidneys, lungs, thyroid, liver, pancreas; lymphomas, leukemias, myeloma.

(3) **Hypersensitivity disease**: Visceral angiitis, disseminated lupus erythematosus, periarteritis nodosa, scleroderma, dermatomyositis, rheumatic fever, drug fever.

(4) **"Periodic fever" or "steroid fever"** associated with high levels of etiocholanolone or other steroid metabolic products.

(5) **Neurogenic or endocrine disorders**: Consider lesions of brain stem and thalamus; encephalitis, hyperthyroidism.

(6) **Factitious fever**: Malingering.

(7) **Miscellaneous**: Consider sarcoidosis, thrombophlebitis, infarctions, poisons, drugs.

RESISTANCE & IMMUNITY

In the preceding section were described various properties of the host which give nonspecific resistance to infection. The term "immunity" signifies all those properties of the host which confer resistance to a specific infectious agent. This resistance may be of all degrees, from almost complete susceptibility to complete insusceptibility. Therefore, "resistance" and "immunity" are relative terms implying only that one host is more or less susceptible to a given infection than another host. No inference can be drawn regarding the possible mechanisms of this resistance.

Immunity may be natural or acquired. Acquired immunity may be passive or active.

NATURAL IMMUNITY

Natural immunity is that which is not acquired through previous contact with the infectious agent (or with a related species). Little is known about the mechanism responsible for this form of resistance.

Species Immunity

A given pathogenic microorganism is often capable of producing disease in one animal species but not in another. The bacillus of avian tuberculosis causes disease in birds but almost never in man; the anthrax bacillus infects man but not chickens (perhaps because of the higher body temperatures of fowl); gonococci infect man but no other animal species.

Racial or Genetic Basis of Immunity

With one animal species there may be marked racial and genetic differences in susceptibility. Some dark-skinned races of man have a 10 times greater chance of developing disseminated coccidioidomycosis following primary infection than light-skinned races. Certain "strains" of mice are highly susceptible to viral and resistant to bacterial infections. With other strains the opposite is true.

In a few instances the biochemical basis of racial (genetic) immunity is known. For example, a hereditary deficiency of glucose-6-phosphate dehydrogenase occurs in the red blood cells of certain individuals. Such persons are markedly less susceptible to *P falciparum* malaria, but more susceptible to red cell hemolysis after certain drugs (sulfonamides, primaquine, nitrofurans) than persons with normal red cell enzyme content.

Individual Resistance

As with any biologic phenomenon, resistance to infection varies with different individuals of the same species and race, following a distribution curve for the host population. Thus certain individuals may be discovered within a "highly susceptible population" who unaccountably cannot be infected with a certain microorganism even though they have had no previous contact with it. Other individuals have genetic defects (see above) in immunologic responsiveness, antibody production, or phagocyte function which make them unusually susceptible to infections. Nutritional status, exposure to ionizing radiation or immunosuppressive drugs, and hormonal balance all greatly influence individual susceptibility.

Differences Due to Age

In general, the very young and the elderly are more susceptible to bacterial disease than persons in other age groups. However, resistance to tuberculosis is higher at 5–15 years than before or after. Many age differences in specific infections can be related to physiologic factors. For example, gonococcal vaginitis occurs mainly in small girls. Near puberty, estrogen production results in epithelial cell cornification and a more acid pH, which induce relative resistance.

Some virus infections damage the fetus severely but otherwise produce only mild disease. Rickettsial infections are, by contrast, more severe with advancing age. Streptococcal infection has a different pattern in the small and the older child. There are many other examples.

Hormonal & Metabolic Influences

Many known hormones influence susceptibility to infection. Only 2 examples are listed here.

In diabetes mellitus there is increased susceptibility to infections of the urinary tract, vagina, and pyogenic infections of tissue. The latter may be due, in part, to altered metabolism, elevated glucose, reduced influx of phagocytic cells, and depression of phagocytosis.

Both in hypoadrenal (Addison's disease) and in hyperadrenal (Cushing's disease) states, susceptibility to infection is increased. Administration of corticosteroids in high doses has similar effects. Bacterial infections are enhanced because of the suppression of the inflammatory response by glucocorticoids. Viral infections (herpes keratitis, varicella) are aggravated perhaps by steroid suppression of interferon production. Huge doses of corticosteroids can directly suppress antibody formation.

Certain clinical associations between an underlying constitutional disorder and a supervening infection are so frequent as to deserve listing:

Sickle cell trait: Salmonella infection
Diabetes mellitus: Mucormycosis
Cirrhosis, nephrosis: Pneumococcal peritonitis
Hypoparathyroidism: Candidiasis
Pulmonary alveolar proteinosis: Nocardiosis
Chronic lymphocytic leukemia: Disseminated herpes zoster

ACQUIRED IMMUNITY

Passive Immunity

By "passive immunity" is meant a state of relative temporary insusceptibility to an infectious agent which has been induced by the administration of antibodies against that agent and which have been formed in another host rather than formed actively by the individual himself. Because the antibody molecules are constantly breaking down while at the same time no new ones are being formed, passive protection lasts only a short time—usually a few weeks at the longest. On the other hand, the protective mechanism is in force immediately upon administration of antibody: There is no lag period such as is required for the formation of active immunity. Antibodies play only a limited role in invasive bacterial infections, and passive immunization (ie, the administration of convalescent serum or globulin) is rarely useful in that type of disease. Where an illness is largely attributable to a toxin, on the other hand (eg, diphtheria, tetanus, botulism), the passive administration of antitoxin is of the greatest use because large amounts of antitoxin can be made immediately available for neutralization of the toxin. In certain virus infections (eg, measles, infectious hepatitis), the administration of specific antibodies (such as gamma globulin) during the incubation period may result in prevention or modification of the clinical disease.

Passive immunity resulting from the in utero transfer to the fetus of antibodies formed earlier in the mother protects the newborn child during the first months of life against some common infections. This passive immunity (acquired from the mother's blood) may be reinforced by antibodies taken up by the child in mother's milk (particularly colostrum), but the immunity wanes at 4–6 months of age.

Active Immunity

Active immunity is a state of resistance built up in an individual following effective contact with microorganisms or their products. "Effective contact" may consist of clinical or subclinical infection, injection with live or killed microorganisms or their antigens, or absorption of bacterial products (eg, toxins, toxoids). In all these instances the host actively produces antibodies and his cells learn to respond to the foreign material. Active immunity develops slowly over a period of days or weeks but tends to persist, usually for years.

A. Mechanisms of Immunity: Of the mechanisms which make up the resistance of acquired active immunity, a few can be defined:

1. Active production of antibodies against antigens of microorganisms or their products. These antibodies may induce resistance because they (1) neutralize toxins or cellular enzymes or products; (2) have direct bactericidal or lytic effect with complement; (3) block the infective ability of microorga-

nisms; (4) agglutinate microorganisms, making them more subject to phagocytosis; or (5) opsonize microorganisms, ie, combine with cellular antigens which normally interfere with phagocytosis and thus contribute to the ingestion of parasites.

Antibody formation is disturbed in certain individuals with agammaglobulinemia or thymic dysfunction.

2. Increased fixation of invading microorganisms at their point of entry. This is a combined effect of humoral and cellular function; hypersensitivity also plays a role (see p 150).

3. Increased ability of phagocytic cells, (see above), particularly those of the reticuloendothelial system, to ingest the particular microorganism and destroy it intracellularly. These functions appear to depend both on specific antibody and on altered cellular behavior. Ingestion of bacteria is specifically enhanced by antibody. The intracellular killing of phagocytized microorganisms may be greatly increased by active immunity. The induction of this cellular resistance is immunologically specific (eg, one certain microorganism), but the subsequent expression is nonspecific (eg, cells resistant to many different microorganisms).

4. Alteration in the biochemical environment in tissue, making it less favorable for spread and multiplication of the parasite.

B. Production of Immunity: Active immunity may be acquired in the following ways, any of which constitute "effective contact."

1. Inoculation of living, virulent microorganisms (1) in doses insufficient to cause disease; (2) by a route unfavorable to progressive infection; and (3) together with antiserum for partial protection.

2. Inoculation of living attenuated infectious organisms which produce infection but no significant disease. These are the most effective immunizations, eg, smallpox, yellow fever, live poliomyelitis and measles vaccines.

3. Repeated injection of microorganisms inactivated by physical or chemical methods.

4. Repeated injection of microbial products (eg, exotoxins) or, preferably, harmless antigenic materials derived therefrom (eg, toxoids).

5. Repeated injection or ingestion of materials derived from microorganisms through disintegration or lysis.

6. Clinical or subclinical infection.

•   •   •

General References

Austen, K.F., & Z.A. Cohn: Contribution of serum and cellular factors in host defense reactions. New England J Med 268:933, 994, 1056, 1963.

Douglas, S.D., & H.H. Fudenberg: Genetically determined defects in host resistance to infection: Cellular aspects. M Clin North America 53:903–922, 1969.

Smith, H.: Biochemical challenge of microbial pathogenicity. Bact Rev 32:164–184, 1968.

12 . . .

Antigens & Antibodies

ANTIGENS

Antigens are substances which when introduced parenterally into a foreign species can elicit the formation of antibodies in the living animal and which, after antibodies are formed, can react with them. Antigens are usually proteins, but some polysaccharides and polypeptides can also act as complete antigens. Lipids or nucleic acids are antigenic only when combined with proteins.

An animal does not commonly produce antibodies against its own proteins. It differentiates between "self" and "nonself." Exceptions to this generalization are sequestered antigens, eg, the thyroid gland as described below. Only immunologically mature animals produce antibodies. When foreign antigens are introduced into the body during fetal life, they often do not give rise to antibodies. (See Immunologic Tolerance.)

The first essential property of an antigen, therefore, is that it be considered "foreign" or "nonself" (by virtue of its chemical composition or physical structure) by immunologically competent cells of the recipient, and the possession on its surface of specific determinant groups. A second essential property of an antigen is a sufficiently large molecular size. Most antigens have a molecular weight of more than 1×10^4 daltons.

Antigenic Specificity

Reactions of antigens with antibodies are highly specific. This means that an antigen will react only with antibodies elicited by its own kind or by a closely related kind of antigen. The majority of antigenic substances are species-specific, and some are even organ-specific within an animal species. Human proteins can easily be distinguished from the proteins of other animals by antigen-antibody reactions and will cross-react only with the proteins of closely related species (eg, anthropoid apes). Within a single species, kidney protein may be distinguished from lung protein, etc. Exceptions to this species-specificity are certain antigens which are widely distributed among animals, particularly protein of the lens of the eye and the so-called **Forssman** or **heterophil antigen** which is present in the organs of the mouse, dog, cat, horse, fish, and chicken as well as in the red cells of sheep and in some bacteria.

Antigenic specificity is a function of the chemical structure of the antigen. Serologically identical proteins appear to be identical in composition, and antigens showing cross-reactions are closely related in chemical structure. Specificity of antigens may be altered by changing small chemical groups on the large protein molecule or by acetylation, methylation, or esterification. Thus the specificity of antigens appears to be determined by the chemical structure of small portions of the molecule. Coupling simple chemical groups like $-COOH$, $-SO_3H$, or $-AsO_3H_2$ on a benzene ring with serum protein (by diazo reactions) showed that each of these groups conferred specificity upon the antigen, depending particularly on the position of the radical (ortho-, meta-, or para-) in the aromatic compound.

A **hapten** is a compound of low molecular weight which cannot by itself elicit the formation of antibodies but which can combine with antibodies elicited by a large molecule which possesses a structural unit similar to or identical with the hapten. The structural unit on the large molecule which determines immunologic specificity is called the antigenic determinant. The latter may be part of, or the whole hapten. Certain substances (eg, drugs or their breakdown products) may act as haptens. They can attach to host proteins to form a complex which is a complete antigen.

The combining sites on the antibodies formed against a given determinant group are not all perfect fits. Any antiserum thus contains some antibodies with very close fit, sharp specificity, and strong binding forces, and some antibodies with poor fit, less specificity, and weak binding forces.

The antigenic site involved in combining with antibody is quite small. With highly charged determinant groups such as the picryl group, the specificity is determined by that group alone. With uncharged polysaccharides such as dextrans, the size of the determinant group is of the order of 3–6 glucose residues. In the case of a simple protein, silk fibroin, the antigenic combining site is probably of the size of 8–12 amino acid residues.

In spite of the very great antigen specificity, cross-reactions occur between determinant groups of closely related structure and their antibodies. The sharing of similar antigenic determinants by molecules of different origin leads to unexpected and unpredictable cross-reactions, eg, between human group A red blood cells and type 14 pneumococci.

When antigenic proteins are denatured by heating or by vigorous chemical treatment, the molecular configuration is somewhat changed. This results usually in the loss of the original antigenic determinants and often leads to the uncovering of new antigenic determinants and new antigenic specificities. Formaldehyde-treated proteins acquire an added antigenicity, and their antisera tend to cross-react with other formaldehyde-treated proteins. However, with gentle formaldehyde treatment the original antigenicity may also be preserved whereas the toxicity of the molecule (eg, exotoxins) may be abolished and the molecule thus converted to a "toxoid" which is immunogenic but nontoxic.

Most microorganisms contain not just one but many antigens to each of which antibodies may develop in the course of infection. Among these antigens may be capsular polysaccharides, somatic proteins or lipoprotein-carbohydrate complexes, protein exotoxins, and enzymes produced by the organism. All enzymes appear to be antigenic, and in some but not all cases that portion of the molecule which combines with specific antibody appears to be distinct from the portion of the molecule responsible for enzymatic activity. Many hormones are also antigenic.

Isoantigens (Blood Group Substances)

In general, antibodies are elicited only by antigens foreign to the injected animal species (heteroantibodies). However, animals may produce "isoantibodies" against "isoantigens," ie, antigens derived from other individuals of the same species. Outstanding among isoantigens are the blood group substances present in the red cells. There are 4 combinations of the 2 antigens present in erythrocytes. Their presence is under genetic control. The serum contains antibody against the absent antigens. As shown in Table 12–1, antigen and corresponding antibody do not coexist in the same blood. To avoid antigen-antibody reactions which would result in serious transfusion accidents, all bloods must be carefully matched for blood transfusion.

In addition to these major isoantibodies, certain red blood cells contain other blood group substances capable of stimulating antibodies. Among them is the Rh substance. Antibodies to Rh are developed when an Rh-negative person is transfused with Rh-positive blood or when an Rh-negative pregnant woman absorbs Rh substance from her Rh-positive fetus. The development of high titer anti-Rh antibodies in this situation can lead to fetal erythroblastosis, abortion, stillbirth, jaundice of the newborn, and other congenital abnormalities.

Apart from certain "sequestered" antigens, eg, thyroid or lens protein, which can definitely serve as autoantigens, it is not clear what may bring about the autoantigenicity of other organ antigens. Perhaps mobilization from the fixed site or slight alteration of structure may predispose to auto-immunization with consequent disease (see Auto-immune Diseases).

TABLE 12–1. Determination of blood group by cross-match.

Group	Antigens in Red Cell	Antibody in Plasma	Determinant Group of Blood Group Antigen
O	. . .	a, b	L-Fucose
A	A	b	α-N-Acetyl-galactosamin-oyl-galactose
B	B	a	α-D-Galacto-syl-galactose
AB	AB	. . .	. . .

ANTIBODIES
(Immunoglobulins)

Antibodies are specialized serum proteins (immunoglobulins), which can react specifically with the antigen that stimulated their production. Antibodies may comprise 1–2% of total serum proteins, and even more in certain abnormal states.

Chemical & Physical Properties of Antibodies

Antibodies may be characterized by their chemical, physical, and (by far the most specific) immunologic properties. Among the prominent physicochemical properties used for classifying antibodies are solubility in salts and solvents, electrophoretic mobility, molecular size, and sedimentation in the ultracentrifuge. Electrophoretically, most antibodies fit into the gamma and beta$_2$ fractions of globulins; a few migrate with alpha globulins.

By ultracentrifugal analysis, antibodies fall into 2 main classes: (1) molecular weight about 1.5×10^5 daltons, sedimentation coefficient 7 S; (2) molecular weight about 9×10^5 daltons, sedimentation coefficient 19 S. However, some immunoglobulins with antibody activity have sedimentation coefficients between 9 S and 11 S. In the solvent temperature fractionation process of human plasma with ethanol (Cohn), most 7 S immunoglobulins appear in fraction II (eg, mumps, influenza, anti-H of *S typhi*); most 19 S immunoglobulins appear in fraction III-1 (eg, isoagglutinins, anti-O of *S typhi*).

In addition to ultracentrifugal determination of molecular weight and electrophoretic separation of proteins through their migration in an electrical field (in paper, starch, gel, etc), immunoelectrophoresis is an important tool in antibody identification. This technic consists of first separating serum proteins by electrophoresis in an agar gel and then permitting an antiserum to that serum to diffuse from a trough cut in the agar along the line of protein migration. As each serum component encounters its specific antibody, a line of precipitate is formed in the agar.

TABLE 12−2. Characteristics of immunoglobulins.

Immuno-globulin	Sedimen-tation Constant	Molecular Weight	Crosses Placenta	Elicit PCA*	Percent Carbohy-drate	Examples	Average Serum Concentration (mg/100 ml)
IgG	7 S	150,000	Yes	Yes	2.5	Many antibodies to bacteria, viruses, toxins, especially late in antibody response.	1000−1500
IgM	19 S	900,000	No	No	5−10	Many early antibodies to infectious agents and other antigens.	60−180
IgA	7 S or 11 S	170,000 or 380,000	No	No	5−10	Isohemagglutinins; antibody in external secretions: 2 mols of 7 S IgA linked by "secretory" piece of molecular weight 60,000.	100−400
IgD	7 S	150,000	No	No	?	Antibody activity not established.	3−5
IgE	8 S	200,000	No ?	No	10	Skin-sensitizing antibody in allergy; reagin.	0.1

*Passive cutaneous anaphylaxis.

Heterogeneity of Antibodies; Classes of Immunoglobulins

The technics mentioned above (and others) have revealed that antibodies are not uniform in their properties. They belong to a family of related proteins, the immunoglobulins, with overlapping physical, chemical, and biologic properties, but exhibit considerable heterogeneity. At present, immunoglobulins are arranged into 5 classes. (See Table 12−2.)

STRUCTURE OF IMMUNOGLOBULINS

From a variety of studies a picture of the probable chemical structure of immunoglobulin molecules is beginning to emerge. A 7 S immunoglobulin molecule consists of 2 "heavy" (H) peptide chains (molecular weight of 5×10^4 daltons) and 2 "light" (L) peptide chains (molecular weight of 2.5×10^4 daltons). These chains are held together by disulfide bonds (Fig 12−1) and can be isolated by reduction (mercaptoethanol) and alkylation followed by chromatography on sephadex G100 at acid pH. The H chains appear to be bonded to each other, and one L chain bound to each of the H chains.

L chains are electrophoretically similar and belong to one of 2 immunologic types, κ and λ, under separate genetic control. Both types occur in all classes of immunoglobulins, but any one molecule contains only one type of L chain. The hereditary human globulin character "Inv" is located on the L chain. H chains are electrophoretically distinct and belong to several different antigenic types. It is probable that both H and L chains contribute to the combining site on the antibody molecule, with most activity on the H chain, and that specific antibody activity is determined by amino acid sequence. The portion of the H chain which is not involved in antibody activity (Fc fragment) carries the chemical sites for complement fixation, skin fixation, placental permeability, the Gm locus reacting with rheumatoid factor, and most of the carbohydrate moiety.

Papain treatment of a 7 S immunoglobulin molecule yields 3 fragments of 3.5 S. Two of these fragments (Fab) each carry one antigen-binding site and consist of one L chain and part of one H chain. The third fragment (Fc) carries the determinants which bind antibody and consist of an H chain with the Gm locus (Fig 12−1).

IgG comprises about 75% of all immunoglobulins in man. It has at least 4 subclasses, IgG 1 to IgG 4, which are recognized on the basis of antigenic differences in their H chains. IgG appears to be the only immunoglobulin which crosses the placenta and can produce passive cutaneous anaphylaxis. The rate of IgG synthesis in man is about 35 mg/kg/day, and its half-life is about 23 days. Adult serum levels (about 1200 mg/100 ml) are reached at 2 years of age. Each IgG molecule can combine with 2 antigen molecules, ie, IgG has a valence of 2.

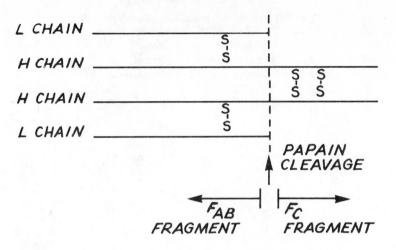

FIG 12—1. Schematic representation of a 7 S immunoglobulin molecule.

IgM comprises about 7% of immunoglobulins in man. Each 19 S IgM molecule consists of 5 subunits. Reducing agents (eg, mercaptoethanol) tend to break the disulfide bonds and dissociate the IgM into monomers of 7 S each. Each monomer consists of 2 L chains and 2 H chains which belong to distinct immunologic classes. Each subunit has at least 1 antigen combining site and thus each IgM molecule can combine with 5 antigen molecules, ie, IgM has a valence of at least 5. IgM antibodies are the earliest antibodies synthesized in response to antigen stimulation. The rate of IgM synthesis is about 8 mg/kg/day, and the half-life is about 5 days. Adult serum levels (about 120 mg/100 ml) are reached at 6—9 months of age, but the fetus synthesizes IgM in utero.

IgA molecules consist of 2 L chains and 2 H chains with specific antigenic subclasses. There appear to be 2 separate systems of IgA antibodies: (1) IgA in the serum, comprising about 15% of circulating immunoglobulins, with serum levels between 100 and 400 mg/100 ml, a rate of synthesis of about 35 mg/kg/day, and rapid catabolism, with a half-life of about 6 days. Serum IgA does not fix complement. (2) Secretory IgA found in tears, saliva, nasal and bronchial fluids, gastrointestinal fluids, and urine. The secretory IgA consists of 11 S molecules which are made up of two 7 S serum IgA molecules linked together by a "secretory" or T piece with a molecular weight of 6 × 10⁴ daltons. This T piece is synthesized in epithelial cells of mucous membranes, whereas the IgA portion of the molecule is synthesized by plasma cells. Secretory IgA possesses many antibody activities, including antibacterial and virus neutralizing activities. Production of secretory IgA appears to be stimulated by infection or antigen administration to the mucous membranes where synthesis occurs, but not by systemic antigen administration.

IgD occurs in minute concentration in serum. Definite antibody activity for IgD has not been established, but some antibodies to penicillin determinants may be IgD. It appears to be rapidly catabolized, so that the half-life is less than 3 days.

IgE immunoglobulins have a molecular weight of 2 × 10⁵ daltons, a sedimentation constant of 8 S, and a carbohydrate content of 10%. They are the skin-sensitizing, "reaginic" antibodies in allergy. In normal individuals, IgE concentrations in serum are negligible, the rate of synthesis is low, and the half-life is 2 days. In allergic persons, substantial serum levels of IgE are found.

One or more immunoglobulins may be present in abnormally high concentration in chronic bacterial or protozoal infections, liver disease, auto-immune diseases, neoplasms of lymphoid or plasma cells, etc. Deficiencies of specific immunoglobulins are usually on a hereditary basis, and can be due either to impaired synthesis or increased catabolism.

Formation of Antibodies

Immunoglobulins are produced in lymphoid tissues in the body. Lymphoid and, especially, plasma cells are most important in antibody synthesis. Lymphoid cells in culture can also produce antibodies. The thymus appears to play an essential role in the development of immunologic competence during fetal and neonatal life, both as a source of lymphoid cells and as a source of humoral substances.

The mechanism by which antibodies are formed is still uncertain, and several hypotheses are being studied. One of the principal uncertainties is whether the presence of antigen is always a prerequisite to the formation of antibody. One theory (clonal selection hypothesis) proposes that immunologic specificity is based on a unique combination of natural globulins rather than on unique globulins created anew to match each possible antigen. Antigens, instead of carrying instructions for the new synthesis of antibody, may merely select out—and greatly stimulate the proliferation of—cells which happen to produce specific matching globulins naturally. Such selected cell lines would subsequently persist indefinitely in the host and could produce antibody in the absence of antigen. This hypothesis has recently fallen somewhat from favor.

Another theory ("instructional" hypothesis) holds that antigen must be present to serve as a direct template for the synthesis of specialized globulin from amino acids or for the folding of a polypeptide chain. Much recent evidence suggests that the initial step in antibody production is the phagocytosis of the antigen by nonantibody-producing macrophages. Subsequently, these cells transmit a ribonuclease-sensitive product to lymphoid cells which are capable of synthesizing specific globulins. The earliest immunoglobulins produced are often 19 S macroglobulins; 7 S globulins appear later.

H chains are synthesized on large polyribosomes (270 S). Each chain is probably synthesized as a unit in 30–60 seconds. L chains occur in a small pool in cells, in association with the polysomes which synthesize H chains. L chains probably combine with H chains on polysomes, and this initiates an orderly release.

Since lymphoid cells are undoubtedly involved in immunoglobulin synthesis, diseases of the lymphoid system often are accompanied by disordered production of immunoglobulins. Thus in multiple myeloma, macroglobulinemia, and similar diseases large quantities of proteins are found which are closely related to one of the Ig classes.

Rate of Production of Antibodies

Depending upon the nature of the antigen and the site of injection, antibody can be detected in the serum several days after the first injection of a minimal dose of antigen. The antibody titer then rises gradually to a low peak, falls slowly, and finally disappears. If a second injection of antigen is given while antibodies from the first stimulus are still present, there is often an immediate drop in titer (negative phase) followed by a rapid rise to a much higher peak than can be attained with only one injection. Following this second stimulus, the antibodies disappear much more slowly than after the first. The rapid rise of antibody titer following a second administration of the antigen ("booster shot") presumably indicates that the antibody-producing cells have been "primed" by the first contact with antigen and can therefore respond more effectively and more quickly when they encounter antigen for a second time (Fig 12–2). In view of the striking ability of lymphoid cells to undergo morphologic transformation, the nature of the cell responsible for "immunologic memory" is not established.

Immunoglobulin synthesis may proceed rapidly. Rates for individual immunoglobulins in man have been given above. The half-lives of immunoglobulins vary because of differences in catabolism.

When 2 or more antigens are injected simultaneously, the host reacts by producing antibodies to each. Competition of antigens for antibody-producing mechanisms has been observed experimentally, but it plays no practical role and combined immunization with several antigens is widely used (eg, diphtheria toxoid + tetanus toxoid + pertussis vaccine). The administration of a specific antibody interferes with the production of antibody against the same specific antigen by the host. A practical application is the injection of human antibody to Rh antigen into Rh negative (Rh–) women with Rh positive (Rh+) husbands and children. If the Rh– woman is permitted to form antibodies to the fetus's Rh+ red cells, these antibodies are likely to produce Rh disease in the fetus or newborn; but if the Rh– woman receives concentrated Rh antibodies before she begins to synthesize Rh antibodies, her antibody production is inhibited and Rh disease of the newborn is prevented.

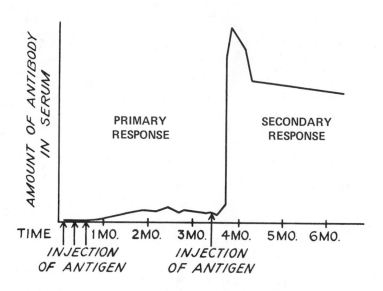

FIG 12–2. Rate of antibody production following initial antigen administration and "booster" injection.

Rate of Absorption & Elimination of Antigen

One of the features which determines the effectiveness of an antigen as a stimulus for antibody production is its rate of absorption and elimination from the site of administration. Antigens differ greatly in their rate of excretion, but the major portion of injected antigen is often eliminated from the host within hours or days. In general, antibody response will be higher and more sustained if the antigen is absorbed slowly from its "depot" at the site of injection. For this reason, many immunizing preparations employ physical methods to delay absorption. Toxoids are often adsorbed onto alum hydroxide or precipitated with alum sulfate. Bacterial or viral suspensions are prepared sometimes with oily media which delay absorption and promote tissue reaction to "fix" the antigen at its site of injection. (Such adjuvants are discussed on p 157.)

Kinds of Antibodies

Antibodies are generally described in terms of their reactions with antigen:

A. Antitoxins: Antibodies to toxins or toxoids which neutralize or flocculate with the antigen.

B. Agglutinins: Antibodies which first immobilize motile organisms and then aggregate cells, forming clumps. Agglutinins can only be demonstrated if the antigen is particulate, or if the antigen is adsorbed onto the surface of a visible particle of uniform size, eg, red blood cell, latex, bentonite.

C. Precipitins: Antibodies which form complexes with antigen molecules in solution, forming precipitates. Precipitins can only be demonstrated if the antigen is soluble.

D. Lysins: Antibodies which, usually together with complement, dissolve the antigenic cells.

E. Opsonins: Antibodies which combine with surface components of microbial and other cells so that they are more readily taken up by phagocytes.

F. Neutralizing (Protective) Antibodies: Antibodies which render their antigenic microorganism (commonly viruses) noninfective.

G. Complement Fixing Antibodies: Detected by the consumption of complement by the antigen-antibody complex. These reactions are discussed in detail in the remainder of the chapter.

H. "Blocking" Inhibitory and Other Nonprecipitating Antibodies: These combine with antigen but are not grossly detectable unless they are shown to inhibit or "block" a reaction or unless the protein species of antibody can be identified.

Characteristics of the Reaction Between
Antigen & Antibody

(1) The reaction is generally specific, although some cross-reactions occur.

(2) Different types of serologic reactions that can be demonstrated with a given antigen and its antiserum probably often reflect different activities of the same antibody molecule. The union between antigen and antibody is probably always the same (unitarian hypothesis). Occasionally there are quantitative differences, one reaction requiring less antibody than another. At times truly different antibody molecules are produced in response to a given antigen, and any one antibody molecule may manifest itself in only a limited fashion.

(3) The union between antigen and antibody is firm but often reversible.

(4) Antigen and antibody combine in varying proportions (see Danysz phenomenon). The combination in multiple proportions depends upon the fact that antibody valence is restricted to 2 (5 for IgM), whereas antigen valence can be 5–10 per molecule or more.

(5) The reaction between antigen and antibody is a chemical one due to the combination of the specific reactant groups of the 2 reagents.

Human Gamma Globulin

Immune serum globulin USP is a preparation of gamma globulin derived from large pools of human plasma by low temperature ethanol fractionation. The preparation contains about 165 mg of gamma globulin per ml of solution, representing a 25-fold concentration of antibody-containing globulins of plasma, glycine as stabilizer, and an antibacterial agent. Such concentrated gamma globulin is injected intramuscularly or subcutaneously, never intravenously. It may be employed clinically in the following conditions:

A. Hypo- or Dysgammaglobulinemia With Recurrent Bacterial Infections: Inject 0.6–1 ml/kg body weight (150 mg gamma globulin per kg) once each month, but twice initially. Antimicrobial drugs must also be used to control active infections.

B. Measles: To prevent clinical disease in nonimmunized children (and interfere with development of active immunity), give 0.2 ml/kg during the first 6 days after exposure. To attenuate the disease (and permit development of active immunity), give 0.04 ml/kg during the first 6 days after exposure, or 0.12 ml/kg between the sixth and tenth days after exposure. Gamma globulin has no effect after the rash has appeared. Attenuation is desirable in all healthy, nonimmune exposed children because it markedly reduces the incidence of complications. Complete prevention is indicated in very young or debilitated children or in institutions. Gamma globulin (0.02 ml/kg) is administered simultaneously with certain live measles virus vaccines to minimize reactions to the vaccine.

C. German Measles: Susceptible women during the first 4 months of pregnancy may be given 0.6 ml/kg. This will prevent disease in up to 50% of exposed women, but it probably does not protect the fetus.

D. Infectious Hepatitis: Use of 0.02 ml/kg once or twice during the incubation period may prevent or modify the disease without interfering with the development of immunity.

E. Serum Hepatitis: Use of 0.14 ml/kg after multiple transfusions given to adults over 40 years of age, to avoid serious disease.

Specific Human Hyperimmune Gamma Globulins

These are obtained from the blood of individuals who have been repeatedly immunized with a given antigen and have acquired high concentrations of specific antibody. A few specific indications are listed below.

A. Tetanus: For prevention of tetanus after injury in nonimmunized individuals, 250–500 units of human hyperimmune tetanus globulin will yield serum levels of 0.03–0.06 unit antitoxin per ml for several weeks (see p 180).

B. Vaccinia: Hyperimmune globulin, 0.6–1 ml/kg, can be used in the rare individual who develops progressive vaccinia gangrenosum after smallpox vaccination. These are often hypogammaglobulinemic persons.

C. Rabies: The prophylactic use of live rabies vaccine in occupationally exposed individuals makes it likely that hyperimmunization of volunteers for globulin production will soon be feasible. Specific human hyperimmune rabies globulin can then be used in severely exposed persons.

D. Mumps: Limited evidence suggests that 20 ml of hyperimmune gamma globulin may prevent orchitis in adult males.

E. Chickenpox: Zoster immune globulin, 2 ml, injected into children within 72 hours of exposure to chickenpox, can prevent the disease.

F. Rh Disease: Specific human anti-Rh immune globulin can be injected into an Rh− mother following delivery of an Rh+ infant. This prevents Rh isoimmunization of the mother and reduces the risk of hemolytic Rh disease in her next Rh+ infant.

SEROLOGIC REACTIONS

Serology is the study of reactions between antigens and antibodies. It attempts to quantitate these reactions by keeping one reagent constant and diluting the other. Some serologic measurements may be made absolutely quantitative by utilizing the technic of immunochemistry.

Serologic reactions are used to identify antigens or antibodies, if either of these reagents is known. They are also employed to estimate the relative quantity of these reactants. Thus the level or titer of antibodies in the serum of man or animal can be determined by means of known antigens, and conclusions can be drawn regarding past contact of the host with the antigen. This is particularly valuable in the diagnosis of infection or of certain forms of hypersensitivity. Conversely, by means of known antibodies the various antigens of a microorganism or other biologic material which characterize it may be identified. Thus serologic technics permit the definitive identification of microorganisms isolated from an individual with an infection or the classification of red blood cells for blood transfusion. Knowledge of antigenic structure

likewise permits proper selection of microorganisms suitable for immunization of man or animals against specific infectious diseases.

The type of antigen-antibody reaction applicable to a given situation depends largely on the physical state of the available antigen (see above). Each of the common types of antigen-antibody reactions is taken up in some detail on the following pages. Because the precipitin reaction permits the most accurate chemical quantitative work, it has been studied in the greatest detail. Some of the characteristics observed in precipitin reactions apply generally to all antigen-antibody reactions.

PRECIPITATION REACTIONS

To demonstrate the presence of antibody against an antigen in solution, the antigen merely has to be layered in a tube over a small volume of antiserum. At the interface of the 2 reagents, precipitation will occur, forming a ring. This gives qualitative evidence of an antigen-antibody reaction but does not indicate whether one or several antigen-antibody systems are present. If, however, the reaction takes place in a semisolid environment (eg, soft agar), then different antigens and antibodies are likely to diffuse at different rates. As a result, optimal proportions for precipitation would occur at different sites in the agar and distinct multiple bands of precipitate would form. Agar diffusion methods based on this principle (Oudin, Ouchterlony) aid in detecting the number of components in mixtures of antigens or in detecting the identity or diversity of different antigens interacting with a single antibody, and vice versa. Agar diffusion can be combined with electrophoretic separation of proteins for their identification (see Immunoelectrophoresis).

In order to perform a titration of the precipitin content of a serum, serial dilutions of the serum are mixed with a constant amount of antigen (as in most other serologic reactions) or a constant amount of serum is mixed with increasing dilutions of antigen. The latter method is generally preferred, because precipitation reactions are markedly inhibited by excess antigen. The precipitin content of the serum is then expressed as the greatest dilution of antigen precipitated. Precipitin reactions require the presence of salt, and pH must be near neutrality. The reaction rate is faster at higher temperatures, but the maximum amount of precipitate is formed in the cold.

Example of Reaction

Serum is obtained from an animal which has been injected repeatedly with a pure antigen in solution (eg, crystalline egg albumin). Equal amounts of serum (eg, 1 ml) are distributed into a series of small tubes. To each tube is added a variable graded amount of the antigen (egg albumin), and the tubes are then left at 0° C for 2 hours. At the end of this period some tubes

TABLE 12–3. Examples of precipitation reactions.

Tube	Serum (ml)	Egg Albumin (mg)	Resulting Precipitation	Test on Supernatant (Zone Formation)	Area of Fig 12–3.
1	1	0.015	Minimal	Excess antibody	A. Zone of antibody excess
2	1	0.030	Slight	Excess antibody	
3	1	0.060	Heavy	Slight excess antibody	B. Zone of equivalence
4	1	0.090	Heavy	Neither antigen nor antibody	
5	1	0.120	Heavy	Slight excess antigen	C. Zone of antigen excess
6	1	0.180	Slight	Excess antigen	
7	1	0.240	None	Large excess antigen	

contain a precipitate and others do not (Table 12–3). This precipitate can be sedimented by centrifugation, washed repeatedly with saline to remove adherent serum, and then analyzed for nitrogen content.

The supernatant from each tube is decanted and distributed into 2 tubes. To one of these is added antigen; to the other, antibody. The occurrence of precipitate in these tubes of supernatant permits distinction of 3 zones.

(1) A zone of antibody excess, in which uncombined antibody is present.

(2) A zone of equivalence, in which both antigen and antibody are completely precipitated and no uncombined antigen or antibody is present.

(3) A zone of antigen excess, in which all antibody has combined with antigen and additional uncombined antigen is present. In this zone precipitation is partly or completely inhibited, because in the presence of excess antigen soluble antigen-antibody complexes form.

Micro-Kjeldahl determinations for total nitrogen are then made on the washed precipitate. The precipitate contains both antibody nitrogen and antigen nitrogen. Therefore the amount of antibody nitrogen contained in the serum (and precipitated completely in the zone of equivalence) can be accurately stated by subtracting the antigen nitrogen added to the tube from the total nitrogen value of the precipitate.

The field of immunochemistry provides methods for absolute quantitative measurement of antibody which can be applied to a large variety of theoretical and practical problems.*

The initial combination of antigen and antibody takes place almost immediately upon mixing of the reactants. The subsequent formation of larger, visible aggregates requires an hour or more and depends somewhat on the temperature and the total volume of the mixture. The reaction is fastest in the zone of equivalence, where optimal proportions between antigen and antibody exist. The speed of gross precipitation is an index of the zone of equivalence, where complete precipitation of both antigen and antibody take place and neither is present in excess.

AGGLUTINATION REACTIONS

The antigen in agglutination reactions is particulate, and commonly consists of suspensions of microorganisms, red blood cells, or uniform particles like latex or bentonite onto which antigens have been adsorbed. When mixed with specific antiserum these cells or particles become clumped; the clumps aggregate and finally settle as large, visible clumps, leaving the supernatant clear. If one of the reagents is known, the reaction may be employed for the identification of either antigen or antibody. Thus the reaction is commonly used to identify, by means of known antisera, microorganisms cultured from clinical specimens. The agglutination reaction is also used to estimate the titer of antibacterial agglutinins in the serum of patients with unknown disease. A rise in antibody titer directed against a specific microorganism occurring during an illness strongly suggests an etiologic relationship.

It must be remembered that microorganisms generally possess a variety of antigens and that antibodies to one or more of these may be present in antiserum. A simple example is provided by the antibody response to infection by flagellated bacteria.

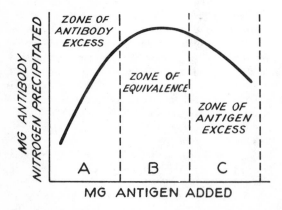

FIG 12–3. The 3 main zones of antigen-antibody interaction.

*The technics, accomplishments, and possibilities of immunochemistry are discussed in E.A. Kabat: *Experimental Immunochemistry,* 2nd ed. Thomas, 1961.

Antibodies may be directed against the flagellar surface antigen, the somatic antigens, or both, with different diagnostic implications (eg, salmonellae). The type of macroscopic agglutination may also be distinctive; the flagellar antigen-antibody complex appears coarse and floccular, whereas the somatic complex appears fine and granular.

The agglutination reaction is aided by elevated temperature (37–56° C) and by movement, which increases the contact between antigen and antibody (eg, shaking, stirring, centrifuging). The aggregation of clumps requires the presence of salts. In the zone of antibody excess (ie, concentrated serum), agglutination is often inhibited. This prozone may give the unwarranted impression that antibodies are absent; this error can be avoided only by using serial dilutions of serum.

The agglutination test may be performed microscopically by mixing a loopful of serum with a suspension of microorganisms on a slide and inspecting the result through the low-power objective. This is done commonly for the identification of unknown cultures. For the estimation of the "titer" of agglutinating antibodies in an unknown serum, a macroscopic tube dilution test is usually done: A suitable fixed amount of antigen is added to each tube of a series of serum dilutions; after thorough shaking, the tubes are incubated at 37° C for 1–2 hours. The result is determined by looking for sedimented clumps and clear supernatant fluid. The "titer" of the serum is the highest dilution with clearly visible agglutination.

The reaction may be carried out by a quantitative absolute procedure resembling that employed in the precipitation reaction. The antigen must then be added in the form of a washed microbial suspension of known nitrogen content. The antibody nitrogen is determined by subtracting the antigen nitrogen from the total nitrogen of the centrifuged and washed agglutinated material.

TOXIN-ANTITOXIN REACTIONS

Many materials of microbial origin are toxic to higher forms of life. The characteristics and properties of such materials cover a wide spectrum from which 2 varieties, endotoxins and exotoxins, are frequently selected because of their clear-cut role in disease. The 2 groups of substances differ as shown in Table 12–4.

The toxin-antitoxin reactions described below apply only to exotoxins, as exemplified by the toxins of diphtheria, tetanus, or botulism. The following examples of definitions of units apply to diphtheria toxin:

MLD (minimum lethal dose): The smallest amount of toxin which will kill a guinea pig weighing 250 gm within 4 days after subcutaneous inoculation.

1 unit of antitoxin (International): The amount of antitoxin in 0.0628 mg of a standard dried antitoxin maintained at the Serum Institute, Copenhagen.

L_0 dose: The greatest amount of toxin which, when mixed with 1 unit of antitoxin and injected subcutaneously into a guinea pig weighing 250 gm, will produce no toxic reaction.

L_+ dose: The smallest amount of toxin which, when mixed with 1 unit of antitoxin and injected subcutaneously into a guinea pig weighing 250 gm, will cause death within 4 days.

L_f dose (flocculating unit): That amount of toxin which flocculates most rapidly with 1 unit of antitoxin in a series of mixtures containing constant amounts of antitoxin and varying amounts of toxin. (This value is calculated from experimental results.)

Antitoxic potency can be measured by the ability to neutralize the toxin when the mixture is injected into animals or to precipitate toxin in vitro.

The MLD of toxin varies with different preparations; furthermore, it is inconstant even with a single preparation because toxic properties deteriorate upon storage. Any preparation of toxin contains some molecules of full toxicity and others of low or no toxicity but persistent antigenicity (toxoid). Dried antitoxin, however, is constant in its ability to combine with toxin or toxoid molecules. For this reason, antitoxin is taken as the constant standard for biologic estimation of toxic or antitoxic potency. The L_0 dose is relatively difficult to determine, and so the L_+ dose is usually relied upon. Because toxin and antitoxin combine in multiple proportions, the L_+ dose is not 1 MLD larger but 10–50 MLD larger than the L_0 unit. The L_f unit is independent of the toxic activity of a given preparation and is only a function of its antigenic combining power. Thus it remains constant when a toxin is converted to toxoid by formalin or heat. It is of great importance in the standardization of antigenic quantities of toxoid.

Toxin-antitoxin flocculations are similar to precipitin reactions, but show a very sharp zone of equivalence. The reaction is inhibited by both antigen excess and antibody excess; soluble complexes result from either.

Danysz Phenomenon

If toxin is added to antitoxin in several fractions with time intervals between them, then more antitoxin (or less toxin) is necessary to give a neutral endpoint in injected animals than if all the toxin had been added at once. This is called the Danysz phenomenon and may be explained by the ability of toxin to combine with antitoxin in multiple proportions. The first fraction of toxin combines with a relatively large amount of the antitoxin present, so that but little antitoxin is left to combine with the second fraction. After some time,

TABLE 12–4. Differentiation of exotoxins and endotoxins.

Exotoxins	Endotoxins
Excreted by living cells; found in high concentration in fluid medium.	Liberated by microbial cell walls only upon their disintegration.
Highly toxic; fatal for laboratory animals in micrograms or less.	Weakly toxic; fatal for laboratory animals in milligrams or more.
Relatively unstable; toxicity usually destroyed rapidly by heat over 60° C.	Relatively stable; withstand heat over 60° C for hours without loss of toxicity.
Converted into antigenic, nontoxic toxoids by formalin, storage, etc.	Not converted into toxoids.
Highly antigenic, stimulating the formation of high titer antitoxin.	Do not stimulate formation of antitoxin.
Heat-labile proteins, molecular weight 10,000 to 900,000.	Lipopolysaccharide complexes.

however, an equilibrium is again reached. The Danysz phenomenon applies similarly to other antigen-antibody reactions.

BACTERICIDAL & LYTIC REACTIONS

When microbial or other foreign cells are injected into a laboratory animal, antibodies are formed which are capable of killing or lysing the type of cells that served as antigen. This was first observed with cholera vibrios, which dissolved upon contact with specific antiserum in the peritoneal cavity of a guinea pig (Pfeiffer phenomenon). Later it was found that following the injection of foreign red blood cells an animal developed antibodies (hemolysins) which were capable of dissolving such red cells.

These reactions depend on 2 components. One is heat-stable, not affected by 56° C for 30 minutes; the other is heat-labile, being inactivated by such exposure. The heat-stable component is a specific antibody elicited by the antigen injected and able to combine with it. It is variously referred to as amboceptor, bacteriolysin, or hemolysin. The heat-labile component is a complex system present in most fresh animal sera and is called **complement.** It is not an antibody but can attach to antigen-antibody complexes, in which case it is said that the "complement is fixed." A cell with attached amboceptor is called "sensitized." Complement can lyse such "sensitized" cells.

Complement (alexin) is a group of proteins found in the normal serum of many animals in inactive form. Fresh guinea pig serum is the usual source of complement. It has to be used fresh or kept frozen; otherwise it deteriorates rapidly. Complement activity depends upon the ionic strength of the medium, pH (optimum, 7.2 to 7.4), volume (inverse relationship), temperature (optimum, 30–37° C), and the presence of Ca^{++} and Mg^{++}.

At present, 9 distinct components of guinea pig complement are recognized: C1, C2, C4, C3, C5, C6, C7, C8, and C9. On heating at 56° C, complement loses activity within a few minutes because of the inactivation of C1, C2, and C8. The remaining components are somewhat more resistant to heat, but all lose much of their activity within 20–30 minutes at 56° C.

When immunoglobulins (IgG or IgM) are aggregated by antigen, C1 is bound and becomes activated as an enzyme (an esterase or protease) which attacks C4 and C2 and mediates their fixation. Other com-

(1) $E + A \longrightarrow EA$

(2) $EA + C1 \xrightarrow{Ca^{++}} EAC1$ ($\overline{C1}^{(a)}$ dissociates readily from this complex)

(3) $EAC1 + C4 \longrightarrow EAC1,4$ ($\overline{C1}^{(a)}$ dissociates fairly readily from this and following complexes)

(4) $EAC1,4 + C2 \xrightarrow{Mg^{++}} EAC1,4,2$ ($\overline{C2}^{(a)}$ moiety unstable at 37° C)

(5) $EAC1,4,2 + C3 \longrightarrow EAC1,4,2,3$ (reactive in immune adherence, phagocytosis)

(6) $EAC1,4,2,3 + C5,6,7 \longrightarrow EAC1,4,2,3,5,6,7$ (stable complex, reactive in leukocyte chemotaxis)

(7) $EAC1,4,2,3,5,6,7 + C8,9 \longrightarrow EAC1,4,2,3,5,6,7,8,9$ (= E*, or cell with one damaged site, leading to lysis)

(a) Activated form of the component.

ponents then react in a biologic chain reaction which can ultimately produce irreversible damage to cell membrane.

For hemolytic and bactericidal activity, all 9 components of complement are required (see scheme on p 144). However, for immune adherence activity and for the enhancement of phagocytosis, only the first 4 components (C1,4,2,3) are essential.

Different animal sera contain different proportions of the various complement components. The component which is lowest in titer in a given serum limits the hemolytic complement activity of that serum.

Complement is commonly titrated by its ability to lyse red blood cells which have been "sensitized" with specific anti-red cell antibodies (hemolysins). The units of hemolysin and of complement are defined in terms of the greatest dilution of serum which will barely cause lysis of a given number of red blood cells in the presence of an excess of the other factor—complement or hemolysin, respectively. Time, volume, and temperature are strictly specified. The end point is either complete and grossly visible lysis or optical estimation of 50% lysis.

An example of immune hemolysis mediated by guinea pig complement is shown in the scheme on p 144. It involves red blood cells (E), specific antibody to red cells (A), all of the components of complement, and metal ions. The reactivity of human complement is similar. All reactions shown can take place at $0°$ C, but most proceed more rapidly at $30-37°$ C. Ultimately, holes are digested in the red blood cell membrane (E*), and the damaged cell lyses. The participation of complement in disease states is being studied. Reactions attributed to "anaphylotoxin" (release of histamine from mast cells) are caused by fragments of complement components C3 or C5. In hereditary angioneurotic edema, there is a deficiency of a normal inhibitor of C1 esterase in serum. In acute glomerulonephritis, systemic lupus erythematosus, and other disorders in which antigen-antibody complexes are being formed, some complement components are greatly depressed in serum.

For optimal ingestion of particles (bacteria, red cells, etc) by phagocytic cells, the C1,4,2,3 complex is necessary. The same complex is required for "complement-dependent" virus neutralization by early antiserum. Fragments of C3 and C5 both (or the C5,6,7 complex) exert chemotactic effects on leukocytes.

Properdin is the name given to a serum protein which neutralizes certain viruses, lyses abnormal erythrocytes (eg, paroxysmal nocturnal hemoglobinuria), destroys some gram-negative bacteria, and may be involved in a variety of other features of resistance or immunity.

There is no general agreement on the properties or biologic role of properdin, nor even on its existence. The observed phenomena attributed to the "properdin system" are explained by some in terms of specific antibody in normal serum. Others believe that properdin is a unique serum protein, distinct from immunoglobulins or complement components.

COMPLEMENT FIXATION REACTIONS

Complement fixation tests depend upon 2 distinct reactions. The first involves antigen and antibody (of which one is known, the other unknown) plus a fixed amount of pre-titrated complement. If antigen and antibody are specific for one another, they will combine; the combination will take up ("fix") the added complement. The second reaction involves testing for the presence of free (unattached) complement. This is done by the addition of red cells "sensitized" with specific hemolysin. If complement has been "fixed" by the antigen-antibody complex, then none will be available for lysis of the sensitized red cells. If the antigen and antibody are not specific for each other, or if one of them is lacking, then complement remains free to attach to the sensitized red cells and lyse them. Therefore, a positive complement fixation test gives no hemolysis; a negative test gives hemolysis. This can be written schematically as follows:

I. Specific antigen X + Complement ⟶ Complement not bound

II. Specific antibody anti-X + Complement ⟶ Complement not bound

III. X + Anti-X + Complement ⟶ Complement bound ("fixed")

To detect whether complement is bound or not bound, a hemolytic system (see above) of red blood cells (RBC) + anti-RBC antibody (Ab) is added to each of the mixtures I, II, and III, with the following results:

I + RBC + Ab ⟶ Lysis of RBC = Negative test

II + RBC + Ab ⟶ Lysis of RBC = Negative test

III + RBC + Ab ⟶ No lysis of RBC = Positive test

A positive test occurs only if X and anti-X have combined to bind available complement. If antigen (X) does not match specific antibody (Y), no complex will be formed, no complement will be consumed, and lysis of added red cells indicates a negative test. If either antigen X alone or antibody anti-X alone (I or II) inactivate complement, they are unsatisfactory for the test and are called anticomplementary. Anticomplementary antigens or sera are detected by suitable controls in the test. Anticomplementary activity can sometimes be removed by heating or dilution.

For the practical performance of the test, it is necessary to control all reagents and environmental conditions carefully. In order to eliminate any complement that might be present in the serum used as source of antibody, all sera must be inactivated by heating for 30 minutes at 56° C. To the antigen and the inactivated serum, a carefully titrated amount of complement is added (usually 1.2–2 units). The mixture is then left at 37° C or in the refrigerator for a specified time to permit interaction of antigen and antibody and "fixation" of complement. Next, the "hemolytic system" is added; this consists generally of a suspension of sheep red cells "sensitized" by the addition of hemolysin (ie, anti-sheep cell rabbit serum). The mixture is then incubated at 37° C for 30 minutes and read for hemolysis.

Specific and detailed directions regarding concentrations and amounts of reagents, time and temperature of "fixation," nature of buffer, etc must be followed for each individual complement fixation test. Complete controls must be included in each test.

If properly controlled, the complement fixation test is among the most sensitive and delicate of all the serologic reactions employed in the diagnostic microbiology laboratory. It is used for the identification of antibody and estimation of its titer (with known antigens) or the identification of antigens (with known antibody). The serologic diagnosis of many viral and fungal infections and of some immunologic disorders rests on complement fixation tests (see Chapter 29).

ABSORPTION REACTIONS

Sera from animals injected with whole microorganisms or from humans who have passed through several infections tend to react with a variety of related antigens. This raises the question of whether the serum contains an antibody specific for a given antigen or merely a related antibody which cross-reacts. Such sera may be rendered specific for one antigen by removing related antibodies through absorption with specific antigens. This is done by mixing the serum with concentrated antigen (eg, a dense bacterial suspension), incubating to permit combination, and then centrifuging the precipitate or agglutinated material and removing the supernatant serum. It is now "absorbed" and should no longer contain antibodies specific for the absorbing antigen. Such absorptions may be performed with a series of antigens, finally leaving a serum which will react only with a single remaining antigen, for which it is highly specific. This is valuable in "antigenic analysis" of bacteria or of any other biologic substances.

INHIBITION REACTIONS

In addition to the various direct methods of demonstrating and measuring antigen-antibody reactions discussed above, some indirect methods exist which, in essence, employ competition for an antibody combining site by 2 antigenic groups, or competition for an antigenic group by 2 antibodies. They are especially useful when there is no visible evidence of direct reaction between antigen and antibody. Several of these methods are yielding important information regarding the size of the antibody combining site and the structure of antigenic groups. *Examples:* Inhibition of precipitation by nonprecipitating antibody or by a fragment of digested antibody; inhibition of viral hemagglutination by antibody; inhibition of the Prausnitz-Küstner reaction by blocking antibody.

IMMUNOFLUORESCENCE
(Fluorescent Antibody Tests, FA)

Certain fluorescent dyes (eg, fluorescein isothiocyanate, rhodamine) can be firmly attached to globulin molecules and thus made visible by using ultraviolet light in the fluorescence microscope. If such fluorescent dyes are conjugated with antibody molecules and all excess is carefully eliminated, such "labeled" antibody may be used to locate and identify specific antigen because of the high specificity of the antigen-antibody bond. By means of such "direct immunofluorescence reactions," bacteria may be identified and viral or other antigens may be located inside cells. In bacteriologic diagnosis, specific direct immunofluorescence is valuable for the rapid identification of group A hemolytic streptococci and of *Treponema pallidum.* In special laboratories, immunofluorescence has been applied to the rapid screening of enteric pathogens, of bacteria causing childhood meningitis, and others.

The "indirect immunofluorescence reactions" involve 3 reagents: Antigen + its antibody A + a fluorescent-labeled antibody to antibody A. Any one of the 3 reagents can be unknown. For example, in the serodiagnosis of syphilis, *T pallidum* antigen fixed to a slide is overlaid with the patient's unknown serum. Fluorescein-labeled antihuman globulin (made in an animal) is then placed on the preparation, which is examined by ultraviolet light. If the patient's serum contains specific antibodies to *T pallidum,* brightly fluorescent spirochetes are seen. If the spirochetes do not fluoresce, no specific antitreponemal antibodies are present. (See FTA test.)

Immunofluorescence can be used for the detection of viral and bacterial antigens or antibodies, tumor antigens, and many others.

OTHER TYPES OF SEROLOGIC REACTIONS

Protection or Neutralization Tests

These are widely employed in the determination of antiviral and a few antibacterial antibodies. They utilize the ability of antibody-containing sera to block the infectivity of these agents upon inoculation of the mixture into susceptible hosts.

Immobilization Tests for *Treponema Pallidum*

These tests (TPI) detect true antibodies against this organism in the serum of infected persons. The test consists of mixing serum with fresh, motile spirochetes from a rabbit chancre and observing their loss of motility in the darkfield microscope. Similar tests can demonstrate the immune adherence of spirochetes to the surface of red blood cells in the presence of specific antibody.

Opsonocytophagic Tests

These have been largely abandoned.

Ferritin-Labeled Antibody Technic

Electron-dense ferritin can be conjugated with antibody molecules, which are thus made visible in the electron microscope. This permits the localization of antigens in cells and ultrathin sections examined by electron microscopy.

Hemagglutination Tests

Red blood cells from various animal species may be clumped by certain viruses. This active hemagglutination can be specifically inhibited by antibody to virus, and the hemagglutination inhibition is a convenient serologic test. In some disease states certain red blood cells are agglutinated by components of serum. Red cells also present a convenient surface onto which many types of antigens can be adsorbed. Such coated cells will clump when mixed with antibodies to these specific antigens, ("passive hemagglutination"). Other convenient particles, eg, latex or bentonite, may substitute for red cells. A macroglobulin (19 S) in the serum of most rheumatoid patients can be measured by a hemagglutination reaction. Red cells coated with 7 S globulin (human) will be clumped by this 19 S "rheumatoid factor." Clinically applicable serologic tests for the diagnosis of infection are listed in Chapter 24.

RECOMMENDED IMMUNIZATION OF ADULTS FOR TRAVEL

Every adult, whether traveling or not, must be immunized with tetanus toxoid. Purified toxoid "for adult use" must be used to avoid reactions. Every adult should also receive primary vaccination for poliomyelitis (oral live trivalent vaccine), for diphtheria (use purified toxoid "for adult use"), and for smallpox. Every traveler must fulfill the immunization requirements of the health authorities of different countries. These are listed in *Immunization Information for International Travel*, USPHS, Division of Foreign Quarantine, 7915 Eastern Ave, Silver Spring, Maryland 20910.

The following are suggestions for travel in different parts of the world.

Tetanus

Booster injection of 0.5 ml tetanus toxoid, for adult use, every 5—7 years, assuming completion of primary immunization. (All countries.)

Smallpox

Revaccination with live smallpox vaccine (vaccinia virus) by multiple pressure method every 3 years. WHO certificate requires registration of batch number of vaccine. The physician should ascertain a "take" by observing vesicle formation after administration of either liquid or freeze-dried effective vaccine. (All countries.)

Typhoid

Suspension of killed *Salmonella typhi.* For primary immunization, inject 0.5 ml subcut (0.25 ml for children under 10 years) twice at an interval of 4—6 weeks. For booster, inject 0.5 ml subcut (or 0.1 ml intradermally) every 3 years. (All countries.)

Paratyphoid vaccines are not recommended and are probably ineffective at present.

Yellow Fever

Live attenuated yellow fever virus, 0.5 ml subcut. WHO certificate requires registration of batch number of vaccine. Vaccination available in USA only at approved centers. Vaccination must be repeated at intervals of 10 years or less. (Africa, South America.)

Cholera

Suspension of killed vibrios, including prevalent antigenic types. Two injections of 0.5 and 1 ml are given IM 4—6 weeks apart. This must be followed by 0.5 ml booster injections every 6 months during periods of possible exposure. Protection depends largely on booster doses. WHO certificate is valid for 6 months only. (Middle Eastern countries, Asia, occasionally others.)

TABLE 12−5. Recommended schedule for active immunization and skin testing of children.

Age	Product Administered	Test Recommended
2−3 months	DPT[1] Oral poliovaccine[2], trivalent, or type 2	
3−4 months	DPT Oral poliovaccine, trivalent or type 1	
4−5 months	DPT Oral poliovaccine, trivalent or type 3	
10−11 months		Tuberculin test
12 months	Measles vaccine[3]	
15−19 months	DPT Oral poliovaccine, trivalent Smallpox vaccine[4]	Read primary take of smallpox often−1 week
2 years	Mumps vaccine[5]	Tuberculin test[6]
3−4 years	DPT Rubella vaccine[7]	Tuberculin test[6]
6 years	TD[8] Smallpox vaccine Oral poliovaccine, trivalent	Tuberculin test[6]
8−10 years		Tuberculin test[6]
12−14 years	TD Smallpox vaccine	Tuberculin test

[1] **DPT**: Toxoids of diphtheria and tetanus, alum-precipated or aluminum hydroxide absorbed, combined with pertussis bacterial antigen. Suitable for young children. Three doses of 0.5 ml IM at intervals of 4−8 weeks. Fourth injection of 0.5 ml IM given about 1 year later.

[2] **Oral live poliomyelitis virus vaccine**: Either trivalent (types 1, 2, and 3 combined) or single type. Trivalent given 3 times at intervals of 6−8 weeks and then as a booster 1 year later. Monovalent type 2, then type 1, then type 3 given at 6-week intervals, and then a booster of trivalent vaccine 1 year later. Inactive (Salk type) trivalent vaccine is available but not recommended. **Note**: The sequence of monovalent vaccines given here (type 2, then 1, then 3) is in accord with the recommendations of the US Public Health Service Advisory Committee on Immunization Practices. The American Academy of Pediatrics recommends the sequence 1, 3, 2.

[3] **Live measles virus vaccine**, 0.5 ml IM. When using attenuated (Edmonston) strain, give human gamma globulin, 0.01 ml/lb, injected into the opposite arm at the same time, to lessen the reaction to the vaccine. This is not advised with "further attenuated" (Schwarz) strain vaccine. Inactivated measles vaccine should not be used.

[4] **Live smallpox vaccine (vaccinia virus)**, usually supplied as calf lymph, must be used fresh, before the expiration date, and must be stored at low temperature. It is administered by multiple pressure technic. Site must be inspected at 7 days for evidence of "primary take" or at 3−4 days for evidence of "accelerated reaction." Some vesicles must be found to indicate immunizing proliferation of virus. Papules without vesication are not acceptable as evidence of "take." Do not vaccinate in the presence of eczema in the child or his siblings, or when there is known immunologic deficiency.

[5] **Live mumps virus vaccine (attenuated)**, 0.5 ml IM.

[6] The frequency with which tuberculin tests are administered depends on the risk of exposure ie, the prevalence of tuberculosis in the population group.

[7] **Rubella live virus vaccine (attenuated)** can be given between age 1 year and puberty, but preferably prior to entry into kindergarten. The entire contents of a single-dose vaccine vial, reconstituted from the lyophilized state, are injected subcutaneously. The vaccine must **not** be given to women who are pregnant or are likely to become pregnant within 3 months of vaccination. Adult women must also be warned that there is a 40% likelihood of developing arthralgias and arthritis (presumably self-limited) within 4 weeks of vaccination.

[8] **Tetanus toxoid and diphtheria toxoid**, purified, suitable for adults.

Plague

Suspension of killed plague bacilli given IM, 2 injections of 0.5 ml each, 4–6 weeks apart, and a third injection 6 months later. (Middle Eastern countries, Asia, occasionally South America and others.)

Typhus

Suspension of inactivated typhus rickettsiae given IM, 2 injections of 0.5 ml each, 4–6 weeks apart. Booster doses of 0.5 ml every 6 months may be necessary. (Southeastern Europe, Africa, Asia.)

Hepatitis

No active immunization available. Temporary passive immunity may be induced by the IM injection of human gamma globulin, 0.02 ml/kg every 2–3 months.

●   ●   ●

General References

Franklin, E.C., & B. Frangione: Immunoglobulins. Ann Rev Med 20:155–174, 1969.

Janeway, C.A., & F.S. Rosen: The gamma globulins. New England J Med 275:826, 1966.

Marcus, D.M.: The ABO and Lewis blood group system. New England J Med 280:994–1006, 1969.

Pensky, J., & others: Properties of highly purified human properdin. J Immunol 100:142–158, 1968.

Schur, P.H., & K.F. Austen: Complement in human disease. Ann Rev Med 19:1–24, 1968.

Tomasi, T.B.: Human immunoglobulin A. New England J Med 279:1327–1330, 1968.

13 ...

Allergy & Hypersensitivity

The term "allergy" denotes an altered reactivity of tissues toward specific substances, ie, reactivity which is different from earlier experiences of the same individual or from experiences of other individuals of the same species. Strictly speaking, this altered reactivity might be increased (hyperergy), diminished (hypoergy), or absent (anergy). In common usage, however, the term "allergy" refers to hyperreactivity, and it is employed here synonymously with "hypersensitivity." Idiosyncrasy, an inherent, qualitatively abnormal reactivity toward physiologically active substances, is excluded from consideration.

Allergic reactions are of great variety, and it is not certain whether the divergent types of reactions share similar mechanisms. However, it is believed that allergic reactions are generally associated with specific immunologic reactions taking place in tissues and resulting in cellular injury. Because of the diversity of phenomena ascribed to hypersensitivity it will be necessary to describe individual types of responses which occur in man or animals and briefly state the available evidence for mechanism of action.

Allergens

The substances which give rise to allergic reactions are called allergens. They fall into a large number of categories. Some are foreign proteins and, as such, complete antigens. Others are polypeptides, lipids or lipoid-soluble extracts of plants or foods, or microbial constituents—all possessing some antigenicity. Still others, like formaldehyde, metal salts, and many drugs such as quinine or penicillin, are compounds of low molecular weight which are not antigens in their own right. It is probable that those substances which are not antigens but allergens combine in the host's body with protein so as to become complete antigens. This complete antigen is then able to elicit the formation of antibodies as well as to induce hypersensitivity. The allergic response may be elicited both by the complete antigen and by the "hapten"-like constituent of low molecular weight.

The development of hypersensitivity in a given individual depends upon his opportunities for repeated contact with the allergen and his capacity for sensitization. The latter is determined genetically.

IMMUNOLOGIC TOLERANCE

Immunologic responses, particularly antibody formation and hypersensitivity reactions, appear to be based on the ability of body mechanisms to distinguish the host's own tissues ("self") from foreign materials ("not self"). These body mechanisms generally do not react to or form antibodies against "self," but do react to "not self" materials. During fetal and early neonatal life the ability to differentiate "self" from "not self" has not yet matured or become fixed. Consequently, if a foreign antigen is administered to a mammal in utero, the same animal, after birth, may be "tolerant" to the same antigen, may not form antibodies to it, and may develop no immunologic responses or hypersensitivity reactions to it. This technic is being widely employed in a multitude of studies, eg, the mechanisms of graft rejection and tissue transplants and in the investigation of "autoimmune diseases."

Some aspects of immunologic tolerance are well established: (1) Tolerance is established most readily to antigens which are relatively closely related to those of the host, but is entirely specific for a given antigen. (2) The induction of tolerance and the time of its persistence are directly related to the dose of antigen initially administered. In addition, it is probable that the maintenance of tolerance depends in many cases upon persistence of the antigen. The mechanism of tolerance appears to depend upon specific suppression of the antibody-forming or other immunologically reactive mechanism. (3) Tolerance varies with species. Human and sheep fetuses are capable of immunologic reactions in utero.

The differentiation of "self" from "not self" must be an important homeostatic function of the animal body. "Autoimmune disease" may be considered a failure of this homeostatic function. Possible mechanisms for the recognition of "self" are discussed by Burnet in New England J Med 264:24, 1961.

The phenomenon of immunologic paralysis appears to be a special form of immunologic tolerance. Immunologic paralysis is produced by injecting into an adult animal a dose of antigen many times larger than that required to stimulate antibody formation. The antigen persists in the recipient's tissues for months, and during this period the animal is incapable of making detectable antibody. Immunologic paralysis is easily induced with polysaccharides but is induced with difficulty with proteins. It is specific for the inducing antigen.

IMMEDIATE VERSUS DELAYED TYPE OF ALLERGIC REACTION

Allergic reactions may be broadly divided into 2 main types: immediate and delayed. Some characteristic features of each type are listed in Table 13—1.

REACTIONS OF THE "IMMEDIATE" TYPE

Immediate reactions may manifest themselves as acute systemic reactions (anaphylactic shock) or localized tissue damage (eg, Arthus reaction, passive cutaneous anaphylaxis). The clinical manifestations may depend largely on the rate and site of the reaction. Systemic anaphylaxis exhibits somewhat different clinical signs in different animal species (see below). The anaphylactic reaction is always the same in a given host species, regardless of the type of antigen involved.

1. ANAPHYLAXIS

Anaphylactic shock characteristically occurs upon injection of a given antigen into a host which is hypersensitive to that antigen. Traditionally, the demonstration of anaphylaxis involves the following steps:

Demonstration of Anaphylaxis

A. Sensitization: An adequate sensitizing dose of antigen must be absorbed. In the guinea pig as little as 0.1 μg of a soluble protein is sufficient, whereas in the rabbit much larger amounts of antigen are necessary. Ease of sensitization in man undoubtedly depends upon genetic background as well as duration, dose, and method of exposure to the antigen.

B. Waiting Period: A waiting period of 2—3 weeks is required. During this period, a rise in antibody titer (IgG) can be demonstrated in serum and antibody (IgE) is bound to leukocytes and mast cells.

C. "Eliciting Injection": The rapid intravenous or intracardiac injection of a massive dose (0.1—10 mg of protein) of the same antigen as was used for the "sensitizing injection" is followed promptly by the onset of typical manifestations of anaphylaxis, as antigen combines with cell-bound antibody to form complexes.

However, anaphylactic shock can be elicited in the normal, previously unsensitized animal by a single injection of soluble antigen-antibody complexes formed in vitro in the zone of antigen excess.

Clinical Reactions to Anaphylaxis

A. Guinea Pig: Within 1 minute there is restlessness, scratching, rubbing of nose with forepaws, cough, convulsions, voiding of urine, cyanosis, and death. At autopsy the lungs are found to be inflated; this is due to extreme spasm of the bronchi. The blood of guinea pigs who have died of anaphylaxis does not coagulate.

B. Rabbit: Irregular respiration, collapse, voiding of urine and feces, convulsions, and death. At autopsy the right heart is found to be dilated; this is due to obstruction to the pulmonary blood flow, attributable to widespread thrombi in pulmonary capillaries.

TABLE 13—1. Immediate and delayed allergic reactions.

	Immediate (Anaphylactic) Type	Delayed (Tuberculin) Type
Clinical examples	Anaphylactic shock; allergy to pollen, with asthma; serum sickness; some allergies to antibiotics.	Tuberculin hypersensitivity, allergy to bacteria (brucella), fungi (histoplasma), parasites (trichina), viruses (mumps), Rhus plants (poison ivy or oak).
Timing	The reaction begins immediately, ie, within minutes after contact with the allergen, and disappears within 1 hour.	The reaction is delayed. It begins within several hours after contact with the allergen and may last for days.
Histology	The main pathologic reaction consists of dilatation of capillaries and arterioles, with prominent erythema and edema but little cellular infiltration.	The main pathologic reaction consists of inflammatory change with predominant mononuclear cell infiltration and tissue induration.
Passive transfer	The reaction is associated with circulating antibodies and can frequently be transferred passively by means of serum.	The reaction is not definitely associated with circulating antibodies and cannot be transferred passively by means of serum. It can sometimes be transferred passively by means of lymphoid cells or their extracts.

C. Dog: Vomiting, diarrhea, collapse, low blood pressure, shock, and death. At autopsy, the liver is found to be enormously distended and congested (hepatic vein spasm).

D. Man: Often there is bronchospasm with labored respiration, asthma, laryngeal edema, itching, giant hives, fall of blood pressure, rapid heart rate, and shock. Death may occur within minutes or hours, or the patient may recover.

Pathologic Physiology of Anaphylaxis

The following physiologic disturbances may be observed in anaphylaxis: (1) Leukopenia as the leukocytes become "sticky" and adhere to the walls of the capillaries in the lungs. (2) Smooth muscle spasm, particularly in bronchioles and arterioles. (3) Edema as a result of injury to vascular endothelium. (4) Liberation of histamine, serotonin, bradykinin, and slow-reacting substance. (5) Liberation of heparin, resulting in diminished coagulability of blood. (6) Fall in normal serum complement, suggesting an antigen-antibody reaction.

Postulated Mechanism of Anaphylaxis

The production of anaphylactic shock in the previously unsensitized animal by a single injection of soluble antigen-antibody complexes strongly suggests that these complexes are responsible for initiating the chain of events which ends in anaphylaxis. It appears that soluble antigen-antibody complexes attach to certain cells; that these complexes injure cells so that they release pharmacologically active substances; and that these substances act on sensitive cells of the "shock organs" which are most intimately involved in anaphylaxis exhibited by different animal species.

The following pharmacologically active substances are known to be liberated during anaphylaxis:

(1) Histamine occurs in tissue mast cells, basophilic leukocytes, and platelets, and is released from them when they are disrupted or degranulated as a result of anaphylaxis. It causes smooth muscle contraction, vasodilatation, and increase in capillary permeability.

(2) Serotonin (5-hydroxytryptamine), derived from tryptophan, is present in most platelets and can be released from them in anaphylaxis. It causes smooth muscle contraction and increases capillary permeability but constricts larger vessels.

(3) Kinins are basic peptides formed by enzymes called kallikreins from precursors in plasma. These peptides (eg, bradykinin) increase in the blood during anaphylaxis, causing smooth muscle contraction, large vessel dilatation, and increased capillary permeability.

(4) Slow-reacting substance (SRS-A) appears to be a lipoprotein of uncertain origin which characteristically induces prolonged contraction of certain smooth muscles, eg, in bronchioles.

These substances are active for only a few minutes after release. Histamine, bradykinin, and serotonin are enzymatically inactivated, whereas SRS-A is removed by adsorption onto tissues.

The mechanism of anaphylaxis postulated on the basis of activity of antigen-antibody complexes is in agreement with earlier studies on mechanism in which the animal was first sensitized and, after a waiting period, shocked by the "eliciting injection" of antigen.

Antibodies are produced in response to the "sensitizing" injection of antigen. Some of these appear to be concentrated in certain tissues, the "shock organs," and may in some fashion be attached to cells ("sessile antibodies"). The massive amount of antigen readministered in the "eliciting" injection combines suddenly with the antibody. This antigen-antibody reaction results in damage to tissue cells and the consequent liberation of the several substances mentioned above. These in turn produce most of the symptoms and signs of anaphylaxis.

It is possible that the essential feature in eliciting anaphylactic shock in the sensitized animal is the sudden production of soluble antigen-antibody complexes on the surface of specialized cells—analogous to the events in the unsensitized animal receiving soluble complexes pre-formed in vitro. The following experimental findings are in agreement with this postulated mechanism:

A. Role of Histamine: Histamine injections reproduce most of the signs and symptoms of anaphylaxis in various species. Administration of antihistaminic drugs (which block the action of histamine) can sometimes prevent anaphylactic reactions.

B. Labeled Antigens and Antibodies: Antigens labeled with radioactive tracers and administered to hypersensitive animals concentrate in "shock organs," indicating a high concentration of antibodies there. Similarly, by means of fluorescent-labeled antibodies (antihuman-globulin), it can be shown that the tissues of animals or man exhibiting "hypersensitivity disease" contain high concentrations of globulin in characteristic sites. It may be that this is antibody globulin, suggesting a local antigen-antibody reaction.

C. In Vitro Anaphylaxis: Tissues from sensitized animals give an anaphylactic reaction in vitro upon contact with the specific antigen. Thus the isolated uterine muscle, intestinal segments, or tracheal rings from a hypersensitive guinea pig, when removed and suspended in a bath, will contract violently upon addition of the specific antigen (Schultz-Dale reaction). This suggests that the antibody attaches to these smooth muscles. This antigen-antibody reaction injures tissue cells and liberates histamine and other substances.

D. Passive Transfer of Anaphylaxis: Serum taken from a hypersensitive animal and injected into a normal animal of the same species renders the recipient subject to anaphylaxis upon injection of the original antigen (passive transfer). Thus, antibodies formed in the first animal can passively transfer a state of hypersensitivity to a second animal which has never been in contact with the antigen. With pure protein antigen-antibody systems, less than 10 μg of antibody globulin per ml of serum can passively transfer susceptibility to systemic anaphylaxis. Less than 0.1 μg of antibody globulin can transfer susceptibility to passive cutaneous anaphylaxis (PCA). To elicit such PCA, a minute amount of antibody is injected intradermally and, after a latent period of 3–4 hours, antigen is introduced systemically (eg, intravenously). There is an immediate reaction (eg, erythema, edema) only at the site of the locally administered antibody.

After the passive transfer of antibody a waiting period of several hours is usually necessary before systemic or local anaphylaxis can readily be elicited. This suggests that fixation of the antibody molecules onto tissue cells of the "shock organ" must take place.

E. Antibody Concentration: An excess of antibody in the circulation tends to combine with the "eliciting" dose of antigen and thus protects the antibody in the shock organ from suddenly combining with antigen.

F. Desensitization: Before anaphylaxis can take place, many antigen molecules must suddenly and simultaneously combine with antibody so as to cause sufficient tissue injury for the liberation of large amounts of vasoactive substances. If a hypersensitive animal is given the antigen in many small doses rather than in one large dose, this massive antigen-antibody reaction will not take place and there will be no anaphylactic shock; the animal has been temporarily desensitized through gradual saturation of "sessile" antibodies with antigen administered in many small injections. The small amounts of vasoactive substances released after each injection are rapidly degraded or eliminated. Such desensitization is employed when a foreign protein must be administered clinically to a person hypersensitive to it (eg, tetanus antitoxin in horse serum). Some days later, however, the hypersensitive state reestablishes itself and the person becomes again susceptible to anaphylaxis. This type of desensitization must be clearly distinguished from the procedure employed in individuals susceptible to recurrent pollen allergy. In the latter, parenteral administration of suitable extracts of the allergen may result in temporary lessening of individual reactivity, probably because a distinct new "blocking" antibody was elicited.

Tests for Hypersensitivity

Because of the danger of fatal anaphylactic shock, foreign proteins and other antigens should never be administered until it has been established that the individual is not hypersensitive to the material contemplated for use. This is done either by means of a skin test or a conjunctival test.

A. Skin Test: 0.1 ml of the antigen (often diluted 1:10) is injected into the skin of the flexor surface of the forearm. Hypersensitive individuals develop the characteristic "wheal and flare" within a few minutes. This consists of an elevated, blanched area of edema, from which pseudopodia may extend, and a surrounding zone of erythema (red "flare"). The reaction may measure 2–10 cm in diameter. It fades in 20–60 minutes. The mechanism of the anaphylactic, immediate type of skin reaction is the following ("triple response" of Sir Thomas Lewis): The histamine released from the cells injured by an antigen-antibody reaction gives (1) local capillary dilatation (initial erythema); (2) a local axon reflex, resulting in widespread dilatation of arterioles (red flare); and (3) increased vascular permeability, resulting in circumscribed edema (wheal).

B. Conjunctival Test: One drop of the antigen (diluted 1:10) is placed in the conjunctival sac of one eye; 1 drop of saline is used in the other eye as a control. The eye in a hypersensitive individual develops reddening, itching, and lacrimation in 5–20 minutes; the control eye remains normal.

Treatment

Anaphylactic reactions can often be prevented or suppressed by the administration of epinephrine, antihistaminic drugs, or cortisone. Antihistamines directly block the action of the released histamine. Corticosteroids do not interfere with the antigen-antibody reaction but probably protect the "shock organ" from injury.

Anaphylactoid Reactions

Reactions resembling anaphylactoid shock are sometimes observed following the injection of colloids or finely suspended material into the blood stream. They have no connection with antigen-antibody reactions and are called anaphylactoid reactions. They may be caused by the liberation of histamine, serotonin, or other vasoactive substances as a consequence of the colloid injection.

2. SERUM SICKNESS

A person receiving an injection of a foreign antigen (eg, tetanus antitoxin) is likely to develop, 7–12 days later, hives, fever; swelling of the lymph nodes, face, and feet; and pain and swelling of the joints. This symptom complex may be transient or may last up to 10 days and is called serum sickness. It is due to an antigen-antibody reaction. The injected antigen (serum) stimulates the production of antibodies, which reach a significant titer in 6–10 days. These antibodies react with traces of the antigen remaining in tissues. The symptoms and signs are associated with the presence of circulating antigen-antibody complexes. Precipitating antibodies against the specific antigen are demonstrable in the serum. When the antigen has been completely eliminated, the reaction ceases.

Serum sickness occurs less frequently now that antibiotics have largely replaced sera for treatment. However, a similar reaction is seen following the use of various drugs, particularly sulfonamides, penicillin, and other antibiotics. These substances presumably form complete antigens by combining with host proteins, and evoke the production of antibodies.

TABLE 13-2. Differentiation of Arthus reaction and systemic anaphylaxis.

	Arthus Reaction	Systemic Anaphylaxis
Can be passively transferred by	Precipitating antibody only	Precipitating or nonprecipitating antibody
Amount of antibody necessary for transfer	Relatively large	Very small
After passive transfer of antibody a latent period is necessary before injection of antigen can give rise to reaction	No	Yes
Injection of histamine can largely duplicate the symptoms of the reaction	No	Yes

3. ARTHUS REACTION

This is an immediate type of reaction which results in localized tissue damage. Animals injected at intervals, intracutaneously or subcutaneously, with the same antigen develop a local reaction which becomes progressively more severe with each injection. The lesion is characterized first by redness and edema; induration appears later and, finally, hemorrhage and necrosis. This reaction is accompanied by changes similar to those of systemic anaphylaxis, eg, leukopenia, increased vascular permeability, thrombosis, edema, and necrosis of the arteriolar wall, with hemorrhage. The intensity of the local reaction varies with the antibody level in the serum, and the reactivity of the tissue can be passively transferred by means of serum. The essential lesion in the Arthus reaction is an inflammatory lesion of blood vessels following the deposition of antigen-antibody complexes in vessel walls. There is fixation of complement, attraction of polymorphonuclear leukocytes, and release of lysosomal enzymes which cause tissue damage. Differences between the Arthus reaction and systemic anaphylaxis are shown in Table 13-2.

4. "SPONTANEOUS" CLINICAL ALLERGY (ATOPY)

This group includes a wide variety of hypersensitivity reactions occurring in persons who have acquired their hypersensitivities through accidental contact with antigens in the environment, eg, asthma or hay fever due to pollen or animal dander; gastrointestinal reactions and skin eruptions due to foods such as fish and nuts; skin eruptions due to contact with plants; and

many others. It must be recognized that so-called "allergic" symptoms may be of multiple origin, including physical, chemical, or emotional stimuli, in addition to antigen-antibody reactions.

Disorders of this type show a marked familial distribution. The susceptibility for sensitization appears to be inherited, but each individual must have effective contact with the respective antigen before hypersensitivity can become established. The specific offending allergen may be determined by immediate reactions with scratch tests performed on the patient's skin. Cross-reactions between related allergens are frequent. The responsible antigens of pollens appear to be large peptides with a high carbohydrate content.

Prausnitz-Küstner Reaction

The serum of allergic patients contains no precipitating antibodies for the specific antigen. It does, however, contain a skin-sensitizing antibody called "reagin" (not related to reagin in syphilis). It is IgE immunoglobulin. This reagin may react with antigen injected intracutaneously to result in an immediate evanescent skin reaction of the "wheal and flare" type. The reagin can be demonstrated more definitely by passive transfer; this is called the Prausnitz-Küstner (PK) reaction. The PK reaction consists of obtaining serum from the allergic individual and injecting it into a skin area of a nonallergic individual. Twenty-four hours later the specific antigen is injected into the prepared skin site of the nonallergic person as well as into another control site. The latter shows no reaction, but at the prepared site the reagin reacts with the antigen to give a marked immediate type of skin test. This provides conclusive proof that the serum donor possesses reagins to the specific antigen and thus permits identification of such an antigen. The PK reaction is much more specific than the direct skin test on the allergic individual, who often tends to give positive reactions to a wide variety of unrelated antigens.

The skin-sensitizing antibodies demonstrated by the PK reaction are IgE immunoglobulins with the following distinctive features: (1) They are heat-labile, being gradually inactivated by heating at 56° C for 1 to several hours; (2) they do not precipitate the specific antigen in vitro; and (3) after being injected into normal human skin they remain fixed there for several weeks, sensitizing the skin to antigen during this period.

Desensitization

It has long been the practice to "desensitize" allergic individuals by frequent repeated injections of minute quantities of the specific allergen identified by skin test or by the Prausnitz-Küstner reaction. Clinical improvement not infrequently follows such a procedure. This improvement is not associated with any change in the circulating reagin, but the injections of allergen elicit the production of another antibody with the following properties: (1) It is relatively heat-stable; (2) it does not sensitize the skin to allergen and does not remain fixed in the skin after injection; (3) if mixed with allergen it inhibits the ability of the allergen to produce a positive skin test in the sensitive individual (therefore called "blocking" antibody); and (4) it is an IgG immunoglobulin which does not precipitate with allergen in vitro.

It is probable (but has not been proved) that this "blocking" antibody combines with allergen in the desensitized allergic person, thus preventing the massive allergen-reagin combination which gives rise to tissue reactions.

Collagen Diseases

The immediate or anaphylactic type of hypersensitivity reactions may take part in a variety of chronic progressive degenerative diseases referred to collectively as "autoimmune" or "collagen" diseases. These diseases are discussed at the end of this chapter.

REACTIONS OF THE "DELAYED" TYPE

Delayed hypersensitive reactions develop more slowly and persist longer than immediate reactions and are not related to serum antibodies; passive transfer of reactivity by means of serum is not possible. Such reactions are often encountered in the "allergy of infection" with bacteria, fungi, viruses, or helminths, and are associated with enhanced host resistance. They also occur following superficial sensitization by skin contact with a variety of simple chemicals ranging from metals (eg, nickel) to catechols (eg, urushiol from the poison ivy plant). The prototype of the delayed type of hypersensitivity reaction is seen in tuberculin hypersensitivity.

1. TUBERCULIN HYPERSENSITIVITY

Koch's Phenomenon

When a tuberculous guinea pig is injected subcutaneously with a suspension of tubercle bacilli there is a massive inflammatory reaction at the injection site which tends to wall off the injected material and often leads to necrosis; this is called the Koch phenomenon. This reaction does not require living tubercle bacilli but occurs similarly both with filtrates of broth in which tubercle bacilli have been grown (Old Tuberculin, OT) or with tuberculoprotein (PPD). These soluble preparations produce local inflammatory reactions, particularly edema, cellular infiltration, hemorrhage, and marked enlargement of the regional lymph nodes; and focal reactions, consisting of marked hemorrhagic inflammation and dense cellular infiltration within existing tuberculous lesions. Because focal reactions may "stir up" tuberculous activity, great caution must be exerted, while performing skin tests, to avoid giving excessive doses of tuberculoprotein to hypersensitive individuals.

Typical Skin Reaction

The typical skin test of the delayed type is exemplified by the tuberculin test. There is no immediate reaction following the intracutaneous injection of tuberculoprotein. After a few hours, redness, edema, and induration develop and tend to increase for 24–48 hours. If the reaction is marked, there may be central blanching, hemorrhage, and necrosis. The redness and edema disappear quickly, but the induration of the skin reaction can be felt for days or weeks. Histologically the lesion of the skin test is characterized by initial vasodilatation, edema, and polymorphonuclear cell infiltration; this is followed soon afterward by marked and persistent focal accumulation and diffuse infiltration with lymphoid and mononuclear cells. The intensity of the tuberculin skin reaction in the hypersensitive individual bears no relationship to the level of antibodies that may be demonstrated by complement fixation or other tests.

Basis of Tuberculin Hypersensitivity

Tuberculin hypersensitivity can be induced not only by infection with tubercle bacilli but also by repeated injection of a mixture of tuberculoprotein with a wax fraction (a peptidoglycolipid) derived from the tubercle bacillus. The importance of this and of similar lipids ("adjuvants") in enhancing the development of delayed hypersensitivity reactions to a variety of substances is discussed below. Tuberculin hypersensitivity is evident not only in the intact animal and tissues but also in individual cells in tissue culture. If dilute tuberculin is added to tissue cultures of cells from tuberculin-hypersensitive individuals, growth and migration of the cells cease and some lymphocytes transform into blast-like cells and divide, whereas in cultures of cells from normal individuals no such effect is observed. Tuberculin-sensitive lymphocytes cultured with tuberculin elaborate a soluble material which causes normal lymphocytes to respond to tuberculin in vitro by transformation to blasts and division.

Delayed type reactions do not require participation of blood vessels and can occur in completely avascular tissue, eg, the cornea.

The fundamental pathogenesis of delayed hypersensitivity reactions appears to be as follows: A small number of specifically sensitized lymphocytes react with antigen and release factors which elicit an inflammatory response and the accumulation of a monocytic infiltrate.

Desensitization

In the tuberculin type of hypersensitivity, desensitization (? "tolerance") is possible by means of the frequently repeated injection of minute amounts of the antigen. The results are only temporary, however, and the injection of the desensitizing doses carries the risk of marked and sometimes quite serious focal reactions.

Passive Transfer

Passive transfer is not possible with serum in the tuberculin type of hypersensitivity. However, if white blood cells are collected from a tuberculin-positive person, disrupted, and injected into the skin of a tuberculin-negative person, that recipient becomes temporarily tuberculin-reactive. This suggests that a special "transfer factor" may be involved in the delayed type of hypersensitivity, and that it—or the capacity to produce it—is transferred in cells from hypersensitive individuals. In rodents, some systemic reactivity to tuberculin has also been transferred by means of viable cells.

Properties of "Transfer Factor"

Transfer factor is stable to repeated freezing and thawing, storage in the lyophilized state, distilled water lysis, and to the action of DNase, RNase, and trypsin. It can be dialyzed, and has a molecular weight near 10,000. Delayed sensitivity begins 1–7 days after injection of the cell extract and may last more than 1 year. The mechanism of "transfer factor" activity is uncertain. It is involved in the passive transfer of specific delayed hypersensitivity to tuberculin, streptococcal antigens, coccidioidin, allograft (homograft) sensitivity, and others.

2. OTHER DELAYED TYPE HYPERSENSITIVITY REACTIONS

The delayed type of hypersensitivity is encountered in many types of infections. It may also be a frequent or even a necessary stage in the development of antibody production. At the stage of delayed type hypersensitivity the sensitized cell may perhaps have the capacity to react with antigen, but it does not yet have the capacity to produce antibody. While these are speculative considerations, delayed type skin reactivity can be a valuable aid in the diagnosis of many infectious processes if it is cautiously interpreted. A positive skin reaction indicates only that the individual has at some time in the past been infected with the specific agent. It provides information about the nature of a specific illness only if conversion from a negative to a positive skin test occurs during the course of illness. Blood transfusion may passively transfer delayed hypersensitivity by means of sensitive lymphocytes. Furthermore, the general skin reactivity declines markedly in far advanced stages of many diseases (anergy). Similar anergy may be encountered during the childhood exanthems (measles, chickenpox), and so a tuberculin-positive child may temporarily give a tuberculin-negative reaction during one of these illnesses. Anergy is also a regular feature of sarcoidosis and Hodgkin's disease, or of patients receiving large doses of corticosteroids or immunosuppressive drugs.

Bacterial Reactions

Among bacterial infections, delayed type skin reactions occur in brucellosis, upon the injection of brucellergen, an antigenic nucleoprotein extract; in tularemia, upon injection of a killed bacterial suspension; in glanders of animals and man, upon injection of mallein (prepared like tuberculin); and in leprosy, upon injection of lepromin (an extract of human leprous tissue). For the diagnosis of chancroid a suspension of Ducrey's bacillus is injected intradermally. This "Ducrey test" gives a delayed reaction in the presence of recent or past infection. Many persons give delayed skin reactions to a variety of streptococcal extracts.

Some people also give delayed reactions to injected diphtheria or tetanus toxoids. This sensitivity is directed against either the toxin-toxoid molecule or constituents of the medium in which the toxin was prepared (eg, peptone).

A skin test (Frei test) for chlamydial infection (eg, lymphogranuloma venereum) determines hypersensitivity to the group antigen.

In the course of delayed hypersensitivity developing with bacterial infections, macrophages become "activated" and contribute markedly to antibacterial immunity. This macrophage "activation" probably results from an interaction with specifically sensitized lymphoid cells.

Viral Reactions

Delayed skin reactions are encountered in many viral infections, including mumps, herpes simplex, and several viral encephalitides, with killed viral suspensions. In persons repeatedly vaccinated against smallpox, the injection of inactive vaccinia virus results in a tuberculin-type skin response (erroneously called an "immune" response) which denotes hypersensitivity of the delayed type to constituents of vaccinia virus.

Fungal Reactions

In fungal infections, delayed reactions resemble the tuberculin reaction in all respects. In coccidioidomycosis a filtrate of culture, coccidioidin, is employed. The usual test strength is 1:100, giving a positive reaction with induration and erythema in 24–48 hours. In histoplasmosis the skin test material is histoplasmin, a concentrated culture medium in which *H capsulatum* has grown for months. It is employed in the usual test strength of 1:100. In blastomycosis, blastomycin, an extract of the yeast phase of *B dermatitidis,* has been used. Cross-reactions occur among the various fungal infections, particularly if very low dilutions of the test materials are employed. A candida skin test is positive in most normal adults. It is used to determine a person's ability to respond with a delayed type reaction. A negative candida skin test suggests anergy.

Helminthic Reactions

Delayed responses are obtained in some infestations with helminths, but in the majority immediate reactions occur when infected individuals are skin-tested with extracts of trichina, filaria, or ascaris. In echinococcus disease, injection of heated fluid from the hydatid cyst gives a tuberculin-type reaction which has diagnostic significance.

Combined Reactions

A combination of immediate and delayed reactions is seen in certain bacterial allergies, eg, streptococcal or pneumococcal hypersensitivity. With pneumococci an immediate reaction occurs with the type-specific polysaccharide early in convalescence. The species-specific pneumococcal nucleoprotein, on the other hand, gives a delayed reaction. A delayed reaction is also observed in many persons with all types of acute infections with the C-polysaccharide of pneumococci. This has no specific meaning and is based on the biologic coincidence that such persons develop a peculiar protein which happens to react in vitro with the somatic C-polysaccharide of pneumococci. It is not an antibody and is called "C-reactive protein." It is found in a variety of disease states.

3. ALLERGY TO DRUGS & SIMPLE CHEMICALS

Many drugs and simple chemicals can give rise to hypersensitivity reactions, both immediate and delayed. Among the most common manifestations of hypersensitivity are fever and various skin eruptions, from transient rashes or hives to serious exfoliative dermatitis.

Drugs usually yield breakdown products which are haptens with a high affinity to serum proteins. The hapten-host protein complex then serves as complete antigen. Thus native penicillin is poorly antigenic, but penicillenic acid and other derivatives are effective haptens which readily combine with host protein and serve as sensitizing antigens. Different drugs yield breakdown products of different allergenic potential. The mode of administration likewise influences the sensitizing potential of the drug. The total amount of drug and the time and route of its administration are important. Lipid vehicles are more likely to enhance sensitization than aqueous ones, perhaps because the lipid acts like an adjuvant. Prolonged application of drugs to the skin is more likely to produce sensitization than parenteral injection, perhaps because of skin lipids.

Simple substances such as nickel or formaldehyde can serve as allergens, presumably by reacting with host proteins to form complete antigens.

A number of plant extracts also produce hypersensitivity which results predominantly in skin reactions. Thus urushiol, a catechol derivative from poison ivy, results in extensive dermatitis on simple contact with the skin of a hypersensitive person. Many persons develop such hypersensitivity to the plants of the Rhus

family (poison ivy, poison oak), but only a few individuals become sensitive to the primrose plants.

Chlorogenic acid, a simple phenolic compound of low molecular weight, is a hapten contained in many different plants, eg, coffee beans, castor beans, fruits, and vegetables. It becomes a complete antigen by combining with host protein, and can induce respiratory or skin allergy in heavily exposed individuals (eg, coffee workers).

A large group of chronic or recurrent lung diseases is caused by allergic reactions to inhaled antigens in persons sensitized to these antigens. Among these diseases are the following: Maple bark disease in paper mill and wood workers inhaling dusts containing the fungus *Cryptostroma corticale;* farmer's lung in agricultural workers exposed to moldy hay containing fungi such as micromonospora or thermopolyspora; sequoiosis from redwood dust inhalation, thresher's lung, mushroom worker's disease, etc. Patients usually have high titers of precipitating antibody against the offending antigen. There is a striking and diffuse infiltration of pulmonary interstitial tissues with lymphoid and epithelioid cells and some poorly defined tubercles.

4. ROLE OF LIPIDS, WAXES, & ADJUVANTS IN THE DEVELOPMENT OF DELAYED HYPERSENSITIVITY

It has been mentioned above that tuberculoprotein stimulates the development of delayed hypersensitivity reactions only if it is administered together with wax from the tubercle bacillus. The same wax permits sensitization of animals with simple chemicals, such as picryl chloride, which does not elicit hypersensitivity if injected alone. It is conceivable that the strongly allergenic properties of substances applied to the skin (compared with other routes of administration) are referable to the many lipids available in the skin. In general it appears that the delayed type of hypersensitivity develops best if the allergen is administered in such a fashion as to elicit a focal inflammatory response. Lipids often elicit focal granulomatous tissue lesions.

When weakly antigenic or allergenic materials are mixed with lipids (eg, lanolin or paraffin) and killed tubercle bacilli, they elicit much greater antibody response and hypersensitivity reactions than the antigens alone, and occasionally result in the production of "autoimmune" diseases. Such enhancing mixtures (often lanolin, paraffin oil, and tubercle bacilli) are referred to as "adjuvants."

5. "AUTOIMMUNE," "AUTOALLERGIC," OR "HYPERSENSITIVITY" DISEASES

Certain disease states are believed to be caused, in part at least, by reactions of hypersensitivity to the host's own tissues. In the majority of the so-called "hypersensitivity diseases" in man, the mechanism of pathogenesis is speculative—often based on circumstantial evidence rather than definitive proof.

In general, the tissue antigens present during fetal and neonatal life are recognized as "self" and so are tolerated by the host. No antibodies or hypersensitivity reactions are developed to them. On the other hand, antigens not present during fetal or neonatal life are rejected as "not self" and antibodies to them are formed.

In certain specialized situations, tolerance may be lost and antibodies to host antigens may be formed. Some possible mechanisms are as follows:

(1) Certain tissues are normally sequestered, so that their antigens have no access to antibody-forming cells. The lens and uveal tract of the eye, sperm, thyroglobulin, and central nervous system tissue are normally isolated from the circulation and are thus not recognized as "self." Entrance of these antigens into the circulation elicits relatively organ-specific antibodies. When these antigens are administered with adjuvant, various disorders such as endophthalmitis, aspermatogenesis, thyroiditis, or encephalitis can be produced experimentally (see below).

(2) Although most antigen-antibody reactions are highly specific, cross-reactions between unrelated antigens do occur. Thus an antibody formed in response to an extrinsic antigen might by chance cross-react with a tissue antigen of the host. Examples are found among vegetable substances which stimulate antibodies reacting with red blood cell antigens, or streptococcal antigens which stimulate antibodies reacting with human heart tissue antigens.

(3) It is possible that in certain circumstances native tissue antigens are slightly altered (perhaps by combination with extrinsic haptens) and thus assume a new antigenic specificity. The antibody forming against the hapten-antigen complex may likewise react with the native antigen. In other circumstances a foreign molecule, eg, a drug, might attach to a cell surface. Antibodies forming to that foreign molecule can combine with it, and the antigen-antibody complex at the cell surface may injure the cell (see Sedormid purpura, p 159).

(4) In still other situations it appears that a genetic abnormality determines the ability of certain individuals and their families to manufacture antibodies to common host tissue constituents. Thus in rheumatoid arthritis the 19 S globulin called "rheumatoid factor" may be an antibody to normal human 7 S globulin. In disseminated lupus erythematosus and related "collagen diseases," antibodies are formed to cell nuclei and other tissue constituents. This may involve an abnormal loss of tolerance.

The following are some oversimplified examples of natural or experimental disorders in which "autoimmune" reactions may be involved.

Chronic Thyroiditis

If rabbits are repeatedly injected with extracts of homologous thyroid gland they develop antibodies against thyroid antigens. These can be demonstrated by serologic technics. At the same time many of the animals develop chronic thyroiditis which histologically resembles the disease in humans. Patients suffering from chronic thyroiditis have in their serum specific antibodies against thyroid antigens, whereas persons not suffering from thyroid disease lack such antibodies. It is probable, therefore, that human thyroiditis develops as an "autoimmune" disease: Through some insult thyroid antigens are no longer recognized as "self" by the host, and consequently it forms antibodies against them. It is likely that lymphoid cells are simultaneously sensitized to thyroid antigens and that these cells provoke the inflammatory process which, in turn, leads to fibrosis and loss of function of the gland.

Allergic Encephalitis

When animal brain substance is mixed with adjuvants (see above) and injected into other members of the same animal species, many of these animals will develop encephalitis. The experiment can even be performed successfully by removing the frontal lobe from a monkey, mixing the ground brain material with adjuvant, and injecting it intramuscularly into the same monkey. Such an animal often develops demyelinating disease of the CNS with disseminated lesions in the brain and cord. Histologically, these lesions greatly resemble "post-vaccinal" encephalomyelitis, which occurs in persons who have been repeatedly injected with animal brain material, as in rabies vaccine.

Experimental allergic encephalitis cannot be transferred passively by serum, but can be passively transferred with lymphoid cells. The severity of lesions bears no relationship to measurable complement-fixing anti-brain antibodies, and such antibodies may even protect against lesions. The likelihood is great that the illness is based on hypersensitivity reactions and that a protein of brain acts as allergen. One such encephalitogenic protein has been isolated in pure form. Some animals developing such encephalitis show a delayed (tuberculin-type) skin reaction to brain substance.

Rheumatic Fever

From epidemiologic evidence it is clear that rheumatic fever in man is regularly preceded by multiple infections with different types of group A beta-hemolytic streptococci. When rabbits are repeatedly injected intradermally with different types of streptococci, a few of them develop heart lesions resembling rheumatic lesions with Aschoff bodies. It may be that the repeated injections permit the development of "chronic anaphylaxis" expressing itself in specific organs. It is possible that "auto-antibodies" form against the host's own tissue and that the subsequent antigen-antibody reaction leads to tissue injury.

An alternative possibility is based on cross-reactions between antigens of human heart and streptococci. Certain group A streptococci contain a cell membrane antigen which cross-reacts with human cardiac muscle fibers, especially the sarcolemma. Thus, antibodies to the streptococci might react with heart muscle.

There is also cross-reactivity between structural glycoproteins of heart valves and streptococcal group-specific carbohydrate.

Glomerulonephritis

From epidemiologic evidence it is known that human glomerulonephritis often follows infection with group A beta-hemolytic streptococci of types 12, 4, or 49. It was proposed that the streptococcal infection in some fashion mobilizes or perhaps slightly modifies kidney antigen; such antigen, perhaps glomerular protein, stimulates antibody production. Alternatively a streptococcal antigen or antigen-antibody complex may localize at the glomerular membrane. Kidney injury may result from an antigen-antibody reaction. The likelihood of an antigen-antibody reaction occurring in acute human glomerulonephritis is suggested by the finding of low levels of complement (suggesting that complement is taken up by antigen-antibody complex). When healing occurs, complement levels rise to normal.

Studies utilizing radioactive or fluorescent labels indicate a high concentration of gamma globulin and streptococcal antigens at the site of the lesion (glomerulus). The globulin may represent localized specific antibody. Immunosuppressive drugs can suppress clinical activity of glomerulonephritis.

Blood Diseases

Various forms of human hemolytic anemias, granulocytopenias, thrombocytopenias, and other blood disorders have been attributed either to the development of auto-antibodies directed against antigens in red blood cells or platelets, or to the attachment of antigen-antibody complexes to the cell surface. As a result of such antigen-antibody reactions, cells would be destroyed. The responsible antibodies have been demonstrated in a number of instances. For example, in the thrombocytopenic purpura caused by Sedormid or quinidine, the sensitive person's serum contains antibody which can lyse platelets onto which the drug has been adsorbed.

Pernicious anemia may represent an "autoimmune" reaction to intrinsic factor.

"Collagen Diseases," "Group Diseases," "Visceral Angiitides"

This is a group of human diseases characterized by collagen degeneration, focal inflammatory reactions around blood vessels, and vascular and cardiac lesions. The group includes rheumatoid arthritis, disseminated lupus erythematosus, polyarteritis (periarteritis) nodosa, scleroderma, dermatomyositis, and probably others. The etiology of these illnesses is not known, but typical cases have occurred following sensitization by sulfonamides or foreign serum. Experimentally, similar lesions have been produced by the repeated injection of foreign proteins into animals. It is believed that these markedly hypersensitive animals developed the lesions as a form of "autoimmune" reaction.

In patients with disseminated lupus erythematosus, a globulin has been demonstrated in the plasma which reacts (by complement fixation, LE cell preparation, or hemagglutination) with nuclei of a variety of human cells, immunofluorescence, and with nucleic acids. It has been suggested that such patients developed autoantibodies to their own nucleoproteins.

In patients with rheumatoid arthritis a 19 S globulin ("rheumatoid factor") can be regularly demonstrated which reacts (eg, by hemagglutination, latex fixation, or precipitation) with human 7 S globulin. It is possible that this 19 S globulin is a true autoantibody. In the blood stream it is often found as a 22 S complex which can dissociate into 19 S rheumatoid factor and 7 S globulin.

•   •   •

TRANSPLANTATION IMMUNITY*

It has long been known that an individual will accept a graft of his own tissue (eg, skin) but not that of another person, except an identical twin. An autograft is a graft of tissue from one individual onto itself, and it "takes" regularly and permanently. An isograft is a graft of tissue from one individual to another genetically identical individual, and it usually "takes" permanently. A heterograft (xenograft) is a graft from one species to another species. It is always rejected. A homograft (allograft) is a graft from one member of a noninbred species to another member, eg, from one human to another human. It is rejected by the homograft reaction. Initial vascularization and circulation of the graft are good, but after 11 to 14 days marked reduction in circulation and infiltration of the bed of the graft with mononuclear cells occur, and the graft eventually becomes necrotic and sloughs. It is highly probable that the mechanism of homograft rejection is similar to that which is operative in delayed type hypersensitivity reactions with competent lymphoid cells of primary importance; but circulating antibodies may also participate in the reaction. If a second homograft from the same donor is applied to a recipient who has rejected the first graft, an accelerated ("second-set") rejection is observed in 5–6 days.

*An excellent review of this subject by P.S. Russell & A.P. Monaco may be found in New England J Med 271:502, 553, 610, 664, 718, 776, 1964.

The problem of tissue transplantation resides in specific "transplantation antigens" which exist in all mammalian cells. These antigens are of a great variety under the control of a number of different "histocompatibility genes." In inbred strains of mice, at least 14 independently segregating genetic loci for transplantation antigens have been recognized. At each of these loci there exist multiple alleles, so that the number and variety of transplantation antigens is enormous. In man, the situation is undoubtedly equally complex. However, transplantation antigens vary in their immunogenic potency, and only the strongest of them may have a marked influence on graft survival.

The closer the genetic make-up of donor and recipient, the greater the probability of partial compatibility in transplantation antigens. The acceptance of grafts in man is aided by close family relationship. In the matching of recipient and donor for tissue transplants, blood group compatibility is important and leukocyte antigen typing is attempted, by means of lymphocyte cytotoxicity tests. This involves mixing purified blood lymphocytes with antiserum and complement and determining the proportion of dead cells after incubation at 37° C. If donor and recipient are well matched, the long-term survival of transplanted organs is enhanced.

To delay or diminish the graft rejection of transplanted tissues or organs, attempts are made to suppress immunologic rejection mechanisms. At present this involves the use of corticosteroids, immuno-suppressive drugs like azathioprine, and antilymphocytic serum, whereas radiation has been largely abandoned. All of these immunosuppressive measures unfortunately enhance the recipient's susceptibility to endogenous or exogenous infections: Even "nonpathogenic" microorganisms (bacteria, fungi, viruses, protozoa) may prove fatal to the immunosuppressed individual. Of the various immunosuppressive measures, antilymphocytic serum (ie, antiserum to heterologous lymphoid cells) appears to provide prolonged survival of homografts without marked toxicity for the recipient and is therefore being investigated intensively.

The longer a tissue or organ graft survives in the recipient, the greater the chance that tolerance to the graft may be established under the cover of immunosuppressive measures. The establishment of tolerance by means of repeated administration of donor cells into recipients has been attempted only rarely.

In certain experimental situations, the transplantation of immunologically competent lymphoid tissue into an immunosuppressed recipient has resulted in a graft-versus-host reaction. The grafted cells appeared to survive and "took over" by rejecting the host. In immunosuppressed mice, lymphoid tissue transplants from normal mice can result in "runting" and death of the recipient as a form of graft-versus-host reaction. A similar occurrence has been observed in immunologically deficient humans implanted with competent lymphoid cells from unrelated donors.

● ● ●

General References

Anthony, B.F., & others: Acute nephritis after type 49 streptococcal infection of skin. J Clin Invest 48:1697–1704, 1969.

Benacerraf, B., & I. Green: Cellular hypersensitivity. Ann Rev Med 20:141–154, 1969.

Ishizaka, K., & T. Ishizaka: Identification of IgE antibodies as a carrier of reaginic activity. J Immunol 99:1187–1198, 1967.

Leskowitz, S.: Tolerance. Ann Rev Microbiol 21:157–180, 1967.

Paterson, R.Y.: Immune processes and infection factors in CNS disease. Ann Rev Med 20:75–100, 1969.

Sadan, N., & others: Immunotherapy of pollinosis in children. New England J Med 280:623–627, 1969.

Sell, S.: Antilymphocytic antibody. Ann Int Med 71:177–193, 1969.

Terasaki, P.I., & D.P. Singal: Human histo-compatibility antigens of leukocytes. Ann Rev Med 20:175–188, 1969.

14 ...

Pyogenic Cocci

THE STAPHYLOCOCCI

The staphylococci are gram-positive spherical cells, usually arranged in irregular clusters. They grow readily on a variety of media and are active metabolically, fermenting many carbohydrates and producing pigments which vary from white to deep yellow. The pathogenic staphylococci often hemolyze blood and coagulate plasma. Some are members of the normal flora of the skin and mucous membranes of man; others cause suppuration, abscess formation, a variety of pyogenic infections, and even fatal septicemia. The most common type of food poisoning is caused by a heat-stable enterotoxin produced by certain staphylococci. Staphylococci rapidly develop resistance to most antimicrobial agents and present difficult therapeutic problems.

Morphology & Identification

A. Typical Organisms: Spherical cells about 1 μm in diameter arranged in irregular clusters. In liquid cultures single cocci, pairs, and chains are also seen. Young cocci stain strongly gram-positive; on aging, many cells become gram-negative. Staphylococci are nonmotile and do not form spores. Under the influence of certain chemicals (eg, penicillin) they are lysed or changed into L forms, but they are not affected by bile salts.

Gaffkya tetragena is characteristically arranged in tetrads, often with a wide capsule.

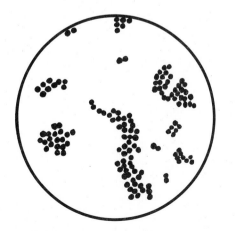

FIG 14–1. Staphylococci from broth culture.

B. Culture: Staphylococci grow readily on most bacteriologic media under aerobic or microaerophilic conditions. They grow most rapidly on 37° C, but form pigment best at room temperature (20° C). Colonies on solid media are round, smooth, raised, and glistening, forming varying pigments: *Staphylococcus aureus* is deep golden yellow; *S albus (S epidermidis)* is porcelain white; intermediate shades also occur. Many colonies develop pigment only upon prolonged incubation at 20° C. No pigment is produced anaerobically or in broth. Various degrees of hemolysis are produced by different strains.

C. Growth Characteristics: Staphylococci are able to ferment slowly many carbohydrates, producing lactic acid but not gas. There are great variations among strains. Proteolytic activity also varies greatly. The extracellular substances produced by pathogenic staphylococci are discussed under Pathogenesis, below.

Staphylococci are relatively resistant to drying and to heat (they will withstand 50° C for 30 minutes), and to 9% sodium chloride, but are readily inhibited by certain dyes, eg, gentian violet in concentrations of 1:100,000–1:2,000,000. Staphylococci are variably sensitive to sulfonamides and antibiotics, and drug-resistant mutants are found in most strains. Many strains are penicillin-resistant by virtue of the production of penicillinase (β-lactamase), an enzyme that destroys penicillins by breaking the β-lactam ring. Its production is controlled by a genetic extrachromosomal element (plasmid) which can be transferred by bacteriophages (transduction). Plasmids also carry genetic control of resistance to other antibiotics. Frequent plasmid transduction may explain the rapid emergence of multiple drug resistance among staphylococci.

D. Variation: Any culture of staphylococci contains certain organisms which differ from the bulk of the population in cultural characteristics (smooth or rough colony type, pigment, hemolysis), in enzyme equipment, in drug resistance, and in pathogenicity.

Antigenic Structure

Staphylococci contain both antigenic polysaccharides and proteins which permit a grouping of strains to a limited extent. Most of the extracellular substances produced by staphylococci are likewise antigenic. While serologic tests have limited usefulness in identifying strains, this can be done by "phage typing." The method is based on the lysis of organisms by one or a series of specific bacteriophages. Such bacteriophage susceptibility (phage type) is a stable genetic characteristic, based on surface receptors. It permits the epidemiologic tracing of strains.

Many staphylococcal strains are lysogenic. Production of some toxins appears to be phage-mediated.

Toxins & Enzymes

Staphylococci can produce disease both through their ability to multiply and spread widely in tissues and through their production of many extracellular substances. Among the latter are the following:

A. "Exotoxin": A filtrable, thermolabile mixture which is lethal for animals on injection, causes necrosis in skin, and contains several soluble hemolysins which can be separated by electrophoresis. The alpha hemolysis, a protein with a molecular weight of 3×10^4 daltons dissolves rabbit erythrocytes, damages platelets, and is probably identical with the lethal and dermonecrotic factors of exotoxin. Alpha hemolysin also has a powerful action on vascular smooth muscle. Beta hemolysin dissolves sheep erythrocytes (but not rabbit cells) upon incubation for 1 hour at 37° C and then 18 hours at 10° C. These hemolysins (and 2 others, the gamma and delta hemolysins) are antigenically distinct and bear no relationship to streptococcal lysins. Exotoxin treated with formalin gives a nonpoisonous but antigenic toxoid which has been used to stimulate antitoxic immunity to staphylococci.

B. Leukocidin: A soluble material which kills exposed white blood cells of a variety of animal species. It is antigenic but more heat-labile than exotoxin. Its role in pathogenesis is uncertain. Pathogenic staphylococci may not kill white blood cells and may be phagocytized as effectively as nonpathogenic varieties. However, they are capable of very active intra-cellular multiplication, whereas the nonpathogenic organisms rapidly die inside the cell. Antibodies to leukocidin may play a role in resistance to recurrent staphylococcal infections.

C. Enterotoxin: A soluble material produced by certain strains of staphylococci, particularly when they are grown in high concentrations of CO_2 (30%) in semi-solid media. Enterotoxin is a protein with a molecular weight of 3.5×10^4 daltons that resists boiling for 30 minutes and the action of gut enzymes, and belongs to one of 4 antigenic types. An important cause of food poisoning, enterotoxin is produced especially when certain staphylococci grow in carbohydrate foods, eg, pastry. Ingestion of 25 μg enterotoxin B results in vomiting and diarrhea in man or monkeys; the same symptoms occur after parenteral injection of 0.1 μg/kg into monkeys or kittens. The emetic effect of enterotoxin is probably the result of CNS stimulation (vomiting center).

D. Coagulase: Most staphylococci pathogenic for man produce coagulase, an enzyme-like substance (a protein) which clots oxalated or citrated plasma in the presence of a factor contained in many sera. The coagulase-reactive factor of serum reacts with coagulase to generate both esterase and clotting activities in a manner similar to the activation of prothrombin to thrombin. Coagulase may deposit fibrin on the surface of staphylococci, perhaps interfering with their ingestion by phagocytic cells or their destruction within such cells. Alternatively, coagulase may neutralize an antistaphylococcal factor in plasma.

E. Other extracellular substances produced by staphylococci include the following: a hyaluronidase, or spreading factor; a staphylokinase resulting in fibrinolysis but acting much more slowly than streptokinase; proteinases, lipases, and penicillinase. Staphylo-

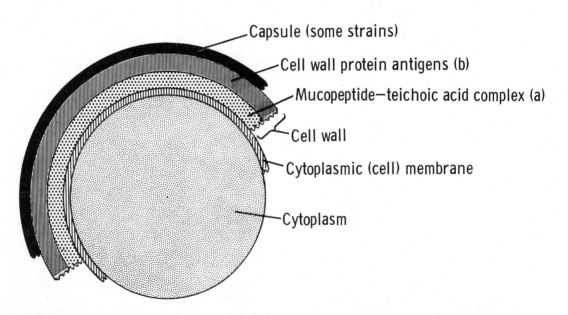

FIG 14–2. Antigenic structure of staphylococci. (a) Site of bacteriophage attachment. Species antigens present (antigenic determinant is N-acetylglucosamine linked to polyribol phosphate). (b) Multiple antigens; several widely distributed.

coccal penicillinase production is under genetic control of a plasmid (see Growth Characteristics, above).

Pathogenesis

Staphylococci (particularly *S albus*) are members of the normal flora of the human skin and of the respiratory and gastrointestinal tracts; they are also found regularly in air and human environments. The pathogenic capacity of a given strain of staphylococci is the combined effect of the above-named extracellular factors and toxins together with the invasive properties of the strain, and it covers a wide scale. At one end is staphylococcal food poisoning, attributable solely to the ingestion of preformed enterotoxin; at the other end, staphylococcal bacteremia and disseminated abscesses in all organs. The potential contribution of the various extracellular factors in pathogenesis is evident from the nature of their individual actions.

Pathogenic, invasive staphylococci (*S aureus*) tend to be hemolytic, produce coagulase and yellow pigment, and ferment mannitol. Nonpathogenic, noninvasive staphylococci (*S epidermidis*) tend to be nonhemolytic, white, coagulase-negative, and do not ferment mannitol. *Gaffkya tetragena* may produce suppuration like other staphylococci and occasionally causes pneumonia.

Pathology

The prototype of a staphylococcal lesion is the furuncle or other localized abscess. Groups of staphylococci established in a hair follicle lead to tissue necrosis (dermonecrotic factor). Coagulase is produced and coagulates fibrin around the lesion and within the lymphatics, resulting in formation of a wall which limits the process and which is reinforced by the accumulation of inflammatory cells and, later, fibrous tissue. Within the center of the lesion, liquefaction of the necrotic tissue occurs (enhanced by delayed hypersensitivity) and the abscess "points" in the direction of least resistance. Drainage of the liquid central necrotic tissue is followed by the slow filling of the cavity with granulation tissue and eventual healing.

Focal suppuration is typical of staphylococcal infection. From any one focus, organisms may spread via the lymphatics and blood stream to other parts of the body. Suppuration within veins, associated with thrombosis, is a common feature of such dissemination.

Staphylococci of low invasiveness are involved in many minor skin infections (eg, acne, impetigo). In osteomyelitis the primary focus of staphylococcal growth is typically in a terminal blood vessel of the metaphysis of long bones, leading to necrosis of bone and chronic suppuration. Staphylococci may be the causative organisms in pneumonia, meningitis, empyema, endocarditis, or sepsis with suppuration in any organ.

Clinical Findings

The picture of a localized staphylococcal infection is that of a "pimple," hair follicle infection, or an abscess—usually an intense, localized, painful inflammatory reaction which undergoes central suppuration and which heals quickly when the pus is drained. The wall of fibrin and cells around the core of the abscess tends to prevent spread of the organisms and should not be broken down by manipulation or trauma. If the organisms become disseminated and bacteremia ensues, the clinical picture resembles that seen with other blood stream infections. The secondary localization within an organ or system is accompanied by the symptoms and signs of organ dysfunction and intense focal suppuration.

Food poisoning due to staphylococcus enterotoxin is characterized by a short (1–6 hours) incubation period, violent nausea, vomiting, and diarrhea, and rapid convalescence. There is no fever.

The suppression of normal bowel flora by antimicrobial drugs favors the development of postoperative staphylococcal enterocolitis which has a high fatality rate.

Diagnostic Laboratory Tests

A. Specimens: Surface swab, pus, blood, sputum, or spinal fluid for culture, depending upon the localization of the process. Antibody studies on serum are not commonly performed.

B. Stained Smears: Typical staphylococci are seen in stained smears of pus or sputum. It is not possible to distinguish saprophytic (*S albus*) from pathogenic (*S aureus*) organisms.

C. Culture: Specimens planted on blood agar plates give rise to typical colonies in 18 hours at 37° C, but hemolysis and pigment production may not occur until several days later, preferably at room temperature. From specimens contaminated with a mixed flora, staphylococci can be grown in media containing 7.5% NaCl. Most human staphylococci are not pathogenic for animals. A staphylococcus is generally considered pathogenic if it produces pigment or coagulase, ferments mannitol, liquefies gelatin, or hemolyzes blood.

D. Coagulase Test: Citrated rabbit (or human) plasma diluted 1:5 is mixed with an equal volume of broth culture and incubated at 37° C. A tube of plasma mixed with sterile broth is included as control. The tubes are frequently inspected for clotting over a period of hours.

Growth on tellurite medium may be substituted for coagulase tests. Most coagulase positive staphylococci reduce tellurite with the production of jet black colonies.

All coagulase positive staphylococci are considered pathogenic for man. Certain types of infections, notably bacterial endocarditis, can be caused by coagulase negative *S albus.*

E. Serologic Tests, Animal Inoculations: These procedures have little practical value. However, phage typing of staphylococci isolated in hospital environments is a useful epidemiologic tool (see below); antibiotic resistance patterns are also helpful.

Treatment

The impression among clinicians that active resistance to staphylococcal infections can be acquired has led to the use of staphylococcal toxoid in persons suffering from recurrent staphylococcal skin infections. While the increase in antitoxin titer which follows toxoid therapy may be associated with diminution in severity of recurrent infections, there is no good evidence for the efficacy of toxoids in treatment. Staphylococcal vaccines are of even more questionable value.

Many antimicrobial agents have some effect against staphylococci in vitro. However, the rapid development of resistance to most agents and the inability of drugs to act in the central necrotic part of the lesions makes it difficult to eradicate pathogenic staphylococci. from infected persons. Drainage of closed suppurating lesions is essential.

Most persons harbor staphylococci on the skin and in the nose or throat. Even if the skin (eg, in eczema) can be cleared of staphylococci, reinfection by droplets will occur almost immediately. Pathogenic organisms are commonly spread from one lesion (eg, furuncle) to other areas of the skin by fingers and clothing. Scrupulous local antisepsis is therefore of considerable aid.

Serious multiple skin infections (furunculosis) occur most often in adolescents and are believed to be favored by hormonal factors. Similar skin infections occur in patients receiving prolonged courses of corticosteroids.

Because of the frequency of resistant variants in most staphylococcal strains and the consequent unpredictability of clinical response to any one antimicrobial drug, all pathogenic staphylococci should be submitted to antibiotic sensitivity testing upon isolation in the laboratory, and adjustments in chemotherapy should be made according to the results. Resistance to drugs of the erythromycin group or novobiocin tends to emerge so rapidly that these drugs should not be used singly for treatment of chronic infection. Tetracycline and penicillin resistance can be transmitted among staphylococci by transducing bacteriophages.

Penicillin G-resistant staphylococci from clinical infections always produce penicillinase. They may be susceptible to β-lactmase-resistant penicillins (eg, methicillin; see p 114), cephalosporins, or vancomycin.

In view of the rapid emergence of drug resistance among staphylococci, hospitals have sometimes restricted the use of an antistaphylococcus drug to the treatment of the most seriously ill patients. Such restriction may greatly prolong the useful period of a new drug.

Epidemiology & Control

Staphylococci are ubiquitous human parasites. The chief sources of infection are accessible human lesions, fomites contaminated from them, and the human respiratory tract and skin. Airborne infection has assumed added importance in hospitals, where a large proportion of the staff and patients carry antibiotic-resistant staphylococci in nose or throat or on the skin. Although cleanliness, hygiene, and aseptic management of lesions ordinarily control the spread of skin infections due to staphylococci, only limited methods are available to prevent the wide dissemination of staphylococci from carriers. Aerosols (eg, glycols) and ultraviolet irradiation of air have little effect. The most endangered areas in hospitals are the newborn nursery and the surgical operating rooms. Massive introduction of "epidemic" pathogenic staphylococci into these areas may lead to serious clinical disease. Persons with active staphylococcal lesions and carriers may have to be excluded from these areas. In such individuals the application of topical antiseptics (eg, neomycin cream) to carriage sites (nostrils, perineum, etc) may diminish shedding of dangerous organisms. Various antiseptics (eg, hexachlorophene) can be used on the skin of the newborn to diminish colonization by staphylococci.

In most hospitals, because antibiotics are used extensively, prevalent staphylococci are resistant to commonly employed antimicrobial drugs. Restriction of new drugs may be advisable (see above). Phage typing provides a valuable tool to establish the transmission of "hospital staphylococci" from personnel and patients to newly admitted patients. During outbreaks of staphylococcal disease among newborns or surgical patients, a single phage type (eg, 80/81) usually prevails. Sporadic infections are often caused by several different types. Certain phage types appear to spread much more readily in the environment and acquire drug resistance more rapidly than others. Most drug-resistant staphylococci of hospitals fall into the series of phage types called "group III."

Experimentally, it is possible to selectively colonize individuals with nonpathogenic staphylococci (eg, 502A) and thereby prevent colonization with pathogenic staphylococci. This "bacterial interference" can also be applied at times to patients whose lesion-causing staphylococci have been temporarily suppressed by drugs. "Bacterial interference" may have a nutritional basis (eg, competition for a metabolite) or may be attributable to the production of an inhibitor.

THE STREPTOCOCCI

The streptococci are spherical microorganisms, characteristically arranged in chains and widely distributed in nature. Some are members of normal human flora; others are associated with important human diseases attributable in part to infection by streptococci, in part to sensitization to them. They produce a variety of extracellular substances and enzymes. Their ability to hemolyze red blood cells to various degrees is one important method of classification.

Morphology & Identification

A. Typical Organisms: Individual cocci are spherical or ovoid and are arranged in chains. The cocci

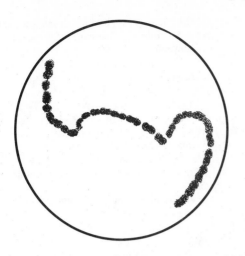

FIG 14−3. Hemolytic streptococcus from broth culture.

divide in a plane perpendicular to the long axis of the chain. The members of the chain often have a striking diplococcal appearance, and rod-like forms are occasionally seen. The lengths of the chains vary widely, conditioned largely by environmental factors.

Some streptococci elaborate a capsular polysaccharide which is comparable to that of pneumococci. The majority of group A and group C strains produce capsules composed of hyaluronic acid. The capsules are most noticeable in very young cultures. They impede phagocytosis. The streptococcal cell wall contains proteins (M, T, R antigens), carbohydrates (group-specific), and mucopeptides (Fig 14−4).

B. Culture: Most streptococci grow in solid media as discoid colonies, usually 1−2 mm in diameter. Group A strains which produce capsular material often give rise to mucoid colonies. Matt and glossy colonies of group A strains are discussed below.

C. Growth Characteristics: Energy is principally obtained from the utilization of sugars. Growth of streptococci tends to be poor on solid media or in broth unless enriched with blood or tissue fluids. Nutritive requirements vary widely among different species. The human pathogens are most exacting, requiring a variety of growth factors. Growth and hemolysis are aided by 10% CO_2:

While most pathogenic hemolytic streptococci grow best at 37° C, group D enterococci grow well between 15° C and 45° C. Enterococci also grow in high (6.5%) sodium chloride concentration and in 0.1% methylene blue. Most streptococci are facultative anaerobes, but some strains from surgical infections are obligate anaerobes. Other characteristics are discussed below.

D. Variation: Variants of the same streptococcus strain may show different colony forms. This is particularly marked among group A strains, giving rise to either matt or glossy colonies. Matt colonies consist of organisms which give rise to much M protein. Such organisms tend to be virulent and relatively insusceptible to phagocytosis by human leukocytes. Glossy colonies tend to produce little M protein and are often nonvirulent.

Antigenic Structure

Hemolytic streptococci can be divided into serologic groups (A−O), and certain groups can be subdivided into types. Several antigenic substances are found:

(1) C Carbohydrate: This substance is contained in the cell wall of many streptococci and forms the basis of serologic grouping (Lancefield A−O). Extracts of C carbohydrate for "grouping" of streptococci may be prepared by extraction of centrifuged culture with hot hydrochloric acid or formamide; by enzymatic lysis of streptococcal cells (eg, with pepsin, trypsin, or enzymes derived from *Streptomyces albus*); or by

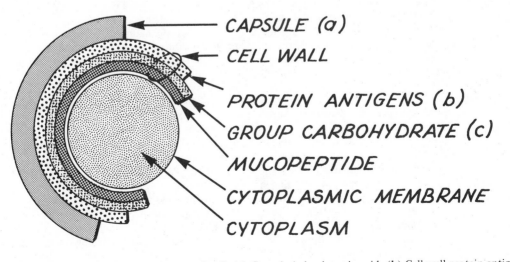

FIG 14−4. Antigen structure of streptococcal cell. (a) Capsule is hyaluronic acid. (b) Cell wall protein antigens M, T, and R. (c) Group carbohydrate for group A streptococci is rhamnose-N-acetylglucosamine.

autoclaving cell suspensions at 15 lb pressure for 15 minutes. The serologic specificity of C carbohydrate is determined by an amino sugar. For group A streptococci this is rhamnose-N-acetylglucosamine; for group C, it is rhamnose-N-acetylgalactosamine; for group F it is glucopyranosyl-N-acetylgalactosamine.

(2) **M Protein:** This substance is closely associated with virulence of group A streptococci and occurs chiefly in organisms producing matt or mucoid colonies. Repeated passage on artificial media may lead to loss of M protein production, which may be restored by rapidly repeated animal passage. M protein interferes with the ingestion of virulent streptococci by phagocytic cells. Growing L forms of streptococci also produce M protein as well as hyaluronic acid.

M protein is present in extracts of group A streptococci made with hot hydrochloric acid. This protein determines the type specificity of group A streptococci as demonstrated by agglutination or precipitation reactions with absorbed type-specific sera. There are more than 50 types in group A. Types are assigned Arabic numbers.

(3) **T Substance:** This antigen has no relationship to virulence of streptococci. It is destroyed by acid extraction and by heat, and thus is separated from M protein. It is obtained from streptococci by proteolytic digestion (which rapidly destroys M proteins) and permits differentiation of certain types. Other types share the same T substance. Yet another surface antigen has been called R protein.

(4) **Nucleoproteins:** Extraction of streptococci with weak alkali yields mixtures of proteins and other substances of little serologic specificity, called P substances, which probably make up most of the streptococcal cell body.

Toxins & Enzymes

More than 20 extracellular products which are antigenic are elaborated by group A streptococci, including the following:

(1) **Streptokinase (fibrinolysin)** is produced by many strains of beta-hemolytic streptococci. It transforms the plasminogen of human serum into plasmin, an active proteolytic enzyme, which digests fibrin and other proteins. This digestion may be interfered with by nonspecific serum inhibitors and by a specific antibody, antistreptokinase, formed in response to previous exposure to streptokinase substance. Streptokinase is employed therapeutically to break down freshly formed adhesions and fibrin barriers.

(2) **Streptodornase (streptococcal deoxyribonuclease)** is an enzyme which depolymerizes deoxyribonucleoprotein and deoxyribonucleic acid (DNA). The enzymatic activity can be measured by the lowering in viscosity of known DNA solutions. Purulent exudates owe their viscosity largely to deoxyribonucleoprotein. Streptodornase is employed therapeutically to liquefy viscous exudates. Mixtures of streptodornase and streptokinase are used in "enzymatic debridement." They help to liquefy exudates and to break down the fibrin barrier. In this way, removal of pus and necrotic tissue is facilitated, antimicrobial drugs gain better access, and infected surfaces recover more quickly.

(3) **Hyaluronidase** is an enzyme which splits hyaluronic acid, an important component of the ground substance of connective tissue. Thus hyaluronidase aids in spreading infecting microorganisms (spreading factor). Hyaluronidases are antigenic and specific for each bacterial or tissue source. Following infection with hyaluronidase-producing organisms, specific antibodies are found in the serum. Purified hyaluronidase is employed in medical therapy to facilitate the spreading and absorption of fluids injected into tissues.

(4) **Erythrogenic toxin** is a soluble toxin which is resistant to heating at 60° C for several hours but is destroyed by boiling for 1 hour. The erythrogenic toxin is responsible for the rash that occurs in scarlet fever. Only strains elaborating this toxin can cause scarlet fever. Erythrogenic toxin is elaborated only by lysogenic streptococci. Strains devoid of the temperate phage genome do not produce toxin. A nontoxigenic streptococcus, after lysogenic conversion, will produce erythrogenic toxin. Erythrogenic toxin is antigenic, giving rise to the formation of specific antitoxin which neutralizes the toxin. Persons possessing such antitoxin are immune to the rash, though susceptible to streptococcal infection. As has been demonstrated by toxin-antitoxin neutralization tests with specific antitoxin sera, there exist some minor qualitative differences between the erythrogenic toxins produced by the different strains. Susceptibility to erythrogenic toxin is demonstrated by the Dick test.

Dick test: 0.1 ml of standardized, diluted, erythrogenic toxin (broth culture filtrate) is injected intradermally. Similar material, heat-inactivated, is used as a control. In the absence of significant concentration of antitoxin in the blood, a positive Dick test is seen, consisting of the appearance in 8–24 hours of an area of erythema and edema measuring more than 10 mm in diameter. In the first few days of scarlet fever the Dick test is generally positive. With recovery the reactions become negative.

The specific nature of the rash of scarlet fever can be demonstrated by means of the *Schultz-Charlton reaction.* This consists of the injection of specific antitoxin into an area of scarlet fever rash. If the rash is caused by erythrogenic toxin of streptococci, the redness will blanch and fade in the injected area where the antitoxin has neutralized the toxin.

(5) Some streptococci elaborate a **diphosphopyridine nucleotidase** into the environment. This enzyme may be related to the organism's ability to kill leukocytes. Proteinases and amylase are produced by some strains.

(6) **Hemolysins:** Many streptococci are able to hemolyze red blood cells in vitro in varying degrees. Complete disruption of erythrocytes with release of hemoglobin is called *beta*-hemolysis. Incomplete lysis of erythrocytes with the formation of green pigment is called *alpha*-hemolysis. "Gamma" sometimes refers to nonhemolytic organisms.

Beta-hemolytic group A streptococci elaborate 2 hemolysins (streptolysins):

Streptolysin O is a protein which is hemolytically active in the reduced state (available –SH groups) but rapidly inactivated when oxidized. It combines quantitatively with antistreptolysin O, an antibody which appears in animals or man following infection with any streptococci that produce streptolysin O. This antibody blocks hemolysis by streptolysin O. This phenomenon forms the basis of a quantitative test for the antibody. An antistreptolysin (ASO) titer of sera in excess of 125 units is considered abnormally high and suggests either recent infection with streptococci or persistently high antibody levels following an earlier exposure.

Streptolysin S is the agent responsible for the hemolytic zones around streptococcal colonies on blood agar plates. It is not antigenic. However, sera of man and animals frequently contain a nonspecific inhibitor which is independent of past experience with streptococci but probably reflects metabolic disturbances associated with variations in phospholipid content of the sera.

Classification of Streptococci

A practical arrangement of streptococci into major categories can be based on (1) action on red blood cells, (2) resistance to physical and chemical factors, and (3) biochemical tests. While individual features for each species have only limited value, their consideration as a group permits separation of streptococci into 4 divisions.

A. Hemolytic Streptococci: Produce soluble hemolysins which result in beta-hemolysis on blood agar. They elaborate group-specific C carbohydrates. Acid extracts containing these C carbohydrates give precipitin reactions with specific antisera which permit the arrangement of hemolytic streptococci into groups A–O. The majority of invasive beta-hemolytic streptococci pathogenic for man fall into group A, but strains of groups B, C, and G are encountered in respiratory infections, bacteremia, and endocarditis.

B. Viridans Streptococci: Do not produce either soluble hemolysins or beta-hemolysis on blood agar. Many species induce alpha-hemolysis, ie, they turn hemoglobin green. Some species have no action on blood and are called indifferent (gamma) streptococci. The effect on blood cells depends on the species of erythrocyte, on environmental conditions (eg, pH, temperature, moisture), and on other factors which are not understood. They do not produce C carbohydrate. In contrast to pneumococci (whose colonies they resemble), they are not bile-soluble. Viridans streptococci are the most prominent members of the normal flora of the human respiratory tract and are ordinarily associated with disease only when they settle on abnormal heart valves (subacute bacterial endocarditis) or establish themselves in the meninges or the urinary tract of man. They also occur widely in nature. Some synthesize large molecular polysaccharides, eg, dextran.

C. Enterococci (*Streptococcus faecalis*): Produce group D-specific C carbohydrate. They are capable of growing at 10° C and 45° C, in 0.1% methylene blue milk, on 40% bile agar, or in 6.5% NaCl concentration. They cause variable hemolysis. They are part of the normal flora of the intestinal tract of man and animals and may cause disease when introduced into tissues, the blood stream, urinary tract, or meninges. Occasionally they are associated with food poisoning. Enterococci are quite resistant to most antibiotic and chemotherapeutic agents. Penicillin often inhibits but does not kill them, unless kanamycin or streptomycin is present.

D. Lactic Streptococci: Elaborate group N-specific C carbohydrate. Their hemolytic ability is variable. They grow on 40% bile agar but not at 45° C or in 6.5% NaCl which differentiates them from enterococci. Lactic streptococci do not produce disease, but they are commonly present in milk and are often responsible for the normal coagulation of milk ("souring").

Pathogenesis & Clinical Findings

A variety of distinct disease processes are associated with streptococcal infections. The biologic properties of the infecting organisms, the nature of the host response, and the portals of entry of the infection all greatly influence the pathologic picture. Infections can arbitrarily be divided into several categories.

A. Diseases Attributable to Invasion by Beta-Hemolytic Group A Streptococci: The portal of entry determines the principal clinical picture. In each case, however, there is a diffuse and rapidly spreading cellulitis which involves the tissues and extends along the lymphatic pathway with only minimal local suppuration. From the lymphatics the infection rapidly extends to the blood stream, whereupon bacteremia supervenes.

1. Erysipelas–If the portal of entry is the skin or superficial mucous membranes, erysipelas results, with massive brawny edema and a rapidly advancing margin.

2. Puerperal fever–If the streptococci enter the uterus after delivery, puerperal fever develops, which is essentially a septicemia originating in the infected wound (endometritis).

3. Sepsis–Infection of traumatic or surgical wounds with streptococci results in streptococcal sepsis, or surgical scarlet fever.

B. Diseases Attributable to Local Infection With Beta-Hemolytic Group A Streptococci and to Their Products:

1. Streptococcal sore throat–The commonest infection due to beta-hemolytic streptococci is streptococcal sore throat. In the infant and small child it occurs as a subacute nasopharyngitis with a thin serous discharge and little fever but with a marked tendency of the infection to extend to the middle ear, the mastoid, and the meninges. The cervical lymph nodes are usually enlarged. The illness may persist for weeks or months. In older children and adults, the disease is more acute and is characterized by intense nasopharyngitis, tonsillitis, and intense redness and edema of the mucous membranes, with purulent exudate; enlarged, tender cervical lymph nodes; and (usually) a high fever. If the infecting streptococci produce erythrogenic toxin and the patient has no antitoxic immunity, scarlet fever rash occurs. Antitoxin to the erythrogenic toxin prevents the rash but does not interfere with the streptococcal infection. With the most intense inflammation, tissues may break down and form peritonsillar abscesses (quinsy) or Ludwig's angina, where massive swelling of the floor of the mouth blocks air passages.

Streptococcal infection of the upper respiratory tract does not usually involve the lungs. Pneumonia due to beta-hemolytic streptococci is most commonly a sequel to viral infections, eg, influenza or measles, which seem to enhance susceptibility greatly.

2. Impetigo—Local infection of the skin's superficial layers, especially in small children, leads to the development of impetigo, superficial blisters which break readily and spread by continuity. The denuded surface is covered with honey-colored crusts. Impetigo is highly contagious in children. Streptococci are usually associated with staphylococci in this infection. Streptococcal skin infection may lead to nonsuppurative poststreptococcal disease, especially nephritis.

C. Bacterial Endocarditis:

1. Acute bacterial endocarditis—In the course of bacteremia, beta-hemolytic streptococci, pneumococci, or staphylococci may settle on normal or previously deformed heart valves, producing acute ulcerative bacterial endocarditis. Rapid destruction of the valves frequently leads to a fatal outcome in days or weeks. Other organisms are encountered occasionally in this disease.

2. Subacute bacterial endocarditis, on the other hand, involves abnormal valves (congenital deformities or rheumatic lesions). Although any organism reaching the blood stream may establish itself on such valves, subacute bacterial endocarditis is most frequently due to microbial constituents of the normal flora of the respiratory or intestinal tract which have accidentally reached the blood. After dental extraction, at least 30% of patients have alpha-hemolytic streptococcal bacteremia. These streptococci, ordinarily the most prevalent members of the upper respiratory flora, are also the most frequent cause of subacute bacterial endocarditis. About 5–10% of cases are due to enterococci. The lesion is slowly progressive, and a certain amount of healing accompanies the active inflammation; vegetations consist of fibrin, platelets, blood cells, and bacteria adherent to the valve leaflets. The clinical course is gradual, but the disease is invariably fatal in untreated cases. The typical clinical picture includes fever, anemia, weakness, a heart murmur, embolic phenomena, an enlarged spleen, and renal lesions.

D. Other Infections: Various streptococci, particularly enterococci, are frequently the cause of urinary tract infections. Anaerobic streptococci occur in the normal female genital tract, in the mouth, and in the intestine. They may give rise to suppurative lesions, either alone or in association with other anaerobes,

particularly bacteroides. Such infections may occur in wounds, postpartum endometritis, following rupture of an abdominal viscus, or in chronic suppuration of the lung. Such pus usually has a foul odor. A variety of other streptococci (groups B–L and O) which are usually found in lower animals may also occasionally produce human infections.

E. Poststreptococcal Diseases (Rheumatic Fever, Glomerulonephritis): Following an acute group A streptococcal infection (especially a "strep throat"), there may be a latent period of 2–3 weeks, after which nephritis or rheumatic fever occasionally develops. The interval of the latent period suggests that these poststreptococcal diseases are not attributable to the direct effect of disseminated bacteria but represent instead a hypersensitivity response which follows streptococcal insult to the affected organs.

1. Acute glomerulonephritis develops in some persons 3 weeks following streptococcal infection, particularly with types 12, 4, or 49. Certain strains are particularly nephritogenic. Thus, 23% of children with a skin infection with a type 49 strain developed nephritis or hematuria. However, after random streptococcal infections, the incidence of nephritis is less than 0.5%.

Glomerulonephritis may be initiated by antigen-antibody complexes on the glomerular basement membrane. The most important antigen is probably in the streptococcal protoplast membrane. In acute nephritis, there is blood and protein in the urine, edema, high blood pressure, and nitrogen retention. A few patients die and some develop chronic glomerulonephritis with ultimate kidney failure, but the majority recover completely.

2. Rheumatic fever is the most serious sequel to hemolytic streptococcal infection because it results in damage to heart muscle and valves. Certain strains of group A streptococci contain a cell wall antigen which cross-reacts with human heart tissue, especially cardiac muscle fibers.

The development of rheumatic fever is generally preceded by a group A streptococcus infection 2 or 3 weeks earlier, although the infection may be mild and may not be detected. Untreated streptococcal infections may be followed by rheumatic fever in up to 3% of military personnel and 0.3% of civilian children.

Typical symptoms and signs of rheumatic fever include fever, malaise, a migratory nonsuppurative polyarthritis, and evidence of inflammation of all parts of the heart (endocardium, myocardium, pericardium). The carditis characteristically leads to thickened and deformed valves and to small perivascular granulomas in the myocardium (Aschoff bodies) which are finally replaced by scar tissue. Erythrocyte sedimentation rates, C-reactive protein, electrocardiograms, and other tests are used to estimate rheumatic activity.

Rheumatic fever has a marked tendency to be reactivated by recurrent streptococcal infections, whereas nephritis does not have this characteristic. The first attack of rheumatic fever usually produces only slight cardiac damage, which, however, increases with each subsequent attack. It is therefore of the utmost importance to protect such patients from recurrent group A hemolytic streptococcal infections by prophylactic sulfonamide or penicillin administration.

In rabbits, repeated skin infections with several types of hemolytic streptococci result in lesions closely resembling those of rheumatic fever in man. In man there is no definite association of selected types of group A streptococci with rheumatic activity.

Diagnostic Laboratory Tests

Specimens to be obtained depend upon the nature of the streptococcal infection. A throat swab, pus, or blood is commonly obtained for culture. Serum is obtained for antibody determinations, particularly antistreptolysin O titer.

A. Stained Smears: Smears from throat swabs or pus often show single cocci or pairs rather than definite chains. Cocci are sometimes gram-negative. If smears of pus show streptococci but cultures fail to grow, anaerobic organisms must be suspected.

Smears from broth cultures of throat swabs 2–3 hours old can be stained with fluorescent group A-specific antibody for the most rapid identification of group A streptococci in clinical disease or carriers.

B. Culture: For rapid identification, all specimens suspected of containing streptococci are cultured on blood agar plates. In addition, if anaerobes are suspected, suitable broth cultures and thioglycollate medium must be inoculated. Blood cultures will grow hemolytic group A streptococci (eg, in sepsis) within hours or a few days. However, because certain alpha-hemolytic streptococci or enterococci may grow very slowly, blood cultures in cases of suspected endocarditis should always be incubated for 2 weeks before being discarded as negative. Blood agar pour plates probably have no significant diagnostic advantages over surface-streaked plates, but incubation in 10% CO_2 often speeds hemolysis. While the degree and kind of hemolysis (and colonial appearance) are sometimes sufficient to place an organism in a definite group, serologic grouping and typing by means of precipitin tests in capillary tubes should be performed, whenever possible, for ultimate classification as well as for epidemiologic reasons. Streptococci belonging to group A may be presumptively identified by empirically determined amounts of bacitracin. A bacitracin disk containing 2 units strongly inhibits growth of group A streptococci.

C. Animal Inoculation: Many streptococci virulent for man are not virulent for laboratory animals. Animal injection is therefore of little help in diagnosis. Serologic tests usually are limited to antistreptolysin O determinations or "bactericidal" tests (see below).

Immunity

Resistance against streptococcal diseases is type-specific. Thus a host who has recovered from infection by one group A streptococcal type is relatively insusceptible to reinfection by the same type but fully susceptible to infection by another type. This resistance is associated with type-specific anti-M antibodies. These are demonstrated in the so-called "bactericidal test"

which exploits the fact that streptococci are rapidly killed after phagocytosis. M protein interferes with phagocytosis, but in the presence of type-specific antibody to M protein streptococci are killed by leukocytes. The changing patterns of streptococcal disease with increasing age suggest that in the course of infections by beta-hemolytic streptococci the general reactivity to all types is altered, with increasing localization and intensity of inflammatory response.

Immunity against the erythrogenic toxin is based on antitoxin in the blood. This antitoxin immunity protects against the rash of scarlet fever but has no effect on infection with streptococci. Antibody to streptolysin O (antistreptolysin) develops following infection but does not indicate immunity to infection. High titers indicate recent or repeated infections and are found more frequently in rheumatic individuals than those with uncomplicated streptococcal infections.

Treatment

Antibiotics have radically changed the prognosis of all types of streptococcal infections. Adequate early treatment with the antibiotic of choice usually leads to recovery.

All beta-hemolytic group A streptococci are sensitive to penicillin G, and for this reason antibiotic sensitivity tests are superfluous. Alpha-hemolytic streptococci and enterococci, on the other hand, vary widely in their susceptibility to chemotherapeutic agents. Particularly in bacterial endocarditis, antibiotic sensitivity tests are essential to determine which drugs (and in what dosage) may be used for optimal therapy. In these cases, laboratory tests should include determinations of both inhibitory and killing power of drugs or drug combinations. Streptomycin or kanamycin often enhances the action of penicillin in killing streptococci, especially enterococci.

Antimicrobial drugs have no effect on established glomerulonephritis and rheumatic fever. However, in acute streptococcal infections, every effort must be made to eradicate streptococci from the patient, eliminate the antigenic stimulus, and thus prevent poststreptococcal disease. Antimicrobial drugs are also very useful in the prevention or early treatment of reinfection with beta-hemolytic group A streptococci in rheumatic subjects.

Anti-erythrogenic antitoxin has been of doubtful value in the treatment of scarlet fever.

Epidemiology, Prevention, & Control

A number of streptococci (viridans streptococci, enterococci, etc) are members of the normal flora of the human body. They produce disease only when established in parts of the body where they do not normally occur (eg, heart valves). To prevent such accidents, particularly in the course of surgical procedures on the respiratory, gastrointestinal, and urinary tracts which result in temporary bacteremia, antimicrobial agents are often administered prophylactically to persons with known heart valve deformity.

For group A beta-hemolytic streptococci, the ultimate source is always a person harboring these organisms. Such an individual may have a demonstrable or subclinical infection, or he may be a permanent carrier. He may distribute streptococci directly to other persons via droplets from the respiratory tract or skin; he may infect clothing, bedding, and utensils; or he may even infect an intermediate, eg, the udder of a cow, whose milk subsequently causes epidemic spread of streptococci. The nasal discharges of a person harboring hemolytic streptococci appear to be the most dangerous source of massive contamination of the environment. Lancefield grouping and typing of group A beta-hemolytic streptococci is a valuable epidemiologic tool for determining the transmission of infection.

Control procedures are directed against the human source and the contaminated environment. Oiling of blankets and floors diminishes the spread of contaminated dust. Ventilation, air filtration, ultraviolet irradiation, and aerosol mists all reduce the frequency of infectious droplets in the air. Milk should always be pasteurized.

Because of the great difficulty of controlling environmental contamination, increasing emphasis has been placed on the following: (1) Eradication of beta-hemolytic streptococci in carriers, when possible, and their elimination from places where they could cause particular damage, eg, obstetric delivery rooms. (2) Early, intensive chemotherapy of streptococcal respiratory infections. (3) Antistreptococcal chemoprophylaxis in persons who have had an attack of rheumatic fever.

Although streptococci are readily suppressed during therapy with penicillin or other antibiotics in chronic carriers, their permanent elimination is not always easy. Such carriers must therefore be removed from danger spots, eg, surgical services in hospitals, children's nurseries.

It has been found that prompt eradication of streptococci from persons with an acute respiratory infection, eg, "strep throat," will effectively prevent the development of poststreptococcal disease. Immediate and prolonged (10 days) penicillin therapy has been shown to prevent the development of rheumatic fever in soldiers suffering from streptococcal pharyngitis. It also suppresses the development of specific antibodies.

The first attack of rheumatic fever infrequently results in significant heart damage. However, such persons are particularly susceptible to streptococcal reinfections, which precipitate relapses of rheumatic activity and give rise to cardiac damage. It is therefore of the greatest importance to protect rheumatic subjects, especially children, from reinfection with hemolytic streptococci. This can be accomplished best by administration of penicillin, which effectively prevents the establishment of streptococci in the body. This chemoprophylaxis has to be continued for years to be maximally effective. No chemoprophylaxis is used for glomerulonephritis because of the small number of nephritogenic types and strains of streptococci.

THE PNEUMOCOCCI

The pneumococci are gram-positive diplococci, often lancet-shaped or arranged in chains, possessing a capsule of polysaccharide which permits easy "typing" with specific antisera. They can be lysed by surface-active agents, eg, bile salts. The organisms are normal inhabitants of the upper respiratory tract of man and can cause pneumonia, sinusitis, otitis, meningitis, and other infectious processes.

Morphology & Identification

A. Typical Organisms: The typical gram-positive, lancet-shaped diplococci (see below) are often seen in specimens of young cultures. In sputum or pus, single cocci or chains are also seen. With age, the organisms rapidly become gram-negative and tend to lyse spontaneously.

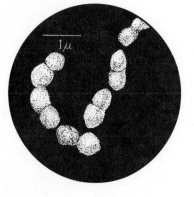

FIG 14—5. Drawing from electron micrograph of pneumococci.

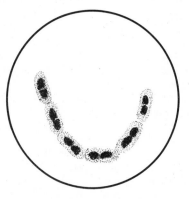

FIG 14—6. Pneumocci in stained smear.

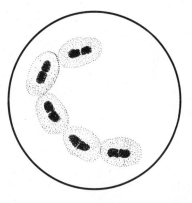

FIG 14—7. Pneumococci mixed with type-specific antiserum (quellung reaction).

Autolysis of pneumococci is greatly enhanced by surface-active agents. Lysis of pneumococci occurs in a few minutes when ox bile (10%) or sodium deoxycholate (2%) is added to a broth culture or suspension of organisms at neutral pH, or when optochin (ethylhydrocupreine hydrochloride, 1:4000) is added to solid media. Viridans streptococci do not lyse. Reliable differentiation between pneumococci and other streptococci can be produced by this "bile solubility test"; this is better than various fermentation reactions (eg, inulin), and important for identification of pneumococci.

B. Culture: Pneumococci form a small round colony, at first dome-shaped and later developing a central plateau with an elevated rim and alpha-hemolysis on blood agar. Routinely they are best grown in meat-infusion blood broth. Ten percent CO_2 aids growth.

Other identifying points include almost uniform virulence for mice when injected intraperitoneally and the "capsule swelling test" or quellung reaction (see below).

C. Growth Characteristics: Most energy is obtained from fermentation of glucose, accompanied by the rapid production of lactic acid, which limits growth. Therefore, neutralization with alkali at intervals results in massive growth.

D. Variation: Any culture (bacterial population) of pneumococci contains a few organisms unable to produce capsular polysaccharide, which gives rise to rough colonies. However, the majority are polysaccharide-producing bacteria, which give rise to smooth colonies. Rough forms can be made to predominate if the culture is grown in type-specific antipolysaccharide serum.

E. Transformation: When a rough (polysaccharide-less) organism of one type is grown in the presence of deoxyribonucleic acid (transforming principle) from another pneumococcus type, smooth cells of the latter type are formed. Similar transformation reactions have been performed which involve changes in drug resistance.

Antigenic Structure

A. Component Structures: The capsular polysaccharide (SSS = specific soluble substance) is immunologically distinct for each of the more than 85 types.

The somatic portion of the pneumococcus contains an M protein which is characteristic for each type and a C carbohydrate which is common to all pneumococci. The C carbohydrate can be precipitated by C-reactive protein, a substance found in the serum of certain patients (see Chapter 24).

B. Quellung Reaction: When pneumococci of a certain type are mixed with an antiserum against that type (specific antipolysaccharide serum) on a microscopic slide, the capsule swells markedly. This reaction is useful for quick identification and for "typing" of the organisms. (See Fig 14–7.)

Pathogenesis

A. Types of Pneumococci: In adults, types I–VIII are responsible for about 80% of cases of pneumococcal pneumonia and for more than half of all fatalities in pneumococcal bacteremia; in children, type XIV is the most frequent cause.

B. Production of Disease: Pneumococci produce disease through their ability to multiply in the tissues. They produce no toxins of significance. The "virulence" of the organism is a function of its capsule, which prevents or delays ingestion of encapsulated cells by phagocytes. A serum which contains antibodies against the type-specific polysaccharide (SSS) protects against infection. If such a serum is absorbed with SSS it loses its protective power. Animals or humans immunized with a given type SSS are subsequently immune to that type and possess precipitating antibodies for that type SSS.

C. Loss of Natural Resistance: Since 40–70% of humans are at some time or other carriers of virulent pneumococci, the normal respiratory mucosa must possess great natural resistance to the pneumococcus. Among the factors that probably lower this resistance and thus predispose to pneumococcal infection are the following:

1. Abnormalities of the respiratory tract—Other infections (eg, viral) which damage surface cells; abnormal accumulations of mucus (eg, allergy), which protects pneumococci from phagocytosis; bronchial obstruction (eg, atelectasis); and respiratory tract injury due to irritating gas or other cause.

2. Alcoholic intoxication, which depresses phagocytic activity, depresses the cough reflex, and facilitates aspiration of foreign material.

3. Abnormal circulatory dynamics (eg, pulmonary congestion).

4. Malnutrition and general debility.

Pathology

Pneumococcal infection causes an outpouring of fibrinous edema fluid into the alveoli, followed by red cells and leukocytes, which results in consolidation of portions of the lung. Many pneumococci are found throughout this exudate. The alveolar walls remain normally intact during the infection. Later, mononuclear cells actively phagocytize the debris, and this liquid phase is gradually reabsorbed. The pneumococci are taken up by phagocytes and digested intracellularly.

Clinical Findings

The onset of pneumococcal pneumonia is usually sudden, with fever, chills, and sharp pleural pain. The sputum is similar to the alveolar exudate, being characteristically bloody or rusty. Early in the disease, when the fever is high, bacteremia is present in at least 25% of cases. Before the days of chemotherapy, recovery from the disease began between the fifth and tenth days and was associated with the development of type-specific antibodies. With antimicrobial therapy, the illness is terminated promptly; if drugs are given early, the development of consolidation is interrupted.

From the respiratory tract, pneumococci may reach other sites. The sinuses and middle ear are most frequently involved. From the blood stream (or through extension from the mastoid), the meninges are reached. With the early use of chemotherapy, acute pneumococcal endocarditis has become rare. Pneumococcal pneumonia must be differentiated from pulmonary infarct, atelectasis, neoplasm, and congestive heart failure. Empyema is the commonest complication and requires aspiration and drainage.

Diagnostic Laboratory Tests

Blood is drawn for culture, and sputum is collected for demonstration of pneumococci by smear and culture. It is impractical to test serum for antibodies.

Sputum may be examined in several ways:

(1) **Stained smears**: Gram-stained film of rusty-red sputum shows typical organisms.

(2) **Capsule swelling tests**: Fresh emulsified sputum mixed with antiserum gives "capsule swelling" for type identification (if specific antiserum is available).

(3) **Culture**: Sputum cultured on blood agar in candle jar.

(4) **Injection of sputum intraperitoneally into white mice**: Animals die in 18–48 hours; heart blood gives pure culture of pneumococci. Peritoneal exudate can be used for quellung reaction.

(5) **Pneumococcal meningitis** may be occasionally diagnosed by demonstrating pneumococcal polysaccharide (SSS) by precipitation with specific antiserum in the spinal fluid, especially when cultures are negative.

Immunity

Immunity to infection with pneumococci is type-specific, incomplete, and of uncertain duration.

Treatment

Type-specific antiserum was formerly administered intravenously to patients who lacked antibodies. Absence of antibodies was determined by the absence of reaction upon intradermal injection of type-specific polysaccharide (Francis test).

Since pneumococci are sensitive to many antimicrobial drugs, early treatment results in rapid recovery, and antibody response seems to play a much diminished role. The penicillins are the drugs of choice. Recently, some drug resistance has appeared: Pneumococci resistant to tetracyclines, erythromycin, and lincomycin have been isolated from patients.

Epidemiology, Prevention, & Control

Pneumococcal pneumonia accounts for ± 80% of all bacterial pneumonias. It is an endemic disease with a high incidence of carriers. The predisposing factors (see above) are more important in the development of illness than exposure to the infectious agent, and the healthy carrier is more important in disseminating infection than the sick patient.

It is possible to immunize individuals with type-specific polysaccharides. However, this may remain impractical. Reliance is placed on the avoidance of "predisposing" factors, prompt diagnosis, and early and adequate chemotherapy. At present, fatalities (5%) from pneumococcal pneumonia are limited to the very young (infants) and the very old, or persons with impaired natural resistance.

THE NEISSERIAE

The neisseriae are a group of gram-negative cocci, usually occurring in pairs. Some members of the group are normal inhabitants of the human respiratory tract and occur extracellularly; others (gonococci, meningococci) are human pathogens and typically occur intracellularly.

Morphology & Identification

A. Typical Organisms: The typical neisseria organism is a gram-negative diplococcus, approximately 0.8 μm in diameter. Neisseriae are nonmotile and nonsporeforming. Individual cocci are kidney-shaped, with the flat or concave sides adjacent. Older cultures or those exposed to antibiotics may contain swollen, distorted organisms. Meningococci and gonococci autolyze quickly, particularly in an alkaline environment.

B. Culture: In 48 hours on enriched media, gonococci and meningococci form convex, glistening, elevated, creamy, mucoid colonies 1–5 mm in diameter. Colonies are transparent, nonpigmented or yellowish, and nonhemolytic. *N flavescens* and *N flava* have a yellowish pigment and are less mucoid. *N sicca* produces opaque, brittle, wrinkled colonies.

C. Growth Characteristics: Neisseriae are strict aerobes. They ferment a variety of carbohydrates, forming acid but not gas. Fermentation reactions are summarized in Table 14–1.

Meningococci and gonococci grow best on media containing complex organic substances such as blood or animal proteins and in an atmosphere containing 10% CO_2 (eg, candle jar). They are easily inhibited by toxic constituents of the medium, such as fatty acids or salts. They are rapidly killed by drying, sunlight, moist heat, and by most disinfectants and chemotherapeutic substances. They produce indophenol oxidase and autolytic enzymes which result in rapid swelling and dissolution of cultures. This process can be inhibited by cyanide or by heating at 65° C for 30 minutes.

NEISSERIA MENINGITIDIS
(*N Intracellularis*, Meningococcus)

Antigenic Structure

By agglutination and agglutinin-absorption tests, meningococci can be classified into 4 main groups,

TABLE 14–1. Fermentation reactions of neisseriae.

	Acid Formed From			Growth on
	Dextrose	Maltose	Sucrose	Plain Nutrient Agar
N meningitidis (meningococcus)	+	+	–	–
N gonorrhoeae (gonococcus)	+	–	–	–
N catarrhalis	–	–	–	+
N sicca	+	+	+	+
N flavescens	–	–	–	+

designated as 1 (A), 2 (B), 2a (C), and 4 (D). Most strains isolated during epidemics fall into group 1 (A), whereas the majority of strains from sporadic cases during interepidemic periods fall into groups 2 and 2a (B and C). Outbreaks of sulfonamide-resistant meningococci were mostly group 2 (B), but also groups 1 (A) and 2a (C). Polysaccharides specific for groups A, B, and C have been isolated and characterized. The nucleoproteins of meningococci (P substance) account for the toxic effect but are not specific for these organisms. Certain nucleic acid extracts are capable of "transformation reactions," inducing streptomycin resistance in meningococci. The composition of cell walls of meningococci resembles that of coliforms; they contain a group-reactive antigen.

Pathogenesis, Pathology, & Clinical Findings

Man is the only natural host for whom meningococci are pathogenic. Mice can be infected intraperitoneally if meningococci are suspended in mucin. The mouse virulence of meningococci is not related to serologic type.

The nasopharynx is the portal of entry of meningococci. There the organisms may cause a local infection or may form part of the transient flora without producing symptoms. From the nasopharynx, organisms reach the blood stream, producing a bacteremia (meningococcemia) with high fever, sepsis, and a hemorrhagic rash. There may be fulminant sepsis, with hemorrhages into the adrenals, and circulatory collapse (Waterhouse-Friderichsen syndrome).

Meningitis is the commonest complication of meningococcemia. It usually begins very suddenly, with intense headache, vomiting, and stiff neck, and progresses to coma within a few hours.

Meningococci in the nasopharynx usually produce no lesions but may produce an exudative pharyngitis. During meningococcemia there is thrombosis of many small blood vessels in many organs, with perivascular infiltration and petechial hemorrhages. In meningitis the meninges are acutely inflamed, with thrombosis of blood vessels and exudation of polymorphonuclear leukocytes so that the surface of the brain is covered with a thick purulent exudate. There may be interstitial myocarditis.

It is not known what transforms an asymptomatic infection of the nasopharynx into meningitis, but this can be prevented by specific bactericidal serum antibodies against the infecting strain. Meningococci are readily phagocytosed in the presence of a specific opsonin.

Diagnostic Laboratory Tests

Specimens of blood are taken for culture, and of spinal fluid for smear, culture, and chemical determinations. Nasopharyngeal swab cultures are suitable for carrier surveys. Puncture material from petechiae may be taken for smear and culture.

A. Smears: Gram's or methylene blue stains of the sediment of centrifuged spinal fluid or of petechial aspirate often show typical diplococci within polymorphonuclear leukocytes or extracellularly. Because meningococci may autolyze rapidly, the fluid must be examined fresh.

B. Culture: Specimens must be promptly plated on heated blood agar (chocolate agar) or Thayer-Martin medium (Public Health Reports 79:49, 1964) and incubated at 37° C in an atmosphere of 5–10% CO_2 (candle jar). Thayer-Martin medium favors the growth of neisseriae and inhibits many other bacteria. Spinal fluid or blood generally yields pure cultures which can be further identified by carbohydrate fer-

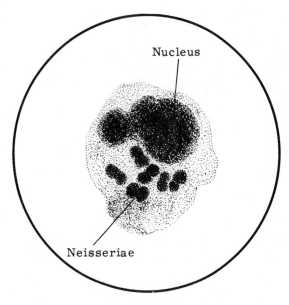

FIG 14–8. Meningococci within a polymorphonuclear leukocyte in spinal fluid.

mentation (dextrose +, maltose +, sucrose −) and agglutination with type-specific (or polyvalent) serum.

Direct incubation of freshly drawn spinal fluid at 37° C may give growth of meningococci. It is also possible to obtain rapid growth by inoculation of the yolk sac of 8- to 10-day-old embryonated eggs.

Colonies of meningococci on solid media, particularly in mixed culture, may be identified by the *oxidase test:* When the plate is sprayed with tetramethylparaphenylenediamine hydrochloride, meningococcus colonies rapidly turn dark. (Other neisseriae behave similarly.)

C. Serology: Agglutinins for meningococci can be estimated some time after infection, but this is rarely done.

Immunity

Immunity to meningococcal infection is associated with the presence of specific bactericidal antibodies in the serum. These antibodies develop after subclinical infections with different strains, or injection of polysaccharides. Infants have passive immunity through IgG antibodies transferred from the mother.

Treatment

Meningococci formerly were uniformly susceptible to sulfonamides, and these were the drugs of choice. Recently, sulfonamide-resistant meningococci have become prevalent. Penicillin G is now the drug of choice. Antimeningococcus serum is no longer employed therapeutically.

Epidemiology, Prevention, & Control

Meningococcal meningitis occurs in epidemic waves and a smaller number of sporadic interepidemic cases. Five to 30% of the normal population may harbor meningococci in the nasopharynx during interepidemic periods. During epidemics the carrier rate goes up to 70 or 80%. A rise in the number of cases is always preceded by an increased number of respiratory "carriers." In the past, widespread chemoprophylaxis with sulfonamides was successful. Since the appearance of many sulfonamide-resistant meningococci, this is no longer possible. Treatment with penicillin or other drugs suppresses meningococci in the nasopharynx but does not eradicate the carrier state. Rifampin may accomplish the latter.

Clinical cases of meningitis present only a negligible source of infection, and isolation has therefore only limited usefulness. More important is the reduction of personal contacts in a population with a high "carrier" rate. This is accomplished by good ventilation and avoidance of crowding. Specific polysaccharides of groups 1 (A) and 2a (C) can stimulate antibody response and protect susceptibles against infection.

NEISSERIA GONORRHOEAE
(Gonococcus)

Morphologically and culturally, the gonococcus resembles the meningococcus; however, it does not ferment maltose.

Antigenic Structure

Gonococci are serologically heterogeneous, although many freshly isolated strains appear to fall into one group. Gonococci possess polysaccharides and nucleoproteins which are similar to those of other neisseriae. Agglutination tests and complement fixation tests are therefore not wholly specific.

Pathogenesis, Pathology, & Clinical Findings

Gonococci attack mucous membranes of the genitourinary tract and the eye, producing acute suppuration which may lead to tissue invasion; this is followed by chronic inflammation and fibrosis. In the male there is usually urethritis, with yellow, creamy pus and painful urination. The process may extend to the prostate and epididymis. As suppuration subsides, there is fibrosis, sometimes leading to urethral strictures. In the female the infection extends from urethra and vagina to cervix, giving rise to mucopurulent discharge. It may then progress to the fallopian tubes, causing pelvic inflammatory disease, fibrosis, and obliteration of tubes with consequent sterility. Chronic gonococcal cervicitis is often asymptomatic.

Blood stream invasion is very rare, and suppurative gonorrheal arthritis uncommon. Ophthalmia neonatorum, an infection of the eye of the newborn, is acquired during passage through an infected birth canal. The initial conjunctivitis rapidly progresses to involve all structures of the eye and commonly results in blindness. To avoid this disaster, the instillation of silver nitrate or penicillin into the conjunctival sac of the newborn has been made compulsory.

Diagnostic Laboratory Tests

Pus and secretions are taken from the urethra, cervix, prostate, and occasionally the rectal mucosa or synovial fluid for culture and smear.

A. Stained Smears: In the acute process Gram's or methylene blue stains of smears reveal many intracellular diplococci within pus cells. These give a presumptive diagnosis. In the later, chronic stages, when the secretions are thinner and contain few pus cells, gonococci are often difficult to find and reliance must be placed on culture. Immunofluorescent staining of smears is more efficient than other stains.

B. Cultures: Immediately after collection, pus or mucus is streaked on plasma hemoglobin agar, infusion chocolate agar, or Thayer-Martin medium and incubated in an atmosphere containing 10% CO_2 (candle jar) at 37° C. Forty-eight hours later, colonies are subjected to the oxidase test (see above). Subcultures of the organisms may be subjected to fermentation reactions (Table 14—1). The gonococcus fails to ferment maltose, and dextrose is the only sugar from which acid is produced.

C. Serology: Complement fixation tests are sometimes performed on persons with negative cultures who are suspected of harboring chronic gonococcal infection. These tests, however, lack specificity and reliability. Antibodies detected by immunofluorescence are promising in gonococcal arthritis.

Immunity

Immunity to gonococci does not develop in the course of infection.

Treatment

Local irrigation of the urethra has little effect. While many strains of gonococci are now resistant to sulfonamides, most strains are still susceptible to penicillin. Two injections of 2.4 million units of procaine penicillin generally result in cure. Recently, strains of gonococci which require 2 units of penicillin per ml for inhibition have been encountered, and some cases of gonorrhea caused by such organisms have failed to respond to the above doses of penicillin. In such instances (or because of hypersensitivity to penicillin), other antibiotics, eg, tetracyclines or erythromycin, can be used. In established chronic infection (prostatitis, cervicitis), prostatic massage may be necessary to open walled-off abscesses, and penicillin, 4.8 million units daily for 10 days, is given.

While antimicrobial therapy usually leads to complete and prompt disappearance of symptoms, cure must be established by repeated cultures. Because syphilis may have been acquired simultaneously, treatment and follow-up must be planned accordingly.

Epidemiology, Prevention, & Control

Gonorrhea is worldwide in distribution, and its incidence has risen steadily since 1955. It is almost exclusively transmitted by sexual contact, principally from women harboring asymptomatic chronic infections. The infectivity of the organism is not very high; experimental inoculation of cultures into volunteers resulted in only 30% infections. The infection rate can be reduced by reduction in sexual promiscuity; rapid eradication of gonococci from infected individuals by means of early diagnosis and treatment; finding of cases and contacts through education and health organizations; and venereal prophylaxis. Mechanical prophylaxis (condoms) is adequate for protection but is rarely employed by individuals having the greatest exposure. Chemoprophylaxis (400,000 units penicillin by mouth immediately prior to or after sexual exposure) can reduce the infection rate.

Ophthalmia neonatorum is prevented by the local application to the conjunctiva of the newborn of a substance bactericidal for gonococci on contact. One percent silver nitrate and penicillin ointment are equally effective.

OTHER NEISSERIAE

N catarrhalis and *N sicca* are normal members of the flora of the respiratory tract, particularly the nasopharynx, and do not produce disease. The pigmented neisseriae (*N flava, N flavescens*) occupy a similar position, but these organisms may on rare occasions cause meningitis or endocarditis.

●   ●   ●

General References

Anderson, M., & others: Lincomycin and penicillin in pneumococcal pneumonia. Am Rev Resp Dis 97:914—918, 1968.

Duma, R.J., & others: Streptococcal infections. Medicine 48:87—128, 1969.

Gotschlich, E., & others: Human immunity to meningococcus. J Exper Med 129:1307—1385, 1969.

Jewett, J.F., & others: Childbed fever. JAMA 206:344—350, 1968.

Kampmeier, R.H.: The rise of venereal diseases. M Clin North America 51:735—751, 1967.

15...
Gram-Positive Bacilli

AEROBIC SPOREFORMING BACILLI

ANTHRAX

The genus Bacillus includes large gram-positive rods occurring in chains. They form spores and are strict aerobes. Most members of this genus are saprophytic organisms prevalent in soil, water, air, and on vegetation, such as *Bacillus cereus* and *B subtilis*. Such saprophytes very rarely produce disease in man (eg, meningitis or endocarditis). *B anthracis* is the principal pathogen of the genus.

Morphology & Identification

A. Typical Organisms: The typical cells, measuring $1 \times 3{-}4$ μm, are arranged in long chains; spores are located in the center of the nonmotile bacilli.

B. Culture: Colonies are round and have a "cut glass" appearance in transmitted light. Hemolysis is uncommon with anthrax but common with the saprophytic bacilli. Gelatin is liquefied, and growth in gelatin stabs resembles an "inverted fir tree."

C. Growth Characteristics: The saprophytic bacilli utilize simple sources of nitrogen and carbon for energy and growth. The spores are resistant to environ-

mental changes, withstand dry heat and certain chemical disinfectants for moderate periods, and persist for years in dry earth. Animal products contaminated with anthrax spores (eg, hides, bristles, hair) can be sterilized by autoclaving.

D. Variation: Variation occurs with respect to virulence, spore formation, and colony form. (In general, virulence is associated with rough colonies.) To minimize variation, living spore suspensions are employed to preserve unstable properties such as virulence.

Antigenic Structure

The capsular substance of *B anthracis*, which consists of a polypeptide of high molecular weight composed of D-glutamic acid, is a hapten. The bacterial bodies contain protein and a somatic polysaccharide, both of which have antigenic properties.

Pathogenesis

Anthrax is primarily a disease of sheep, cattle, and horses; man is affected only rarely. The infection is usually acquired by the entry of spores through injured skin or mucous membranes, rarely by inhalation of spores into the lung. In animals the portal of entry is the mouth and gastrointestinal tract. The spores from contaminated soil find easy access when ingested with spiny or irritating vegetation. In humans, scratches in the skin favor infection.

The spores germinate in the tissue at the site of entry, and the growth of the vegetative organisms results in formation of a gelatinous edema and congestion. Bacilli spread via lymphatics to the blood stream, and bacteria multiply freely in the blood and tissues shortly before and after the death of the animal. In the plasma of animals dying from anthrax a lethal factor has been demonstrated. This material kills mice or guinea pigs upon inoculation and is specifically neutralized by anthrax antiserum. Its nature is still uncertain.

The exudate in anthrax contains a polypeptide, identical with that in the capsule of the bacillus, which is able to evoke histologic reactions similar to those of anthrax infection. Other proteins isolated from exudate stimulate solid immunity to anthrax upon injection into animals. From culture filtrates ("anthrax toxin"), 3 substances have been separated by glass filtration and chromatography: (1) "protective antigen" (a protein), (2) "edema factor," and (3) "lethal factor." Mixtures of (1), (2), and (3) are

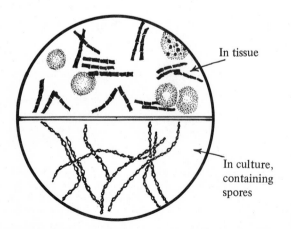

FIG 15-1. Anthrax bacilli in a smear from tissue or culture.

In tissue

In culture, containing spores

more toxic in animals, and such mixtures are more immunogenic than single substances.

Pathology

In susceptible animals the organisms proliferate at the site of entry. The capsules remain intact, and the organisms are surrounded by a large amount of proteinaceous fluid containing few leukocytes from which they rapidly disseminate and reach the blood stream.

In resistant animals the organisms proliferate for a few hours, by which time there is massive accumulation of leukocytes. The capsules gradually disintegrate and disappear. The organisms remain localized.

Clinical Findings

In man anthrax gives rise to an infection of the skin (malignant pustule). A papule first develops within 12–36 hours after entry of the organisms or spores through a scratch. This papule rapidly changes into a vesicle, then a pustule, and finally into a necrotic ulcer from which the infection may disseminate, giving rise to septicemia. Another type of disease, a primary pneumonia, results from inhalation of spores from the dust of wool, hides, and hair ("woolsorter's disease").

Diagnostic Laboratory Tests

A. Specimens: Fluid or pus from local lesion; blood, sputum.

B. Stained Smears: From the local lesion or blood of dead animals; chains of large gram-positive rods are often seen.

C. Culture: When grown on blood agar plates, the organisms produce nonhemolytic gray colonies with typical microscopic morphology. Carbohydrate fermentation is not useful. In semi-solid medium anthrax bacilli are always nonmotile, whereas related nonpathogenic organisms (*B cereus*) exhibit motility by "swarming." Virulent anthrax cultures kill mice upon intraperitoneal injection.

D. Ascoli Test: Extracts of infected tissues show a ring of precipitate when layered over immune serum.

E. Serologic Tests: These are of little value at the present time.

Resistance & Immunity

Some animals are highly susceptible (guinea pig) and others are very resistant (rat) to anthrax infection. This fact has been attributed to a variety of defense mechanisms: leukocytic activity, body temperature, and the bactericidal action of the blood. Certain basic polypeptides which kill anthrax bacilli have been isolated from animal tissues. A synthetic polylysine has a similar action.

Active immunity to anthrax can be induced in susceptible animals by vaccination with live attenuated bacilli, with spore suspensions, or with protective antigens from culture filtrates (see above). Immune serum is sometimes injected, together with live bacilli, into animals. Anthrax immunization is based on the classical experiments of Louis Pasteur, who in 1881 proved that cultures which had been grown in broth at 42–52° C for several months lost much of their virulence and could be injected live into sheep and cattle without causing disease; subsequently, such animals proved to be immune. There are great variations in the efficacy of various vaccines, and protection is often far from complete or lasting.

Treatment

Many antibiotics are effective against anthrax in man, but treatment must be started early. Penicillin in moderate doses is satisfactory.

Epidemiology, Prevention, & Control

Soil is contaminated with anthrax spores from the carcasses of dead animals. These spores remain viable for decades. Grazing animals, infected through injured mucous membranes, serve to perpetuate the chain of infection. Contact with infected animals or with their hides, hair, and bristles is the source of infection in man. Control measures include (1) disposal of animal carcasses by burning or by deep burial in lime pits, (2) decontamination (usually by autoclaving) of animal products, (3) the use of protective clothing and gloves when handling potentially infected materials, and (4) active immunization of domestic animals and of persons with high occupational risk.

ANAEROBIC SPOREFORMING BACILLI

THE CLOSTRIDIA

The clostridia are anaerobic, gram-positive rods which form spores. Many decompose proteins or form toxins, and some do both. Their natural habitat is the soil or the intestinal tract of animals and man. Most species are saprophytic organisms in the soil. Among the pathogens are the organisms causing botulism, tetanus, and gas gangrene.

Morphology & Identification

A. Typical Organisms: All species of clostridia are large, gram-positive rods, and all can produce spores. The spores are usually wider than the diameter of the rods in which they are formed. In *Cl tetani* the spore is located at one end of the rod, giving it a drumstick appearance. In the various species the spore is placed centrally, subterminally, or terminally. Most species are motile and possess peritrichous flagella.

B. Culture: Clostridia grow only under anaerobic conditions, established by one of the following means:

1. Agar plates or culture tubes are placed in an airtight jar from which air is removed and replaced by nitrogen with 10% CO_2, or oxygen may be removed by other means.

2. Fluid media in deep tubes containing either fresh animal tissue (eg, chopped meat), or 0.1% agar and a reducing agent such as thioglycollate. Such tubes can be handled like aerobic media, and growth will occur from the bottom up to within 15 mm of the surface exposed to air.

C. Colony Forms: Some organisms produce large raised colonies with entire margins (eg, *Cl perfringens*); others produce smaller colonies which extend in a meshwork of fine filaments (eg, *Cl tetani*). Most species produce a zone of hemolysis on blood agar.

D. Growth Characteristics: The outstanding characteristic of anaerobic bacilli is their inability to utilize oxygen as the final hydrogen acceptor. They lack cytochrome and cytochrome oxidase and are unable to break down hydrogen peroxide because they lack catalase and peroxidase. Therefore it has been suggested that hydrogen peroxide tends to accumulate to toxic concentrations in the presence of oxygen. It has been postulated that such anaerobes can carry out their metabolic reactions only at a negative oxidation-reduction potential (Eh), ie, in an environment which is strongly reducing.

Clostridia can ferment a variety of sugars; many can digest proteins. Milk is turned acid by some, digested by others, and undergoes "stormy fermentation" (ie, clot torn by gas) with a third group (eg, *Cl perfringens*). Various enzymes are produced by different species (see below).

E. Antigenic Characteristics: Clostridia share antigens but also possess specific soluble antigens which permit grouping by means of precipitin tests.

CLOSTRIDIUM BOTULINUM

This microorganism is worldwide in distribution; it is found in soil, and occasionally in animal feces.

Types of *Cl botulinum* are distinguished by the antigenic type of toxin they produce. Spores of the organism are highly resistant to heat, withstanding 100° C for at least 3–5 hours. Heat resistance is diminished at acid pH or high salt concentration.

Toxin

During the growth of *Cl botulinum* and during autolysis of the bacteria, toxin is liberated into the environment. Six distinct antigenic varieties of toxin— A, B, C, D, E, and F—are known. Types A, B, and E are most commonly associated with human illness. Type C produces limberneck in fowl; type D, botulism in cattle. Type A, B, and E toxins have been purified and fractionated to yield toxic peptides with a molecular weight of about 150,000. These are among the most highly toxic substances known: One mg contains approximately 20 million mouse lethal doses. The lethal dose for man is not known but is probably less than 1 μg. The toxins are destroyed by heating for 10 minutes at 100° C.

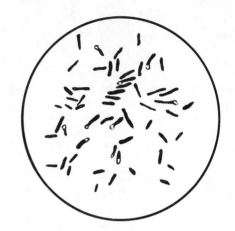

FIG 15–2. *Cl botulinum* from broth grown under anaerobic conditions.

Pathogenesis

While *Cl botulinum* types A and B have been implicated in a few rare cases of wound infection, they generally do not produce infection in man. Botulism is an intoxication resulting from the ingestion of food in which *Cl botulinum* has grown and produced toxin. The most common offenders are spiced, smoked, or home canned alkaline foods which are eaten without cooking. In such foods, spores of *Cl botulinum* germinate; under anaerobic conditions vegetative forms grow and produce toxin.

The toxin probably acts by blocking acetylcholine release or production at the neuromuscular junction.

Clinical Findings

Symptoms begin 18–96 hours after ingestion of the toxic food, with visual disturbances (incoordination of eye muscles, double vision), inability to swallow, and speech difficulty; signs of bulbar paralysis are progressive, and death occurs from respiratory paralysis or cardiac arrest. Gastrointestinal symptoms are not prominent. There is no fever. The patient remains fully conscious until shortly before death. The fatality rate is high. Patients who recover do not develop antitoxin in the blood.

Diagnostic Laboratory Tests

Specimens from the patient are rarely useful. Occasionally toxin can be demonstrated in serum. The proof of diagnosis rests on the demonstration of the toxin in leftover food. Mice injected intraperitoneally die rapidly. The antigenic type of toxin is identified by neutralization with specific antitoxin. Mice protected with a specific type of antitoxin survive injection of that toxin, while controls not so protected die. *Cl botulinum* may be grown from food remains and tested for toxin production, but this is rarely done and is of questionable significance. Botulinus toxin can occasionally be demonstrated in food by agglutination of red cells coated with specific antiserum.

Treatment

Potent antitoxins to the different types of botulism toxins have been prepared. Since the type responsible for an individual case is usually not known, polyvalent antitoxin, 80,000 units, is administered intravenously as early as possible. Patients are occasionally saved by this measure.

Epidemiology, Prevention, & Control

Since spores of *Cl botulinum* are widely distributed in soils, they often contaminate vegetables, fruits, and other materials. When such foods are canned or otherwise preserved, they must be either sufficiently heated to ensure destruction of spores or must be boiled before consumption. Strict regulation of commercial canning has largely overcome the danger of large outbreaks. At present the chief danger lies in home canned foods, particularly string beans, corn, spinach, olives, peas, and smoked fish or vacuum packed fresh fish in plastic bags. Toxic foods may be spoiled and rancid, and cans may "swell"; or the appearance may be innocuous. Home canned foods should be boiled for more than 10 minutes before consumption. Toxoids are used for active immunization of cattle in South Africa.

CLOSTRIDIUM TETANI

Cl tetani is worldwide in distribution in the soil and in the feces of horses and other animals. Several types of *Cl tetani* can be distinguished by specific flagellar antigens. All share a common O (somatic) antigen, which may be masked, and all produce the same toxin. L forms of *Cl tetani* also produce toxin.

Toxin

Good yields of toxin are obtained when the organism is grown in a semisynthetic medium containing

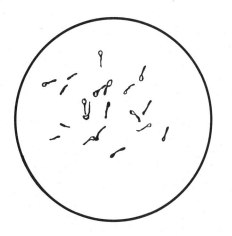

FIG 15–3. *Cl tetani* from blood agar grown under anaerobic conditions.

casein hydrolysate, tryptophan, cystein, phosphates, trace elements, and growth factors, provided the concentration of iron is held within sharp limits. The toxin is a heat-labile protein, being inactivated by 5 minutes' exposure to 65° C and rapidly destroyed by proteolytic enzymes, eg, of the digestive tract. Purified crystalline toxin contains more than 6 million mouse lethal doses per mg.

Pathogenesis

Cl tetani is not an invasive organism. The infection remains strictly localized in the area of devitalized tissue (wound, burn, injury, umbilical stump, surgical suture) into which the spores have been introduced. The volume of infected tissue is small, and the disease is almost entirely a toxemia. Germination of the spore and development of vegetative organisms which produce toxin are aided by (1) necrotic tissue, (2) calcium salts, and (3) associated pyogenic infections, all of which aid establishment of low oxidation-reduction potentials. The action of the toxin is partly on the nervous tissue in the spinal cord, increasing reflex excitability; and partly on peripheral nerves, resulting in muscle spasm (perhaps because of accumulation of acetylcholine at the motor nerve endings). The receptor for toxin in the CNS appears to be a water-soluble ganglioside which in tissue forms insoluble complexes with cerebrosides and sphingomyelins.

Clinical Findings

The incubation period may range from 4–5 days to as many weeks. The disease is characterized by convulsive tonic contraction of voluntary muscles. Muscular spasms often involve first the area of injury and infection and then the muscles of the jaw (trismus, lockjaw), which contract so that the mouth cannot be opened. Gradually, other voluntary muscles become involved, resulting in tonic spasms. Any external stimulus may precipitate a convulsion. Drug reaction to phenothiazine may simulate tetanus.

Diagnostic Laboratory Tests

In clinical cases diagnosis rests on the clinical picture and a history of injury. Anaerobic culture of tissues from contaminated wounds may yield *Cl tetani*, but neither preventive nor therapeutic use of antitoxin should ever be withheld pending such demonstration. Proof of isolation of *Cl tetani* must rest on production of toxin and its neutralization by specific antitoxin.

Treatment

A. Antitoxin: Prevention of tetanus depends upon (1) active immunization with toxoids, (2) proper care of wounds contaminated with soil, etc, (3) prophylactic use of antitoxin, and (4) administration of penicillin. Tetanus antitoxin, prepared in various animals or in man, can neutralize the toxin, but only before it becomes fixed onto nervous tissue. One International Unit of antitoxin is defined as 10 times the smallest amount of serum necessary to maintain life for 96 hours in a 350 gm guinea pig inoculated with a standard test dose of toxin furnished by the National Institutes of Health. One unit of tetanus antitoxin neutralizes about 1000 MLD of toxin.

Because of the frequency of hypersensitivity reactions to foreign serum, and because of the rapidity with which foreign serum is eliminated, the administration of human antitoxin is much preferable. The intramuscular administration of 250—500 units of human antitoxin probably gives adequate systemic protection (0.01 unit per ml of serum or more) for 2—4 weeks. Human tetanus-immune globulin is now commercially available. Only if human antitoxin is not available should heterologous (horse, sheep, rabbit) antitoxin be used in a prophylactic dose of 1500—6000 units. Whenever heterologous antitoxin is to be administered, tests for hypersensitivity to the foreign serum protein must be done. Active immunization with tetanus toxoid should always accompany antitoxin prophylaxis.

Patients who develop symptoms of tetanus sometimes are given very large doses of antitoxin intravenously in an effort to neutralize toxin which has not yet been bound to nervous tissue. However, the efficacy of antitoxin for treatment is doubtful except in neonatal tetanus, where it may be lifesaving.

B. Surgical Measures: Surgical debridement is vitally important because it removes the necrotic tissue which is essential for proliferation of the organisms. Hyperbaric oxygen has no proved effect.

C. Antibiotics: Penicillin strongly inhibits the growth of *Cl tetani* and stops further toxin production. Antibiotics may also control associated pyogenic infection.

D. "Booster" Shot: When a previously immunized individual sustains a potentially dangerous wound, an additional dose of toxoid may be injected to restimulate antitoxin production. This "recall" injection of toxoid may be accompanied by antitoxin injected into a different area of the body, to provide immediately available antitoxin for the period during which antitoxin levels may be inadequate.

Prevention & Control

Tetanus toxoid is produced by detoxifying the toxin with formalin and then concentrating it. Fluid toxoid or alum-precipitated toxoid is employed. Three injections comprise the initial course of immunization; this should be followed by a "booster" dose, about 1 year later, for longer lasting and higher blood levels of antitoxin. Initial immunization should be carried out in all children during the first year of life. A fifth injection of toxoid is given upon entry into school. Thereafter, "boosters" can be spaced 10 years apart to maintain serum levels of 0.01 unit antitoxin per ml. Tetanus toxoid is often combined with diphtheria toxoid and pertussis vaccine. (For schedule of immunizations, see Table 12—5.)

Control measures are not possible because of the wide dissemination of the organism in the soil and the long survival of its spores. Narcotic addicts are a high risk group.

THE CLOSTRIDIA OF GAS GANGRENE

The 3 most common species of clostridia to be found in gas gangrene are *Cl perfringens (Cl welchii), Cl novyi (Cl oedematiens),* and *Cl septicum.* In addition to these, other species are sometimes present in cases of gas gangrene, particularly *Cl bifermentans, Cl histolyticum,* and *Cl fallax.*

Toxins

The clostridia produce a large variety of toxins and enzymes which result in a spreading infection. *Cl perfringens, Cl novyi, Cl septicum, Cl histolyticum, Cl bifermentans,* and others produce specific toxins. Many of these toxins have lethal necrotizing and hemolytic properties. In some cases these are different properties of a single substance; in other instances they are due to different chemical entities. The alpha toxin of *Cl perfringens* type A is a lecithinase, and its lethal action is proportionate to the rate at which it splits lecithin (an important constituent of cell membranes) to phosphocholine and diglyceride. The theta toxin has similar hemolytic and necrotizing effects but is not a lecithinase. A collagenase which digests collagen of subcutaneous tissue and muscle, hyaluronidase, and DNase are also produced. Some gas gangrene clostridia produce a specific nontoxic antigen ("bursting factor") which enhances infectivity and can immunize animals to gas gangrene.

Pathogenesis

If necrotic tissue is present, gas gangrene develops following the introduction into a wound of soil or fecal matter containing spores. As the organisms multiply, they ferment carbohydrates present in tissue and produce gas. The distention of tissue and interference with blood supply, together with the secretion of necrotizing toxin and hyaluronidase, favor the spread of infection. Tissue necrosis extends, providing an opportunity for increased bacterial growth, hemolytic anemia, and, ultimately, severe toxemia and death.

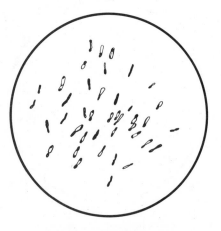

FIG 15—4. Gas gangrene bacilli.

In gas gangrene a mixed infection is the rule. In addition to the toxigenic clostridia, proteolytic clostridia and various cocci and gram-negative organisms are also usually present. *Cl perfringens* occurs in the genital tract of 5% of normal women. Clostridial uterine infections may follow instrumental abortions. Clostridial bacteremia is frequent in patients with neoplasms.

Clinical Findings

From a contaminated wound (eg, a compound fracture, postpartum uterus), the infection spreads in 1–3 days to produce crepitation in the subcutaneous tissue and muscle, foul-smelling discharge, rapidly progressing necrosis, fever, toxemia, shock, and death. Until the advent of specific therapy, early amputation was the only treatment. At times the infection results only in anaerobic cellulitis. *Cl perfringens* can produce serious food poisoning and fatal intestinal or uterine infections.

Diagnostic Laboratory Tests

A. Specimens: Material from wounds, pus, tissue.

B. Smears: The presence of large gram-positive, sporeforming rods in gram-stained smears suggests gas gangrene clostridia. However, spores are not always seen.

C. Culture: Material is inoculated into cooked chopped meat medium, thioglycollate medium, and onto blood agar plates incubated anaerobically. The growth from one of the media is transferred into milk. A clot torn by gas in 24 hours is suggestive of *Cl perfringens*. Once pure cultures have been obtained by selecting colonies from anaerobically incubated blood plates, they are identified by biochemical reactions (various sugars in thioglycollate, action on milk), hemolysis, and colony form. Lecithinase activity is evaluated by the precipitate formed around colonies on egg yolk media. Final identification rests on toxin production and neutralization by specific antitoxin, in vivo and in vitro.

D. Serologic tests are not useful.

Treatment

The most important aspect of treatment is prompt and extensive surgical debridement of the involved area and excision of all devitalized tissue, in which the organisms are prone to grow. Administration of antimicrobial drugs, particularly penicillin, is begun at the same time. Hyperbaric oxygen may be of great help in the medical management of clostridial tissue infections. It is said to "detoxify" patients rapidly.

Antitoxins are available against the toxins of *Cl perfringens, Cl novyi, Cl histolyticum,* and *Cl septicum,* usually in the form of concentrated immune globulins. Since the clinical picture is similar with all species of toxin-forming clostridia, polyvalent antitoxin (containing antibodies to several toxins) is usually relied on. While such antitoxin is often administered to individuals with contaminated wounds containing much devitalized tissue, the efficacy of the antitoxin is uncertain. Antitoxin in very large doses is being administered to patients who have developed gas gangrene, but surgical management and antibiotics are probably more important and more effective than antitoxin.

Prevention & Control

Early and adequate cleansing of contaminated wounds and surgical debridement, together with the administration of antimicrobial drugs directed against clostridia (eg, penicillin), are the best available preventive measures. Antitoxins should not be relied on. While toxoids for active immunization have been prepared, they have not as yet come into practical use.

Control of the source of contamination is not possible because of the wide dissemination of the organisms and their spores.

•   •   •

General References

Brown, H.: Tetanus. JAMA 204:614–617, 1968.
Lamanna, C., & C.J. Carr: The botulinal, tetanal and enterostaphylococcal toxins: A review. Clin Pharmacol Therap 8:286–332, 1967.
Maclennan, J.D.: The clostridia of gas gangrene. Bact Rev 26:177–276, 1962.
Peebles, T., & others: Tetanus: Toxoid emergency boosters. New England J Med 280:575–581, 1969.

16 . . .

Corynebacteria

Corynebacteria are gram-positive rods, nonmotile and nonsporeforming, which often possess club-shaped ends and irregularly staining granules. They are often in characteristic arrangements, resembling "Chinese letters" or palisades. They form acid but not gas in certain carbohydrates. Several species form part of the normal flora of the human respiratory tract, other mucous membranes, and skin. *C diphtheriae* produces a powerful exotoxin which causes diphtheria in man.

Morphology & Identification

A. Typical Organisms: Corynebacteria are 0.5–1 μm in diameter and several μm long. Characteristically they possess irregular swellings at one end, which gives them a "club-shaped" appearance. Irregularly distributed within the rod (often near the poles) are granules staining deeply with aniline dyes (metachromatic granules, Babes-Ernst bodies), which give the rod a beaded appearance.

Individual corynebacteria in stained smears tend to lie parallel or at acute angles to one another. True branching is rarely observed in cultures.

B. Culture: On Löffler's coagulated serum medium the colonies are small, granular, and gray, with irregular edges. On McLeod's blood agar containing potassium tellurite, the colonies are gray to black because the tellurite is reduced intracellularly. The 3 types of *C diphtheriae* typically have the following appearance on such media: (1) var *gravis*—nonhemoly-

tic, large, gray, irregular, striated colonies; (2) var *mitis*—hemolytic, small, black, glossy, convex colonies; (3) var *intermedius*—nonhemolytic small colonies with characteristics between the 2 extremes. In broth, var *gravis* strains tend to form a pellicle, var *mitis* strains grow diffusely, and var *intermedius* strains settle as a granular sediment.

C. Growth Characteristics: Corynebacteria grow on most ordinary laboratory media. On Löffler's serum corynebacteria grow much more readily than other respiratory pathogens, and the morphology of organisms is typical in smears. Acid, but not gas, is formed from some carbohydrates as shown in Table 16–1.

D. Variation & Conversion: Corynebacteria tend to pleomorphism in microscopic and colonial morphology. Variation from smooth to rough forms has been described. Variants from toxigenic strains often are nontoxigenic. When some nontoxigenic (avirulent) diphtheria organisms are exposed to bacteriophage from certain toxigenic (virulent) diphtheria bacilli, the offspring of the exposed bacteria are lysogenic and toxigenic (virulent), and this trait is subsequently hereditary. (See Chapter 4, Genetics; and Chapter 9, Bacteriophage.) When toxigenic diphtheria bacilli are serially subcultured in specific antiphage serum (antiserum against the temperate phage that they carry), they tend to become nontoxigenic. Thus acquisition of phage leads to toxigenicity (lysogenic conversion). The actual production of toxin occurs perhaps only when the prophage of the lysogenic *C diphtheriae* becomes induced and lyses the cell. While toxigenicity is under control of the phage gene, virulence (invasiveness) is under control of the bacterial gene.

Antigenic Structure

Serologic differences have been observed between types and within each type of *C diphtheriae*, but no satisfactory or useful classification is available. Serologic tests are not generally employed in identification.

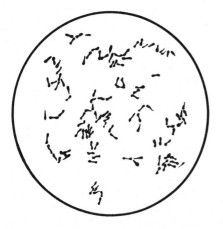

FIG 16–1. *C diphtheriae* from Löffler's medium.

TABLE 16–1.

	Starch	Glucose	Sucrose
C diphtheriae, gravis	+	+	−
C diphtheriae, mitis	−	+	−
C pseudodiphtheriticum	−	−	−
C xerose	−	+	+

Diphtheria toxin contains at least 4 antigenic determinants.

Pathogenesis

Some corynebacteria, notably *C pseudodiphtheriticum* and *C xerose,* are commonly called "diphtheroids." They are normal inhabitants of the mucous membranes of the respiratory tract and the conjunctiva and do not cause disease. A number of other diphtheroids cause infections in animals and, rarely, in man. Anaerobic diphtheroids regularly reside in normal skin. They may participate in the pathogenesis of acne. They produce lipases, which split off free fatty acids from skin lipids. These fatty acids can produce tissue inflammation and contribute to acne.

The principal human pathogen of the group is *C diphtheriae.* In nature *C diphtheriae* occurs in the respiratory tract, in wounds, or on the skin of infected persons or normal carriers. They are spread by droplets or contact to susceptible individuals; virulent bacilli then grow on mucous membranes and start producing toxin.

All toxigenic *C diphtheriae* are capable of elaborating the same disease-producing exotoxin. In vitro production of this toxin depends largely on the concentration of iron. Toxin production is optimal at 0.14 μg of iron/ml of medium, but is virtually suppressed at 0.5 μg/ml. Other factors influencing the yield of toxin in vitro are osmotic pressure, amino acid concentration, pH, and availability of suitable carbon and nitrogen sources. The factors which control toxin production in vivo are not well understood.

Diphtheria toxin is a homogeneous, heat-labile protein of molecular weight 70,000 which has been crystallized. It can be lethal for animals in a dose of 0.2 μg/kg.

The mechanism of action of diphtheria toxin is not fully understood. It arrests protein synthesis and rapidly kills susceptible cells. The structural resemblance to cytochrome b is of uncertain significance.

Corynebacterium minutissimum (Nocardia minutissima) is the cause of erythrasma, a superficial infection of axillary and pubic skin. The organism produces bright pink fluorescence under ultraviolet light on Mueller-Hinton agar.

Pathology

The toxin is absorbed into the mucous membranes and causes destruction of epithelium and a superficial inflammatory response. The necrotic epithelium becomes embedded in exuding fibrin and red and white cells, so that a grayish "pseudomembrane" is formed—commonly over the tonsils, pharynx, or larynx. Any attempt to remove the pseudomembrane exposes and tears the capillaries and thus results in bleeding. The regional lymph nodes in the neck enlarge, and there may be marked edema of the entire neck. The diphtheria bacilli within the membrane continue to produce toxin actively. This is absorbed and results in distant toxic damage, particularly parenchymatous degeneration, fatty infiltration, and necrosis in heart muscle, liver, kidneys, and adrenals, sometimes accompanied by gross hemorrhage. The toxin also produces nerve damage, resulting often in paralysis of the soft palate, eye muscles, or extremities.

Wound or skin diphtheria is limited chiefly to the tropics. A membrane may form on an infected wound which fails to heal. However, absorption of toxin is usually slight and the systemic effects negligible. The "virulence" of diphtheria bacilli is due to their capacity for establishing infection, growing rapidly, and then quickly elaborating toxin which is effectively absorbed. *C diphtheriae* does not actively invade deep tissues and practically never enters the blood stream.

Clinical Findings

When diphtheritic inflammation begins in the respiratory tract, sore throat and fever usually develop. Prostration and dyspnea soon follow because of the obstruction caused by the membrane. This obstruction may even cause suffocation if not promptly relieved by tracheostomy. Irregularities of cardiac rhythm indicate damage to the heart muscle. Later there may be difficulties with vision, swallowing, or movement of the arms or legs. All of these symptoms and signs tend to subside spontaneously.

There is a broad correlation between the type of *C diphtheriae* and the severity of the disease. In general, var *gravis* infections tend to be more severe than var *mitis,* with a correspondingly higher mortality.

Diagnostic Laboratory Tests

These serve to confirm the clinical impression and are of epidemiologic significance. **Note:** Specific treatment must never be delayed for laboratory reports if the clinical picture is strongly suggestive of diphtheria.

A. Specimens: Swabs from the nose, throat, or other suspected lesions must be obtained before antimicrobial drugs are administered.

B. Smears: Smears stained with alkaline methylene blue, Gram's stain, or certain special stains (eg, Albert's) show beaded rods in typical arrangement.

C. Culture: Inoculate a blood agar plate (to rule out hemolytic streptococci), a Löffler slant, and a tellurite plate, and incubate all 3 at 37° C. Unless the swab can be inoculated promptly it should be kept moistened with sterile horse serum so the bacilli will remain viable. In 12–18 hours the Löffler'slant may yield organisms of typical "diphtheria-like" morphology. In 36–48 hours the colonies on tellurite medium are sufficiently definite for recognition of the type of *C diphtheriae.*

Any diphtheria-like organism cultured must be submitted to a "virulence" test before the bacteriologic diagnosis of diphtheria is definite. Such tests are really tests for toxigenicity of an isolated diphtheria-like organism. They can be done in one of 3 ways:

1. Intracutaneous test—Culture is prepared as for the subcutaneous test (see below) and injected intracutaneously so that each guinea pig (rabbits may be used) receives 0.1 ml in 2 different skin areas. One control guinea pig is protected with 500 units antitoxin (see subcutaneous test below); the other is given 50 units of antitoxin intraperitoneally 4 hours after the skin test to prevent abrupt death. Inflammatory lesions at the site of injection progress to necrosis in 48–72 hours in the unprotected animal, whereas the control guinea pig must remain completely well to rule out the possibility of other invasive bacteria.

2. Subcutaneous test–The growth is scraped from a Löffler plate or slant, emulsified in broth, and 0.3 ml of the emulsion is injected into each of 2 guinea pigs, one of which has received 500 units of diphtheria antitoxin 18–24 hours previously. The unprotected animal should die in 2–3 days. This test is little used because it is wasteful of animals.

3. In vitro test–A strip of filter paper saturated with antitoxin is placed on an agar plate containing 20% horse serum. The cultures to be tested for toxigenicity are streaked across the plate at right angles to the filter paper. After 48 hours' incubation the antitoxin diffusing from the paper strip has precipitated the toxin diffusing from toxigenic cultures and resulted in lines radiating from the intersection of the strip and the bacterial growth.

Resistance & Immunity

Since diphtheria is principally the result of the action of the toxin formed by the organism rather than invasion by it, resistance to the disease depends largely on the availability of specific neutralizing antitoxin in the blood stream and tissues. Although this correlation is not absolute it is generally true that diphtheria occurs only in persons who possess no antitoxin or only very low levels of it. Similarly, the treatment of diphtheria rests largely on the early administration of specific antitoxin against the toxin formed by the organisms at their site of entry and multiplication. Thus there may be active or passive antitoxic immunity to diphtheria. Recovery from the disease is usually followed by a lasting immunity The relative amount of antitoxin that a person possesses at a given time (it tends to fluctuate greatly) can be estimated in one of 2 ways:

A. Titration of Serum for Antitoxin Content: (Too complex for routine use.) Serum is mixed with varying amounts of toxin and the mixture injected into susceptible animals. The greater the amount of toxin neutralized, the higher the concentration of antitoxin in the serum.

B. Schick Test: This test is based on the fact that diphtheria toxin is very irritating and results in a marked local reaction when injected intradermally unless it is neutralized by circulating antitoxin. A standard dose of toxin (1/50 of the minimum lethal dose for guinea pigs) is injected into the skin of one forearm and an identical amount of heated toxin is injected into the other forearm as a control. (Heating for 15 minutes at 60° C destroys the effect of the toxin.) The test should be read at 24 and 48 hours and again in 6 days. Results are interpreted as follows:

1. Positive reaction (susceptibility to diphtheria toxin, ie, absence of adequate amounts of neutralizing antitoxin)–Toxin produces redness and swelling which increase for several days and then slowly fade, leaving a brownish pigmented area. The control site shows no reaction.

2. Negative reaction (adequate amount of antitoxin present)–Neither injection site shows any reaction.

3. Pseudoreaction–Schick test reactions may be complicated by hypersensitivity to materials other than the toxin contained in the injections. A pseudoreaction shows redness and swelling on both arms which disappear simultaneously on the second or third day. It constitutes a negative reaction.

4. Combined reaction–A combined reaction begins like a pseudoreaction, with redness and swelling at both injection sites; the toxin later continues to exert its effects, however, whereas the reaction at the control site subsides rapidly. This denotes hypersensitivity as well as relative susceptibility to toxin.

Treatment

Diphtheria antitoxin is produced in various animals (horses, sheep, goats, and rabbits) by the repeated injection of purified and concentrated toxoid. Treatment with antitoxin is mandatory when there is strong clinical suspicion of diphtheria. From 10,000–100,000 units are injected IV after suitable precautions have been taken (skin or conjunctival test) to rule out hypersensitivity to the animal serum employed. The antitoxin should be given on the day the clinical diagnosis of diphtheria is made and need not be given again. Intramuscular injection may be used in mild cases.

Antimicrobial drugs (penicillin, tetracyclines, erythromycin) inhibit the in vitro growth of diphtheria bacilli but have virtually no effect on the disease process. Their chief usefulness is the more rapid elimination of *C diphtheriae* from the respiratory tracts of patients than might occur spontaneously.

Antibiotic administration (tetracycline) in acne may inhibit the lipolytic action of anaerobic diphtheroids; this reduces tissue inflammation. Variable benefit has been claimed for this treatment of acne.

Epidemiology, Prevention, & Control

Before artificial immunization diphtheria was mainly a disease of small children. The infection occurred either clinically or subclinically at an early age and resulted in the widespread production of antitoxin in the population. An asymptomatic reinfection during adolescence and adult life served as a stimulus for maintenance of high antitoxin levels. Thus most members of the population, except children, were immune.

With the introduction of artificial active immunization the situation has changed. After active immunization during the first few years of life, antitoxin levels are generally adequate until adolescence. However, there are very few cases or carriers of diphtheria in the population, so that the stimulus of minimal subclinical infections is lacking. Consequently many adolescents and adults have no significant amounts of antitoxin and thus are again susceptible to the disease.

Following either natural infection or active immunization, antitoxin levels last only a limited period of time and are subject to great fluctuations. Since the degree of individual resistance varies with the antitoxin titer, all degrees, from complete susceptibility to complete immunity, are likely to be present. This situation is further complicated by the fact that certain Schick-negative individuals may contract the disease, whereas some Schick-positive individuals may be resistant.

The principal aim of prevention therefore must be to limit the distribution of toxigenic diphtheria bacilli in the population and to maintain as high a level of active immunization as possible.

A. Isolation: To limit contact with diphtheria bacilli to a minimum, patients with diphtheria must be isolated and every effort made to rid them of the organisms. Without treatment a large percentage of infected persons continue to shed diphtheria bacilli for weeks or months after recovery (convalescent carriers). This danger may be greatly reduced by active early treatment with antibiotics. However, there are some healthy carriers from whom diphtheria bacilli cannot be eradicated with the measures now available. Tonsillectomy is sometimes performed.

B. Active Immunization: The following preparations have been employed:

1. Fluid toxoid—A filtrate of broth culture of a toxigenic strain is treated with 0.3% formalin and incubated at 37° C until toxicity has disappeared. Toxoid is standardized in terms of flocculating units (Lf), often as 30 Lf/ml. Three doses of 0.5—1 ml are injected subcutaneously.

2. Alum-precipitated toxoid—Toxoid prepared as above is precipitated with 1—2% potassium alum. This is a somewhat better antigen and remains longer in the subcutaneous tissue. Only 2 injections are required for initial immunization, but the alum-precipitated toxoid may induce hypersensitivity more frequently than fluid toxoid. It is commonly combined with tetanus toxoid and pertussis vaccine in a single injection. Toxin can also be adsorbed onto aluminum hydroxide or aluminum phosphate for delayed absorption.

Children should receive an initial course of toxoid injections during the first year of life and should have recall ("booster") inoculations at 3—4 and 6—8 years. Adolescents should receive another recall injection. In adults the incidence of hypersensitivity reactions to toxoids is very high, and random injections in the older age groups are undesirable. Persons likely to have such reactions can be detected by the Moloney test, which consists of the intradermal injection of 1:10 diluted toxoid. If this test is positive (redness and swelling in 24 hours), only purified fluid toxoid in small doses can be used.

3. Toxin-antitoxin mixtures—These have been abandoned because of the danger of dissociation of the "neutral" mixture and the serious reactions to the free toxin.

•   •   •

General References

Belsey, M.A., & others: *Corynebacterium diphtheriae* skin infections. New England J Med 280:135—141, 1969.

Kaplan, K., & L. Weinstein: Diphtheroid infections of man. Ann Int Med 70:919—929, 1969.

Rosenberg, E.W.: Bacteriology of acne. Ann Rev Med 20:201—206, 1969.

17 . . .

Mycobacteria

The mycobacteria are rod-shaped bacteria which do not stain readily but which, once stained, resist decolorization by acid or alcohol and are therefore called "acid-fast" bacilli. In addition to many saprophytic forms, the group includes pathogenic organisms (*M tuberculosis, M leprae*) which cause chronic diseases producing lesions of the infectious granuloma type.

MYCOBACTERIUM TUBERCULOSIS

Morphology & Identification

A. Typical Organisms: In animal tissues, tubercle bacilli are thin straight rods, measuring about 0.4 × 3 µm. On artificial media, coccoid and filamentous forms are seen. Mycobacteria cannot be classified either as gram-positive or gram-negative. Once stained by basic dyes they cannot be decolorized by alcohol, regardless of treatment with iodine. True tubercle bacilli are characterized by "acid-fastness," eg, ethyl alcohol containing 3% hydrochloric acid (acid-alcohol) quickly decolorizes all bacteria except the mycobacteria. Acid-fastness depends on the integrity of the cellular structure. The Ziehl-Neelsen technic of staining is employed for identification of acid-fast bacteria.

B. Culture: Three types of media are employed.

1. Simple synthetic media—Large inocula grow on simple synthetic media in several weeks. Small inocula fail to grow in such media because of the presence of minute amounts of toxic fatty acids. The toxic effect of fatty acids can be neutralized by animal serum or albumin, and the fatty acids may then actually promote growth. Activated charcoal aids growth.

2. Oleic acid-albumin media support the proliferation of small inocula, particularly if Tweens (water-soluble esters of fatty acids) are present. Ordinarily, mycobacteria grow in clumps or masses due to the hydrophobic character of the cell surface. Tweens wet the surface of the tubercle bacilli and thus permit dispersed growth in liquid media. Growth is often more rapid than on complex media.

3. Complex organic media—Small inocula traditionally were grown on media containing complex organic substances, eg, egg yolk, animal serum, tissue extracts. These now have little advantage over media containing Tween 80. Penicillin containing blood agar is also useful.

C. Growth Characteristics: Mycobacteria are strict aerobes and derive energy from the oxidation of many simple carbon compounds. Increased CO_2 tension enhances growth. Biochemical activities are not characteristic, and the growth rate is much slower than that of most bacteria. Saprophytic forms grow more rapidly, proliferate well at 22° C, produce more pigment, and are less acid-fast than the pathogenic forms.

D. Reaction to Physical and Chemical Agents: Mycobacteria tend to be more resistant to chemical agents than other bacteria because of the hydrophobic nature of the cell surface and their clumped growth. In the presence of wetting agents (eg, Tween 80), which result in dispersed growth and better surface contact, the organisms become quite susceptible to a variety of chemicals. Nevertheless, concentrations of dyes (eg, malachite green) or antibacterial agents (eg, penicillin) which are bacteriostatic to other bacteria can be incorporated into media without inhibiting the growth of tubercle bacilli. Acids and alkalies permit the survival of some exposed tubercle bacilli and are used for "concentration" of clinical specimens and partial elimination of contaminating organisms. Tubercle bacilli are fairly resistant to drying, and survive for long periods in dried sputum.

E. Variation: Variation occurs in colony appearance, virulence, and cellular characteristics of tubercle bacilli. "Eugonic" organisms grow luxuriantly on egg media and form rough colonies with irregular edges. Their growth can be enhanced by glycerin. This is the usual appearance of human strains on first isolation. "Dysgonic" cultures grow more slowly, forming flat, circular colonies with entire edges. They are inhibited by the presence of glycerin. This is the usual appearance of bovine strains. "Dysgonic" cultures may assume "eugonic" characteristics of growth. Non-virulent strains treated with nonionic surface-active agents may acquire virulence and "cord" formation (see below).

F. Types of Tubercle Bacilli: Differences between the 3 main species of tubercle bacilli are particularly evident in their virulence for laboratory animals (Table 17–1).

Human and bovine strains are equally pathogenic for man by either the respiratory or the gastrointestinal route. The route of primary infection determines the pattern and location of tuberculous lesions. Some "anonymous" mycobacteria are often associated with tuberculosis-like disease in man; others are pre-

TABLE 17-1. Virulence of tubercle bacilli.

Virulent For	Mycobacterium			
	tuber-culosis	bovis	avium	Anonymous
Guinea pigs	+++	+++	—	— to +
Rabbits	+	+++	+++	—
Mice*	+++	+++	—	— to +++
Cattle	—	+++	—	?
Fowl	—	—	+++	?
Man	+++	+++	—	— to +++

*Certain strains.

sumed to cause disease rarely. They are described below.

Constituents of Tubercle Bacilli

The constituents listed below are are found large-ly in cell walls. Mycobacterial cell walls can induce delayed hypersensitivity, induce some resistance to infection, increase reactivity of mice to endotoxin, and replace whole mycobacterial cells in Freund's adjuvant. Protoplasm does none of these things, but can provoke delayed hypersensitivity reactions in previously sensitized animals.

A. Lipoid Fraction: Virulent eugonic strains of tubercle bacilli form microscopic "serpentine cords" in which acid-fast bacilli are arranged in parallel chains. Cord formation is correlated with virulence. A "cord factor" which inhibits migration of leukocytes has been extracted from virulent bacilli with petroleum ether. It is probably trehalose-6,6'-dimycolate. It is not found in avirulent organisms.

B. Protein Fraction: Each type of tubercle bacillus contains several proteins which elicit the tuberculin reaction. Proteins bound to a wax fraction can, upon injection, induce tuberculin sensitivity. They can also elicit the formation of a variety of antibodies.

C. Polysaccharides: Tubercle bacilli contain a variety of polysaccharides. Their role in the pathogenesis of tuberculosis is uncertain. They can induce the immediate type of hypersensitivity, and can interfere with some antigen-antibody reactions in vitro.

D. Lipids: Mycobacteria are rich in lipids, and many complex lipids, fatty acids, and waxes have been isolated from them. In the cell the lipids are largely bound to proteins and polysaccharides. Some such complexes have been isolated. Lipids are probably responsible for most of the cellular tissue reactions to tubercle bacilli. Phosphatide fractions have been used to produce tubercle-like cellular responses and caseation necrosis. Lipids are to some extent responsible for acid-fastness. When tubercle bacilli are defatted with ether, this staining property is lost. Analysis of the lipids by gas chromatography may reveal species-specific patterns, and aids classification.

Pathogenesis

Tubercle bacilli produce no recognized toxins. The disease results from establishment and prolifera-

tion of virulent organisms and interactions with the host. Virulence can be correlated with colonial characteristics ("cord formation"). Avirulent bacilli do not survive for long in the normal host. Resistance and hypersensitivity of the host greatly influence the development of the disease. Pathogenicity for guinea pigs and catalase production by tubercle bacilli are often parallel.

Pathology

The production and development of lesions and their healing or progression are determined chiefly by (1) the number of tubercle bacilli in the inoculum and their subsequent multiplication, and (2) the resistance and hypersensitivity of the host.

A. Two Principal Lesions:

1. Exudative type—This consists of an acute inflammatory reaction, with edema fluid, polymorphonuclear leukocytes, and, later, monocytes around the tubercle bacilli. This type is seen particularly in lung tissue, where it resembles bacterial pneumonia. It may heal by resolution, so that the entire exudate becomes absorbed; it may lead to massive necrosis of tissue; or it may develop into the second (productive) type of lesion.

2. Productive type—When fully developed, this lesion, a chronic granuloma, consists of 3 zones: (1) a central area of large, multinucleated giant cells containing tubercle bacilli; (2) a mid-zone of pale epithelioid cells, often arranged radially; and (3) a peripheral zone of fibroblasts, lymphocytes, and monocytes. Later, peripheral fibrous tissue develops and the central area undergoes caseation necrosis. Such a lesion is called a tubercle. A caseous tubercle may break into a bronchus, empty its contents, and form a cavity. It may heal by fibrosis or calcification.

B. Spread of Organisms in the Host: Tubercle bacilli spread in the host by direct extension, through the lymphatic channels and blood stream, and via the bronchi and gastrointestinal tract.

In the first infection, tubercle bacilli always spread from the initial site via the lymphatics to the regional lymph nodes. From there the thoracic duct and the blood stream are occasionally reached, which in turn distribute bacilli to all organs (miliary distribution). The blood stream can be invaded also by erosion of a vein by a caseating tubercle or lymph node. If a caseating lesion discharges its contents into a bronchus, they are aspirated and distributed to other parts of the lungs or are swallowed and passed into the stomach and intestines.

C. Intracellular Site of Growth: Once tubercle bacilli establish themselves in tissue they reside principally intracellularly in monocytes, reticuloendothelial cells, and giant cells. The intracellular location is one of the features which makes chemotherapy difficult and favors microbial persistence. Within the cells of immune animals, multiplication of tubercle bacilli is greatly inhibited.

TABLE 17—2. Diagnosis of acid-fast organisms in sputum specimens.

(1) Digest sputum by adding an equal volume of 4% sodium hydroxide, shaking with glass beads for 20 minutes at room temperature.

(2) Restore neutral pH by adding 25% hydrochloric acid, drop by drop.

(3) Inoculate Loewenstein-Jensen medium and incubate at 37° C. Inspect at 5-day intervals. When colonies appear, make smears and acid-fast stains. If acid-fast organisms are present, follow key as shown below.

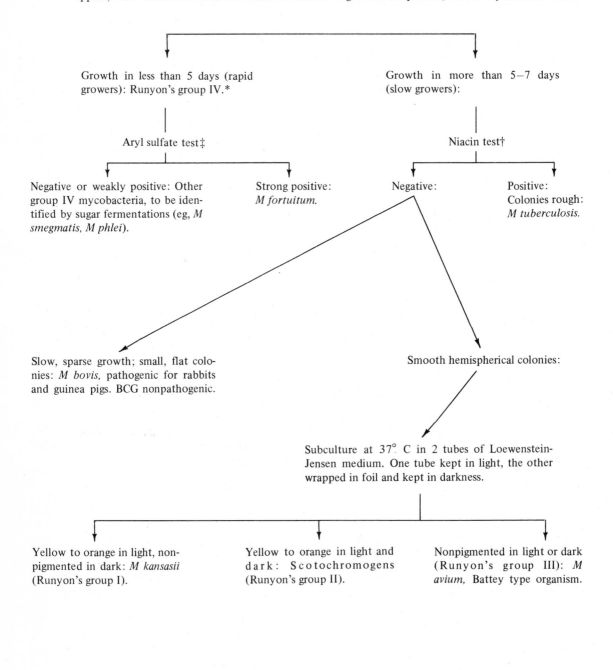

*Runyon, E.H.: M Clin North America 43:273, 1959.

†Runyon, E.H., & others: Am Rev Tuberc 79:663, 1959.

‡Kubica, G.P., & Bestal, A.L.: Am Rev Resp Dis 82:737, 1961.

First Infection & Reinfection Types of Tuberculosis

When a host has first contact with tubercle bacilli, the following features are usually observed: (1) An acute exudative lesion develops and rapidly spreads to the lymphatics and regional lymph nodes. The "Ghon complex" is the primary tissue lesion (in lung or intestine) together with the involved lymph nodes. The exudative lesion in tissue often heals rapidly. (2) The lymph node undergoes massive caseation, which usually calcifies.

This first-infection type occurred in the past usually in childhood, but now is seen frequently in adults who have remained free from infection and therefore tuberculin-negative in early life. In first infections the involvement may be in any part of the lung, but is most often at the base.

The reinfection type may be caused by tubercle bacilli which have survived in the primary lesion (endogenous reinfection) or by bacilli newly inhaled from the environment (exogenous reinfection). Reinfection tuberculosis is characterized by a more chronic tissue lesion and a predominantly "productive" type of tissue response (the formation of tubercles, caseation, and fibrosis). Regional lymph nodes are only slightly involved, and caseation never occurs. Reinfection almost always begins at the apex of the lung.

The contrast between first infection and reinfection is shown experimentally in the "Koch phenomenon." When a guinea pig is injected subcutaneously with virulent tubercle bacilli, the puncture wound heals quickly but a nodule forms at the site of injection in 2 weeks. This nodule ulcerates, and the ulcer does not heal. The regional lymph nodes develop tubercles and caseate massively. When the same animal is later injected with tubercle bacilli in another part of the body, the sequence of events is quite different: There is rapid necrosis of skin and tissue at the site of injection, but the ulcer heals rapidly. Regional lymph nodes do not become infected at all, or only after a delay.

These differences between first infection and reinfection are attributed to (1) resistance and (2) hypersensitivity induced by the first infection of the host with tubercle bacilli. It is not clear to what extent each of these components participates in the modified response in reinfection tuberculosis.

Immunity & Hypersensitivity

Unless a host dies during the first infection with tubercle bacilli, he acquires a certain resistance (see Koch phenomenon, above). He has an increased capacity to localize tubercle bacilli, to retard their multiplication, and even to destroy them, limit their spread, and reduce lymphatic dissemination. This can be largely attributed to the ability of mononuclear cells to limit the multiplication of ingested organisms and perhaps to destroy them. Mononuclear cells acquire this characteristic in the course of initial infection of the host.

Antibodies form against a variety of the cellular constituents of the tubercle bacilli, but none of them are believed to play a role in acquired resistance to infection. Antibodies have been determined by precipitation and complement fixation tests and by a hemagglutinating reaction in which sera of tuberculous animals or man clump red cells which have adsorbed tuberculin. None of these serologic reactions bears any definite relation to the state of resistance of the host.

In the course of first infection the host also acquires hypersensitivity to the tubercle bacilli. This is made evident by the development of a positive tuberculin reaction (see below). Tuberculin sensitivity can be induced by whole tubercle bacilli or by tuberculoprotein in combination with the chloroform-soluble wax of the tubercle bacillus, but not by tuberculoprotein alone. Hypersensitivity and resistance appear to be separate aspects of the same cellular reaction. However, in man it is not clear what factors determine whether hypersensitivity will aid or hinder the manifestations of resistance.

Tuberculin Test

A. Material: Old tuberculin (OT) is a concentrated filtrate of broth in which tubercle bacilli have grown for 6 weeks. In addition to the reactive tuberculoproteins, this material contains a variety of other constituents of tubercle bacilli and of growth medium. A purified protein derivative (PPD) can be obtained by chemical fractionation of OT and is the preferred material for skin testing. Both OT and PPD are standardized in terms of their biologic reactivity as "tuberculin units" (TU) (Table 17–3).

B. Dose of Tuberculin: A large amount of tuberculin injected into a hypersensitive host may give rise to severe local reactions and a flare-up of inflammation and necrosis at the main sites of infection (focal reactions). For this reason tuberculin tests in surveys employ 5 TU; in persons suspected of hypersensitivity, skin testing is begun with 1 TU. More concentrated material (250 TU) is administered only if the reaction to the more dilute material is negative. The volume is usually 0.1 ml injected intracutaneously.

C. Reactions to Tuberculin: In an individual who has not had contact with tubercle bacilli, there is no reaction to OT or PPD. An individual who has had a first infection with tubercle bacilli develops induration exceeding 10 mm in diameter, edema, erythema in 24–48 hours, and, with very intense reactions, even central necrosis. The skin test should be read in 48 or 72 hours. It is considered positive if the injection of 5 TU is followed by induration 10 mm or more in diameter. Positive tests tend to persist for several days. Weak reactions may disappear more rapidly.

The tuberculin test becomes positive within 4–6 weeks after infection (or injection of avirulent bacilli). It may be negative in the presence of tuberculous infection when "anergy" develops due to overwhelming tuberculosis, measles, Hodgkin's disease, sarcoidosis, or immunosuppressive drugs. A positive tuberculin test may revert to negative on the isoniazid

TABLE 17–3. Approximate tuberculin equivalents based on comparative skin test potency.

TU	"Strength"	PPD* mg/dose†	OT mg/dose‡	OT Dilution
1	First	0.00002	0.01	1:10,000
5	Intermediate	0.0001	0.05	1:2,000
250§	Second	0.005	1.0	1:100

*International Standard Tuberculin adopted by World Health Organization in 1952.
†Based on mg of protein.
‡Based on 1 ml of concentrated OT = 1 gm.
§On the basis of OT weight this represents 100 TU. The excess reactivity may be due to cross reactions.

treatment of a recent converter. After BCG vaccination, a positive test may last for only 3–7 years. In either case, the elimination of viable tubercle bacilli results in reversion of the tuberculin test to negative. The reactivity to tuberculin can only be transferred by cells—not by serum—from a tuberculin-positive to a tuberculin-negative person.

D. Interpretation of Tuberculin Test: A positive tuberculin test indicates only that an individual has been infected with tubercle bacilli in the past; it does not indicate present active disease. It is believed that tuberculin-positive healthy individuals are less susceptible to superinfection with resulting serious widespread disease than tuberculin-negative ones.

PPD's from other mycobacteria have been prepared. They exhibit some species specificity in low concentrations and marked cross-reactions in higher concentrations.

Clinical Findings

Since the tubercle bacillus can involve every organ system, its clinical manifestations are protean. Fatigue, weakness, weight loss, and fever may be signs of tuberculous disease. Pulmonary involvement giving rise to chronic cough and spitting of blood usually is associated with far-advanced lesions. Meningitis can occur in the absence of other signs of tuberculosis.

Diagnostic Laboratory Tests

Neither the tuberculin test nor any now available serologic test gives evidence of active disease due to the tubercle bacillus. Only isolation of tubercle bacilli gives such proof.

Specimens consist of fresh sputum, gastric washings, urine, pleural fluid, spinal fluid, joint fluid, biopsy material, or other suspected material.

A. Stained Smear: Sputum, or sediment from gastric washings, urine, exudates, or other material is stained for acid-fast bacilli by the Ziehl-Neelsen technic or a comparable method. If such organisms are found, this is presumptive evidence of tuberculosis. However, saprophytic, nonpathogenic acid-fast bacilli must be ruled out by culture or animal inoculation.

B. Concentration for Stained Smear: If a direct smear is negative, sputum may be liquefied by addition of Chlorox (hypochlorite solution), centrifuged, and the sediment stained and examined microscopically. This "digested material" is unsuitable for culture.

C. Culture: Urine, spinal fluid, and materials not contaminated with other bacteria may be cultured directly. Sputum is first treated with sodium hydroxide, sulfuric acid, or other agents bactericidal for contaminating microorganisms but less so for tubercle bacilli. The liquefied sputum is then neutralized and centrifuged and the sediment inoculated into egg media or oleic acid-albumin media (Dubos). Incubation of the inoculated media is continued for 2–8 weeks.

D. Animal Inoculation: Part of the cultured material may be inoculated subcutaneously into young guinea pigs, which are tuberculin tested after 3–4 weeks and autopsied after 6 weeks to search for evidence of tuberculosis. In competent hands cultures are just as reliable. The use of both procedures, however, ensures the highest number of positive results. Isoniazid-resistant tubercle bacilli are often nonpathogenic for guinea pigs but grow on artificial media.

E. Serology: Complement fixation and hemagglutination tests have little diagnostic or prognostic value.

Treatment

Physical and mental rest, nutritional buildup, and various forms of collapse therapy have long been employed. The most widely used antituberculosis drugs at present are streptomycin, isoniazid (isonicotinic acid hydrazide, INH), and aminosalicylic acid (PAS). Unfortunately, resistant variants of tubercle bacilli against each of these drugs emerge rapidly. Treatment is most successful when the drugs are used concomitantly (eg, streptomycin + INH; INH + PAS; streptomycin + PAS + INH), thus delaying the emergence of resistant forms. Other drugs (eg, ethionamide, pyrazinamide, ethambutol, viomycin, and cycloserine) are less frequently employed because of their more pronounced side-effects. The available chemotherapeutic drugs result in suppression of tuberculous activity but usually do not eradicate all organisms. Host factors are important in control.

The following explanations have been advanced for the particular resistance of chronic tuberculosis to chemotherapy: (1) Most bacilli are intracellular, and some drugs (eg, streptomycin) penetrate cells poorly. (2) The caseous material in lesions, although it is itself inimical to bacterial proliferation, interferes with drug action. (3) Many lesions, particularly cavities, have avascular fibrous walls which interfere with penetration of drugs. (4) In chronic lesions tubercle bacilli are nonproliferating, metabolically inactive "persisters" which are not susceptible to drug action.

Epidemiology

The most frequent source of infection is the human who excretes, particularly from the respiratory tract, large numbers of tubercle bacilli. Close contact (eg, in the family) and massive exposure (eg, in medical personnel) make transmission by droplet nuclei most likely. The milk of tuberculous cows is an important source of infection where bovine tuberculosis is not well controlled.

Relative susceptibility to the development of tuberculosis is greatly influenced by constitutional factors, as is best illustrated by studies on identical twins living in different environments. The American Indian and Negro appear to be more susceptible than the American white, but a racial element in resistance has been proved conclusively only in experimental animals. Small infants tend to develop more serious disease than older children or adults. Death rates vary with sex and age. In women, death from tuberculosis is highest between 15 and 25, whereas in men the rate rises later and increases more rapidly with age. Nutrition is believed to have some effect.

Infection occurs at an earlier age in urban than in rural populations. Disease occurs only in a small proportion of infected individuals. Tuberculosis is especially severe when introduced into populations that have never before harbored the organisms.

Prevention & Control

(1) Public health measures designed for early detection of cases and sources of infection (tuberculin test, x-ray) and for their isolation and treatment until noninfectious.

(2) Eradication of tuberculosis in cattle ("test and slaughter") and pasteurization of milk.

(3) Drug treatment of asymptomatic tuberculin "converters" in the age groups most prone to develop complications (eg, young children).

(4) **Immunization**: Various living avirulent tubercle bacilli, particularly BCG (bacille Calmette Guérin, an attenuated bovine organism) have been used to induce a certain amount of resistance in those heavily exposed to infection. Vaccination with these organisms is a substitute for primary infection with virulent tubercle bacilli, without the danger inherent in the latter. The available vaccines are inadequate from many technical and biologic standpoints. Their use is suggested only in tuberculin-negative persons who are heavily exposed (members of tuberculous families, medical personnel, etc). Statistical evidence indicates that an increased resistance for a limited period follows BCG vaccination.

The possible immunizing value of nonliving bacterial fractions, especially one derived from bacilli disrupted in oil, is under investigation.

(5) **Individual Host Resistance**: Nonspecific factors may reduce host resistance, thus favoring the conversion of asymptomatic infection into disease. Among such "activators" of tuberculosis are starvation, gastrectomy, and massive corticosteroid administration.

OTHER MYCOBACTERIA

Many acid-fast organisms other than *M tuberculosis* are encountered in man's environment. Many are free-living saprophytes and tend to grow rapidly on simple bacteriologic media. Some are associated with animals, eg, Johne's bacillus (*M paratuberculosis*), which produces a chronic enteritis in cattle and results in severe economic losses; or *M balnei (M marinum)*, which occurs in water, may infect cold-blooded animals, and occasionally produces stubborn "swimming pool granuloma" in man. The preference of that organism for the cool body surface is shared by *M ulcerans*, which produces chronic skin ulcers in man and grows in vitro at 31° C. Other mycobacteria (eg, *M smegmatis*) are regularly found in the sebaceous secretions of the skin of man but are not known to cause disease. They may give rise to confusion with tubercle bacilli.

From human sputum, and occasionally from other sites also, acid-fast mycobacteria are recovered at times which resemble tubercle bacilli in certain respects but are atypical in others. The taxonomic position and the medical significance of many of these organisms are unsettled, but it is clear that some produce unequivocal disease closely resembling tuberculosis. The tentative grouping of Runyon (M Clin North America 43:273, 1959) is widely accepted at present. These "anonymous" mycobacteria are divided into groups according to pigmentation and growth rate.

Group I consists of photochromogens (growing colonies which produce little pigments in the dark but, after exposure to light for 1 hour, turn yellow-orange in 48 hours), requiring complex media and growing a little faster than tubercle bacilli. The most important representative is *M kansasii* (originally described from Kansas as the "yellow bacillus"), which definitely produces human pulmonary infection indistinguishable clinically or histologically from tuberculosis.

Group II, scotochromogens (colonies are yellow-orange in either light or dark) are a very heterogeneous group, most members of which are probably not involved in human disease. They do not grow on plain nutrient agar.

Group III consists of buff or light tan colonies of softer consistency than most *M tuberculosis* and grow somewhat faster. A prominent member of this group is the so-called Battey bacillus; it definitely causes human lung disease and appears to be similar to the avian variety of tubercle bacilli.

Group IV consists of organisms producing nonpigmented colonies which grow very rapidly on simple media. Many such organisms (eg, *M phlei*) are definite saprophytes, but *M fortuitum* can be associated with progressive pulmonary pathology.

Of great practical concern is the relative resistance of most "anonymous" mycobacteria to antituberculosis drugs, particularly streptomycin, isoniazid, and aminosalicylic acid. Extracts equivalent to PPD prepared from such mycobacteria give delayed skin reactions in many persons, including some who are tuberculin-negative.

M LEPRAE

Although this organism was described by Hansen in 1878 (4 years before Koch's discovery of the tubercle bacillus), it has never been cultivated with certainty.

Typical acid-fast bacilli—singly, in parallel bundles, or in globular masses—are regularly found in smears or scrapings from skin or mucous membranes (particularly the nasal septum) in lepromatous leprosy. The bacilli are often found within the endothelial cells of blood vessels or in mononuclear cells. The organisms have not been grown on artificial media with certainty. Limited multiplication through a spheroplast stage has been claimed for leprosy bacilli maintained for weeks at pH 5.5 in a complex medium. When bacilli from human leprosy (ground tissue, nasal scrapings) are inoculated into foot pads of mice, local granulomatous lesions develop with limited multiplication of bacilli. Animals have not been infected by other routes, and the role of leprosy bacilli as the sole etiologic agent of human leprosy is still not completely established.

Clinical Findings

The disease usually progresses slowly over many years. Two types of changes occur: (1) a nodular form, causing nodular granulomas in the skin, mucous membranes, and many organs; and (2) an anesthetic form (involvement of peripheral nerves), which results in loss of sensation and favors injury and mutilation of the hands and feet.

Leprosy may manifest itself in the "lepromatous" or the "tuberculoid" form at different times in the same patient. In the lepromatous form there appears to be a defect in delayed type hypersensitivity: Macrophages are filled with bacilli. There is rapid progression of disease. The lepromin (extract of lepromatous tissue) and other skin tests are negative. By contrast, in the tuberculoid form there are few bacilli, lesions tend to heal by fibrosis, and skin tests are positive.

Diagnosis

Scrapings with a scalpel blade from the nasal mucosa, or from a biopsy of ear lobe skin, are smeared on a slide and stained by the Ziehl-Neelsen technic. No serologic tests are of value. Serologic tests for syphilis frequently yield false biologic positive results in leprosy.

Treatment

Several specialized sulfones (eg, dapsone [diaminodiphenylsulfone, DDS]) suppress the growth of *M leprae* and the clinical manifestations of leprosy if given for many months.

Epidemiology

The mode of transmission of leprosy is uncertain. It is believed that suceptibility to infection is greatest in childhood, that the incubation period may extend over many years, and that the infected persons develop symptoms and signs only in adult life. Infection is most likely contracted by children from other infected members of the family.

Prevention & Control

In endemic areas, removal of young children from infected families is employed with some success. Chemotherapy of active cases is good prophylaxis for the community. Chemoprophylaxis with sulfones in close family contacts has been employed. Experimentally, BCG vaccination engenders some resistance to *M leprae* infections or to the development of disease.

•   •   •

General References

Mackaness, G.B.: The immunology of antituberculous immunity. Am Rev Resp Dis 97:337–344, 1968.

Mitchell, R.S.: Control of tuberculosis. New England J Med 276:842–848, 905–911, 1967.

Sheagren, J.N., & others: Immunologic reactivity in patients with leprosy. Ann Int Med 70:295–303, 1969.

Shepard, C.C.: Chemotherapy of leprosy. Ann Rev Pharmacol 9:37–50, 1969.

18 . . .

Enteric Gram-Negative Microorganisms

The enteric organisms are a large group of gram-negative, nonsporeforming rods whose natural habitat is the intestinal tract of man and animals. Some (eg, *Escherichia coli* and *Aerobacter aerogenes*) form part of the normal flora of the intestinal tract; others (eg, salmonellae, shigellae) are regularly pathogenic for man. Enteric bacteria are aerobes, ferment a wide range of carbohydrates, and possess a complex antigenic structure.

Most gram-negative bacteria possess complex lipopolysaccharides in their cell wall. These substances, endotoxins, have a variety of pathophysiologic effects which are summarized below. Subsequent sections deal with coliform bacteria, proteus, and pseudomonas organisms. Salmonellae and shigellae are discussed separately.

ENDOTOXINS OF GRAM-NEGATIVE BACTERIA

The endotoxins of gram-negative bacteria are complex lipopolysaccharides derived from the walls of the bacterial cell, and often liberated when bacteria lyse. The substances are heat-stable, with molecular weights variously estimated between 100,000 and 900,000. It is probable that a high molecular weight aggregate (perhaps in the form of micelles) is necessary for manifestation of toxicity, but toxicity has also been claimed for the isolated lipid A. The physiopathologic effects of all endotoxins are similar (whatever their origin), but antigenically they appear to be distinct. The sequence of monosaccharide units imparts antigenic specificity to the molecule. The specific antibody combines with the polysaccharide portion of the molecule. There is no correlation between the disease-producing potential of a gram-negative organism and its endotoxin content.

After introduction into the mammalian body, endotoxins are removed ("cleared") largely by cells of the reticuloendothelial (RE) system after initial temporary adsorption onto leukocytes in the circulation. Factors in serum perhaps contribute to the inactivation of endotoxin. The adrenal steroids reduce certain toxic effects of endotoxins, perhaps by altering membrane permeability.

Physiopathologic Effects of Endotoxins

Among the many physiopathologic effects of endotoxins are the following:

A. Pyrogenicity (Fever Production): After intravenous injection of endotoxin in microgram amounts, fever occurs in rabbits and man. (In the mouse endotoxin produces a fall in temperature.) After injection there is a latent period of 30 minutes or more, then a short rise in temperature and a marked decrease in the number of circulating polymorphonuclear leukocytes. This is followed by a more prolonged second rise in temperature, probably caused by an "endogenous pyrogen" released from white blood cells under the influence of endotoxin.

B. Tolerance: Repeated daily injections of endotoxin result in progressive diminution of febrile and other responses to any endotoxin. Active infection with gram-negative bacteria (eg, pyelonephritis) can induce similar tolerance. Tolerance has been attributed to enhanced removal of endotoxin from the circulation by a stimulated RE system; to neutralization of endotoxin by specific antibodies; or to a "desensitization" at the level of reactive cells. The serum of tolerant animals can passively confer partial specific tolerance on normal recipients. Tolerance can be abolished by RE "blockade" with particles of carbon, thorium dioxide, or saccharated iron.

C. Lethal Shock: Bacterial endotoxin injected in large doses produces (in 1–2 hours) weakness, lethargy, diarrhea, hypotension, irreversible shock, and death. Gastrointestinal hemorrhage is usually the only gross autopsy finding. By immunofluorescence, endotoxin is found in the walls of blood vessels and throughout the RE system. The presence of large numbers of gram-negative bacteria in the blood stream (eg, sepsis, or transfusion of contaminated blood) produces similar lethal shock. There is much evidence to suggest that reversible shock (eg, from blood loss) may be converted into irreversible shock by endotoxin absorbed from the gastrointestinal tract. This can be prevented or treated with corticosteroids and removal of the source of endotoxin (treatment of sepsis, suppression of gastrointestinal flora by antimicrobial drugs).

D. Shwartzman Phenomenon: If a rabbit is injected with endotoxin intradermally on one day and intravenously on the next, hemorrhagic necrosis of the prepared skin site follows in a few hours. This phenomenon is probably unrelated to hypersensitivity or antigen-antibody reactions. After the intradermal "preparatory" injection, polymorphonuclear cells accumulate in and around dermal blood vessels and there is some vascular endothelial damage. After the intravenous "provoking" dose leukocyte-platelet thrombi form in the area, fibrin precipitates, vessels are occluded, and there is necrosis of blood vessel walls with hemorrhage and subsequent tissue necrosis. The phenomenon can be inhibited either by first making the animal leukopenic or by inhibiting its clotting mechanism (eg, with heparin). In the Shwartzman phenomenon lesions also occur in kidneys and other organs. These are much more prominent if, instead of a "preparatory" injection of endotoxin, the animal receives corticosteroid systemically. Under such circumstances bilateral hemorrhagic renal necrosis occurs. It is uncertain whether the Shwartzman phenomenon ever participates in human disease.

E. Tumor Damage: Endotoxin can elicit hemorrhagic necrosis in tumor tissue, largely through the production of vascular thrombosis. This has no practical value in the treatment of neoplastic diseases because the effect is limited by the development of tolerance.

F. Abortion and Prematurity: In pregnant animals endotoxin can produce decidual hemorrhage, uterine contractions and abortion. Pregnant women with active urinary tract infections caused by gram-negative bacteria may have premature labor and a consequently high perinatal mortality. This may be caused by endotoxin originating in the urinary tract.

G. Resistance to Infection: Small doses of endotoxin given experimentally may stimulate the phagocytic activity of leukocytes, enhance the filtering capacity of the reticuloendothelial system, and induce rises in the serum concentration of "properdin" and of opsonins active against gram-negative bacteria.

H. Resistance to Ionizing Radiation: Mammals exposed to excessive amounts of radiation commonly die from overwhelming gram-negative infection. This increased susceptibility to infection is counteracted, in part, by prior repeated administration of endotoxin, although the mechanism (humoral substances, reticuloendothelial proliferation) is uncertain.

THE COLIFORM BACTERIA

The coliform bacteria are a large and heterogeneous group of gram-negative rods resembling, to some extent, *Escherichia coli*. The complexity of the group, the variations in biochemical test results, and the changing ecologic relationships have led to a confusing profusion of names. Besides *E coli*, derived from the intestinal tract, the following groups of organisms are often included among the "coliforms":

(1) The Klebsiella-Aerobacter-Hafnia-Serratia group: Typical *Klebsiella pneumoniae*, originally known as a respiratory pathogen, is now the most com-

monly encountered member, especially in hospital infections. It is characterized by mucoid growth, large polysaccharide capsules, and lack of motility. Aerobacter aerogenes is often motile, exhibits less mucoid growth, has small capsules, and may be found free-living as well as in the intestinal tract, in urinary tract infections, and in sepsis. (Aerobacter has recently been renamed enterobacter but, for the time being, the term aerobacter will be used here.) *Serratia marcescens* is a small, usually free-living gram-negative rod which may produce an intense red pigment in culture. Serratia usually ferments lactose very slowly and was therefore included with the "paracolon" bacteria. Hafnia are "paracolon" organisms sometimes associated with gastroenteritis.

(2) The Arizona-Edwardsiella-Citrobacter group: These organisms ferment lactose very slowly, if at all, and were called "paracolon bacteria." They resemble salmonellae both in biochemical features and, occasionally, in pathogenicity for man.

(3) Organisms of the "Providence" group, formerly included with "paracolon bacteria," are biochemically related to proteus, deaminate amino acids (eg, lysine), and are encountered free-living or in urinary tract infections, sepsis, etc.

From a practical medical standpoint, there is some utility in retaining the term "paracolon" organisms to designate slow lactose fermenters that often have low pathogenicity and produce infections in debilitated hosts or organ systems with impaired function.

Morphology & Identification

A. Typical Organisms: The coliform bacteria are short gram-negative rods which may form chains. Under unfavorable conditions of culture (eg, exposure to antibiotics), long filamentous forms occur. Capsules are rare in *E coli*, more frequent in aerobacter, and large and regular in klebsiella. Motility is present in most strains of *E coli* and some strains of aerobacter; it is absent in klebsiella.

B. Culture: *E coli* forms circular, convex, smooth colonies with distinct edges. Aerobacter colonies are similar but somewhat more mucoid. Klebsiella colonies are large, very mucoid, and tend to coalesce with prolonged incubation. Hemolysis on blood agar is produced by some strains of *E coli*.

C. Growth Characteristics: Escherichia and aerobacter break down many carbohydrates with the production of acid and gas. Escherichia produces approximately equal amounts of CO_2 and H_2 from dextrose; aerobacter produces twice as much CO_2 as H_2. Paracolon bacteria characteristically ferment lactose slowly or not at all and differ in other biochemical features. Klebsiella also ferments many carbohydrates, but variations among strains are great. For some typical reactions, see Table 18–4.

The following special tests (IMViC) are employed for differentiation of typical *E coli* and *A aerogenes*:

1. Indole test—*E coli* produces indole in peptone broth.

2. **Methyl red test**—This test indicates pH of culture in 0.5% glucose broth after 4 days at 37° C. *E coli* will be below pH 4.5 and is therefore methyl red-positive.

3. **Voges-Proskauer reaction**—Depends upon production of acetylmethylcarbinol from dextrose. In the presence of alkali it is oxidized to diacetyl and gives a pink color (aerobacter).

4. **Citrate test**—Utilization of citrate as sole source of carbon (free-living organisms).

IMViC, the mnemonic formula for these four tests, is for *E coli* ++−−; for *A aerogenes,* −−++. There are many intermediate forms between the typical intestinal *E coli* and the typical free-living *A aerogenes.* The formula for *E freundii,* a free-living organism, is ±+−+.

D. Variation: All cultures contain variants and stable mutants with respect to colonial morphology (rough or smooth), antigenic characteristics, biochemical behavior, and virus resistance. *E coli* strain K-12 has been extensively studied from the standpoint of genetics, and sexual recombination of inherited characteristics has been demonstrated.

Antigenic Structure

Coliform organisms have a complex antigenic structure, and strains are divergent in their serologic behavior. They are classified by heat-stable somatic O antigens (more than 120 different ones), by heat-labile capsular K antigens, and by flagellar H antigens. The K antigens occur on surfaces and often interfere with O agglutination unless they are destroyed by heating. The antigenic formula of an *E coli* might be O55:K5:H21.

Klebsiellae form large capsules consisting of polysaccharides (K antigens) covering the somatic (O or R) antigens. Klebsiellae can be identified by capsular swelling tests with specific antisera. Human infections of the respiratory tract are caused particularly by capsular types 1 and 2; those of the urinary tract, by types 8, 9, 10, and 24.

Certain O antigens are found in representatives of coliforms, salmonellae or shigellae. A single organism commonly carries several O antigens. The type 2 capsular polysaccharide of klebsiellae is very similar to the polysaccharide of type 2 pneumococci. There are many other examples of overlapping antigenic structures.

Colicins (Bacteriocins)

Many gram-negative organisms produce bacteriocins (colicins, pyocins). These are antibiotic-like bactericidal substances produced by certain strains of bacteria active against some other strains of the same or closely related species of bacteria. Their production is controlled by episomes. Colicins are produced by coliform organisms; pyocins by pseudomonas. Bacteriocin production is accompanied by death and lysis of the producing cell. Bacteriocin producing strains are resistant to their own bacteriocin; consequently, bacteriocins can be used for "typing" of organisms.

Pathogenesis & Pathology

The coliform bacteria constitute a large part of the normal intestinal flora. Within the intestine, they do not cause disease and may even contribute to normal function and nutrition. These organisms become pathogenic only when they reach tissues outside the intestinal tract, particularly the urinary tract, the biliary tract, the peritoneum, or the meninges, causing inflammation at these sites. When normal host defenses are inadequate, particularly in early infancy, old age, in the terminal stages of other diseases, or after exposure to ionizing radiation, coliform bacteria may reach the blood stream and cause sepsis. In the neonatal period, high susceptibility to coliform sepsis may be caused by the absence of bactericidal 19 S globulins which cannot pass the placenta. *E coli,* especially O serotypes 1, 2, 4, 6, 7, 50, and 75, is the commonest cause of urinary tract infections.

Certain strains of *E coli* belonging to several distinct serologic types (eg, O55, O111, O127) appear to be related to infantile diarrhea in certain outbreaks, particularly in newborn nurseries.

Certain "paracolon bacteria" (Arizona-citrobacter) resemble salmonellae and can cause enteritis and sepsis. Others (Providence, Hafnia groups) are encountered in normal intestinal flora and occasionally in diarrheal disorders. Citrobacter and serratia are common in hospitalized patients as "superinfections." Serratia (usually nonpigmented) can cause pneumonia and sepsis. All cause urinary tract infections at times and frequently are resistant to antimicrobial therapy.

Klebsiella pneumoniae occurs in the respiratory tract and in the feces of about 5% of normal individuals and is the etiologic agent responsible for a small proportion (about 2%) of bacterial pneumonias. *K pneumoniae* produces extensive hemorrhagic consolidation of the lung, which, if untreated, has a high mortality rate (40–90%). Occasionally it produces urinary tract infection or enteritis in children. Other coliform organisms may also produce pneumonia. Two other klebsiella organisms are associated with inflammatory conditions of the upper respiratory tract: *K ozaenae* has been isolated from the nasal mucosa in ozena, a fetid, progressive atrophy of mucous membranes; and *K rhinoscleromatis* from rhinoscleroma, a destructive granuloma of the nose and pharynx.

Donovania (Calymmatobacterium) granulomatis is related to the klebsiellae. It causes granuloma inguinale, a venereal disease. In vitro, it is grown with difficulty on media containing egg yolk.

Clinical Findings

The clinical manifestations of infections with coliform bacilli depend entirely on the site of the infection and cannot be differentiated by symptoms or signs from processes caused by other bacteria. Coliform bacteremia is often associated with vascular collapse and shock. Gram-negative rod bacteremia has greatly increased in persons with impaired host defenses who are subjected to drugs and surgical procedures.

TABLE 18–1. Identification of gram-negative enteric bacteria.

Lactose Fermented Rapidly	Lactose Fermented Slowly	Lactose Not Fermented
E coli: Metallic sheen on differential media; motile; flat, nonviscous colonies. **Aerobacter-enterobacter:** Raised colonies, no metallic sheen; often motile; more viscous growth. Resistant to cephalosporins.	**Paracolon bacilli** (including serratia, citrobacter, Hafnia, Arizona, Providence, etc)	**Shigella species:** Nonmotile; no gas from dextrose. **Salmonella species:** Motile; acid and usually gas from dextrose.
Klebsiella: Very viscous, mucoid growth; nonmotile. Some strains susceptible to cephalosporins.		**Proteus species:** "Swarming" on agar; urea rapidly decomposed (smell of ammonia). **Pseudomonas species:** Soluble pigments, blue-green, and fluorescing; sweetish smell.

Diagnostic Laboratory Tests

A. Specimens: Urine, blood, pus, spinal fluid, sputum, or other material, as indicated by the localization of the process.

B. Stained Smears: Because gram-negative rods of the coliform group all resemble each other, only the presence of large capsules (klebsiella) is diagnostic. Direct capsule-swelling tests can be performed on klebsiellae visible in fresh specimens.

C. Culture: Specimens are plated both on ordinary agar and blood agar and on "differential" media which contain special dyes and carbohydrates; this permits the rapid recognition of lactose-fermenting and nonlactose-fermenting colonies (Table 18–1). On such media, eg, McConkey's or eosin methylene blue agar, *E coli* colonies have a distinct metallic sheen. Organisms isolated on "differential" media are further identified by biochemical and serologic tests (Table 18–4). Rapid preliminary identification of gram-negative enteric bacteria is often possible (Table 18–1).

Treatment

No single specific therapy is available. The sulfonamides, ampicillin, chloramphenicol, tetracyclines, polymyxins, and aminoglycosides have marked antibacterial effects against the coliform group, but variation in strain susceptibility is great and laboratory tests for antibiotic sensitivity are essential. Typically, aerobacter is resistant to cephalosporins, and some klebsiellae are susceptible. Serratia is often resistant to all available systemic antimicrobials except gentamicin. Certain conditions predisposing to infection by these organisms must be corrected surgically, eg, by relief of urinary tract obstruction, closure of perforation in an abdominal organ, or resection of a bronchiectatic portion of lung.

Epidemiology, Prevention, & Control

Coliform bacteria establish themselves in the normal intestinal tract within a few days after birth and from then on constitute a main portion of the normal microbial flora of the body. *E coli* is the prototype of these intestinal bacteria. Finding *E coli* in water or milk is accepted as proof of fecal contamination. *A aerogenes* occurs in the intestinal tract in much smaller numbers, and this species is found free-living on vegetation. Since the aerobacter-klebsiella group of organisms may be present in water in the absence of fecal contamination, tests have been employed to separate them from *E coli* for the purpose of sanitary control. This is a questionable practice because the presence of either escherichia or aerobacter species, or their intermediates, in large numbers in drinking water suggests surface contamination.

Control measures are not feasible as far as the normal endogenous flora is concerned. Enteropathogenic *E coli* serotypes and certain paracolon bacteria should be controlled like salmonellae. Coliforms constitute a principal problem in hospital infection at present. Rigorous asepsis and disinfection are helpful.

Immunity

In systemic infections, specific antibodies develop; but it is uncertain whether significant immunity follows infections due to these organisms.

THE PROTEUS GROUP

The proteus organisms are gram-negative, motile, aerobic bacilli. Most species are free-living in water, soil, and sewage. *P vulgaris* commonly occurs in the normal fecal flora of the intestinal tract, and *P morganii* has been incriminated in summer diarrhea in children. Proteus does not ferment lactose, rapidly liquefies gelatin, decomposes urea with the liberation of ammonia, and tends to "swarm," spreading rapidly over the surface of solid media. "Swarming" can be inhibited by incorporation of chloral hydrate or phenylethyl alcohol into the medium. It does not grow well at an acid pH (Table 18–4).

Motile strains of proteus contain H antigen in addition to the somatic O antigen. Certain strains labeled OX share specific polysaccharides with some rickettsiae. The OX strains are agglutinated by sera from patients with rickettsial diseases (Weil-Felix test).

P vulgaris, like the coliform bacilli, produces infections in humans only when it leaves its normal habitat in the intestinal tract. It is a frequent cause of urinary tract infections. Because of the remarkable resistance of proteus to most antimicrobial agents, its numbers tend to increase when the more susceptible coliforms are suppressed. There are great variations among strains of proteus in antibiotic sensitivity. Nitrofurantoin and kanamycin are at present the most active drugs against proteus. *Proteus mirabilis* is often inhibited by penicillin G and ampicillin.

PSEUDOMONAS AERUGINOSA
(Bacillus Pyocyaneus)

The pseudomonas group is composed of gram-negative, motile rods which produce water-soluble pigments that diffuse through the medium. They occur widely in soil, water, sewage, and air.

Pseudomonas aeruginosa is frequently present in small numbers in the normal intestinal flora. Its prevalence there increases greatly when coliform organisms are suppressed. It is also found on the human skin.

It grows readily on culture media, does not ferment lactose, and forms smooth round colonies with a fluorescent greenish color and a sweetish aromatic odor. From the colonies, bluish-green pigment diffuses into the medium. Some strains hemolyze blood. Among the pigments produced by *Ps aeruginosa* are pyocyanin, a bluish material soluble in chloroform and water and possessing some antimicrobial activity; and fluorescein, a greenish, fluorescent, water-soluble (but not chloroform-soluble) material (Table 18–4).

Ps aeruginosa is a pathogen only when introduced into areas devoid of normal defenses or when participating in mixed infections. It produces infection of wounds, giving rise to blue-green pus; meningitis, when introduced by lumbar puncture; urinary tract infection, when introduced by catheters and instruments or in irrigating solutions. Involvement of the respiratory tract is uncommon, but the organism is often found in otitis externa. Infection of the eye, which may lead to rapid destruction of the eyeball, occurs most commonly after injury or surgical procedures. *Ps aeruginosa* is resistant to most antimicrobial agents (it produces a potent β-lactamase) and therefore becomes dominant and important when more susceptible bacteria of the normal flora are suppressed. In debilitated persons or infants, it may invade the blood stream and

result in fatal sepsis. This occurs commonly in patients with leukemia or lymphoma who have received antineoplastic drugs or radiation, and in severe burns. In pseudomonas sepsis, verdoglobin (a breakdown product of hemoglobin) or fluorescent pigment can be detected in wounds, burns, or urine by ultraviolet fluorescence. For epidemiologic purposes, strains can be typed by bacteriophage or by pyocins (antibiotic-like substances produced by some strains under genetic control acting on other strains). (See Colicins, above.)

Polymyxins and gentamicin are the antimicrobial agents most commonly effective against *Ps aeruginosa*.

THE SALMONELLAE

Salmonellae are gram-negative motile aerobic rods which characteristically fail to ferment lactose and are pathogenic for man or animals by the oral route. The different species are closely related antigenically.

Morphology & Identification

Salmonellae are gram-negative, nonsporeforming bacilli which vary in length. Most species are motile with peritrichous flagella (except *S pullorum* and *S gallinarum*). Salmonellae grow readily on ordinary media but do not ferment lactose, sucrose, or salicin; they form acid and usually gas from glucose, maltose, mannitol, and dextrin (Table 18–4). Fermentations of sugars form a method of differentiating various species, but this is not as reliable as antigenic analysis. Salmonellae are resistant to freezing in water and to certain chemicals, eg, brilliant green, sodium tetrathionate, and sodium deoxycholate; such compounds inhibit coliform bacilli and are, therefore, useful for isolation of salmonellae from feces.

Salmonella species can be identified by biochemical tests and antigenic analysis. Strains within a single species may be identified by lysis by a specific bacteriophage. This "phage typing" is of epidemiologic significance.

Antigenic Structure

A. Antigens: There are 3 main antigens:

1. "H" or flagellar antigens are inactivated by heating over 60° C and also by alcohol and acids. They are best prepared for serologic testing by adding formalin to young motile broth cultures. With sera containing anti-"H" antibodies, such antigens agglutinate rapidly in large fluffy clumps. These "H" antigens contain several immunologic constituents. Within a single Salmonella species, flagellar antigens may occur in either or both of 2 forms called phase 1 and phase 2. The organisms tend to mutate from one phase to the other; this is called phase variation. Antibodies to H antigens are predominantly 7 S globulins.

2. "O" or somatic antigens occur on the surface of the bacterial body in both motile and nonmotile forms and are resistant to prolonged heating at 100° C,

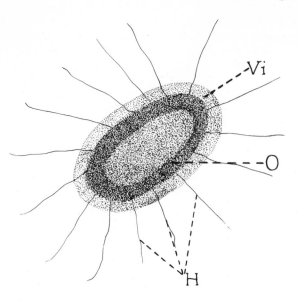

FIG 18—1. Antigenic structure of *Salmonella typhi*.

to alcohol, and to dilute acids. "O" antigens are prepared from nonmotile bacilli or by treatment with heat and alcohol. With sera containing anti-"O" antibodies, such antigens agglutinate slowly in granular masses. Antibodies to O antigens are predominantly 19 S globulins. Certain somatic O antigens are lipopolysaccharides free from protein.

3. The "Vi" antigen present at the extreme periphery of the body often interferes with agglutination of freshly isolated strains by antisera containing mainly anti-"O" agglutinins. It is destroyed by heating for 1 hour at 60° C and by acids and phenol. Cultures possessing "Vi" antigen may be more virulent for mice than those lacking it.

The Kauffmann-White classification of salmonellae is based on agglutination tests with absorbed sera, so that the content of "O" antigens and of phase 1 and phase 2 "H" antigens can be determined in an unknown organism. In the resulting "formula of antigenic constitution," "O" antigens and nonspecific phase 2 "H" antigens are given in Arabic numerals; phase 1 and specific phase 2 antigens are given in lower case letters. Examples are as follows: *S typhi:* 9, 12, Vi:d; *S typhimurium:* 1, 4, 5, 12:i-1, 2. The formula for *S typhi* shows that it contains O antigens 9 and 12; Vi antigen; and phase 1 H antigen d.

B. Variation: Organisms may lose "H" antigens and become nonmotile. Loss of "O" antigen is associated with change from smooth to rough colony form. "Vi" antigen may be lost partially or completely. Antigens may be acquired (or lost) in the process of transduction (see Chapter 4).

Toxins

Like those of other gram-negative bacteria, the cell walls of salmonellae contain lipopolysaccharides. These are liberated upon lysis of the cell and act as endotoxins.

Pathogenesis & Pathology

In all forms of salmonella infection, the organisms enter via the oral route and may produce either clinical or subclinical infection. Salmonellae may produce 3 main types of disease, but mixed forms are frequent.

A. The "Enteric Fevers": Typhoid (*S typhi* [formerly *S typhosa*]) and paratyphoid (*S paratyphi, S schottmülleri,* etc). Organisms ingested with contaminated food or drink reach the small intestine, from which they enter (perhaps within plasma cells) the intestinal lymphatics. They then travel via the thoracic duct into the blood stream and are thus disseminated into many organs, including the kidney and the intestines, where organisms multiply in lymphoid tissue and are excreted in the stool.

The outstanding lesions are hyperplasia and necrosis of lymphoid tissue (eg, Peyer's patches), focal necrosis in liver, inflammation in the gallbladder and occasionally of other sites (eg, periosteum, lungs).

B. Septicemias: Eg, due to *S choleraesuis.* Early invasion of the blood stream follows infection by the oral route, although intestinal involvement is often absent. The organisms are widely disseminated and tend to cause focal suppuration, abscesses, meningitis, osteomyelitis, pneumonia, and endocarditis, especially in debilitated hosts.

C. Gastroenteritis: (Often called "food poisoning.") Eg, due to *S typhimurium, S enteritidis,* or *S derby.* Symptoms appear after only 1—3 days' incubation, which suggests that ingestion of large numbers of organisms liberates toxin which results in a local violent irritation of mucous membranes; there is, however, no invasion of blood stream and no distribution to other organs.

Diagnostic Laboratory Tests

Blood for culture must be taken repeatedly. In enteric fevers and septicemias, blood is often positive in the first week of the disease. Bone marrow cultures may be useful.

Stool specimens also must be taken repeatedly. In enteric fevers the stools are positive from the second or third week on; in gastroenteritis, during the first week.

Duodenal drainage establishes the location of the organisms in the biliary tract in carriers.

Repeated specimens of blood serum for serology should be taken to demonstrate a rise in titer.

A. Bacteriologic Methods for Isolation of Salmonellae:

1. Enrichment cultures—Put specimen (usually stool) into selenite F or tetrathionate broth, both of which inhibit normal intestinal bacteria and permit multiplication of salmonellae. After incubation for 1—2 days, this is plated on differential and selective media or examined by direct immunofluorescence.

2. Selective medium cultures—The specimen is plated on SS (salmonella-shigella) agar or on deoxycholate citrate agar, which favors growth of salmonellae and shigellae over coliform organisms.

3. Differential medium cultures—Eosinmethylene blue, McConkey's, or deoxycholate medium permit

TABLE 18–2. Clinical diseases induced by salmonellae.

	Enteric Fevers	Septicemias	Gastroenteritis
Incubation period	7–20 days	Variable	8–48 hours
Onset	Insidious	Abrupt	Abrupt
Fever	Gradual, then high plateau, with "typhoidal" state.	Rapid rise, then spiking "septic" temperature.	Usually low
Duration of disease	Several weeks	Variable	2–5 days
Gastrointestinal symptoms	Often early constipation; later, bloody diarrhea.	Often none	Nausea, vomiting, diarrhea at onset.
Blood cultures	Positive in 1st–2nd week of disease.	Positive during high fever.	Negative
Stool cultures	Positive from 3rd week on; negative earlier in disease.	Only occasionally positive.	Positive soon after onset

rapid detection of lactose nonfermenters (which include not only salmonellae and shigellae but also proteus, pseudomonas, and other organisms). Gram-positive organisms are somewhat inhibited. Bismuth sulfite medium permits rapid detection of *S typhi,* which forms black colonies due to H_2S production.

4. Final identification—Suspected colonies from solid media are picked and identified by biochemical tests (Table 18–4) and by agglutination tests with specific sera.

B. Serologic Methods: Serologic technics are used for identification of an unknown culture with a known serum (see above), and detection of antibody titer in patients with unknown illness. Serum agglutinins rise sharply during the second and third week of salmonella infection. At least 2 serum specimens should be obtained at intervals of 7–10 days to prove rise in titer.

1. The rapid slide agglutination test is performed by mixing undiluted serum and unknown culture on a slide and observing the mixture under the low power objective. Clumping, when it occurs, can be observed within a few minutes. This test is particularly useful for preliminary identification of cultures.

2. The tube dilution agglutination test (Widal test)—Serial (2-fold) dilutions of unknown serum are tested against antigens from representative salmonellae, particularly "H," "O," and "Vi." The results are interpreted as follows: (1) High titer "O" (1:160 or more), low titer "H" suggests that active infection is present. (2) High titer "H" (1:160 or more), low titer "O" suggests past vaccination or past infection. (3) High titer "Vi" suggests the subject is a carrier.

Immunity

Infection due to *S typhi, S paratyphi,* and *S schottmülleri* usually confers a certain degree of immunity. Reinfection may occur, but is often milder. A heat-labile protective antigen has been partially purified. Circulating antibodies to O, H, or Vi are not clearly related to immunity.

Treatment

In severe diarrhea, replacement of fluids and electrolytes is essential. Opiates may be needed. Many anti-microbial agents are effective against salmonellae. Chloramphenicol or ampicillin is most successful in suppressing the disease but not necessarily in eradication of the organisms, which remains a function of immune processes. Multiple drug resistance transmitted genetically by an episome-like resistance transfer factor (RTF) among enteric bacteria plays a role in the increasing treatment problems of salmonella infections.

In carriers, the organisms may reside in the intestine or in the gallbladder and biliary ducts. Intestinal carriers can sometimes be treated successfully with ampicillin. Biliary carriers require cholecystectomy in addition to ampicillin. While enteric fever can be effectively treated, salmonella gastroenteritis is usually not shortened by antimicrobial drugs and excretion of organisms may even be prolonged.

Epidemiology

A. Sources of Infection: The sources of infection are food and drink which have been contaminated with salmonellae. The following sources are important:

1. Water—Contamination with feces often results in explosive epidemics.

2. Milk and other dairy products (ice cream, cheese, custard)—Contamination with feces or due to inadequate pasteurization or improper handling. The disease usually occurs in limited outbreaks traceable to source of supply.

3. Shellfish—Contaminated water.

4. Dried or frozen eggs—From infected fowl or contamination during processing.

5. Dried coconut.

6. Meats and meat products—Either from infected animals (poultry) or contaminated with feces by rodents or man. Corned beef has been involved.

7. Animal dyes (eg, carmine) used in drugs, foods, and cosmetics.

8. Household pets, eg, turtles, dogs, and cats.

B. Origin of Contamination: The feces of unsuspected subclinical cases or carriers are a more important source of contamination than frank clinical cases who are promptly isolated. Fecal contamination of this sort is especially dangerous if food handlers are "shedding" organisms. Many animals, cattle, rodents, and fowl are naturally infected with a variety of salmonellae and have the bacteria in their tissues (meat), excreta, or eggs. The incidence of typhoid fever has decreased, but the incidence of other salmonella infections has increased markedly in the USA.

C. Carriers: After manifest or subclinical infection, some individuals continue to harbor organisms in their tissues for variable lengths of time (convalescent carriers or healthy permanent carriers). Three percent of survivors with typhoid become permanent carriers, harboring the organisms in the gallbladder, the intestine, or, rarely, the urinary tract.

Prevention & Control

Sanitary measures must be taken to prevent contamination of food and water by rodents or other animals which excrete salmonellae. Infected poultry, meats, and eggs must be thoroughly cooked. Carriers must not be allowed to work as food handlers and should observe strict hygienic precautions. Cholecystectomy or ampicillin may eliminate the carrier state.

Two injections of acetone-killed bacterial suspensions of *S typhi*, followed by a booster injection some months later, give partial resistance to small doses of typhoid bacilli but not to large doses. The vaccines against other salmonellae give even less protection and are not recommended.

THE SHIGELLAE

Shigellae are nonmotile, gram-negative, aerobic rods which, with a few exceptions, do not ferment lactose but which do ferment other carbohydrates, producing acid but not gas. Many species share common antigens with one another and with other enteric bacteria. The natural habitat of shigellae is limited to the intestinal tracts of man and other primates where a number of species produce bacillary dysentery.

Morphology & Identification

A. Typical Organisms: Slender, unencapsulated, nonmotile, nonsporeforming, gram-negative rods. Coccobacillary forms may occur in young cultures.

B. Culture: Shigellae are facultative anaerobes but grow best aerobically. Convex, circular, transparent colonies with intact edges reach a diameter of about 2 mm in 24 hours. They are commonly recognized on differential media by their inability to ferment lactose, thus remaining colorless while lactose fermenters turn red.

C. Growth Characteristics: All shigellae ferment glucose; none ferment salicin. With the exception of *S sonnei* and *S dispar,* they do not ferment lactose. They form acid from carbohydrates but, with the exception of *S newcastle* and *S manchester,* do not produce gas. Shigellae may also be divided into those which ferment mannitol (eg, *S sonnei* and *S flexneri*) and those which do not (eg, *S dysenteriae*) (Table 18–3).

D. Variation: Mutants with different biochemical, antigenic, and pathogenic properties emerge frequently from the parent strains. Variation from smooth (S) to rough (R) colony form is associated with loss of endotoxin.

Antigenic Structure

Shigellae have a complex antigenic pattern. There is great overlapping in the serologic behavior of different species, and most of them share O antigens with other enteric bacilli.

The somatic O antigens of shigellae are lipopolysaccharide-protein complexes. Their serologic specificity appears to be a function of the polysaccharide component. The classification of shigellae relies on a combination of biochemical and antigenic characteristics. The principal pathogenic species are shown in Table 18–3.

Pathogenesis & Pathology

The natural habitat of dysentery bacilli is the large intestine of man. *S alkalescens* and *S dispar* are almost never associated with bowel disease and are now called escherichiae. The other shigellae can cause bacillary dysentery. Shigella infections are practically always limited to the gastrointestinal tract; blood stream invasion is quite rare. The essential pathologic process is an inflammation of the wall of the large intestine and terminal ileum, leading to necrosis of the mucous membrane, superficial ulceration, bleeding, and formation of a "pseudomembrane" on the ulcerated area. This consists of fibrin, leukocytes, cell debris, a necrotic mucous membrane, and bacteria. As the process subsides, granulation tissue fills the ulcers and scar tissue forms. This series of events is probably caused by the release of toxin from the autolyzing shigellae.

Toxins

All shigellae release, upon autolysis, their toxic somatic antigen. This endotoxin probably accounts for the intense irritation of the bowel wall.

In addition, *S dysenteriae* (type 1) produces a heat-labile potent toxin which can easily be separated from the cell bodies and is sometimes referred to as "exotoxin." It is a protein, highly lethal for experimental animals, antigenically distinct from the endotoxin, and stimulates the production of a specific antitoxin. This antitoxin neutralizes the lethal properties of the toxin. The toxin of *S dysenteriae* is probably responsible for some of the clinical severity and "intoxication" of the dysentery due to the shiga bacillus, and may also cause some CNS reactions (meningismus, coma) seen in severe cases.

Clinical Findings

After a short incubation period (1–4 days) there is a sudden onset of abdominal pain, cramps, diarrhea, and fever. The stools are liquid and contain mucus and blood after the first few movements. Their passage is accompanied by much straining and tenesmus (rectal

TABLE 18–3. Pathogenic species of shigella.

	Group and Type	Present Designation	Earlier Designation
Mannitol-negative	A (1) A (2) A (3–7)	*S dysenteriae* *S schmitzii* *S arabinotarda*	*S shigae*, Shiga's bacillus *S ambigua* *S large-sachsii*, parashiga group
Mannitol-positive	B (1–6) C (1–15) D (1–2)	*S flexneri* *S boydii* *S sonnei*	*S paradysenteriae*, Flexner subgroup *S paradysenteriae*, Boyd subgroup Sonne bacillus

spasms). Spontaneous recovery generally occurs in a few days, but small children sometimes succumb to dehydration and acidosis. The disease caused by *S dysenteriae* is particularly severe.

Most persons, on recovery, shed dysentery bacilli for only a short period, but a few remain chronic intestinal carriers and may have recurrent bouts of the disease. Upon recovery from the infection, most persons develop antibodies to shigellae in their blood, but these do not protect against reinfection. Injection of killed dysentery bacilli likewise stimulates the production of antibodies but fails to protect humans against the infection.

Diagnostic Laboratory Tests

Specimens consist of fresh stool, mucus flecks, and rectal swabs for culture. Serum specimens, if desired, must be taken 10 days apart to demonstrate rise in titer of agglutinating antibodies.

A. Culture: The materials are streaked on differential selective media (eg, McConkey's or eosin-methylene-blue agar) and on SS thiosulfate-citrate-bile agar, which suppress coliform and gram-positive organisms. Colorless (lactose-negative) colonies are inoculated into double sugar medium or triple sugar iron medium (Table 18–4). Organisms producing acid on the slant and acid and gas in the butt should be discarded; they are either coliforms or paracolon bacilli. Proteus is ruled out by the rapid formation of red color in Christensen's urea medium. Organisms which fail to produce H_2S, which produce acid but not gas in the butt and an alkaline slant, and are nonmotile should be subjected to slide agglutination by specific shigella antisera.

B. Serology: Serologic diagnosis with a single specimen of the patient's serum is impractical because normal persons often have agglutinins against several Shigella species. However, serial determinations of antibody may be useful, showing a rise of specific antibody.

Immunity

A type-specific serologic response occurs with infection, but little resistance develops to subsequent attacks.

Treatment

A potent specific antitoxin against *S dysenteriae* exotoxin is available, but convincing proof of its clinical efficacy is lacking. Therapy with bacteriophages specific for shigellae has likewise been disappointing. Sulfonamides, ampicillin, streptomycin, tetracyclines, and chloramphenicol are often bacteriostatic for shigellae and can suppress acute clinical attacks of dysentery promptly. They occasionally fail to eradicate the organisms from the intestinal tract, however, and permit the carrier state to establish itself. Multiple drug resistance can be genetically transmitted by an episome, and resistant infection is widespread.

Epidemiology, Prevention, & Control

Shigellae are transmitted by "food, fingers, feces, and flies" from man to man. Vaccines are not successful. Mass chemoprophylaxis for limited periods of time (eg, in military personnel) is practical, but resistant strains of shigellae tend to emerge rapidly. Since man is the main recognized host of pathogenic shigellae, control efforts must be directed at eliminating the organisms from this reservoir by (1) isolation of patients and disinfection of excreta; (2) prevention of the carrier state by adequate and prolonged chemotherapy of the acute phase; (3) detection of subclinical cases, particularly in food handlers; and (4) sanitary control of water, food, and milk, sewage disposal, and fly control.

THE VIBRIOS

Vibrios are curved, gram-negative, aerobic rods; they are motile, possessing a single polar flagellum. *V cholerae* (formerly *V comma*) and related vibrios produce cholera in man.

Morphology & Identification

A. Typical Organisms: Upon first isolation vibrios are comma-shaped, curved rods about 2–4 μm long and are very actively motile by means of a single polar flagellum. They do not form spores. On prolonged cultivation vibrios may become straight rods, resembling other gram-negative enteric bacteria.

B. Culture: Vibrios produce convex, smooth, round colonies, opaque and granular in transmitted light. Some variants form folded colonies. *V cholerae* grows readily on the usual laboratory media.

TABLE 18–4. Biochemical reactions.

Organism	Motility	Glucose	Lactose	Sucrose	Mannitol	Xylose	H_2S Prod.	Triple Sugar Iron Agar or Russel's Double Sugar Agar	
								Slant	Butt
E coli	+	AG	AG	±	AG	AG	−	A	AG
A aerogenes	±	AG	AG	AG	AG	AG	−	A	AG
Paracolon bacteria	±	AG	d±	−	AG	AG	±	±A	AG
K pneumoniae	−	AG	±	±	±	±	−	±	AG
S typhi	+	A	−	−	A	±	±	Alk	A
S paratyphi (A)	+	AG	−	−	AG	−	−	Alk	AG
S paratyphi (B) (*schottmülleri*)	+	AG	−	−	AG	AG	+	Alk	AG
S typhimurium	+	AG	−	−	AG	±	+	Alk	AG
S choleraesuis	+	AG	−	−	AG	AG	±	Alk	AG
S enteritidis	+	AG	−	−	AG	AG	+	Alk	AG
Sh dysenteriae	−	A	−	−	−	−	−	Alk	A
Sh flexneri	−	A	−	±	±	−	−	Alk	A
Sh sonnei	−	A	dA	dA	A	−	−	Alk	A
P vulgaris	+	AG	−	AG	−	±	+	±A	AG
Ps aeruginosa	+	±	−	±	−	−	−	Alk	±A
Alcaligenes faecalis	+	−	−	−	−	−	−	Alk	Alk

(±) Variable   (−) Negative   (AG) Acid and gas   (d) Delayed
(+) Positive   (A) Acid (Yellow)   (Alk) Alkaline

C. Growth Characteristics: Vibrios grow well at 37° C on defined media containing mineral salts and asparagin as sources of carbon and nitrogen. Characteristically, these organisms grow at very high pH (8.5–9.5) but are rapidly killed by acid. Cultures containing fermentable carbohydrates therefore quickly become sterile.

V cholerae regularly ferments sucrose and mannose but not arabinose. When these organisms are grown in a peptone medium containing adequate amounts of tryptophan and nitrate, indole is produced and nitrate reduced. Upon addition of sulfuric acid a red color develops (nitroso-indol reaction, "cholera red test"). Glucose inhibits this reaction.

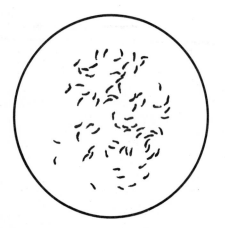

FIG 18–2. Typical organisms of *V cholerae* from broth.

Some vibrios (eg, *El Tor*) produce soluble hemolysins. Others (*V cholerae*) digest red blood cells without liberating a soluble hemolysin. They remove myxovirus receptors from the red cell surface by means of a receptor destroying enzyme (RDE), neuraminidase.

In culture (and probably in vivo also), vibrios elaborate "choleragen." This is an unconjugated protein with electrophoretic characteristics similar to 7 S globulin. After ingestion, choleragen causes marked increase in intestinal vascular permeability and diarrhea. Choleragen elaborated by different vibrios is probably of a single antigenic type.

D. Variation: The colonial variation from smooth to rough is associated with antigenic changes. Rough variants agglutinate in physiologic saline solution or acriflavine.

Antigenic Structure

Vibrios have a single heat-labile flagellar H antigen. Antibodies to the H antigen are probably not involved in the protection of susceptible hosts. The H antigen is the same in many vibrios. Cholera vibrios possess somatic O antigens, which can be extracted. These are complex toxic molecules and possess polysaccharide fractions that confer serologic specificity which places the O antigen in one of 6 groups. Antibodies to the O antigens tend to protect laboratory animals against infections with *V cholerae*. Both group-specific and type-specific O antigens have been found. H antigen, with its corresponding antibody, agglutinates in loose flocculi. Agglutination of O antigen by its corresponding antibody results in fine granular complexes; bacteriolysis occurs in the presence of complement. If immunized guinea pigs are intraperitoneally injected with living suspensions of cholera vibrios, lysis of the organisms can be observed within the peritoneal cavity (Pfeiffer phenomenon). In vitro, vibrios are converted to a protoplast-like, osmotically fragile form in the presence of specific antibody and complement. Lysis occurs unless osmotic protection is provided (eg, 0.5 M lactose).

Choleragen is antigenic and probably of a single type.

Pathogenesis & Pathology

Under natural conditions, cholera vibrios are pathogenic only for man. However, when organisms suspended in mucin are injected intraperitoneally into mice, the mice may die.

Cholera is not an invasive infection. The organisms never reach the blood stream but remain localized within the intestinal tract. There they multiply and liberate endotoxin, mucinases, and choleragen. These materials are intensely irritating to the mucous membranes, damage the epithelium, and stimulate hypersecretion. As a result, there is an outpouring of fluid and salts with resulting diarrhea, dehydration, acidosis, shock, and death.

The feces of animals or men who have recovered from the infection contain antibodies which agglutinate *V cholerae* (coproantibodies). These are secretory IgA and have protective activity.

Clinical Findings

After an incubation period of 2–5 days there is a sudden onset of nausea and vomiting and profuse diarrhea with abdominal cramps. The stools resemble "rice water" and contain mucus, epithelial cells, and large numbers of vibrios. There is rapid loss of fluids and salts, which leads to profound dehydration, circulatory collapse, and anuria. The death rate is between 25 and 50%. *El Tor* vibrios produce a similar diarrheal disease.

Several other members of the genus Vibrio produce disease in animals, eg, horses and cattle. These localize in the genital tract and may cause abortion. *Vibrio fetus* may produce sepsis and abortion in humans.

The diagnosis of a full-blown case of cholera presents no problem in the presence of an epidemic. However, sporadic or mild cases are not readily differentiated from other diarrheal diseases.

Diagnostic Laboratory Tests

Specimens for culture consist of mucus flakes from stools and, occasionally, vomitus. Growth is rapid on peptone agar, Dieudonné blood agar (pH near 9.0), or alkaline hemoglobin agar, and typical colonies can be picked in 18 hours. For enrichment, a few drops of stool can be incubated for 6–8 hours in peptone water (pH 8.0–9.0), and the pellicle on the surface can be stained.

Organisms resembling vibrios are further identified by slide agglutination tests, fermentation reactions, and a positive cholera-red reaction.

Immunity

An attack of cholera is followed by immunity to reinfection, but the duration and actual degree of immunity are not known. In experimental animals, specific antibodies in the lumen of the intestine (secretory IgA, "coproantibodies") may be protective. Similar antibodies appear in man after infection. Vibriocidal antibodies in serum develop also after infection but last only a few months.

Treatment

The most important part of therapy consists of water and electrolyte replacement to correct the severe dehydration and salt depletion. Many antimicrobial agents are effective against *V cholerae*. Oral tetracycline or furazolidone tends to reduce stool output in cholera and may shorten the period of excretion of vibrios.

Epidemiology, Prevention, & Control

Cholera is endemic in India and southeast Asia. From these centers it is carried along shipping lanes, trade routes, and pilgrim migrations. The disease is spread by individuals with mild or early illness and by water, food, flies, and person-to-person contact. The carrier state seldom exceeds 3 or 4 weeks, and true chronic carriers are rare. Vibrios survive in water for up to 3 weeks.

Control rests on education and improvement of sanitation, particularly of food and water. Patients should be isolated, their excreta disinfected, and contacts quarantined. Chemoprophylaxis with antimicrobial drugs may have a place. Repeated injection of a vaccine containing either lipopolysaccharides extracted from vibrios or dense vibrio suspensions can confer significant protection.

●　●　●

General References

Aserkoff, B., & others: Effect of antibiotic therapy in acute salmonellosis. New England J Med 281:636–640, 1969.

Edmondson, E.B., & J.P. Sanford: The Klebsiella-Enterobacter-Serratia group. Medicine 46:323–340, 1967.

Fields, B.N., & others: The so-called "paracolon" bacteria. A bacteriologic and clinical reappraisal. Am J Med 42:89–106, 1967.

Nelson, J.D., & others: Endemic shigellosis. Am J Epid 86:683–694, 1967.

Phillips, R.A.: Asiatic cholera. Ann Rev Med 19:69–80, 1968.

Prost, E.: Food-borne salmonellosis. Ann Rev Microbiol 21:495–528, 1967.

Wahab, M.F., & others: Paratyphoid A fever. Ann Int Med 70:913–917, 1969.

19...
Small Gram-Negative Rods

THE BRUCELLAE

The brucellae are small, aerobic, gram-negative coccobacilli which are nonmotile, nonsporeforming, and relatively inactive metabolically. They are obligate parasites of animals and man and are characteristically located intracellularly. *Br melitensis* typically infects goats; *Br suis*, swine; and *Br abortus*, cattle. The disease in man, brucellosis (undulant fever, Malta fever), is characterized by an acute septicemic phase followed by a chronic stage which may extend over many years and may involve many tissues.

Morphology & Identification

A. Typical Organisms: The appearance in young cultures varies from cocci to rods 0.8 μm in length, with short coccobacillary forms predominating. The organisms are gram-negative but often stain irregularly. Capsules can be demonstrated on smooth and mucoid variants. The organisms are nonmotile and nonspore-forming.

C. Culture: On enriched media small, convex, smooth colonies appear in 24—48 hours. The colonies are at first translucent; later they often become brownish.

C. Growth Characteristics: Brucellae are adapted to an intracellular habitat, and their nutritional requirements are complex. Some strains have been cultivated on defined media of 18 amino acids, vitamins, salts, and glucose. Fresh specimens from animal or human sources are usually inoculated on trypticase soy or liver infusion agar. On primary isolation various constituents of the medium may be toxic to the organisms (eg, toxic amounts of sulfur may be liberated from sulfur-containing amino acids in the medium). Other constituents of the medium must neutralize these toxic effects to permit growth of brucellae. *Br abortus* requires 5—10% CO_2 for growth, whereas the other 2 species grow in the presence of air.

Brucellae utilize carbohydrates but produce neither acid nor gas in amounts sufficient for classification. Catalase is produced by some strains and may have some correlation with virulence. Hydrogen sulfide is produced by many strains, and nitrates are reduced to nitrites.

Brucellae are moderately sensitive to heat and acidity. They are killed in milk by pasteurization.

D. Variation: Smooth, mucoid, and rough variants are recognized by colonial appearance and virulence. The typical virulent organism forms a smooth, transparent colony; it tends to mutate to the rough form, which is avirulent. These avirulent (rough) cells agglutinate in 1% acriflavine solution, whereas virulent (smooth) forms do not.

The selection of mutants in vivo appears to be influenced by materials in the environment. Thus the serum of susceptible animals contains a globulin and a lipoprotein which suppress growth of nonsmooth, avirulent types and favor the growth of virulent types. Resistant animal species lack these factors, so that rapid mutation to avirulence can occur. D-Alanine has been shown in vitro to have a similar selective effect.

Antigenic Structure

Different species of brucellae cannot be differentiated by agglutination tests but can be distinguished by agglutinin absorption reactions. It is probable that 2 antigens, A and M, are present in different proportions in the 3 species. In addition, a superficial L-antigen has been demonstrated which resembles the Vi antigen of salmonellae.

Species differentiations among the 3 Brucella species is made possible by their characteristic sensitivity to dyes. (See Table 19—1.)

Bordetella bronchiseptica is a small gram-negative rod often found in the respiratory tracts of canines. It is related both to brucellae and to *Hemophilus influenzae*.

Pathogenesis & Pathology

Although each species of Brucella has a preferred host, all can infect a wide range of animals, including man.

The common routes of infection in man are the intestinal tract (ingestion of infected milk), mucous membranes (droplets), and skin (contact with infected tissues of animals). The organisms progress from the portal of entry, via lymphatic channels and regional lymph nodes, to the thoracic duct and the blood stream, which distributes them to the parenchymatous organs. In lymphatic tissue, liver, spleen, bone marrow, and other parts of the reticuloendothelial system, granulomatous nodules form which may develop into abscesses. In such lesions the brucellae are principally intracellular. There is also occasionally osteomyelitis, meningitis, or cholecystitis. The main histologic reac-

TABLE 19–1. Dye sensitivity of brucellae.

| | Growth in Presence of | | H_2S Production | CO_2 Requirement |
	Thionine (1:50,000)	Basic Fuchsin (1:25,000)		
Br abortus	--	+	++	+
Br melitensis	+	+	+	–
Br suis	+	–	+++	–

tion in brucellosis consists of proliferation of mono-nuclear cells, exudation of fibrin, coagulation necrosis, and fibrosis. The granulomas consist of epithelioid and giant cells, with central necrosis and peripheral fibrosis.

Persons with active brucellosis react more markedly (fever, myalgia) to injected brucella endo-toxin than normal persons. Sensitivity to endotoxin thus may play a role in pathogenesis.

Fetal membranes of many animals contain erythritol, a growth factor for brucellae. This may explain the particularly high susceptibility of pregnant animals.

Clinical Findings

The incubation period is 1–6 weeks. The onset is insidious, with malaise, fever, weakness, aches, and sweats. The fever usually rises in the afternoon; its fall during the night is accompanied by drenching sweat. There may be gastrointestinal and nervous symptoms. Lymph nodes enlarge, and the spleen becomes palpable. Hepatitis may be accompanied by jaundice. Deep pain and disturbances of motion, particularly in vertebral bodies, signify osteomyelitis. These symptoms of generalized brucella infection generally subside in weeks or months, although localized lesions and symptoms may continue.

Following the initial infection, a chronic stage may develop characterized by weakness, aches and pains, low-grade fever, nervousness, and other nonspecific manifestations compatible with psychoneurotic symptoms. Brucellae cannot be isolated from the patient at this stage, but the agglutinin titer may be high. The diagnosis of "chronic brucellosis" is difficult to establish with certainty unless local lesions are present.

Diagnostic Laboratory Tests

Take blood for culture, biopsy material for culture (lymph nodes, bone marrow, etc), and serum for serologic tests.

A. Culture: Blood or tissues are incubated in trypticase-soy broth with 1% citrate. At intervals of several days, subcultures are made on solid media of similar composition or on liver infusion agar. All cultures are incubated in 10% CO_2 and should be observed and subcultured for 6 weeks before being discarded as negative.

If organisms resembling brucellae are isolated, they are typed by H_2S production, dye inhibition, and agglutination by absorbed sera. As a rule, brucellae can be cultivated from patients only during the acute phase of the illness.

B. Serology: Early in the disease agglutinating antibodies appear, somewhat later precipitating and blocking antibodies. The latter tend to persist without relation to activity of the infection, but precipitating antibodies disappear when the active infection is terminated spontaneously or by therapy.

1. Agglutination test—To be reliable, agglutination tests must be performed with standardized heat-killed, phenolized, smooth brucella antigens available from brucellosis centers and should be incubated at 37° C for 48 hours. Agglutinin titers above 1:80 indicate past or present infection. Lower titers may be significant if they can be attributed to mercaptoethanol-resistant 7 S agglutinins. Individuals injected with cholera vaccine may develop agglutinin titers to brucellae. Skin tests with brucella antigen may give a rise in brucella agglutinin titer. If the serum agglutination test is negative in patients with strong clinical evidence of brucella infection, tests must be made for the presence of incomplete, "blocking" antibodies. This can be done most simply by using 5% NaCl or albumin solution as diluents for the patient's serum instead of 0.85% NaCl solution in the agglutination test.

2. Opsonocytophagic test—This test is subject to great variations and is probably not reliable.

3. Precipitin test—Sera from patients with active brucellosis contain a precipitin for brucella extracts after the initial acute stage of the disease. These precipitating antibodies disappear when activity of the infection subsides. Thus precipitins appear to be the best indicator of active infection after the acute stage.

4. Blocking antibodies manifest themselves by inhibiting other serologic reactions. They are responsible for prozone inhibition, ie, failure of serologic tests to be positive in low serum dilutions although positive in higher dilutions. These antibodies appear at the same time as precipitins, during the subacute stage of infection, but tend to persist for many years independently of activity of infection.

C. Skin Test: When "brucellergen" or a crystalline polypeptide brucella extract is injected intradermally, erythema, edema, and induration develop within 24 hours in individuals hypersensitive to brucellae. Most infected individuals are skin test-positive, but a negative test does not rule out infection. The skin test is therefore of limited diagnostic usefulness. Application of the skin test may stimulate the agglutinin titer.

Immunity

An antibody response occurs with infection, and it is probable that some resistance to subsequent attacks is produced. In immunogenic fractions from brucella cell walls, there is a high phospholipid content, lysine predominates among 8 amino acids, and there is no heptose (thus distinct from endotoxin).

Treatment

Brucellae are quite sensitive to streptomycin and the tetracycline antibiotics. Symptomatic relief may occur within a few days after treatment with these drugs is begun. However, because of their intracellular location, the organisms are not readily eradicated completely from the host. For best results treatment must be prolonged. Combined treatment with streptomycin and one of the tetracyclines is advocated, but tetracycline alone may be satisfactory.

Epidemiology, Prevention, & Control

Brucellae are essentially animal pathogens transmitted in animal populations by contact with feces, urine, milk, and infected tissues. Infection of man is accidental, through contact with these same infected materials. The common sources of infection for man are unpasteurized milk and milk products and occupational contact (eg, farmers, veterinarians, slaughterhouse workers) with infected animals. Occasionally the airborne route may be important. Because of occupational contact, brucella infection is much more frequent in men. The majority of infections remains asymptomatic (latent).

Infection rates vary greatly with different animals and in different countries. In the USA about 4% of all cattle are infected, and about 15% of herds contain infected animals. Eradication of brucellosis in cattle can be attempted by test and slaughter, active immunization of heifers with avirulent live strain 19, or combined testing, segregation, and immunization. Cattle are examined by agglutination tests and skin tests.

Active immunization of humans is still in the experimental stage. Control rests on limitation of spread and possible eradication of animal infection, pasteurization of milk and milk products, and reduction of occupational hazards wherever possible.

THE PASTEURELLAE

Pasteurellae are short, gram-negative rods showing bipolar staining by special methods. They are nonsporeforming, aerobic or microaerophilic organisms. All are nonmotile except *P pseudotuberculosis.* Different species attack a variety of carbohydrates, producing acid but not gas. Some species produce hemorrhagic septicemia in various animals (*P multocida*); others infect animals and also produce serious disease in man (*P pestis,* plague; *P [Francisella] tularensis,* tularemia).

Morphology & Identification

A. Typical Organisms: The typical short, ovoid, plump, gram-negative rods are predominant in cultures and in smears from infected tissues. *P pseudotuberculosis* possesses flagella; other species are nonmotile. Wayson's stain (methylene blue with carbolfuchsin) brings out the bipolar appearance of these organisms, causing them to resemble safety pins. Capsules or "envelopes" around the bacterial body are frequently present. Upon prolonged incubation or in an unfavorable environment, the rods are pleomorphic, varying greatly in size and shape. Long filamentous rods are occasionally seen.

B. Culture: All pasteurellae except *P tularensis* grow on ordinary bacteriologic media, but they grow more rapidly on media containing tissue fluids or blood. Gray, viscous colonies are formed from virulent tissue inocula, but irregular rough colonies occur frequently. *P tularensis* grows from small inocula only on complex media containing blood or tissue extracts and cystine, forming minute drop-like colonies in 48–76 hours at 37° C. All pasteurellae grow readily in the yolk sacs of embryonated eggs.

C. Growth Characteristics: Pasteurellae ferment carbohydrates, forming acid but not gas. There is great variation among strains, and species are not uniform in their biochemical reactions. The temperature for optimal rate of growth is 30° C for *P pestis* and 37° C for *P tularensis,* but the production of certain antigenic components (eg, the protein-carbohydrate complex of fraction I in *P pestis*) is greater at 37° C than at 30° C. *P pseudotuberculosis* grown at 22° C is motile; at 37° C it is nonmotile. Catalase activity is greater in virulent than in avirulent strains of *P pestis.*

D. Variation: Variants and stable mutants occur commonly with respect to appearance, morphology (eg, motility in *P pseudotuberculosis*), biochemical characteristics, antigenic makeup, virulence, and drug resistance. Stable, avirulent mutants have been widely employed for vaccination against plague.

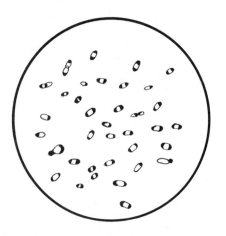

FIG 19–1. Typical organisms of *P pestis* from smear of lymph node.

Antigenic Structure

The members of each species of Pasteurella fall into certain antigenic patterns; even within each species, however, there are antigenic differences among strains, and different species may appear interrelated by serologic tests. All pasteurellae possess somatic O antigens which are toxic for animals and which chemically are polysaccharide-lipoprotein complexes. These have been subdivided by chemical fractionation into components of varying immunologic and serologic activity. In *P pestis,* for example, fraction I, precipitated by 33% saturation of ammonium sulfate from aqueous extracts of acetone-dried bacilli, is largely responsible for stimulating antibacterial immunity. This fraction is produced by virulent and by certain avirulent strains at 37° C but is produced only to a limited extent at 30° C; it appears to be located in the outer "envelope" of the plague bacillus. Organisms virulent for guinea pigs produce, in addition to fraction I, a V-W antigen which makes them resist phagocytosis even in the absence of a visible "envelope." V-W alone suffices for full mouse virulence. A pure toxin has been isolated from *P pestis* which is homogeneous protein with a molecular weight of 74,000 and an LD_{50} for mice of 1 µg. The "toxin" for mice is a mixture of at least 2 proteins and is distinct from the "toxin" for guinea pigs.

P pseudotuberculosis carries an H antigen in its flagella when grown at 22° C. At 37° C this antigen does not form and the organisms are universally nonmotile. At least one of the O antigens of *P pseudotuberculosis* cross-reacts with that of *P pestis.* Bacteriophages specific for *P pestis* tend to lyse many strains of *P pseudotuberculosis,* but they usually do not lyse *P multocida* or *P tularensis.* Bacteriophages that lyse *P pseudotuberculosis* also lyse certain strains of shigellae or salmonellae. *P tularensis* strains are relatively homogeneous serologically but cross-react with some brucellae. All this indicates close relationship of antigenic constituents among many gram-negative bacilli.

Pathogenesis & Pathology

Some Pasteurella species have narrow host ranges, producing disease in only a few types of animals; others affect a large variety of hosts. Pasteurellae generally produce disease by rapid invasion of the host body, multiplying in many tissues until overwhelming sepsis supervenes. When the population of pasteurellae reaches a high level, autolysis probably liberates sufficient "toxin" to be harmful to the host tissues.

Purified plague toxins depress respiration of heart mitochondria in vitro, affecting different animal species in different degrees.

Hemorrhagic Septicemia of Animals

There are varieties of *P multocida* which are pathogenic for one or more of the following animals: rabbits, rats, horses, sheep, fowl, dogs, cats, and swine. The organisms are usually normal inhabitants of the respiratory tracts of animals and may suddenly assume pathogenicity when the host-parasite balance is disturbed. This occurs either (1) when there is unusually rapid passage from one host to another (eg, in the experimental passage of tissue in series), or (2) when host resistance is impaired through drastic environmental changes or intercurrent infections (particularly those due to viruses). Under such circumstances there may be acute septicemia with rapid proliferation of bacilli in tissues and blood stream, high fever, prostration, diarrhea, and death within 12–48 hours. Pathologically there are serous and hemorrhagic inflammatory changes in all organs and vast numbers of bacilli in the blood. In the subacute and chronic disease necrotic foci form in various organs, and the animals often survive. Human infections with *P multocida* are very rare.

Plague

P pestis is a parasite of various rodents, eg, rats and squirrels. It is transmitted from one rodent to another through the bites of fleas who have become infected by sucking the blood of an infected animal. The plague bacilli proliferate vastly in the intestinal tract of the flea and eventually block the lumen of the proventriculus completely so that no food can pass through. The hungry flea bites ferociously, and the aspirated blood is regurgitated, with an admixture of plague bacilli, into the bite wound. Thus, plague infection is transmitted from rodent to rodent and, occasionally, from rodent to man. It is not transmitted from man to man by fleas. When in the course of human infection pneumonia develops, droplets containing plague bacilli are coughed up. Such droplets are highly infectious by the airborne route and result in primary pneumonic plague in man, which is always fatal without chemotherapy and is readily transmitted from person to person. Some plague strains are so highly virulent that infection with a single organism may be lethal.

When plague bacilli enter the host via the mucous membranes or through the bite of a flea, they extend via the lymphatic channels to the regional lymph node. Along the lymphatics and in the lymph nodes there is a rapidly spreading hemorrhagic inflammation and the node becomes greatly enlarged, forming a "bubo." Such buboes are usually located in the groin or axilla and may undergo necrosis and become fluctuant. In the lesser forms of plague the infective process stops there. Often, however, organisms progress via efferent lymphatics and the thoracic duct to the blood stream, which rapidly disseminates them to all organs, especially to the spleen, liver, and lungs. In parenchymatous organs hemorrhagic inflammation is followed by development of focal necrosis. There are serosanguinous effusions in the pleura, the peritoneum, and the pericardium, and there may be (plague) meningitis. Terminally, plague bacilli may proliferate freely in the blood stream.

Pseudotuberculosis

P pseudotuberculosis produces an infection of birds, rodents, and other animals which is rarely transmitted to man. The route of transmission has not been established, but it is probable that animals become infected through ingestion of contaminated droppings. Typical lesions consist of whitish nodules, grossly resembling tubercles, in the intestines and the parenchymatous organs. They consist of a necrotic center surrounded by inflammatory cells, but there are no giant or epithelioid cells. The disease tends to be chronic and to progress slowly, but there may be sepsis with rapidly fatal outcome. One clinical form in man presents as appendicitis with enteritis and regional lymphadenitis, all of which tend to subside spontaneously.

Pasteurella X (*Yersinia enterocolitica*) is an occasional member of the human gut flora also encountered in ileocecal inflammation and endocarditis.

Tularemia

P tularensis (Francisella tularensis) is essentially a parasite of rodents which is adapted to transmission by biting flies (Chrysops), ticks (Dermacentor and others), and a rabbit louse, all of which transmit the infection among the rodent population and thus maintain the reservoir of infection. Hares, rabbits, and muskrats are the main sources of disease in man. Handling, skinning, or eating such infected animals may result in human infection. *P tularensis* may enter the host via the skin or mucous membranes, through the bites of arthropods, or via the respiratory or gastrointestinal tracts. An ulcerating papule often develops at the site of penetration of the skin or mucous membranes, and the regional lymph nodes enlarge and suppurate. Transitory bacteremia establishes the organisms in various parenchymatous organs, where granulomatous nodules form which often undergo necrosis. As the disease progresses, tularemic pneumonia and septicemia develop which are fatal if untreated. Often the localizing signs are limited to the portal of entry. Thus the clinical picture may be "oculoglandular," following infection via the conjunctivas; "ulceroglandular," following entry through the skin; or "pneumonic," following primary inhalation of infectious droplets. At other times there may be no localizing symptoms whatever and only a febrile systemic illness.

Clinical Findings

Sporadic cases of pasteurella infection usually present difficult diagnostic problems, whereas in epidemics (eg, of plague) the diagnosis is readily apparent. Usually the clinical features of a local lesion, adenopathy, and a bubo in a febrile illness with a history suggestive of exposure warrant the performance of laboratory procedures which can establish the diagnosis unequivocally.

Diagnostic Laboratory Tests

Blood for culture should be collected repeatedly, as well as blood serum for serologic tests; after an initial specimen in the acute stage, subsequent specimens should be obtained at 12- to 21-day intervals. Sputum for smear and culture must be obtained when pulmonary involvement is probable, and material from local lesions or aspirated material from a suppurating lymph node will be required for smear, culture, and animal inoculation. Strict aseptic precautions must be maintained because some pasteurellae are highly infective.

A. Stained Smears: Gram-stained films often show pleomorphic gram-negative organisms ranging from coccal forms to long rods. When plague is suspected, immunofluorescent staining can identify the organism rapidly.

B. Cultures: Materials are cultured in rich blood culture media and on blood agar (plates), incubated both aerobically and with 10% CO_2. If tularemia is suspected, specimens should also be cultured on blood-glucose-cystine agar. If growth occurs, bacteria may be identified by biochemical and serologic tests, susceptibility to specific bacteriophages, subculture at 20° C for motility (*P pseudotuberculosis*), and animal inoculation. **Note:** Great caution is necessary in handling highly infectious cultures. Sometimes it is difficult or impossible to assign a species designation to a pasteurella organism recovered from clinical or pathologic material because they do not always fit rigidly into the described species characteristics. The pasteurellae may be thought of as a broad group of organisms in which host affinity and susceptibility and ecologic relationships influence the behavior of the "strains" recovered from a given host at a given time.

C. Animal Inoculations: One of the important classifying characteristics of the pasteurella group is its ability to cause disease and specific lesions in a variety of laboratory animals (eg, *P pestis* is pathogenic for white rats and guinea pigs; *P pseudotuberculosis* for guinea pigs but not for rats). Laboratory animals must be kept in strict isolation and must be rid of ectoparasites before being injected. Animal inoculation is particularly valuable when the specimen is contaminated with other organisms which tend to outgrow pasteurellae in culture. Such organisms frequently are nonpathogenic for laboratory animals and thus permit pasteurellae to produce specific lesions.

D. Serology: In subacute or chronic infections with pasteurellae, recovery of the organism in culture is rarely possible. Diagnosis often depends on the outcome of serologic tests. To be reliable the antigen must be obtained from a standard source, eg, a state health department. A rise in titer is more significant in establishing diagnosis than is a single high titer.

Agglutination and complement fixation tests can be performed for antibodies to each of the pasteurellae. Very low serum titers are of questionable significance, since some cross-reactions occur with different types of organisms (brucellae, shigellae). A single high titer indicates only that infection has occurred at some time in the past; it does not establish the etiology of the current disease. Only by a definite rise in serum titer in 2 specimens taken 2 weeks apart can the diagnosis be established. Antiplague sera agglutinate *P pseudotuberculosis,* but anti-pseudotuberculosis sera usually do not agglutinate plague bacilli. Precipitin tests with chemical fractions of *P tularensis* and *P pestis* can be performed. Precipitins appear in humans after infection but not after injection of killed vaccines. Such precipitins may be associated with immunity. Their development may be suppressed by antimicrobial therapy early in the infection.

E. Skin Tests: In some cases of tularemia the intradermal injection of a killed suspension of *P tularensis* gives a tuberculin-type reaction during the first week of the disease. This reaction is not reliable as a diagnostic aid.

Immunity

A solid immunity to plague and tularemia follows infection and recovery in each case.

Treatment

Most pasteurellae are sensitive to sulfonamides, streptomycin, tetracyclines, and other antimicrobial drugs. Streptomycin, either alone or in combination with one of the tetracyclines, is rapidly curative in most patients if treatment is begun early in the disease.

Prevention

Vaccines have been prepared from various pasteurellae for the protective inoculation of exposed hosts. Attenuated cultures of killed suspensions of *P multocida* are sometimes employed in the hope of preventing hemorrhagic septicemia in domestic animals. Vaccines against plague can be prepared from (1) avirulent live bacteria; (2) heat-killed or formalin-inactivated suspensions of virulent bacteria; or (3) chemical fractions of the bacilli. The first 2 of these have been used on millions of persons in endemic areas and have given some protection which, however, is incomplete and of relatively short duration. Therefore, repeated vaccination of exposed individuals is essential in maintaining effective resistance. Reinfection following recovery from natural plague is quite rare, and immunity is thus presumed to be solid.

No practical or useful vaccines are available for pseudotuberculosis. A living, avirulent vaccine against tularemia has been used in Russia on a large scale.

In endemic areas plague can be efficiently prevented (even in persons exposed to patients with pneumonic involvement) by the daily administration of 2–4 gm of a sulfonamide. No spontaneously emerging sulfonamide-resistant plague bacilli have as yet been discovered.

Epidemiology & Control

Pasteurella infections are animal diseases and are only accidentally transmitted to man. The risk to man can be reduced if the animal infection rate can be kept low. This is the principle of control measures. Infections of man with *P multocida* and *P pseudotuberculosis* are so rare that active measures against the animal reservoir of infection are not carried out. Tularemia is maintained in wild rodents away from human habitation. Proper precautions when dealing with wild rabbits, and thorough cooking, are adequate safeguards in the majority of instances. In some parts of the world (eg, Russia, USA), water, grain, or hay contaminated by infected wild rodents may convey *P tularensis* to man.

Plague, on the other hand, presents an enormous epidemiologic problem. It is essentially an infection of wild rodents (squirrels, field mice, voles, gerbilles, etc) and occurs in many parts of the world. The chief enzootic areas are India, East Asia, South Africa, South America, and the western states of North America and Mexico. In these regions reservoirs of infection are always present in wild rodents and, intermittently, many animals die from the infection. The infection is transmitted by infective fleas among wild rodents. When the rate of infection rises in wild rodents, rats in urban environments become infected; the rat flea (*Xenopsylla cheopis*) is the chief vector in transmitting the disease to man. Once plague pneumonia occurs in man, direct man-to-man transmission through droplets constitutes a serious threat. From cities and harbors infected rats are transported across oceans on ships to start new outbreaks in other seaports.

Control measures are directed toward breaking the infection chain at several points: (1) Reduction of wild rodent populations and continuous survey of the rate of plague infection. Practical measures include shooting, trapping, and poisoning. (2) Reduction of rat populations in cities and continuous survey for plague infection in trapped rats. Measures are directed against rats on ships and in harbors. (3) Widespread application of insecticides to kill fleas, eg, DDT. (4) Chemoprophylaxis (sulfonamides) in all contacts whenever plague is suspected. (5) Prompt and efficient chemotherapy of cases. (There are probably no human plague carriers.) (6) Active immunization as a supplementary measure in highly endemic areas, in troops, and in persons who may be forced into situations of potential exposure. (7) Strict isolation of plague cases and observation for pneumonic involvement.

THE HEMOPHILIC BACTERIA

This is a heterogeneous group of small, gram-negative, aerobic bacilli which are nonmotile and nonsporeforming and which require enriched media, usually containing blood or its derivatives, for isolation. Some are among the normal flora of the mucous membranes; others (*H influenzae, B pertussis*) are important human pathogens.

HEMOPHILUS INFLUENZAE
(Pfeiffer's Bacillus)

Morphology & Identification

A. Typical Organisms: In specimens from acute infections the organisms are short (1.5 μm) coccoid bacilli, sometimes occurring in short chains. Long rods and large spherical bodies are also found. In cultures the morphology depends both on age and on the medium employed. At 6–8 hours in rich medium, coccobacillary forms predominate. Later there are longer rods, lysed bacteria, and very pleomorphic forms.

Organisms in young cultures (6–18 hours) on rich medium have a definite capsule. This capsule is rapidly dissolved by autolytic enzymes and therefore is poorly seen in older cultures. Capsule swelling tests are employed for "typing" *H influenzae* (see below).

B. Culture: On "Levinthal agar" (brain-heart-infusion agar with blood, heated and filtered), small, round, convex colonies with a strong iridescence develop in 24 hours. The colonies on "chocolate" (heated blood) agar take 36–48 hours to develop diameters of 1 mm. There is no hemolysis. Around staphylococcal (or other) colonies, the colonies of *H influenzae* grow much larger ("satellite phenomenon").

C. Growth Characteristics: Identification of organisms of the hemophilus group depends in part upon demonstrating the need for certain growth factors called X and V. Factor X acts physiologically as hemin; factor V can be replaced by coenzyme I or II or by nicotinamide nucleoside. The requirements for X and V factors of various Hemophilus species are listed in Table 19–2. Carbohydrates are fermented poorly and irregularly.

D. Variation: In addition to morphologic variation, *H influenzae* has a marked tendency to lose its capsule and the associated type specificity. Nonencapsulated variants give colonies lacking iridescence.

E. Transformation: Under proper experimental circumstances the deoxyribonucleic acid (DNA) extracted from a given type of *H influenzae* is capable of transferring that type specificity to other cells. Antibiotic resistance has been similarly transmitted by DNA.

Antigenic Structure

Encapsulated *H influenzae* contains capsular polysaccharides of one of 6 types (a–f); these polysaccharides resemble the specific soluble substance of pneumococci in behavior and chemical makeup and, in some instances, give serologic cross-reactions with pneumococcal types 6, 29, and others.

The somatic antigen of *H influenzae* consists of at least 2 proteins: The P substance constitutes much of the bacterial body, whereas the M substance is a labile surface antigen. Filtrable endotoxins can be derived from many fluid cultures of *H influenzae,* but their antigenic nature is not clear.

Encapsulated *H influenzae* can readily be typed by a capsule swelling test with specific antiserum; this test is identical in all respects with the "quellung test" for pneumococci.

Pathogenesis

H influenzae produces no exotoxin, and the role of its toxic somatic antigen in natural disease is not clearly understood. The nonencapsulated organism is a regular member of the normal respiratory flora of man. The encapsulated forms of *H influenzae,* particularly type b, produce suppurative respiratory infections (sinusitis, laryngotracheitis, epiglottitis, otitis) and, in young children, meningitis. Over the age of 3 years, the blood of most individuals has strong bactericidal power for *H influenzae,* and clinical infections are rare.

The role of *H influenzae* in human influenza of the pandemic type (particularly as occurred in 1918–1919) is not definitely known. This organism may well have been only a secondary invader producing pneumonitis in the respiratory tract already damaged by influenza virus. On the other hand it may have been definitely contributory to pandemic influenza in man, just as *H suis* is an essential etiologic component of swine influenza. Swine influenza is caused by a virus related to influenza type A but requires in addition the presence of *H suis* for the development of clinical symptoms. *H influenzae* is not pathogenic for laboratory animals.

Clinical Findings

H influenzae type b enters by way of the respiratory tract in small children and produces a nasopharyngitis, often with fever. Other types rarely produce disease. There may be local extension with involvement of the sinuses or of the middle ear. The organisms may reach the blood stream and be carried to the meninges or, less frequently, may establish themselves in the joints. The meningitis thus induced does not differ clinically from other forms of bacterial meningitis in children under 3 years of age, and diagnosis rests on bacteriologic demonstration of the organism.

Occasionally, a fulminating obstructive laryngotracheitis with swollen, cherry-red epiglottis develops in babies and requires prompt tracheostomy as a lifesaving procedure. Pneumonitis and epiglottitis due to *H influenzae* may follow upper respiratory tract infec-

TABLE 19–2. Characteristics and growth requirements of some hemophilic organisms.

Organism	Hemolysis	Requires X	Requires V	Capsule
H influenzae	−	+	+	+
H parainfluenzae	−	−	+	+
H hemolyticus	+	+	+	−
H suis	−	+	+	+
H hemoglobinophilus	−	+	−	−
Bordetella pertussis	+	−	−	+

tions in small children and old or debilitated people.

Diagnostic Laboratory Tests

Specimens consist of nasopharyngeal swabs, pus, blood, and spinal fluid for smears and cultures.

A. Direct Identification: When organisms are present in large numbers in specimens, they may be identified by immunofluorescence or may be mixed directly with specific rabbit antiserum (type b) and a capsule swelling test performed. A direct precipitin test may be done on spinal fluid in which no bacteria can be seen. This test is performed by layering the spinal fluid over specific type b rabbit antiserum in a small test tube. A precipitate developing rapidly at the interface constitutes a positive test. It indicates that the fluid contains high concentrations of specific polysaccharide from *H influenzae* type b.

B. Culture: Specimens are grown in meat infusion blood broth or on enriched "chocolate" agar until typical colonies can be identified with the capsule swelling test (in 36–48 hours). *H influenzae* is differentiated from related gram-negative bacilli by observing the requirements for X and V factors and hemolysis on blood agar (Table 19–2).

Immunity

No methods are available for active immunization. Most persons over the age of 3–4 years are immune to infection because of the bactericidal activity of their blood against *H influenzae.*

Treatment

Rabbit antiserum to *H influenzae* type b was moderately effective in reducing the mortality (90% in untreated cases) of influenzal meningitis. However, with the highly efficient chemotherapeutic agents now available, it is little used. Most strains of *H influenzae* type b are very susceptible to ampicillin, chloramphenicol, or tetracyclines. These drugs are effective in therapy. Greatest emphasis must be placed on early diagnosis and treatment, for if there is a delay in chemotherapy the incidence of late neurologic and intellectual impairment is high. Prominent among late complications of influenzal meningitis is the development of a localized subdural accumulation of fluid which requires surgical removal.

Epidemiology, Prevention, & Control

Encapsulated *H influenzae* type b is transmitted from person to person by the respiratory route. The patient with influenzal meningitis is not an important source of infection.

BORDETELLA (HEMOPHILUS) PERTUSSIS
(Whooping Cough Bacillus)

Morphology & Identification

A. Typical Organisms: Short, ovoid, gram-negative bacilli, resembling but less pleomorphic than *H influenzae.* With toluidine blue stain, bipolar metachromatic granules can be demonstrated. A capsule is present.

B. Culture: Primary isolation of *B pertussis* requires complex, enriched media. Commonly employed is Bordet-Gengou's medium (potato-blood-glycerol-agar), on which small, convex, smooth colonies with a pearl-like luster develop in 36–72 hours. The colonies are mucoid and tenacious, and on blood agar there is a narrow zone of hemolysis.

C. Growth Characteristics: The organism is not very active metabolically and forms acid but not gas in glucose and lactose. It does not require X and V factors on subculture.

D. Variation: When isolated from patients and cultured on enriched media, *B pertussis* is in the smooth, encapsulated, virulent phase I. Phase IV is the designation for a rough, nonencapsulated, avirulent form. Phases II and III are intermediates.

Antigenic Structure

B pertussis cells possess many antigens. Most external are an agglutinogen and a hemagglutinin. The cell wall contains a heat-stable toxin, the protective antigen, and a histamine-sensitizing factor (the last 2 may be identical). Upon disruption of the cell, the protoplasm contains a heat-labile endotoxin, which is destroyed by 56° C for 30 minutes, and several other antigens. Phase I variants contain larger amounts of the protective and other antigens than other variant phases.

Pathogenesis & Pathology

B pertussis survives for only brief periods outside the human host. There are no vectors. Transmission is largely by the respiratory route from early cases and possibly via carriers. The organism multiplies rapidly on the surface of the epithelium in the trachea and bronchi and interferes with ciliary action. The blood is not invaded. Disintegrating organisms liberate an endotoxin which irritates surface cells, giving rise to catarrhal symptoms and causing marked lymphocytosis. Later there may be necrosis of parts of the epithelium and polymorphonuclear infiltration with peribronchial inflammation and interstitial pneumonia. Secondary invaders like staphylococci or *H influenzae* may give rise to bacterial pneumonia. Obstruction of the smaller bronchioles by mucous plugs results in atelectasis and diminished oxygenation of the blood. This probably contributes to the frequency of convulsions.

Clinical Findings

After an incubation period of about 2 weeks the "catarrhal stage" develops, with mild coughing and sneezing. During this stage large numbers of organisms are sprayed in droplets and the patient is highly infectious but not very ill. During the "spasmodic" stage the cough develops its explosive character and the characteristic "whoop" upon inhalation. This leads to rapid exhaustion and may be associated with vomiting, cyanosis, and convulsions. The WBC is high (16,000–30,000/cu mm), with an absolute lymphocytosis. Convalescence is slow. Rarely, whooping cough is followed by encephalitis of unknown origin.

Diagnostic Laboratory Tests

Specimens consist of nasopharyngeal swab or cough droplets for culture. "Cough plate" (Bordet-Gengou) is held 6 inches from the mouth of the patient during paroxysm.

A. Culture: The swab is passed through a drop of penicillin solution (1000 units/ml) before streaking. This tends to inhibit other microorganisms but permits growth of *B pertussis* in 2–4 days. Typical colonies are identified by agglutination with specific antiserum.

B. Serology: During the third week of the disease, agglutinating and complement-fixing antibodies develop for phase I *B pertussis.* A positive skin test to the agglutinogen also develops.

Immunity

Recovery from whooping cough or adequate vaccination is followed by immunity. Second infections may occur but are mild; reinfections occurring years later in older adults usually are severe.

Treatment

Hyperimmune globulin (prepared from the sera of immune persons repeatedly injected with pertussis vaccine) administered early in the course of the illness can modify its course and make it milder. *B pertussis* is susceptible in vitro to many antimicrobial agents, and there is some evidence that the antibiotics shorten the course of the disease or diminish the frequency and severity of the paroxysms. However, the response is not striking.

Prevention

During the first year of life every infant should receive 3 injections of killed phase I organisms in proper concentration. This vaccine is usually administered in combination with toxoids of diphtheria and tetanus. An infant exposed to whooping cough without prior immunization can obtain temporary passive protection with hyperimmune gamma globulin.

Epidemiology & Control

Whooping cough is endemic in most densely populated areas all over the world and also occurs intermittently in epidemic outbreaks. The source of infection is usually a patient in the early catarrhal stage of the disease. The communicability is high, ranging from 30% to 90%. The majority of cases occur in children under 5 years of age; most deaths occur during the first year of life.

Control of whooping cough rests mainly on adequate active immunization of all infants.

OTHER ORGANISMS OF THE HEMOPHILUS GROUP

Bordetella (Hemophilus) Parapertussis

May produce a disease similar to whooping cough even though it differs from typical *B pertussis* in certain bacteriologic criteria and resembles *B bronchiseptica* bacteriologically. Infection is often subclinical.

Hemophilus Parainfluenzae

Resembles *H influenzae* and is a normal inhabitant of the human respiratory tract; it has been encountered in disease only in bacterial endocarditis. (Am J Clin Path 37:319, 1962.)

Hemophilus Hemoglobinophilus

Requires X but not V factor and has been found in dogs but not in human disease.

Hemophilus Suis

Resembles *H influenzae* bacteriologically. Acts synergistically with swine influenza virus to produce the disease in hogs.

Hemophilus Hemolyticus

The most markedly hemolytic organism of the group in vitro; it occurs both in the normal nasopharynx and associated with rare upper respiratory tract infections of moderate severity in childhood.

Hemophilus Aphrophilus

This organism is encountered rarely in bacterial endocarditis and pneumonia, and is also probably present in the normal respiratory tract flora. It is related to *Actinobacillus actinomycetemcomitans,* and occasionally mistaken for actinomyces. Tiny colonies adhere to the sides of broth tubes.

Hemophilus Aegyptius (Koch-Weeks Bacillus, *Hemophilus Conjunctivitidis*)

Resembles *H influenzae* closely and is associated with a highly communicable form of conjunctivitis.

Moraxella Lacunta (Morax-Axenfeld Bacillus)

A gram-negative diplobacillus which is grown with difficulty from purulent exudates in eye infections and which perhaps occurs in association with virus infections.

Hemophilus Ducreyi

The causative organism of chancroid (soft chancre), a venereal disease. The chancroid consists of a ragged ulcer on the genitalia, with marked swelling and tenderness. The regional lymph nodes are enlarged and painful.

The small gram-negative rods occur in strands in the lesions, usually in association with other pyogenic microorganisms. They are grown with considerable difficulty and only in the presence of blood. Injection of pure cultures into the skin of rabbits or humans results in local ulcerative lesions. Suspensions of killed *H ducreyi* serve as a useful skin-test antigen for the diagnosis of chancroid (Ducrey's skin test). The test may become positive 1–2 weeks after infection and may remain positive for years. There is no permanent immunity following chancroid infection.

Hemophilus Vaginalis

A serologically distinct organism isolated from the female genitourinary tract, associated with vaginitis. Serum is essential for growth; X and V factors stimulate growth.

Bordetella Bronchiseptica

A small gram-negative bacillus which inhabits the respiratory tracts of canines and may be associated with pneumonitis. It resembles *B parapertussis* bacteriologically.

●   ●   ●

General References

Finegold, M.J.: Pathogenesis of plague. Am J Med 45:549–554, 1968.

Johnson, W.D., & others: *Hemophilus influenzae* pneumonia in the adult. Am Rev Resp Dis 97:1112–1117, 1968.

Page, M.I., & E.O. King: Infection due to *Actinobacillus actinomycetemcomitans* and *Haemophilus aphrophilus.* New England J Med 275:181–188, 1965.

Young, L.S., & others: Tularemia epidemic, Vermont 1968. New England J Med 280:1253–1260, 1969.

20...
Miscellaneous
Pathogenic Microorganisms

MYCOPLASMAS (PPLO) & L FORMS

Mycoplasmas (previously called pleuropneumonia-like organisms, or PPLO) are a group of organisms with the following characteristics: (1) The smallest reproductive units have a size of 100–125 nm. (2) They are highly pleomorphic because they lack a rigid cell wall, and instead are bounded by a triple-layered "unit membrane." (3) They are completely resistant to penicillin but inhibited by tetracycline. (4) They can reproduce in cell-free media; on agar the center of the whole colony is characteristically embedded beneath the surface. (5) Growth is inhibited by specific antibody. (6) Mycoplasmas do not revert to or from bacterial parental forms.

L forms have properties similar to the mycoplasmas but characteristically arise from, and revert to, bacterial parent forms. Laboratory methods which induce L form production include penicillin under hypertonic environmental conditions. Some mycoplasmas cause disease in man (eg, Eaton agent pneumonia), or plants (eg, yellows), animals (eg, pleuropneumonia in cattle). Others are part of the normal flora of mucous membranes.

Morphology & Identification

A. Typical Organisms: Mycoplasmas cannot be studied by the usual bacteriologic methods because of the small size of their colonies, the plasticity and delicacy of their individual cells (due to the lack of a rigid cell wall), and their poor staining with aniline dyes. The morphology appears different according to the method of examination (eg, darkfield, Giemsa-stained films from solid or liquid media, agar fixation).

Growth in fluid media gives rise to many different forms, including rings, bacillary and spiral bodies, filaments, and granules. Growth on solid media consists principally of plastic protoplasmic masses of indefinite shape, easily distorted and often appearing as disks or globules which contain "chromatin bodies" and dense granules. All of these structures vary greatly in size, ranging from 50–300 nm in diameter.

B. Culture: Many strains of mycoplasma grow in heart infusion peptone broth of 2% agar (pH 7.8) to which about 30% human ascitic fluid or animal serum (horse, rabbit) has been added. Following incubation at 37° C for 48–96 hours, there may be no turbidity; but Giemsa stains of the centrifuged sediment show the characteristic pleomorphic structures, and subculture on solid media yields minute colonies.

After 2–6 days on special agar medium incubated in a Petri dish which has been sealed to prevent evaporation, isolated colonies measuring 20–500 μm can be detected with a hand lens. These colonies are round, with a granular surface and a dark center nipple typically buried in the agar. They can be subcultured by cutting out a small square of agar containing one or more colonies and streaking this material on a fresh plate or dropping it into liquid medium. The organisms can be stained for microscopic study by placing a similar square on a slide and covering the colony with a coverglass onto which an alcoholic solution of methylene blue and azure has been poured and then evaporated (agar fixation). Such slides can also be stained with specific fluorescent antibody.

C. Growth Characteristics: Mycoplasmas are unique in microbiology because of (1) their extremely small size and (2) their growth on complex but cell-free media.

Filtration studies with gradocol membranes indicate that the smallest reproductive unit measures about 100–125 nm and thus is in the range of magnitude of the larger viruses.

All parasitic strains of mycoplasma require for growth a protein from serum or yeast extract as well as cholesterol, but are resistant to thallium acetate, 1:10,000. Many human mycoplasmas produce peroxides and hemolyze red blood cells. In cell cultures mycoplasmas develop predominantly at cell surfaces. Many established cell lines carry mycoplasmas as contaminants.

D. Variation: The extreme pleomorphism of mycoplasmas is one of their principal characteristics. There appears to be no genetic relationship between mycoplasmas, L forms, and their parent bacteria. The characteristics of L forms are quite similar to those of mycoplasmas but, by definition, mycoplasmas do not revert to parent bacteria or originate from them. L forms may continue to synthesize some antigens which are normally located in the cell wall of the parent bacteria (eg, streptococcal L forms produce M protein and capsular polysaccharide; see Chapter 11). Reversion of L forms to the parent bacteria is enhanced by growth in the presence of 15–30% gelatin or 2.5% agar, whereas reversion is inhibited by inhibitors of protein synthesis. The essential feature of L forms, their loss of septum-forming and wall-forming ability, may be associated with a loss of mesosomes.

Antigenic Structure

From animals (eg, mice, chicken, turkeys), many antigenically distinct species of mycoplasmas have been isolated. In man, 6 distinct antigenic types are presently recognized: *M hominis* type 1, *M hominis* type 2, *M salivarium*, *M orale*, *M fermentans*, and *M pneumoniae*. The first and last named are known to be capable of causing human disease. The complement fixing antigens of mycoplasmas are carbohydrate-containing lipids.

Diseases Due to L Forms & Mycoplasmas

It is doubtful that L forms cause tissue reactions resulting in disease. However, L forms may be important for the persistence of microorganisms in tissues and recurrence of infection after termination of antimicrobial treatment.

The parasitic mycoplasmas appear to be strictly host-specific, being communicable and potentially pathogenic only within a single host species. In vivo mycoplasmas appear to be intracellular parasites with a predilection for mesothelial cells (pleura, peritoneum, synovia of joints). Several extracellular products are known to be elaborated, eg, hemolysins and at least one neurotoxin. In human respiratory tract infections, mucous membranes are inflamed and there may be interstitial pneumonia and necrotizing bronchiolitis.

A. Diseases of Animals: Bovine pleuropneumonia is a contagious disease of cattle producing pulmonary consolidation and pleural effusion, with occasional deaths. The disease probably has an airborne spread. Mycoplasmas are found in inflammatory exudates.

Agalactia of sheep and goats in the Mediterranean area is a generalized infection with local lesions in the skin, eyes, joints, udder, and scrotum; it leads to atrophy of lactating glands in females. Mycoplasmas are present in blood early; in milk and exudates later.

In poultry, several economically important respiratory diseases are caused by mycoplasmas. The organisms can be transmitted from hen to egg and chick. Swine, dogs, rats, mice, and other species harbor mycoplasmas which can produce infection involving particularly the pleura, peritoneum, joints, and respiratory tract.

B. Diseases of Man: Mycoplasmas have been cultivated from human mucous membranes and tissues, particularly from the genital, urinary, and respiratory tracts and from the mouth. Some mycoplasmas are inhabitants of the normal genitourinary tract, particularly in females, but are found with somewhat greater frequency in association with inflammatory processes, eg, cervicitis, urethritis, or prostatitis. The possible etiologic role of these agents remains uncertain, but the T strains (tiny colonies, requiring 10% urea for growth) probably cause certain cases of nongonococcal urethritis. Infrequently, mycoplasmas have been isolated from brain abscess and pleural or joint effusion. Mycoplasmas are part of the normal flora of the mouth and have been grown frequently from normal saliva, oral mucous membranes, sputum, or tonsillar tissue. By means of volunteer inoculation, 2 species of mycoplasmas *(M hominis* type 1 and *M pneumoniae)* have now been unequivocally proved to cause human disease.

M hominis type 1 can produce an acute, febrile respiratory illness with sore throat and tonsillar exudate. The frequency of natural infection with clinical disease is uncertain, but over half of normal adults have specific antibodies to this agent.

M pneumoniae is one of the causative agents of the syndrome "primary atypical pneumonia" (see below). The effects in man of infection with *M pneumoniae* range from inapparent infection to mild or severe upper respiratory disease, ear involvement (myringitis), and bronchial pneumonia.

C. Diseases of Plants: Aster yellows, corn stunt, and other plant diseases appear to be caused by mycoplasmas. They are transmitted by insects and can be suppressed by tetracyclines.

Diagnostic Laboratory Tests

Specimens consist of throat swab, sputum, inflammatory exudates, and respiratory or urethral secretions.

A. Microscopic Examination: Direct examination of a specimen is useless. Cultures are examined as described above.

B. Culture: The material is inoculated onto special solid media (above) and incubated for 3–10 days at 37° C (often under anaerobic conditions), or into special broth (above) incubated aerobically. One or 2 transfers of media may be necessary before growth appears, suitable for microscopic examination by staining or immunofluorescence. Colonies may have a "fried egg" appearance on agar.

C. Serology: Antibodies develop in humans infected with mycoplasmas and can be demonstrated by several methods. Complement fixation tests can be performed with antigens extracted with chloroform-methanol from cultured mycoplasmas. Hemagglutination inhibition tests can be applied to tanned red cells with adsorbed mycoplasma antigens. Indirect immunofluorescence may be used. Most specific is the test which measures growth inhibition by antibody. With all these serologic technics, there is adequate specificity for different human Mycoplasma species, but a rising antibody titer is required for diagnostic significance because of the high incidence of positive serologic tests in normal individuals.

Treatment

Many strains of mycoplasma are inhibited by a variety of antimicrobial drugs, but virtually all strains are resistant to penicillins, bacitracin, polymyxins, and sulfonamides. Tetracyclines and erythromycins are effective both in vitro and in vivo and are, at present, the drugs of choice.

Epidemiology, Prevention, & Control

Isolation of infected livestock will control the highly contagious pleuropneumonia and agalactia in limited areas. No vaccines are available. It has been suggested that nonbacterial urethritis in the human male might be acquired through sexual contact with a female carrying T strains asymptomatically in the genital tract. This remains to be proved. Primary atypical pneumonia caused by *M pneumoniae* behaves like a communicable viral respiratory disease (see below), and experimental vaccines have been made.

Primary Atypical Pneumonia & Mycoplasma (Eaton Agent) Pneumonia

Primary atypical pneumonia (PAP) is an acute, usually self-limited respiratory syndrome characterized by malaise, fever, cough, and pulmonary infiltration demonstrated far more readily by x-ray than by physical signs. It is a syndrome of multiple etiology; adenoviruses, influenza viruses, respiratory syncytial virus, parainfluenza type 3 virus, the agent of psittacosis, and the rickettsia of Q fever have been implicated as important causes. However, the single most prominent etiologic agent is *M pneumoniae*. Especially in military recruit populations, up to 65% of cases of PAP have been associated with mycoplasmal infection in some years.

In addition to the features described above, *M pneumoniae* has the following characteristics: Colonies are usually less than 0.5 mm in diameter and grow into the agar. There is a nutritional requirement for a protein from horse serum or fresh yeast extract. The organism grows slowly, aerobically or anaerobically; ferments glucose, maltose, xylose, and other sugars; and produces acid. *M pneumoniae* lyses erythrocytes from many mammalian species. It is most markedly inhibited by tetracyclines or erythromycins.

Infection in man may range from asymptomatic to serious bronchial pneumonia. An association between *M pneumoniae* infection and Stevens-Johnson syndrome has been noted. Typical cases in epidemics and in volunteers experimentally infected with *M pneumoniae* showed the following picture:

The incubation period varies from 1–3 weeks. The onset is usually insidious, with malaise, fever, headache, sore throat, and cough. Initially the cough is nonproductive. Later there may be mucopurulent or blood-streaked sputum and chest pain. Early in the course, the patient appears only moderately ill, and physical signs of pulmonary consolidation are often negligible even when x-rays reveal it strikingly. Later, when the infiltration is at a peak, the illness may be severe. Resolution of pulmonary infiltration and clinical improvement occur slowly for 1–4 weeks. While the course of the illness is exceedingly variable, death is very rare, usually attributable to cardiovascular dysfunction. Complications are uncommon, but involvement of almost every organ system has been reported. Myringitis has occurred in many inoculated volunteers. The most common pathologic findings are interstitial and peribronchial pneumonitis and necrotizing bronchiolitis.

The following laboratory and diagnostic findings are common in *M pneumoniae* pneumonia: The white and differential counts are within normal limits. The etiologic mycoplasma can be recovered by culture early in the disease from the pharynx and from sputum. Immunofluorescent stains of mononuclear cells from the throat may reveal the agent. There is a rise in specific antibodies to *M pneumoniae* which is demonstrable by complement fixation, immunofluorescence, passive hemagglutination, and growth inhibition.

A variety of nonspecific reactions can be observed. Cold hemagglutinins for group O human erythrocytes appear in about 50% of untreated patients, in rising titer, with the maximum reached in the third or fourth week after onset. A variable proportion of patients also develop agglutinins to streptococcus MG (apparently quite unrelated to the illness).

Tetracyclines or erythromycins in full systemic doses (2 gm daily for adults) are the drugs of choice. Penicillin has no effect.

M pneumoniae infections are endemic all over the world. In populations of children and young adults where close contact prevails, and in families, the infection rate may be high (50–90%), but the incidence of pneumonitis is variable (3–15%). For every case of frank pneumonitis, there exist several cases of milder respiratory illness. *M pneumoniae* is apparently transmitted mainly by direct contact involving respiratory secretions. Second attacks are infrequent. The presence of antibodies to *M pneumoniae* is associated with resistance to infection. Experimental vaccines have been prepared from agar-grown *M pneumoniae*. Certain preparations have induced a degree of protection, but others have aggravated subsequent disease.

STREPTOBACILLUS MONILIFORMIS

Streptobacillus moniliformis is an aerobic, gram-negative, highly pleomorphic organism which forms irregular chains of bacilli interspersed with fusiform enlargements and large round bodies. It grows best at 37° C in media containing serum protein, egg yolk, or starch, but ceases to grow at 22° C. In most cultures of the organism, L-forms can easily be demonstrated. Subculture of pure colonies of L-forms in liquid media often yields the streptobacillus again. All strains of streptobacilli appear to be antigenically identical.

S moniliformis is a normal inhabitant of the throats of rats, and humans can be infected by rat bites. The human disease (rat bite fever) is characterized by septic fever, blotchy and petechial rashes, and polyarthritis. Diagnosis rests on cultures of blood, joint fluid, or pus; on mouse inoculation, and on serum agglutination tests.

This organism can also produce infection after being ingested in milk—a disease called Haverhill fever which has occurred in epidemics. Penicillin, streptomycin, and perhaps other antibiotics are therapeutically effective.

LISTERIA MONOCYTOGENES

Listeria monocytogenes is a short, gram-positive, nonsporeforming, motile rod in its smooth form; in its rough form it is long and filamentous. Growth on simple media is enhanced by the presence of blood, ascitic fluid, or glucose. Listeria is isolated more readily from pathologic specimens if the tissue is kept at 4° C for some days before inoculation into bacteriologic media. The organism is a facultative anaerobe and is catalase-positive. Most strains produce a zone of hemolysis on blood agar plates. Listeria produces acid but not gas in a variety of carbohydrates. There are at least 4 antigenic types.

Spontaneous infection occurs in many animals (domestic and wild) and in man. In smaller animals (rabbits, chickens) there is a septicemia with focal abscesses in liver and heart muscle and marked monocytosis. A glyceride extracted from listeria can likewise induce monocytosis in rabbits. This cellular reaction, however, is not related to human infectious mononucleosis. Listeria infection leads to the production of cold agglutinins for human and sheep red cells as well as specific agglutinating antibodies.

In man and in ruminants (eg, sheep), listeria may produce meningoencephalitis with or without bacteremia. Listeriosis may be superimposed on lymphoma. The diagnosis rests on isolation of the organism in cultures of blood and spinal fluid. A second form of human listeriosis, granulomatosis infantiseptica, is an intrauterine infection with a high mortality for the fetus or the newborn child. There is generalized infection with focal necroses in many organs. The route of infection for adults is sometimes the genital tract. It is probable that asymptomatic infection is rather widespread. Penicillin, erythromycin, the tetracyclines, and chloramphenicol are effective in experimental infections, and tetracyclines have had clinical success.

ERYSIPELOTHRIX INSIDIOSA
(RHUSIOPATHIAE)

This organism resembles listeria bacteriologically but produces an entirely different disease. In its smooth form it grows as clear, minute colonies in which short, nonsporeforming, nonmotile rods are arranged in short chains; in its rough form, long filaments predominate.

Growth is aided by blood and glucose in the medium. On blood agar only slight hemolysis is produced. Carbohydrates are fermented irregularly, and catalase is not produced. The antigenic pattern is not established.

Infection with *E rhusiopathaie* occurs in worldwide distribution in a variety of animals, especially hogs. Infection in man follows skin abrasions from contact with fish, shellfish, meat, or poultry. The infection, called erysipeloid, is limited to the skin. There is pain, edema, and purplish erythema with sharp margins which extends peripherally but clears centrally. Relapses and extension of the lesions to distant areas are common, but there is usually no fever. Rare cases of endocarditis have occurred. There is no permanent immunity following an attack. The diagnosis rests on isolation of the organism in cultures from a skin biopsy. The fragment should be incubated in glucose broth for 24 hours, then subcultured on blood agar plates. Typical clinical appearance in a person with occupational exposure is highly suggestive of infection due to this organism.

Penicillin appears to be the antibiotic of choice.

MIMEAE

A group of aerobic gram-negative bacteria, often resembling neisseriae on smears because diplococcal forms predominate on solid media, have been recovered from meningitis and have been confused with meningococci. They also have been isolated from blood, sputum, skin, pleural fluid, and urine, but their pathogenic role is not entirely established. In patients with burns or with immunologic deficiency, these organisms can produce sepsis. By precipitin tests with enzymatic digests of organisms and specific antisera, mimeae can be grouped into at least 10 antigenic types. They are fairly inactive metabolically and often are antibiotic-resistant, responding most commonly to tetracyclines, kanamycin, or gentamicin. Herrellea and Mima are the most frequently encountered genera. Infections are occasionally induced in hospitals, but the source of sepsis is uncertain.

BARTONELLA BACILLIFORMIS

This is a gram-negative, very pleomorphic, motile organism which causes Oroya fever, a serious infectious anemia, and verruga peruana, a skin disorder in man. The infection is limited to the mountainous areas of the American Andes in tropical Peru, Columbia, and Ecuador, and is transmitted by the sandfly Phlebotomus.

Bartonella grows in semisolid nutrient agar containing 10% rabbit serum and 0.5% hemoglobin. After about 10 days' incubation at 28° C, some turbidity develops in the medium and rod-shaped and granular organisms can be seen in Giemsa-stained smears.

Human infection is characterized by the rapid development of severe anemia due to blood destruction, enlargement of spleen and liver, and hemorrhage into the lymph nodes. Masses of bartonella fill the cytoplasm of cells lining the blood vessels, and endothelial swelling may lead to vascular occlusion and thrombosis. The mortality of untreated Oroya fever is about 40%. The diagnosis is made by examining stained blood smears and blood cultures in semisolid medium.

Verruga peruana is a vascular granulomatous skin lesion which occurs in successive crops, lasts for about 1 year, and produces little systemic reaction and no fatalities. Bartonella can be seen in the granuloma; blood cultures are often positive, but there is no anemia. Verruga often occurs in persons who have recovered from Oroya fever.

Penicillin, streptomycin, and chloramphenicol are dramatically effective in Oroya fever and greatly reduce the fatality rate, particularly if blood transfusions are also given. Control of the disease depends upon the elimination of the sandfly vectors. Insecticides, DDT insect repellents, and elimination of breeding areas are of value. Prevention with antibiotics may be useful.

BACTEROIDES

Bacteroides constitutes a large group of nonspore-forming, strictly anaerobic, usually gram-negative bacteria which are very pleomorphic. They may be tapered "fusiform bacilli," slender rods, branching forms, or round bodies. They grow most readily on complex media containing blood or tissue extracts (eg, 25% ascitic fluid) and neomycin or vancomycin.

Bacteroides are normal inhabitants of the respiratory, genital, and intestinal tracts. They constitute 95% or more of the normal fecal flora. They may be associated with ulcerative lesions of mucous membranes and can produce suppuration in surgical infections such as localized peritonitis after bowel operations, lung abscesses, and similar clinical situations. Pus is usually foul-smelling. Bacteremia and even endocarditis occasionally occur. In pathologic processes bacteroides usually are part of a mixed flora. Tetracyclines or massive doses of penicillin are often curative.

The most commonly encountered bacteroides are *B fragilis, B funduliformis, B nigrescens* (melaninogenicus), *B oralis,* and Fusobacterium species. Classification is based on colonial and biochemical features.

Veillonella are small, anaerobic, gram-negative cocci which ferment few sugars. They are part of the normal mouth flora.

PSEUDOMONAS (ACTINOBACILLUS) MALLEI & PSEUDOMONAS PSEUDOMALLEI

Pseudomonas mallei is a small, nonmotile, gram-negative, aerobic rod which grows readily on most bacteriologic media and does not ferment lactose. It causes glanders, a disease of horses transmissible to man. Human infection (often fatal) usually begins as an ulcer of the skin or mucous membranes followed by lymphangitis and sepsis. Inhalation of the organisms may lead to primary pneumonitis.

The disease has been controlled by slaughter of infected horses and mules, and at present is very rare. In many countries laboratory infections are the only source of the disease.

The diagnosis is based on rising agglutinin titers, the mallein skin test, or culture of the organism from local lesions of man or horse. Human cases can be treated effectively with sulfonamides.

Melioidosis, a disease resembling glanders in man, occurs in Burma, Vietnam, Guam, the Philippines, and perhaps also in the Western Hemisphere. It is caused by *Pseudomonas pseudomallei,* which resembles other nonpigmented pseudomonads but is antigenically distinct. The infection occurs spontaneously in rats, guinea pigs, and rabbits, and may be transmitted to man by arthropod vectors or by food and water contaminated by rodent excreta. The epidemiology of this disorder is still uncertain, and there is no known treatment.

Melioidosis may manifest itself as an acute or a chronic lung disease, and has a high fatality if untreated. *Pseudomonas pseudomallei* is susceptible to many antibiotics in vitro. Chloramphenicol (2 gm daily), alone or in combination with kanamycin, may be the treatment of choice. Drug resistance emerges frequently.

AEROMONAS HYDROPHILA

Aeromonas hydrophila is a motile gram-negative rod isolated commonly from water, soil, or foods, and rarely from the human intestinal tract. It can be found in bacteremia in persons with seriously impaired host defenses. Aeromonas is occasionally isolated from the feces of patients with diarrhea. Most strains are susceptible to tetracyclines, aminoglycosides, and polymyxins.

General References

Buchner, L.H., & S.S. Schneierson: *Listeria monocytogenes* infections. Am J Med 45:904–921, 1968.

Gravenitz, A., & A.H. Mensch: The genus Aeromonas in human bacteriology. New England J Med 278:245–249, 1968.

Razin, S.: Structure and function in mycoplasma. Ann Rev Microbiol 23:317–356, 1969.

Rotheram, E.B., & others: Nonclostridial anaerobes in septic abortion. Am J Med 46:80–93, 1969.

Steinberg, P., & others: Ecology of *Mycoplasma pneumoniae*. Am J Epidem 89:62–73, 1969.

21 . . .

Spirochetes &
Other Spiral Microorganisms

The spirochetes are a large, heterogeneous group of spiral, motile organisms. (See Chapter 3 for general morphologic characteristics.)

One family (Spirochaetaceae) of the order Spirochaetales includes 3 genera of free-living, large spiral organisms. The other (Treponemataceae) includes 3 genera pathogenic for man: (1) Treponema, which causes syphilis, bejel, yaws, and pinta; (2) Borrelia, which causes relapsing fever; and (3) Leptospira, which causes systemic infections with fever, jaundice, and meningitis.

TREPONEMA PALLIDUM

Morphology & Identification

A. Typical Organisms: Slender spirals measuring about 0.2 μm in width and 5–15 μm in length. The spiral coils are regularly spaced at a distance of 1 μm from each other. The organisms are actively motile, rotating steadily around their long axes. The long axis of the spiral is ordinarily straight, but may sometimes bend so that the organism forms a complete circle for moments at a time, returning then to its normal straight position.

The spirals are so thin that they are not readily seen unless darkfield illumination or immunofluorescent stain is employed. They do not stain well with aniline dyes, but they do reduce silver nitrate to metallic silver which is deposited on the surface so that treponemes can be seen in tissues (Levaditi silver impregnation).

Treponemes ordinarily reproduce by transverse fission, and divided organisms may adhere to one another for some time. The formation of cyst-like structures suggestive of a reproductive cycle with several distinct shapes has been described.

B. Culture: *Treponema pallidum* pathogenic for man has never been cultured with certainty on artificial media, in fertile eggs, or in tissue culture. The strains of purported *T pallidum* (eg, Reiter) cultured anaerobically in vitro are probably merely saprophytes, but they appear to be related to *T pallidum.*

C. Growth Characteristics: Because *T pallidum* cannot be grown, no studies of its physiology have been made. The growth requirements for one cultured probably saprophytic strain (Reiter) have, however, been established. A defined medium of 11 amino acids, vitamins, salts, minerals, and serum albumin supports its growth.

In proper suspending fluids and in the presence of reducing substances *T pallidum* may remain motile for 3–6 days at 25° C. In whole blood or plasma stored at 4° C, organisms remain viable for at least 24 hours, which is of potential importance in blood transfusions.

D. Reactions to Physical and Chemical Agents: Drying kills the spirochete rapidly, as does elevation of the temperature to 42° C also. This fact formed, in part, the basis for fever therapy of syphilis. Treponemes are rapidly immobilized and killed by trivalent arsenicals, mercury, and bismuth. This killing effect is accelerated by high temperatures and can be partially reversed, and the organisms reactivated by compounds containing —SH (eg, cysteine, BAL). Penicillin is treponemicidal in minute concentrations, but the rate of killing is slow, presumably because of the metabolic inactivity and slow multiplication rate of the organism (estimated division time is 30 hours).

E. Variation: A life cycle has been postulated for *T pallidum,* including granular stages and cyst-like spherical bodies in addition to the spirochetal form. The occasional ability of *T pallidum* to pass through bacteriologic filters has been attributed to the filtrability of the granular stage.

FIG 21–1. Typical organism of *Treponema pallidum* from tissue fluid in dark field.

Antigenic Structure

The antigens of *T pallidum* are unknown. In the human host the spirochete stimulates the development of antibodies capable of immobilizing and killing live motile *T pallidum* and of fixing complement in the presence of suspensions of *T pallidum*. The spirochetes also cause the development of a distinct antibody-like substance, reagin, which gives positive complement fixation and flocculation tests with aqueous suspensions of lipids extracted from normal mammalian tissues. Either reagin or true antibody is used for the serologic diagnosis of syphilis.

Pathogenesis, Pathology, & Clinical Findings

A. Acquired Syphilis: Natural infection with *T pallidum* is limited to the human host. Experimentally, rabbits and monkeys can also be infected. Human infection is usually transmitted by sexual contact and the infectious lesion is found on the skin or mucous membranes of the genitalia. In about 10% of cases, however, the primary lesion is extragenital (usually oral). *T pallidum* can probably penetrate intact mucous membranes, or it may enter through a break in the epidermis.

Spirochetes multiply locally at the site of entry, and some also spread to nearby lymph nodes and thus reach the blood stream. In 2–10 weeks after infection a papule develops at the site of infection which breaks down to form an ulcer with a clean, hard base ("hard chancre"). The inflammation is characterized by a predominance of lymphocytes and plasma cells. This "primary lesion" always heals spontaneously, but 2–10 weeks later the "secondary" lesions appear. These consist of a red maculopapular rash anywhere on the body, and moist, pale papules (condyloma) in the anogenital region, axillas, and mouth. There may also be syphilitic meningitis, chorioretinitis, or periostitis. The secondary lesions also subside spontaneously. Both the primary and the secondary lesions are rich in spirochetes and are highly infectious. Contagious lesions may recur within the first 5 years after infection, but thereafter the individual is no longer infectious. Syphilitic infection may remain subclinical, with the patient passing through the primary or secondary stage (or both) without symptoms or signs. Yet such persons may develop tertiary lesions.

In about 25% of cases early syphilitic infection progresses spontaneously to complete cure without treatment. In another 25% the infection remains latent (principally evident by positive serologic tests). In the remainder the disease progresses to the "tertiary stage," characterized by the development of granulomatous lesions (gummas) in skin, bones, and liver, degenerative changes in the CNS (paresis, tabes), or syphilitic cardiovascular lesions, particularly aortitis (sometimes with aneurysm formation) and aortic valve insufficiency. In all tertiary lesions treponemes are very rare, and the exaggerated tissue response must be attributed to some form of hypersensitivity to the organisms. However, treponemes can occasionally be found in the eye or CNS of late cases.

B. Congenital Syphilis: A pregnant syphilitic woman can transmit *T pallidum* to the fetus through the placenta. Some of the infected fetuses die and miscarriages result; others are stillborn at term. Others are born live but develop the signs of congenital syphilis in childhood: interstitial keratitis, Hutchinson's teeth, saddle nose, periostitis, and a variety of CNS anomalies. Adequate treatment during the first half of pregnancy prevents congenital syphilis. The reagin titer in the blood of the child rises if he is infected but falls with time if antibody was passively transmitted from the mother. In congenital infection the child makes IgM antibody.

C. Experimental Disease: Rabbits can be experimentally infected in the skin, testis, and eye with human *T pallidum*. The animal develops a chancre rich in spirochetes, and organisms persist in lymph nodes, spleen, and bone marrow for the entire life of the animal, although there is no progressive disease.

Diagnostic Laboratory Tests

A. Specimens: Tissue fluid expressed from early surface lesions for demonstration of spirochetes; blood serum for serologic tests.

B. Darkfield Examination: A drop of tissue fluid or exudate is placed on a slide and a coverslip pressed over it to make a thin layer. The preparation is then examined under oil immersion with darkfield illumination for typical motile spirochetes. Many fields in several preparations may have to be scanned before positive results are obtained. The finding of characteristic spirochetes in material from a clinically typical lesion of early syphilis establishes the diagnosis. A fluorescent antibody method for *T pallidum* is more sensitive than ordinary darkfield tests and permits the use of acetone-fixed smears. Treponemes disappear from lesions within a few hours after the beginning of antibiotic treatment.

C. Serologic Tests for Syphilis (STS): These are basically of 2 kinds: the detection of reagin or of specific antibody.

1. Reagin test—Qualitative and quantitative estimation of reagin in the patient's serum after the second or third week of infection, or in the spinal fluid after the fourth to eighth week of infection. The "antigens" for estimation of reagin are lipids extracted with alcohol from mammalian tissues. The purified cardiolipin from beef heart is a diphosphatidyl-glycerol. It requires the addition of lecithin and cholesterol or other "sensitizers" to react with syphilitic reagin. The most commonly used tests are flocculation tests and complement fixation tests.

a. Flocculation tests (Hinton, Kahn, Kline, Mazzini, VDRL [Venereal Disease Research Laboratory], etc) are based on the fact that the particles of the lipid antigen remain dispersed in normal serum but combine with reagin to form visible aggregates, particularly when shaken or centrifuged.

b. Complement fixation tests (Wassermann, Kolmer) are based on the fact that reagin-containing sera fix complement in the presence of cardiolipin "antigen." It is necessary to ascertain that the serum is not "anticomplementary" (ie, that it does not destroy complement in the absence of antigen). An estimate of the amount of reagin present in a serum can be made by performing a serologic test with 2-fold dilutions of serum and expressing the "titer" as the highest dilution which still gives a positive result.

Biologic false-positive (BFP) results may occur (1) because of the technical complexities of the tests and (2) because certain sera regularly give positive flocculation or complement fixation tests in the absence of syphilitic infection. BFP occur with other infections (eg, malaria, leprosy, measles), smallpox vaccination, in collagen diseases (disseminated lupus erythematosus, polyarteritis nodosa), and other conditions.

"Reagin" appears to be a mixture of 19 S and 7 S globulins, with antibody characteristics. The specificity appears to be directed against some tissue antigens which are widely distributed.

The ultimate diagnosis often depends upon the results of the *Treponema pallidum* immobilization test (TPI) or the FTA-ABS test (see below).

2. TPI tests—Demonstration of *T pallidum* immobilization (TPI) by specific antibodies in the patient's serum after the second week of infection. Dilutions of serum are mixed with live, actively motile *T pallidum* extracted from the testicular chancre of a rabbit and complement, and the mixture is observed under the microscope. If specific antibodies are present, the spirochetes will be immobilized; in normal serum, active motion continues. This test is difficult to perform and requires live treponemes from infected animals.

3. Fluorescent treponemal antibody (FTA-ABS) test—A test employing indirect immunofluorescence (killed *T pallidum* + patient's serum + labeled anti-human gamma globulin) shows good specificity and sensitivity for syphilis antibodies. This test appears to be as reliable as the TPI (above) if the patient's serum, prior to the FTA test, has been absorbed with sonicated Reiter spirochetes. The FTA-ABS test often remains positive long after effective treatment of early syphilis. The test cannot be used to judge the efficacy of the treatment.

4. *Treponema pallidum* complement fixation test—Spirochetes extracted from syphilomas of rabbits form specific antigens for complement fixation tests which probably measure the same antibody as the TPI test, above. Such spirochetal suspensions are difficult to prepare and have not been widely adopted. Antigens prepared from cultured Reiter spirochetes are occasionally employed in the Reiter complement fixation test.

STS can also be performed on spinal fluid. Antibodies do not reach the CSF from the blood stream but are probably formed in the CNS in response to syphilitic infection.

Immunity

A person with active syphilis or yaws appears to be resistant to superinfection with *T pallidum*. How-ever, if early syphilis or yaws is treated adequately and the infection is eradicated, the individual becomes again fully susceptible.

Treatment

Arsenicals and bismuth salts were the drugs of choice for the treatment of syphilis until the advent of antibiotics. However, they have now been abandoned. Penicillin in concentrations of 0.003 unit/ml has definite treponemicidal activity, and penicillin is now the treatment of choice. In early syphilis, penicillin levels are maintained for 2 weeks; in late syphilis, for 4–6 weeks. Other antibiotics can occasionally be substituted. Prolonged follow-up is essential.

Epidemiology, Prevention, & Control

With the exceptions of congenital syphilis and the rare occupational exposure of medical personnel, syphilis is acquired through sexual exposure. An infected person may remain contagious for 4–5 years during "early" syphilis. "Late" syphilis, of more than 5 years' duration, is usually not contagious. Consequently, control measures depend on (1) prompt and adequate treatment of all discovered cases; (2) follow-up on sources of infection and contacts so they can be treated; (3) sex hygiene; and (4) prophylaxis at the time of exposure. At present, mechanical prophylaxis (condoms) is more reliable than chemoprophylaxis (eg, penicillin after exposure). The application of disinfectants to the genitalia after exposure has been abandoned.

DISEASES RELATED TO SYPHILIS

These diseases are all caused by treponemes indistinguishable from *T pallidum*. All give biologic true-positive serologic tests for syphilis, and some cross-immunity can be demonstrated in experimental animals and perhaps in man. All are nonvenereal diseases and are commonly transmitted by direct contact. None of the etiologic organisms have been cultured on artificial media.

Bejel

Bejel occurs in Arabia, particularly among children, and produces highly infectious skin lesions; late visceral complications are rare. Penicillin is the drug of choice.

Yaws (Frambesia)

Yaws is endemic, particularly among children, in many humid, hot tropical countries. It is caused by *Treponema pertenue.* The primary lesion, an ulcerating papule, occurs usually on the arms or legs. Transmission is by person-to-person contact in children under the age of 15. Transplacental, congenital infection does not occur. Scar formation of skin lesions and bone destruction are common, but visceral or nervous system complications are very rare. It has been debated whether yaws represents a variant of syphilis adapted to nonvenereal transmission in hot climates. There appears to be cross-immunity between yaws and syphilis. Diagnostic procedures and therapy are similar to those for syphilis. The response to penicillin treatment is dramatic.

Pinta

Pinta is caused by *Treponema carateum* and occurs endemically in all age groups in Mexico, Central and South America, the Philippines, and some areas of the Pacific. The disease appears to be restricted to dark-skinned races. The primary lesion, a nonulcerating papule, occurs on exposed areas. Some months later, flat, hyperpigmented lesions appear on the skin; depigmentation and hyperkeratosis take place years afterward. Late cardiovascular and nervous system involvement probably occurs. Transmission is nonvenereal, either by direct contact or through the agency of a fly (Hippelates). Diagnosis and treatment are the same as for syphilis.

Rabbit Syphilis

Rabbit syphilis (*Treponema cuniculi*) is a natural venereal infection of rabbits producing minor lesions of the genitalia. The etiologic organism is morphologically indistinguishable from *T pallidum* and may lead to confusion in experimental work.

OTHER SPIROCHETAL DISEASES

BORRELIA RECURRENTIS

Morphology & Identification

A. Typical Organisms: *B recurrentis* is an irregular spiral 10–30 μm long and 0.3 μm wide. The distance between turns varies from 2–4 μm. The organisms are highly flexible and move both by rotation and by twisting. *B recurrentis* stains readily with bacteriologic dyes as well as with blood stains such as Giemsa's or Wright's stain.

B. Culture: The organism can be cultured in fluid media containing blood, serum, or tissue, but it rapidly loses its pathogenicity for animals when transferred repeatedly in vitro. Multiplication is rapid in chick embryos when blood from patients is inoculated into the chorioallantoic membrane.

C. Growth Characteristics: Virtually nothing is known of the metabolic requirements or activity of borreliae. At 4° C, the organisms survive for several months in infected blood or in culture. In some ticks (but not in lice), spirochetes are passed from generation to generation.

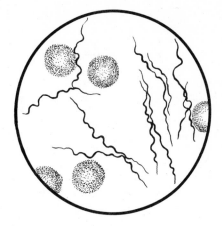

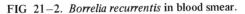

FIG 21–2. *Borrelia recurrentis* in blood smear.

D. Variation: The only significant variation of borrelia is with respect to its antigenic structure.

Antigenic Structure

Many strains of *B recurrentis* have been isolated from different parts of the world (erroneously given different names), from different hosts, and from different vectors (lice or ticks). Some strains grow preferentially in one vector and some in another, but these are not stable differences.

Agglutinins, complement fixing antibodies, and lytic antibodies develop in high titer after infection with borreliae. Apparently the antigenic structure of the organisms changes in the course of a single infection. The antibodies produced initially may act as a selective factor which permits the survival only of antigenically distinct variants. It has been suggested that the relapsing course of the disease is due to the multiplication of such variants, against which the host must then develop new antibodies. Ultimate recovery (after 3–10 relapses) might, if this is true, be associated with the presence of antibodies against several antigenic variants.

Pathology

Fatal cases show spirochetes in great numbers in the spleen and liver, necrotic foci in other parenchymatous organs, and hemorrhagic lesions in the kidneys and the gastrointestinal tract. Spirochetes have been occasionally demonstrated in the spinal fluid and brains of persons who have had meningitis. In experimental animals (guinea pigs, rats), the brain may serve as a reservoir of borreliae after they have disappeared from the blood.

Pathogenesis & Clinical Findings

The incubation period is 3–10 days. The onset is sudden, with chills and an abrupt rise of temperature. During this time spirochetes abound in the blood. The fever persists for 3–5 days and then declines, leaving the patient weak but not ill. The afebrile period lasts from 4–10 days and is followed by a second attack of chills, fever, intense headache, and malaise. There are from 3–10 such recurrences, generally of diminishing severity. During the febrile stages (especially when the temperature is rising), organisms are present in the blood; during the afebrile periods they are absent. Organisms appear less frequently in the urine.

Antibodies against the spirochetes appear during the febrile stage, and it is possible that the attack is terminated by their agglutinating and lytic effects. These antibodies may select out antigenically distinct variants which multiply and cause a relapse. Several distinct antigenic varieties of borreliae may be isolated from an individual patient's several relapses, even following experimental inoculation with a single organism.

Diagnostic Laboratory Tests
A. Specimens: Blood obtained during the rise in fever, for smears and animal inoculation.
B. Stained Smears: Thin or thick blood smears stained with Wright's or Giemsa's stain reveal large, loosely coiled spirochetes among the red cells.
C. Animal Inoculation: White mice or young rats are inoculated intraperitoneally with blood. Stained films of tail blood are examined for spirochetes 1–4 days later.
D. Serology: Spirochetes grown in culture can serve as antigens for complement fixation tests, but the preparation of satisfactory antigens is difficult. Patients suffering from epidemic (louse-borne) relapsing fever may develop high titers of agglutinins for proteus OXK.

Immunity
Immunity following infection is usually of short duration.

Treatment
The great variability of the spontaneous remissions of relapsing fever makes evaluation of chemotherapeutic effectiveness difficult. Arsenicals were used in the past, and penicillin, streptomycin, and the tetracyclines have been claimed to be beneficial in terminating individual attacks and preventing relapses.

Epidemiology, Prevention, & Control
Relapsing fever is endemic in many parts of the world. Its main reservoir is the rodent population, which serves as a source of infection for ticks of the genus Ornithodorus. The distribution of endemic foci and the seasonal incidence of the disease are largely determined by the ecology of the ticks in different areas. In the USA, infected ticks are found throughout the West, especially in mountainous areas, but clinical cases are rare. In the tick, borrelia may be transmitted transovarially from generation to generation.

Spirochetes are present in all tissues of the tick and may be transmitted by the bite or by crushing the tick. The tick-borne disease is not epidemic. However, when an infected individual harbors lice, the lice become infected by sucking blood; 4–5 days later,

they may serve as a source of infection for other individuals. The infection of lice is not transmitted to the next generation, and the disease is the result of rubbing crushed lice into bite wounds. Severe epidemics may occur in louse-infested populations, and transmission is favored by crowding, malnutrition, and cold climate.

In endemic areas human infection may occasionally result from contact with the blood and tissues of infected rodents. The mortality of the endemic disease is low, but in epidemics it may reach 30%.

Prevention is based on avoiding exposure to ticks and lice and on delousing (cleanliness, DDT, insecticides). No vaccines are available.

LEPTOSPIRAE

Morphology & Identification
A. Typical Organisms: Tightly coiled, thin, flexible spirochetes 5–15 μm long, with very fine spirals 0.1–0.2 μm wide. One end of the organism is often bent, forming a hook. There is active rotational motion, but no flagella have been discovered. Electron micrographs show a thin axial filament and a delicate membrane. The spirochete is so delicate that in the dark field it may appear only as a chain of minute cocci. It does not stain readily but can be impregnated with silver.
B. Culture: Leptospirae grow best aerobically at 30° C in peptone broth with 10% inactivated serum. On semisolid media, round colonies 1–3 mm in diameter develop if agar contains 10% serum and hemoglobin. Leptospirae also grow on chorioallantoic membranes of embryonated eggs.
C. Growth Requirements: Metabolic activity or requirements have not been studied. The organisms are able to survive for long periods in water, particularly at an alkaline pH.

Antigenic Structure
The main strains of leptospirae isolated from man or animals in different parts of the world and designated as different species (Table 21–1) are all serologically related and exhibit marked cross-reactivity in serologic tests. This indicates considerable overlapping in antigenic structure, and quantitative tests and antibody absorption studies are necessary for a specific serologic diagnosis. From many strains of leptospirae, a serologically reactive lipopolysaccharide has been extracted which has group reactivity.

Pathogenesis & Clinical Findings
Human infection results usually from ingestion of water or food contaminated with leptospirae. More rarely, the organisms may enter through mucous membranes or breaks in the skin. After an incubation period of 1–2 weeks, there is a variable febrile onset during which spirochetes are present in the blood stream. They then establish themselves in the paren-

TABLE 21–1. Principal leptospiral diseases.

Leptospiral Species*	Source of Infection	Disease in man	Clinical Findings	Distribution
L icterohaemorrhagiae	Rat urine, water	Weil's disease	Jaundice, hemorrhages, meningitis	Worldwide
L canicola	Dog urine	Infectious jaundice	Influenza-like illness, meningitis	Worldwide
L grippotyphosa	Rodents, water	Marsh fever	Fever, prostration, meningitis	Europe, USA, Africa
L pomona	Swine, cattle	Swineherd's disease	Fever, prostration, aseptic meningitis	Europe, USA, Australia
L hebdomadis	Rats, mice	Seven day fever	Fever, jaundice	Japan, Europe
L mitis	Swine	—	Meningitis	Australia
L bovis	Cattle, voles	—	Fever, prostration	USA, Israel, Australia
L autumnalis	?	Pretibial fever or Ft. Bragg fever	Fever, rash over tibia	USA, Japan

*In the view of some investigators *L canicola* and the others listed beneath it are not different species but serotypes of *L icterohaemorrhagiae.*

chymatous organs (particularly liver and kidneys), producing hemorrhage and necrosis of tissue and resulting in dysfunction of those organs (jaundice, hemorrhage, nitrogen retention). The CNS is frequently invaded, and this results in a clinical picture resembling "benign aseptic meningitis." There may be lesions in skin and muscles also. Often there is episcleral injection of the eye. The degree and distribution of organ involvement vary in the different diseases produced by different leptospirae in various parts of the world (Table 21–1). Many infections are mild or subclinical.

Kidney involvement in many animal species is chronic and results in the elimination of large numbers of leptospirae in the urine; this is probably the main source of contamination and infection of man. Human urine also may contain spirochetes in the second and third weeks of disease.

Agglutinating, complement fixing, and lytic antibodies develop during the infection. Serum from convalescent patients protects experimental animals against an otherwise fatal infection. Immunity resulting from infection in man and animals appears to be specific for leptospirae. Dogs have been artificially immunized with killed cultures of leptospirae.

Diagnostic Laboratory Tests

Specimens consist of blood for microscopic examination, culture, and inoculation of young hamsters or guinea pigs; and serum for agglutination tests.

A. Microscopic Examination: Darkfield examination or thick smears stained by Giemsa's technic occasionally show leptospirae in fresh blood from early infections. Darkfield examination of centrifuged urine may also be positive.

B. Culture: Whole fresh blood can be cultured in diluted serum (large inoculum).

C. Animal Inoculation: A sensitive technic for the isolation of leptospirae consists of the intraperitoneal inoculation of young hamsters or guinea pigs with fresh plasma or urine. Within a few days, spirochetes become demonstrable in the peritoneal cavity; on the death of the animal (8–14 days), hemorrhagic lesions with spirochetes are found in many organs.

D. Serology: Agglutinating antibodies attaining very high titers (1:10,000 or higher) develop slowly in leptospiral infection, reaching a peak at 5–8 weeks after infection. For agglutination tests, cultured leptospirae are used live or fixed with formalin. With live suspensions, agglutination is often followed by lysis. Complement fixation tests may also be performed. Leptospiral extracts sensitize sheep erythrocytes in the presence of specific antibodies, so that these sheep red blood cells are lysed by complement. Reactions are group-specific.

Immunity

A solid species-specific immunity (directed against individual serotypes) follows leptospiral infection.

Treatment

In very early infection, antibiotics (penicillin, tetracycline, and streptomycin) have some therapeutic effect but do not eradicate the infection.

Epidemiology, Prevention, & Control

The leptospiroses are essentially animal infections; human infection is only accidental, following contact with water or other materials contaminated with the excreta of animal hosts. Rats, mice, wild rodents, dogs, swine, and cattle are the principal sources of human infection. They excrete leptospirae in urine and feces both during the active illness and during the asymptomatic carrier state. Leptospirae remain viable in stagnant water for several weeks; drinking, swimming, bathing, or food contamination may lead to human infection. Persons most likely to come in contact with water contaminated by rats (eg, miners, sewer workers, farmers, fishermen) run the greatest risk of infection. Children acquire the infection from dogs more frequently than do adults. Control consists of preventing exposure to potentially contaminated water and reducing contamination by rodent control. Vaccination of dogs has been proposed.

SPIRILLUM MINUS
(Spirillum Morsus Muris)

Spirillum minus causes one form of ratbite fever (sodoku). This very small (3–5 μm) and rigid spiral organism is carried by rats all over the world. The organism is inoculated into humans through the bite of a rat and results in a local lesion, regional gland swelling, skin rashes, and fever of the relapsing type. The frequency of this illness depends upon the degree of contact between humans and rats. The spirillum can be isolated by inoculation of guinea pigs or mice with material from enlarged lymph nodes or blood. In the USA and Europe, this disease has been recognized only infrequently. Several other motile gram-negative spiral aerobic organisms can produce spirillum fever. (J. Kowal: New England J Med 264: 123, 1961.)

SPIROCHETES OF THE NORMAL MOUTH & MUCOUS MEMBRANES

A number of spirochetes occurs in every normal mouth. Some of them have been named (eg, *Borrelia buccalis*), but neither their morphology nor their physiologic activity permits definitive classification. On normal genitalia, a spirochete called *Borrelia refringens* is occasionally found which may be confused with *T pallidum*. These organisms are harmless saprophytes under ordinary conditions. Most of them are strict anaerobes which can be grown in petrolatum-sealed meat infusion broth tubes to which some tissue has been added.

FUSOSPIROCHETAL DISEASE

Under certain circumstances, particularly injury to mucous membranes, nutritional deficiency, or concomitant infection (eg, with herpes simplex virus) of the epithelium, the normal spirochetes of the mouth, together with cigar-shaped, banded, anaerobic fusiform bacilli, find suitable conditions for vast increase in numbers. This occurs in ulcerative gingivostomatitis (trench mouth), often called Vincent's stomatitis or Vincent's infection. When this type of process produces ulcerative tonsillitis and massive tissue involvement, it is often called Vincent's angina. It also occurs in lung abscesses where pyogenic microorganisms have broken down tissue; in bronchiectasis, where anatomic and physiologic disturbances interfere with normal drainage; in leg ulcers with mixed infection and venous stasis; and similar situations.

In all of these instances, necrotic tissue provides the anaerobic environment required by the fusospirochetal flora. The latter in turn prevents rapid healing and may contribute to tissue breakdown. Fusiform bacilli are a form of bacteroides (see Chapter 20). The fusospirochetal flora is readily inhibited by antibiotics. Thus antibiotic therapy may control gingivostomatitis or angina. However, the fusospirochetal organisms are not primary pathogens. Effective treatment must direct itself against the initial cause of tissue breakdown.

Fusospirochetal disease is generally not transmissible through direct contact, since everybody carries the organisms in his mouth. However, outbreaks occur occasionally in children or young adults. This is attributed to poor hygiene and nutrition ("trench mouth") or to the transmission of a viral agent (eg, herpes simplex virus) in a susceptible population group.

● ● ●

General References

Harner, R.E., & others: The FTA-ABS test in late syphilis. JAMA 203:545–548, 1968.

Southern, P.M., & J.P. Sanford: Relapsing fever. Medicine 48:129–170, 1969.

22...

Medical Mycology

For purposes of convenience, fungal infections of man are divided into superficial and deep (or systemic) mycoses. Superficial fungal infections of skin, hair, and nails are often chronic and resistant to treatment but rarely affect the general health of the patient. The deep mycoses, on the other hand, often produce systemic involvement and are sometimes fatal.

Fungi are frequent causes of plant diseases, but only about 50 of the thousands of known species of fungi cause disease in man or animals and only the superficial mycoses (dermatophytoses) are readily transmitted from man to man.

Most of the deep mycoses are caused by organisms that live free in nature. Infection is frequently limited to certain geographic areas. In such areas, a majority of inhabitants may acquire the fungal infection; most infected persons, however, develop no (or only minor) symptoms, and only a small minority progress to the full-blown serious or fatal disease.

Pathogenic fungi generally produce no toxins. In the host they induce hypersensitivity to their chemical constituents with great regularity. In systemic mycoses, the typical tissue reaction is a chronic granuloma with varying degrees of necrosis and abscess formation.

With few exceptions, most of the fungi pathogenic for man are classified as *fungi imperfecti,* so named because they produce only asexual spores and have no known sexual spore development in the highly specialized structures that are found in other classes of fungi. Recently, the sexual form of some of the dermatophytes has been discovered, thereby causing these fungi to be reclassified.

The general morphology of fungi has been described in Chapter 1. Some typical structures of pathogenic fungi are mentioned below; others are given with the descriptions of specific disease entities.

STRUCTURES OF FUNGI

When grown on suitable media, many fungi produce long branching filaments. Each filament is called a *hypha.* Hyphae may become divided into a chain of cells by the formation of transverse walls, or septa. These are called septate hyphae. As the hyphae continue to grow and branch a mat of growth develops called a *mycelium.* That part of the growth which projects above the surface of the substrate is called an *aerial* mycelium; the part which penetrates into the substrate and absorbs food is known as the *vegetative* mycelium.

Fungi reproduce by spores of various types, many of which develop on the aerial mycelium, which is then called the *reproductive* mycelium. Spores are called *asexual* when no fusion of nuclei takes place in their formation; when such fusion does take place, they are called *sexual.* The majority of fungi of medical importance have no known sexual spore development. The following sexual spores are encountered in fungi of medical interest:

A. **Zygospores:** In certain phycomycetes the tips of approximating hyphae come together and their contents fuse, thus developing large, thick-walled bodies called zygospores.

B. **Ascospores:** Usually 4 spores form within a specialized cell called an ascus in which nuclear fusion has taken place.

Other Common Types of Spores in Fungi of Medical Interest

A. **Blastospore:** A simple asexual spore which develops by budding and subsequent separation of the bud from the parent cell (eg, in candida, cryptococcus).

B. **Chlamydospores:** Cells in a hypha enlarge and develop thick walls. These asexual spores are resistant to unfavorable environmental conditions and germinate when conditions become more favorable for vegetative growth.

C. **Arthrospores:** Asexual spores resulting from a hypha fragmenting into individual cells (eg, in coccidioides).

D. **Conidia:** Spores produced on specialized hyphae (called conidiophores) by "pinching off" at the point of attachment. When more than one kind of conidia is produced within a colony, small, single-celled conidia are called microconidia. Large, often multicelled conidia are called macroconidia.

THE ACTINOMYCETES

The actinomycetes are a heterogeneous group of filamentous microorganisms clearly related to "true bacteria" (corynebacteria and mycobacteria), while superficially resembling fungi. The characteristic growth is a branched mycelium which tends to fragment into bacteria-like pieces. Some actinomycetes are acid-fast. Many are free-living, particularly in soil. The anaerobic species *Actinomyces israelii* and some of the aerobic Nocardia and Streptomyces species produce disease in man and animals.

ACTINOMYCES ISRAELII (& *A BOVIS*)

Morphology & Identification

A. **Typical Organisms:** In culture, *A israelii* is a gram-positive, nonacid-fast, nonmotile, filamentous organism which shows characteristic branching. The filaments break easily into short bacillary fragments with observable branching in the form of a **V** or **Y**. In

FIG 22–1. Ascospores in an ascus.

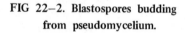

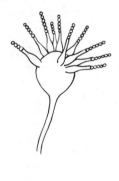

FIG 22–2. Blastospores budding from pseudomycelium.

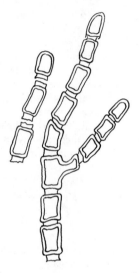

FIG 22–3. Arthrospores.

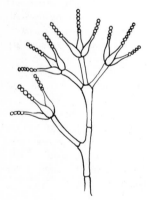

FIG 22–4. Chains of conidia on conidiophores.

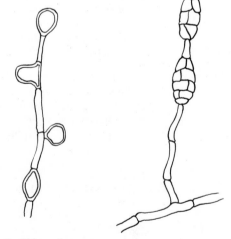

FIG 22–5. Chlamydospores.

FIG 22–6. Macroconidia.

[Figs 22–1 to 22–6 redrawn, with permission, from Conant, N.F., & others: *Manual of Clinical Mycology,* 2nd ed. Saunders, 1954.]

tissues, "sulfur granules" are formed which consist of a central mass of filamentous mycelia. A peripheral array of swollen eosin-staining "clubs" may be present.

A israelii differs in certain respects from *A bovis,* eg, *A bovis* hydrolyzes starch whereas *A israelii* does not, and the cell wall composition of the 2 species differs significantly. However, from a medical and bacteriologic standpoint, they are sufficiently similar to be considered together.

B. Culture: Rough, heaped-up, small, irregular, dead-white colonies form on blood agar or brain-heart infusion agar with 1% glucose after 48 hours of anaerobic incubation. Smooth, glossy colonies are formed less frequently. Thioglycollate medium or chopped-meat infusion broth are the best liquid media. In these, *A israelii* grows as small fluffy balls below the surface of the medium. Strains can be maintained best if grown alternately in different media.

C. Growth Characteristics: Fermentation of carbohydrates varies with different strains, but the presence of sugars favors growth. Most strains are anaerobic but may grow under microaerophilic conditions, particularly if reducing substances are present. Most strains are nonhemolytic and nonproteolytic.

D. Variation: Rough forms are most commonly isolated from actinomycosis in man. Smooth colonial forms isolated from lesions in cattle have been called *A bovis.* Occasionally this form has been isolated from man.

Antigenic Structure

By gel diffusion technics, *A israelii* can be differentiated from *A bovis.* Species-specific antigens (mainly polysaccharides from cell wall) occur in acetone concentrates of culture fluid supernate. There are at least 2 serotypes of *A israelii.*

Pathogenesis & Pathology

Single injections of cultures of *A israelii* do not regularly produce disease in laboratory animals. Perhaps hypersensitivity is necessary for the development of lesions.

Typical *A israelii* can be recovered from the teeth (especially the calculus deposits), pharynx, and tonsils of many normal persons. It is uncertain whether trauma (eg, tooth extraction), pyogenic infection, or hypersensitivity precipitate disease due to these organisms.

The typical lesion consists of an abscess with central necrosis, surrounded by granulation tissue and fibrous tissue; the pus often contains sulfur granules and an abundance of leukocytes. Histologically, the lesions are not typical unless "sulfur granules" can be found.

Clinical Findings

The characteristic appearance of actinomycosis is a hard, red, relatively nontender swelling which usually develops slowly. It becomes fluctuant, points to a surface, and eventually drains, forming a chronic sinus tract which has little tendency to heal. The lesion tends to extend locally, and there may also be dissemination via the blood stream.

In about half the cases of actinomycosis the initial lesion is cervicofacial, involving the tissues of the face, neck, tongue, and often the mandible. About 1/5 of cases show predominant involvement of the lungs with abscesses and empyema (thoracic actinomycosis). An equal number have abdominal actinomycosis, where the primary lesion is in the cecum, appendix, or in the pelvic organs; multiple draining fistulas may develop.

Diagnostic Laboratory Tests

Animal inoculation, skin tests, and serologic procedures are not useful in diagnosis.

Specimens consist of pus from lesion or sinus tract, discharge from fistula, and sputum; biopsy specimens are occasionally taken.

A. Microscopic Examination: Every effort must be made to find "sulfur granules" in the specimen. Wash one in saline, place it on a slide, and crush with a coverglass for wet mount examination. The appearance of the central mycelium and peripheral clubs is charac-

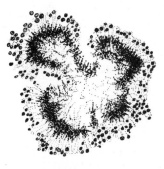

Sulfur Granule in Pus

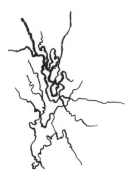

Branching Filaments in Pus

Diphtheroid-like Branching in Culture

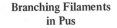

FIG 22–7. *Actinomyces israelii*

teristic. If no "sulfur granules" are found, the demonstration of branching rods and filaments is suggestive.

B. Culture: Material is inoculated into thioglycollate medium, streaked onto blood agar or brain-heart infusion agar plates, and incubated anaerobically for at least 2 weeks. The small, heaped-up opaque colonies of *A israelii* (or the "fluff-ball" colonies in thioglycollate) can then be examined microscopically for branching mycelia or "twiglike" gram-positive rods.

Immunity

It is uncertain whether any immunity is produced by infection with actinomycetes.

Treatment

Prolonged administration of sulfonamides, penicillin, and the tetracycline antibiotics, alone or in combination, has been found effective in many cases. However, drugs may penetrate poorly into the abscesses and some of the tissue destruction may be irreversible. Surgical drainage and surgical removal are accepted forms of treatment.

Epidemiology

Because of the many free-living actinomycetes and the occurrence of "lumpy jaw" in cattle, it was at one time believed that actinomycosis in man was acquired from grasses, straws, etc, which acted by traumatizing the mucous membranes and introducing the etiologic organism. However, it has now been well established that potentially pathogenic *A israelii* is a common inhabitant of mucous membranes in the mouth, so that no introduction from the outside need be postulated. The disease is never communicable.

Virtually all isolates from human sources are *A israelii;* most isolates from bovine sources are *A bovis.*

NOCARDIA ASTEROIDES & RELATED SPECIES

Morphology & Identification

A. Typical Organisms: Nocardia and Streptomyces species have narrow, gram-positive, branching filaments which may fragment into bacillary or coccal forms. Some are acid-fast. Bacillary and filamentous forms may be seen in tissue exudates or in pus; white or colored (yellow, red, or black) mycelial granules which may not have peripheral clubs may also be seen.

B. Culture: These actinomycetes grow aerobically very slowly, on many simple media. Colonies are most often dry, wrinkled, and crumbling, resembling acid-fast bacilli, but are sometimes soft and mucilaginous. Varying pigmentation, ranging from yellow to red, is produced by different strains. In liquid media a wrinkled surface pellicle is produced.

C. Growth Characteristics: Most strains of aerobic actinomycetes ferment no carbohydrates; some (but not *N asteroides*) coagulate milk and liquefy gelatin.

D. Variation: Variation among strains is great with regard to all cultural and biologic properties. However, 5 species have been proposed: *N asteroides, S madurae, S pelletieri, N brasiliensis,* and *N paraguayensis.*

Antigenic Structure

Serologic tests demonstrate at least one antigen which is shared by all aerobic actinomycetes, but species cannot be differentiated by serologic means. Rabbits infected with *N asteroides* give specific delayed skin reactions to protein and polysaccharide fraction of the organism. Guinea pigs inoculated with *N asteroides* in water-in-oil emulsion also develop tuberculin sensitivity.

Pathogenesis

N asteroides injected intravenously into rabbits causes a generalized infection with miliary abscesses in many organs. Guinea pigs injected intraperitoneally develop diffuse, fatal peritonitis.

Pathology & Clinical Findings

In man, either localized or generalized infection may occur. *N asteroides* may occasionally reside on skin or in the respiratory tract without producing disease. Nocardiosis occurs frequently as a complication of underlying disease.

(1) A localized, chronic suppurating granuloma of subcutaneous tissues and bones, with draining sinuses which discharge pus containing the pigmented "granules." This occurs particularly in the extremities (*Madura foot,* or mycetoma) and leads to progressive bone destruction and deformity but little systemic illness. The clinical picture is indistinguishable from maduromycosis (Madura foot) caused by *Monosporium apiospermum.*

Nocardia minutissima (Corynebacterium minutissimum) causes a superficial skin infection, erythrasma.

(2) A systemic infection with infiltration and suppuration of the lungs extending via the blood stream to the meninges, brain, or other organs. The presenting symptoms may be fever without localizing manifestations; headache, nausea, and vomiting, suggestive of brain abscess; or fever, night sweats, cough and sputum, and weight loss similar to those of tuberculosis.

Diagnostic Laboratory Tests

Serologic tests are unreliable at present. A polypeptide extracted from nocardia cells gives a specific positive skin test (delayed) experimentally.

Specimens consist of pus from sinus, biopsy material, sputum, or spinal fluid, depending upon type of localization.

A. Microscopic Examination: Pigmented granules should be looked for. They may resemble the actinomycotic "sulfur granules" or may consist only of a tangled mass of hyphae. Wet mounts in 10% potassium hydroxide and Gram's stains should be examined. The latter may contain only coccal forms and short, branching gram-positive rods. Acid-fast stains are also indicated.

B. Culture: Both aerobic and anaerobic cultures must be made, and Sabouraud's glucose agar slants should be inoculated to detect other fungi. Intravenous inoculation of rabbits or intraperitoneal injection of guinea pigs may be useful to determine pathogenicity.

Treatment

Treatment is similar to that for actinomycosis (see above). However, the pulmonary disease caused by aerobic nocardia responds less satisfactorily than that caused by anaerobic actinomyces. The sulfonamides are currently the drugs of choice, occasionally in combination with cycloserine.

Epidemiology

Potentially pathogenic nocardia of all types live free in nature and probably enter the body by the respiratory route or through trauma. Nocardiosis is not communicable.

SUPERFICIAL MYCOSES (DERMATOPHYTOSES)

The dermatophytes are a group of closely related fungi, now classified into 3 genera: Epidermophyton, Microsporum, and Trichophyton. They infect only superficial keratinized tissues, particularly the skin, hair, and nails, but do not invade deeper tissues and do not become disseminated. In keratinized tissues they form only hyphae and arthrospores. In culture on Sabouraud's glucose agar at 20° C, they develop char-

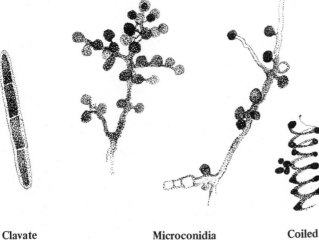
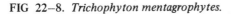
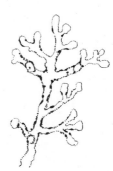

Clavate Macroconidium   Microconidia   Coiled Hypha   FIG 22–9. *Trichophyton schoenleini* showing "favic chandeliers."

FIG 22–8. *Trichophyton mentagrophytes.*

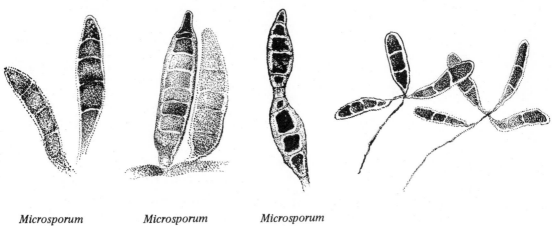

Microsporum gypseum   *Microsporum canis*   *Microsporum audouini*   *Epidermophyton floccosum*

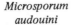
FIG 22–10. Macroconidia.

acteristic colonies and spore forms, and it is by means of these that they are classified. Sexual spores of some species have been found.

Most dermatophytes are worldwide in distribution, but some species show a higher incidence in certain regions than in others (eg, *T schoenleini* in the Mediterranean area, *T rubrum* in tropical climates). Many domestic and other animals have dermatophyte infections, and a few of them (eg, *M canis*) are transmitted from dogs or cats to children.

Morphology & Identification

The representative colony forms on Sabouraud's agar and the predominant spore forms seen in slide culture are listed in Table 22–1. Some generic characteristics are as follows:

A. Trichophyton: Colonies may be powdery, velvety, or waxy, with pigmentation ranging from white, pink, red, and purple to brown and yellow. Microconidia are the predominant spore forms. They may be arranged in clusters on the sides of hyphae or on conidiophores (see below). Macroconidia are few, elongated, with blunt ends. Fungus invades hair, skin, and nails.

B. Microsporum: Colonies are white to tan or brown in color. Macroconidia are the predominant spore forms. They are single, large, multicellular, and spindle-shaped, and occur on the ends of hyphae (Fig 22–10). This fungus invades hair and skin but rarely the nails.

C. Epidermophyton: Colonies are velvety to powdery and greenish-yellow in color. Oval or club-shaped macroconidia having 2–6 cells are typically arranged in clusters (Fig 22–10). Thus, fungus invades skin and nails but not hair.

Antigenic Structure

Dermatophytes contain both group-specific and species-specific antigens. Both of these are contained in trichophytin, a preparation derived from cultures of dermatophytes which is analogous to tuberculin. A positive trichophytin test (a delayed reaction) merely indicates present or past infection and is of no diagnostic value. The skin test is positive in those individuals who manifest hypersensitivity by developing "dermatophytids."

TABLE 22–1. Cultural and clinical features of dermatophytes.

| Organism | Characteristics of Culture | | Clinical Features and Epidemiology |
	Colonies	Morphology	
Trichophyton mentagrophytes	White to tan; powdery or cottony.	Coiled hyphae; spherical microconidia in grape-like clusters or along sides of hyphae.	Common cause of athlete's foot; also infections of hair, nails, skin, beard. Worldwide.
T rubrum	Velvety, white, reddish, or purple. Pigmentation on reverse of colony.	Club-shaped microconidia along sides of hyphae.	Chronic, treatment-resistant lesions of skin and nails. Worldwide. Very common in tropics. Griseofulvin is useful.
T tonsurans	Cream or yellow, with central furrows.	Elongated microconidia along sides of hyphae.	Endothrix infections, common in Mexico, increasing incidence in USA.
T schoenleini	Smooth, waxy, irregularly folded; brownish.	Hyphal swellings, chlamydospores; "favic chandelier," ie, antler-like processes on ends of hyphae.	Favus on scalp and skin. Common in Europe and Near East; rare in USA.
T concentricum	Similar to *T schoenleini*.		Tinea imbricata. In tropics only.
T violaceum	Violet; otherwise similar to *T schoenleini*.		Ringworm in Eastern Europe and Asia.
T ferrugineum	Orange; otherwise similar to *T schoenleini*.		Ringworm in Far East and Eastern Europe.
Microsporum audouini	Velvety, brownish, with light orange pigmentation in agar.	Rare macroconidia; microconidia club-shaped.	Epidemic ringworm of scalp. In humans only.
M canis	Cottony white mycelium, with brilliant orange pigmentation in agar.	Many large macroconidia, spindle-shaped, multicelled; thick-walled.	Infects dogs, cats, horses, man. About half of ringworm in USA.
M gypseum	Fast-growing, powdery, cinnamon-colored colony.	Many macroconidia, spindle-shaped, multicelled.	Ringworm. Frequently isolated from soil.
Epidermophyton floccosum	Greenish, powdery colony.	Club-shaped macroconidia in clusters predominate.	Skin and nail infections.

Clinical Findings

A. Tinea Pedis (Athlete's Foot): This is the most prevalent of all dermatophytoses. The toe webs are infected with a Trichophyton species or with *Epidermophyton floccosum.* Initially there is itching between the toes and the development of small blisters which rupture and discharge a thin fluid. The skin of the toe webs becomes macerated and peels, whereupon cracks appear which are prone to secondary bacterial infection. When secondary infection does occur, lymphangitis and lymphadenitis develop. When the fungal infection becomes chronic, peeling and cracking of the skin are the principal manifestations. Sometimes the nails become brittle, thickened, yellow, and irregular (tinea unguium).

In the course of a chronic dermatophytosis the individual becomes hypersensitive to constituents or products of the fungus and may develop allergic manifestations, called dermatophytids (usually vesicles), elsewhere on the body (most often on the hands). The trichophytin skin test is markedly positive in such persons.

B. Tinea Corporis (T Glabrosa) (Ringworm): This is a dermatophytosis of the nonhairy skin of the body which gives rise commonly to the annular lesions of ringworm, with a clearing, scaly center surrounded by a raised, red, advancing border which often contains vesicles.

C. Tinea Capitis (Ringworm of the Scalp): This occurs in childhood and heals spontaneously at puberty, perhaps because of the elaboration, during adult life, of higher fatty acids which are fungistatic. The dermatophytes grow in or on the hair and the keratinized epithelium of dead skin. They produce inflammatory changes, with redness, edema, scaling, vesicle formation, and thickening of the keratinized layer. The deeper layers of the epidermis show vasodilatation and cellular infiltration. The gross appearance varies with the infecting microorganism: In microsporum infections, the hair is broken off a short distance from the surface of the scalp, resulting in circumscribed spots of discolored hair stubs. There may also be a pronounced inflammation of the scalp, even resembling pyogenic infection, called kerion (especially with *M canis* or *M gypseum*).

In some trychophyton infections the hair shaft itself is invaded and the hair broken off at the surface of the scalp. The follicle is left with a black hair stub center surrounded by scaling skin. Scalp infection with *T schoenleini* gives cuplike structures (scutula) formed by crusts around infected follicles. Microsporum-infected hairs (except with some strains of *M gypseum*) fluoresce and take on a green color under Wood's light. Trichophyton-infected hairs do not fluoresce.

Trichophyton species may involve the bearded region of man (tinea barbae); they closely resemble pyogenic infections of that area.

D. Tinea Versicolor: An infection of the skin which usually produces brownish-red scaling patches on the neck, trunk, and arms. It is caused by *Malassezia furfur,* a fungus which appears microscopically in the skin as clusters of round, budding cells intermixed with short fragments of hyphae.

E. Piedra: An infection of the hair resulting in hard black nodules (*Piedraia hortai*) or soft white nodules (*Trichosporon beigelii*) attached to hair.

F. Erythrasma: A superficial infection of axillary or pubic skin caused by *Nocardia minutissima (Corynebacterium minutissimum).*

Diagnostic Laboratory Tests

Specimens consist of scrapings of skin and nails and hair plucked from involved areas. Microsporum infected hairs are best located by observing the fluorescent areas under Wood's light in a darkened room.

A. Microscopic Examination: Specimens are placed on a slide in a drop of 10–20% potassium hydroxide, covered with a coverslip, and examined immediately as well as after 10–30 minutes. In skin or nails, branching hyphae only are seen. In hairs, microspora often form dense sheaths of spores in a mosaic pattern around the hair; trichophyta form parallel rows of spores outside (ectothrix) or inside (endothrix) the hair shaft.

B. Culture: All final identification of dermatophytes must be made in cultures. Specimens are inoculated onto Sabouraud's glucose agar slants, incubated for 2–3 weeks at room temperature, and then further examined in slide cultures if necessary.

Treatment

Therapy consists of adequate removal of infected and dead epithelial structures and application of a topical antifungal chemical. Harmful overtreatment must be avoided, and attempts must be made to prevent reinfection. In serious or widespread involvement, oral administration of griseofulvin for 2–4 weeks has been strikingly effective.

A. Scalp Infections: In scalp infections, if griseofulvin is not given, the hair should be either plucked manually, clipped, or sometimes epilated by x-ray. Frequent thorough washing with soap, application of ointments containing salicylic acid, salicylanilide, or undecylenates; and the wearing of cotton stocking caps to prevent shedding of infected hair—all have their place in adequate therapy. Treatment must be continued for months. Systemic griseofulvin has been particularly useful in *T rubrum* infections.

B. Body Infections: Use antifungal ointments, eg, ammoniated mercury, 5%; undecylenic acid, 5%; salicylic acid, 3%; benzoic acid, 5%. In tinea versicolor, sodium thiosulfate is also effective.

C. Foot Infections:

1. Acute phase—Soak in potassium permanganate, 1:4000, until the acute inflammation subsides. Then use antifungal chemicals as mentioned below.

2. Subacute or chronic phases—Apply antifungal chemicals as creams (at night) and powders (during the day), eg, undecylenic acid, 5%, and zinc undecylenate, 20%; salicylic acid, 3%, and benzoic acid, 5%. Many other preparations may be used with comparable success.

Epidemiology & Control

Only sporadic cases of ringworm infection come from cats or dogs (*M canis*). The majority of cases arise from contact with infected children or infected hair and skin. Epidemics of *M audouini* infection in children have been traced to the use of common barber shop clippers and the transfer of infected hairs on theater seats as well as to person-to-person contact. Only a concerted public health approach involving proper treatment of children, sterilization of instruments (hot paraffin oil), and reduction of contacts can accomplish control.

Athlete's foot spreads through the use of common showers and dressing rooms, where infected, desquamated skin serves as a source of infection. No really effective control measures (other than widespread use of local treatment) are available. In many persons, chronic athlete's foot is asymptomatic and becomes activated only in excessive heat, moisture, or with unsuitable footwear.

DEEP MYCOSES

CANDIDA ALBICANS

Candida (Monilia) albicans is an oval, budding, yeastlike fungus which produces a pseudomycelium both in culture and in tissues and exudates. It is a member of the normal flora of the mucous membranes in the respiratory, gastrointestinal, and female genital tracts. In these and other locations it may gain dominance and be associated with pathologic conditions. Very rarely it produces systemic progressive disease.

Morphology & Identification

In smears of exudates, candida appears as a gram-positive, oval, budding yeast, measuring 2–3 X 4–6 μm, and gram-positive, elongated budding cells resembling hyphae. On Sabouraud's glucose agar incubated at room temperature, soft, cream-colored colonies develop which have a yeast-like odor. The surface growth consists of oval budding cells. The submerged growth consists of pseudomycelium. This is composed of long budding cells adherent to one another, forming blastospores at the nodes and sometimes chlamydospores terminally. *C albicans* ferments glucose and maltose, producing both acid and gas, produces acid from sucrose, and does not attack lactose. These carbohydrate fermentations, together with colonial and morphologic characteristics, differentiate *C albicans* from the other species of Candida (*C krusei, C parakrusei, C stellatoidea, C tropicalis, C pseudotropicalis,* and *C guilliermondii*), which are also occasionally members of normal human flora but are rarely implicated in disease.

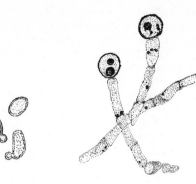

Budding Cells in Sputum

Pseudomycelium and Chlamydospores in Culture (Corn Meal Agar)

FIG 22–11. *Candida albicans.*

Antigenic Structure

By agglutination tests with absorbed sera, all *C albicans* strains fall into 2 distinct groups: A and B. Group A appears to be antigenically identical with *C tropicalis;* group B, with *C stellatoidea.*

Pathogenesis & Pathology

Upon intravenous injection into rabbits dense suspensions of *C albicans* result in widespread abscesses, particularly in the kidney, and death in less than one week.

Histologically the various skin lesions in man show inflammatory changes. Some resemble abscess formation; others resemble chronic granulomata. Large numbers of candida are sometimes found in the intestinal tract following administration of oral antibiotics, but this usually causes no symptoms. Candida may be carried by the blood stream to many organs, including the meninges, but in general is not able to establish itself and cause miliary abscess formation except in a grossly debilitated host. Dissemination occurs sometimes in lymphoma or immunosuppression, and is enhanced by antibacterial antibiotics, eg, tetracyclines.

Clinical Findings

Among the principal predisposing factors to *C albicans* infection are the following: diabetes mellitus, general debility, immunosuppression, nutritional deficiency, and disturbances in the normal flora with the absence of those bacterial components that ordinarily keep candida in check. Imbalance of these components is often brought about by prolonged administration of antimicrobial agents.

A. Mouth: Infection of the mouth (thrush) occurs, mainly in children, as white adherent patches on the buccal mucous membranes which consist largely of pseudomycelium and desquamated epithelium with only minimal erosion of the membrane.

B. Female Genitalia: Vulvovaginitis resembles thrush but produces irritation, intense itching, and discharge.

C. Skin: Infection of the skin occurs principally in moist, warm parts of the body, such as the axilla, intergluteal folds, groin, or inframammary folds; it is most common in obese and diabetic individuals. These areas become red, weeping, and may develop vesicles.

D. Hands: Candida infection of the hands and nails is seen most frequently following repeated prolonged immersion in water; it is most common in maids, housewives, cooks, vegetable and fish handlers, etc. There is swelling of the nailbed, resembling a pyogenic paronychia, and thickening and transverse grooving of the nails.

E. Lungs and Other Organs: Candida infection may be a secondary invader of lungs or kidneys where a preexisting disease is present (eg, tuberculosis or cancer). In uncontrolled leukemia and in immunosuppressed patients, candidal lesions may occur in many organs.

Diagnostic Laboratory Tests

Many normal adults possess agglutinating antibodies to candida, so that serologic findings are of no value in diagnosis.

Specimens consist of swabs and scrapings from surface lesions, sputum, and exudates.

A. Microscopic Examination: Sputum or exudates may be examined in wet smears or Gram's stains for yeastlike cells. Skin or nail scrapings are first placed in a drop of 10% potassium hydroxide.

B. Culture: All specimens are cultured on Sabouraud's glucose agar at room temperature and at 37° C; typical colonies are examined for yeastlike cells and pseudomycelia. Production of chlamydospores of *C albicans* is an important differential test: These can be produced on either corn meal agar or the chlamydospore agar of Nickerson and Mankowski.

C. Serology: A carbohydrate extract of group A candida gives positive precipitin reactions with sera of 50% of normal persons and of 70% of persons with mucocutaneous candidiasis. A sonicate of candida cells precipitates with sera of 85% of patients with systemic candidiasis and only 10% of normals.

D. Skin Test: A candida skin test is almost universally positive in normal adults. It is used therefore as an indicator of the ability to respond with a delayed hypersensitivity reaction.

Immunity

Animals can be immunized actively and are then resistant to disseminated candidiasis. Human sera often contain IgG antibody which clumps candida in vitro, and may be candidacidal.

Treatment

Orally administered nystatin does not reach tissues and thus is of no avail in disseminated candida infections. Soluble amphotericin B has been successful in some patients.

Local lesions are best treated by removing the cause: Avoid moisture; keep areas cool, powdered, and dry; and withdraw antibiotics. Both serum and vaccine therapy have been advocated, but there is no convincing evidence of their effectiveness. Various chemicals have been employed with more or less success, eg, 1% gentian violet for thrush, and parahydroxybenzoic acid esters or sodium propionate for vaginitis. Nystatin suppresses intestinal and vaginal candidiasis which follows tetracycline administration.

Epidemiology & Control

The most important preventive measure is to avoid interfering with the normal balance of microbial flora and with normal host defenses. Candida infection is not communicable, since most individuals harbor the organism under normal circumstances.

CRYPTOCOCCUS NEOFORMANS
(Torula Histolytica)

Cryptococcus neoformans is a yeastlike, budding fungus characterized by a wide capsule both in culture and exudates. It is free-living in the soil and is found frequently in pigeon feces. In man, primary pulmonary infection is occasionally followed by meningitis.

Morphology & Identification

In spinal fluid or tissue, the organism is spherical or ovoid, 5–12 μm in diameter, often budding, and enclosed in a wide capsule. On Sabouraud's agar at room temperature, the colonies are glistening and mucoid, and cream-colored organisms appear as in tissue. No mycelium is produced. Cultures produce no gas from carbohydrates. However, they assimilate glucose, maltose, sucrose, and galactose (but not lactose). They hydrolyze urea. In contrast to nonpathogenic cryptococci, *C neoformans* grows readily at 37° C on most laboratory media. A selective medium employs creatinine as N source and diphenyl and chloramphenicol as inhibitors for molds and bacteria.

Antigenic Structure

At least 3 serologic types of capsular polysaccharide material—A, B, and C—have been identified among different strains. Some of the capsular material is dissolved in spinal fluid and gives a precipitate with specific anticryptococcal serum. Such serum also gives a capsular swelling reaction. Patients with progressive cryptococcal infection may develop specific antibodies. Antipolysaccharide antibodies are not associated with increased resistance.

Pathogenesis

Intraperitoneal or intracerebral injection of *C neoformans* into mice leads to a fatal infection from which organisms can be recovered in pure culture. Infection in man occurs through the respiratory tract. Primary pulmonary disease may be followed by systemic dissemination and establishment of the infection in the CNS.

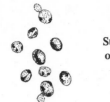

Suspension
of Culture

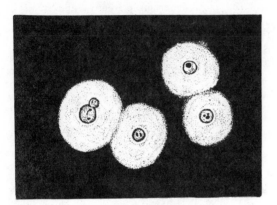

India Ink Preparation
of Spinal Fluid

FIG 22–12. *Cryptococcus neoformans.*

Histologically, the reaction varies from mild inflammation to typical granulomas.

Clinical Findings

In man the most common clinical consequence of infection with *C neoformans* is a slowly developing, chronic meningitis with frequent spontaneous remissions and relapses. The meningitis may resemble a brain tumor, brain abscess, syphilitic or tuberculous meningitis, or degenerative disease of the CNS. The pressure and protein content of the spinal fluid may be greatly increased; the cell count may be mildly elevated; the spinal fluid sugar is normal or low. In addition, there may be lesions of skin and of the lungs or other organs.

The course of cryptococcal meningitis may extend over many years, often with long remissions, but ultimately all untreated cases appear to be fatal. The disease is not communicable. Pathogenic cryptococci have been isolated from soil, but bird feces are the main source of infection.

Diagnostic Laboratory Tests

Specimens consist of spinal fluid, exudates, and sputum.

A. Microscopic Examination: Specimens are examined in wet mount, either directly or after mixing with India ink (which makes the large capsules stand out clearly around the budding yeast cells), or by immunofluorescence.

B. Culture: Growth is rapid at 20–37° C on both Sabouraud's glucose agar and other laboratory media. Urea is hydrolyzed. Cultured cells should be injected into mice to determine their pathogenicity. Direct inoculation of specimens is also desirable. In mice injected either intraperitoneally or intracerebrally, organisms can be demonstrated microscopically.

C. Serology: Tests for both antigen and antibody can be performed on CSF and serum. The latex slide agglutination test reveals antigen. Cryptococcal antibody agglutinates whole cells. No serologic test is highly sensitive or completely specific.

Treatment

Most antimicrobial agents have been ineffective, but amphotericin B (100 mg/day), although toxic, has resulted in several apparent cures. 5-Fluorocytosine (200 mg/day) has also been effective.

Epidemiology & Control

Soil or bird droppings containing *C neoformans* are the source of infection for both animals and man. The organism grows luxuriantly in bird feces, but the birds do not appear to be infected. At present, the only method of control is reduction of the pigeon population and site decontamination with alkali.

BLASTOMYCES DERMATITIDIS

Blastomyces dermatitidis is a yeastlike fungus which consists of thick-walled, budding spherical forms in tissues or when cultured at 37° C but which shows filamentous growth at room temperature. It causes a chronic granulomatous disease, North American blastomycosis, which may be limited to the skin or lung or may be widely disseminated in the body.

Morphology & Identification

In tissues, pus, or exudates, the organism appears as a round, budding sphere, 8–20 μm in diameter, with a thick, doubly refractile wall. Each cell shows only a single bud. Colonies on blood agar at 37° C are wrinkled, waxy, and soft, and the cells are morphologically similar to the tissue stage, although short hyphal segments may also be present. When grown at room temperature on Sabouraud's glucose agar, a white to brownish filamentous colony develops which consists of branching, septate hyphae with lateral spherical or pear-shaped spores (Fig 22–13). The organism ferments no sugars. The yeast phase produces a hemolysin. The sexual stage of *B dermatitidis* has recently been discovered.

Antigenic Structure

Carbohydrates and proteins isolated from the yeast phase of *B dermatitidis* give positive skin tests in infected patients or animals. A delayed tuberculin-like reaction is also shown to blastomycin, a skin-test mate-

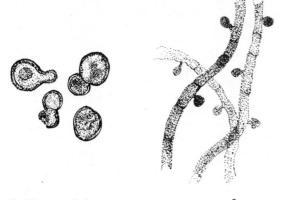

In Tissue or Culture at 37° C	Culture at 20° C on Sabouraud's Agar

FIG 22–13. *Blastomyces dermatitidis.*

rial prepared from the filtrate of a synthetic medium in which the organism has grown. Complement fixing antibodies can be demonstrated only in individuals with widespread or progressive infection.

Pathogenesis & Pathology

Many laboratory animals can be experimentally infected. The mechanism and route of human infection are not known, but the organism probably enters via the respiratory tract. Dissemination usually involves the skin, bones, viscera, and meninges.

Histologically, there are both small abscesses and distinct granulomas resembling tubercles. The budding, thick-walled spheres are commonly seen in pus or tissues.

Clinical Findings

A. Skin: The primary skin lesion is a pustule which breaks down in the center and spreads peripherally, forming an irregular ulcer with a raised red border studded with small abscesses. This lesion may occur anywhere on the body but occurs most frequently on exposed areas.

B. Metastases: The lungs, bones, and other organs may be involved through blood stream dissemination. Apparent primary pulmonary blastomycosis occurs and may remain limited to the lungs.

C. Skin Test: The blastomycin skin test is positive in many patients but is positive also in some persons without any disease; this suggests either subclinical exposure or cross-reaction with other fungal infections.

Diagnostic Laboratory Tests

Specimens consist of sputum, pus, exudates, and biopsy from skin lesions.

A. Microscopic Examination: Wet mounts of specimens may show budding, thick-walled, yeast-like organisms which may also be apparent in histologic sections.

B. Culture: Colonial and cellular morphology is typical on blood agar at 37° C and on Sabouraud's glucose agar at 20° C.

C. Animal Inoculation: Massive doses of yeast phase cultures injected intravenously or intraperitoneally into mice, guinea pigs, or rabbits are fatal in 3–20 days.

D. Serology: Serologic tests are undependable.

Treatment

Sulfonamides and antibiotics have very little effect on the course of the disease. However, the aromatic diamidines (eg, dihydroxystilbamidine) induce prolonged remissions even of extensive lesions and may result in permanent cure. Vaccines are of some value. Amphotericin B injected intravenously for many weeks can be curative. Surgical removal of lesions is occasionally valuable.

Epidemiology

Infection with *B dermatitidis* probably occurs only in the USA and Canada. The organism has recently been isolated from soil, and spontaneously infected dogs have been found.

It is probable that *B dermatitidis* occurs in soil or on vegetation. Infection probably follows inhalation or trauma. The disease is not communicable from person to person.

BLASTOMYCES BRASILIENSIS

Blastomyces brasiliensis is a yeast-like fungus which causes South and Central American blastomycosis (paracoccidioidal granuloma). This organism occurs only in South America, the majority of cases being noted in Brazil. In tissues and in culture at 37° C, it forms thick-walled spheres with both single and multiple buds. At room temperature, cultures develop an aerial mycelium.

Morphology & Identification

B brasiliensis resembles *B dermatitidis* in both tissue and culture; the principal difference is that *B brasiliensis* forms thick-walled cells (10–60 μm in tissue, 6–30 μm in culture) which characteristically have multiple buds.

Pathogenesis & Clinical Findings

Members of the white and Oriental races develop South American blastomycosis more commonly than do Negroes, perhaps indicating a difference in racial susceptibility.

The disease begins with papillary granulomas on the mucous membranes of the mouth and adjacent skin and then spreads to regional and distant lymph nodes. These enlarge greatly.

A different form of the infection begins in the lymphoid tissue of the intestine and spreads first to the

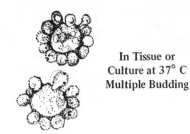

In Tissue or
Culture at 37° C
Multiple Budding

FIG 22–14. *Blastomyces brasiliensis.*

mesenteric lymph nodes and then to other abdominal viscera. Histologically, there is either abscess formation or granuloma with central caseation. Organisms are frequently seen in tissue, giant cells, or pus and are always characterized by their multiple budding.

Skin tests with "paracoccidioidin" are analogous to those with blastomycin in the North American disease. The same material can be used as antigen for complement fixation tests which are positive in extensive or progressive involvement.

Diagnostic Laboratory Tests

These are essentially the same as for *B dermatitidis.* Animal inoculation is best carried out by the intratesticular injection of guinea pigs and culture of the developing lesion.

Treatment

South American blastomycosis responds strikingly to prolonged administration of sulfonamides. All forms of the disease have shown improvement. Amphotericin B has proved curative in some patients.

Epidemiology

South American blastomycosis occurs mainly in rural areas, particularly among farmers. The disease is much more frequent in males than females, which suggests that the men acquire the infection while working in the fields. The fungus has not yet been isolated from nature. The disease is not communicable.

HISTOPLASMA CAPSULATUM

Histoplasma capsulatum is a yeast-like fungus which causes histoplasmosis. In tissues and on blood agar at 37° C, it is seen as a small, ovoid, budding organism. In cultures at room temperature, it produces filamentous colonies.

Morphology & Identification

Within phagocytic cells and on sealed blood agar slants incubated at 37° C, *Histoplasma capsulatum* forms oval, yeast-like budding cells measuring 2–4 μm. On blood agar at 37° C, colonies are smooth and white. On Sabouraud's glucose agar incubated at room temperature, white, cottony colonies develop, with large (8–20 μm), thick-walled, spherical spores having finger-like projections. The appearance of these tuberculate spores is diagnostic of *H capsulatum* infection.

Antigenic Structure

Patients with histoplasmosis give positive skin tests with histoplasmin, a filtrate of broth in which *H capsulatum* has been grown. The reaction is delayed and tuberculin-like. From yeast phase or mycelium, polysaccharides with precipitating and complement fixing activity can be isolated.

Pathogenesis & Clinical Findings

Infection with *H capsulatum* usually occurs through the respiratory tract. It is often asymptomatic, in which case the small inflammatory or granulomatous foci in the lungs heal with calcification. Such miliary calcification has been observed in many tuberculin negative, histoplasmin positive individuals in the endemic area in the USA. With heavy respiratory exposure, clinical pneumonia and protracted illness can develop.

Disseminated histoplasmosis develops in a small minority of infected individuals, but more frequently in white than in dark-skinned persons. The reticuloendothelial system is particularly involved, with lymphadenopathy, enlarged spleen and liver, high fever, anemia, and a high fatality rate. Tumor-like ulcers of the nose, mouth, tongue, and intestine can occur. In such individuals the histologic lesion shows focal areas of necrosis in small granulomas in many organs. Phagocytic cells (mononuclear or polymorphonuclear leukocytes of the blood, fixed reticuloendothelial cells of liver, spleen, and bone marrow) contain the small, oval yeast-like cells.

Many animals, including dogs and rodents, are spontaneously infected in endemic areas. Mice and guinea pigs can be infected experimentally with cultures.

Diagnostic Laboratory Tests

Specimens consist of sputum, scrapings from lesions, and blood smears; biopsies from sternal marrow, skin, lymph nodes; and blood for serology.

A. Microscopic Examination: In histologic sections, the small ovoid cells may be detected intracellularly. The same is true for smears of blood or bone marrow.

B. Culture: All specimens must be cultured both at 37° C and at room temperature on blood and Sabouraud's agar; cultures must be kept for 3 weeks.

C. Serology: Latex agglutination, complement fixation, or precipitin tests are positive within a few weeks after infection, reach a peak titer in 2–3 months, and then fall to low levels if the disease is inactive. With progressive disease, the complement fixation test remains positive in high titer (1:32). Two precipitin bands can be formed in serum. One (H) connotes active histoplasmosis; the other (M) may arise from repeated skin testing.

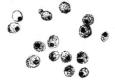

| Yeast Phase in
Culture at 37° C | Tuberculate Spores in
Culture at 20° C | Showing
Intracellular Bodies |

FIG 22–15. *Histoplasma capsulatum.*

D. Skin Test: The histoplasmin skin test becomes positive soon after infection and remains positive if the disease is arrested. It may be negative in disseminated, progressive disease.

Immunity

Some degree of immunity appears to follow infection with histoplasma.

Treatment

Symptomatic therapy in primary pulmonary histoplasmosis suffices for the recovery of most infected persons. No definitive treatment for disseminated histoplasmosis has been discovered, although claims for amphotericin B have been made.

Epidemiology & Control

The endemic area for *H capsulatum* in the USA includes the central and eastern states, where small epidemics have occurred and where the fungus has been recovered from the soil, from animals, and from certain locations on farms (eg, silos). The fungus grows abundantly in bird feces (chicken houses) and bat guano (caves). Exposure in such places may result in massive infection with severe disease (eg, cave disease). In endemic areas it must be assumed that very small infective inocula are spread by dust. A large proportion of inhabitants (about 65%) apparently become infected, without symptoms, during childhood, develop positive histoplasmin skin tests, and occasionally have healed miliary calcifications in the lungs. The disease is not communicable. Spraying of formaldehyde on infected soil may destroy histoplasma.

COCCIDIOIDES IMMITIS

Coccidioides immitis is a fungus which is endemic in the southwestern USA and causes coccidioidomycosis. In tissue it is a large, thick-walled spherule filled with endospores. Cultured at room temperature, it produces a cottony colony with hyphae which fragment into highly infectious arthrospores.

Morphology & Identification

In histologic sections of tissues or in pus or sputum, *C immitis* appears as a spherule, 15–75 μm in diameter, with a thick, doubly refractile wall. The spherule is filled with minute endospores which occasionally can be seen to have erupted into surrounding tissues. Spherules can be produced in vitro by using specialized culture media. When grown at room temperature on common laboratory media or on Sabouraud's glucose agar, a fluffy, cottony white colony develops. The hyphae of this growth contain rectangular arthrospores, which are freed in old cultures through fragmentation of the hyphae. These spores are very light, float readily in air, and are highly infectious. When inoculated into tissues or into the yolk sacs of developing chick embryos, these spores develop into spherules.

Antigenic Structure

Coccidioidin is produced from the filtrate of a broth culture in which *C immitis* has been grown. It gives positive skin tests (in dilutions up to 1:10,000) in infected persons and acts as antigen in precipitin and complement fixation tests. A polysaccharide has been isolated from it which also gives positive skin and precipitin tests. In low dilutions of coccidioidin (1:10), there are cross-reactions with histoplasmin and perhaps with the antigens of other fungi.

Pathogenesis & Clinical Findings

Infection is acquired through the inhalation of air- and dust-borne arthrospores. There follows a respiratory infection which may be asymptomatic and may manifest itself only by the development of a positive coccidioidin skin test in 3 weeks. Otherwise, the individual may have an influenza-like illness, with fever, malaise, cough, aches, pains, and sweats, from which he recovers. About 3–5% of individuals who have had

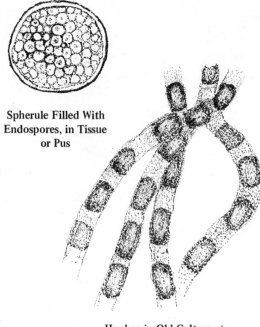

Spherule Filled With
Endospores, in Tissue
or Pus

Hyphae in Old Culture at
Room Temperature Breaking
Up into Arthrospores

FIG 22–16. *Coccidioides immitis.*

such an illness develop, 1–2 weeks later, hypersensitivity reactions in the form of erythema nodosum or erythema multiforme. This symptom complex is referred to as "valley fever" or "desert rheumatism" and is self-limited. Thin-walled cavities occasionally develop in the lungs at this time; these also tend to subside spontaneously.

Fewer than 1% of persons who have been infected progress to the disseminated, highly fatal form called "coccidioidal granuloma." This occurs 10 times more frequently in dark-skinned than in light-skinned individuals. Dissemination, when it occurs, develops almost always within one year or less of the initial infection, either by direct extension of the process or by endogenous reinfection. It denotes some defect in the individual's ability to localize and control infection with *C immitis*. Most individuals can be considered immune to the organism once their skin test has become positive.

Disseminated coccidioidomycosis is entirely comparable to tuberculosis, with lesions in all organs and in the CNS. Histologically, these lesions are typical granulomas which are indistinguishable from tuberculosis unless spherules can be detected in them. The clinical course often involves remissions and exacerbations.

Diagnostic Laboratory Tests

Specimens consist of sputum, pus, gastric washings, spinal fluid, biopsy specimens, and blood for serology.

A. Microscopic Examination: All materials should be examined fresh (after centrifuging, if necessary) for typical spherules; histologic sections must be stained.

B. Cultures: Culture should be carried out on blood agar at 37° C and on Sabouraud's agar at room temperature.*

C. Animal Inoculations: Mice injected intraperitoneally develop progressive disease.

D. Serology: Precipitating antibodies (19 S) in titers of diagnostic significance develop soon after infection, then diminish. Complement fixing antibodies (7 S) become positive in high titer only in progressive disseminated disease; when this happens the prognosis is poor.

Immunity

Immunity usually follows infection with *C immitis*. Experimental vaccines are under study.

Treatment

For the primary infection, because most persons recover completely, only symptomatic treatment and rest are necessary. For coccidioidal granuloma, no uniformly effective treatment is available. Recoveries have occasionally been attributed to the use of ethyl vanillate. Amphotericin B injected intravenously is the most promising agent at present.

Epidemiology & Control

The endemic area of *C immitis* in the USA includes the dry, arid regions of the southwestern states, particularly the San Joaquin Valley of California, the area around Tucson and Phoenix in Arizona, and west Texas. Some spread of the endemic area is being noted. It also occurs in Central and South America in a "lower sonoran life zone." In those areas the fungus is found in the soil and in rodents, and the majority of residents (up to 90%) give evidence, by positive coccidioidin skin tests, of past infection. The infection rate is highest during the dry months of summer and autumn, when dust is most prevalent.

Infection can be diminished by dust control measures: paving roads and airfield runways, planting lawns, and using oil sprays. The disease is not communicable, and there is no evidence that infected animals contribute to its spread.

GEOTRICHUM CANDIDUM

Geotrichum candidum is a yeast-like fungus which produces geotrichosis, an infection of bronchi, lungs, and mucous membranes.

*A special medium may also be employed that consists of sodium acetate, 1%; ammonium chloride, 1%; tribasic potassium phosphate, 0.8%; cupric sulfate, 0.04%; and agar, 2%. Add cupric sulfate (1 ml of 4% solution per 100 ml) after the remainder has been autoclaved for 10 minutes at 15 lb. This medium must be prepared fresh for each culture.

Morphology & Identification

In sputum, *G candidum* appears as rectangular arthrospores 5 × 10 μm or thick-walled, ovoid, yeast-like cells. Characteristically, both are present. Cultures on Sabouraud's agar produce slow-growing, membranous, flat, soft, white colonies. The hyphae segment into arthrospores.

Pathogenesis & Clinical Findings

The natural habitat of the fungus is not known. In man, it is associated with chronic bronchitis with the x-ray appearance of diffuse peribronchial thickening, diffuse pulmonary infiltration resembling tuberculosis, or thrush-like lesions in the mouth. The sputum is mucoid and occasionally blood-streaked and contains the organisms. The prognosis is generally good.

Diagnostic Laboratory Tests

Examination of sputum by microscopy and culture.

Treatment

Potassium iodide by mouth is claimed to result in improvement. One percent gentian violet suppresses oral lesions. Polymyxins may inhibit geotrichum.

SPOROTRICHUM SCHENCKII

Sporotrichum schenckii is a fungus producing a leathery colony with typical clusters of pear-shaped conidia on the hyphae. It causes sporotrichosis, a chronic granulomatous infection of skin, lymphatics, and other tissues in animals and man.

Morphology & Identification

The organisms are only rarely seen in pus and tissues from human infections but may appear as small, spindle-shaped, single, gram-positive budding cells. In cultures on Sabouraud's agar, cream-colored to black, folded, leathery colonies develop within 3–5 days. (The pigment formations of different strains of *S schenckii* are variable.) They consist of thin, septate, branching hyphae which carry clusters of pear-shaped conidia at the ends of lateral branches.

Antigenic Structure

Heat-killed saline suspensions of cultures (or carbohydrate fractions from them) give positive delayed skin tests in infected man or animals. A variety of antibodies is also produced.

Pathogenesis & Clinical Findings

The fungus is introduced into the skin of the extremities through trauma. A local lesion develops as a pustule, abscess, or ulcer, and the lymphatics leading from it become thickened and cord-like. Multiple subcutaneous nodules and abscesses occur along the

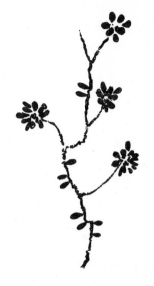

FIG 22–17. *Sporotrichum schenckii* in culture, showing clusters of conidia on conidiospores.

lymphatics. Usually there is little systemic illness associated with these lesions, but dissemination of the infection sometimes occurs. Rarely, primary infection in man occurs through the lung. A variety of animals (rats, dogs, mules, and horses) are found naturally infected.

Histologically, the lesions show both chronic inflammation and specific granulomas which undergo necrosis.

Diagnostic Laboratory Tests

Specimens consist of pus or biopsy from lesions.

A. Microscopic Examination: In human lesions, the organism can rarely be seen, whereas the fusiform cells are common in experimental infections of rats or mice.

B. Culture: On Sabouraud's agar, typical colonies and clusters of conidia are diagnostic. The organism will grow on most laboratory media.

C. Serology: Not helpful in diagnosis.

Immunity

No immunity develops to this infecting organism.

Treatment

In the majority of cases the infection is self-limited although very chronic. Potassium iodide administered orally for weeks—or amphotericin B—has a therapeutic effect.

Epidemiology & Control

S schenckii occurs worldwide in nature on plants, thorns, and timber; in dust, and on infected animals. In the USA, the principal endemic area is the Mississippi Valley. Occupational exposure of gardeners, miners, and persons in contact with animals accounts for the majority of cases. Prevention of trauma in these occupations is effective, since the organism must be passively introduced into the skin to produce disease.

CHROMOBLASTOMYCOSIS

Chromoblastomycosis is a chronic, slowly progressive, granulomatous infection of skin and lymphatics caused by the fungi *Hormodendrum (Cladosporium) pedrosoi, Hormodendrum (Cladosporium) compactum, Phialophora verrucosa,* and others.

Morphology & Identification

In exudates and tissues, these fungi produce dark brown septate bodies, 6–12 μm in diameter, which reproduce by splitting. On Sabouraud's glucose agar the following characteristics are noted:

A. *H Pedrosoi:* Colonies are dark green to brown or black, with felt-like aerial mycelia. Conidia may be in branching chains, may surround the swollen ends of hyphae, or may be produced from flask-shaped conidiophores.

B. *H Compactum:* Colonies are brittle, heaped-up, and black, with a coarse aerial mycellium. Spherical conidia are arranged in compact sporulating heads.

C. *P Verrucosa:* Colonies are brown or black with a short, felt-like, gray aerial mycelium. Conidia are produced within the ends of flask-shaped conidiophores which are laterally attached to hyphae.

Pathogenesis & Clinical Findings

The fungus is introduced by trauma into the skin, usually of the lower extremities. Slowly, over a period of weeks or months, wart-like growths develop and extend gradually along the lymphatics. Cauliflower-like nodules eventually cover part of the leg, and elephantiasis may result from fibrosis and obstruction of lymph channels. Dissemination to other parts of the body is very rare.

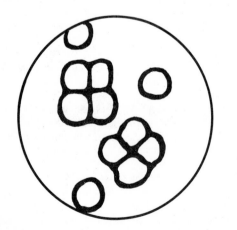

FIG 22–18. *Hormodendrum (Cladosporium) pedrosoi in tissue.*

Histologically, the lesions are granulomas; within leukocytes or giant cells the dark-brown, round fungus bodies may be seen.

Diagnostic Laboratory Tests

Specimens consist of scrapings or biopsy from the lesions.

A. **Microscopic Examination:** Specimens are placed in a 10% potassium hydroxide solution and examined for the dark, round, splitting fungus bodies.

B. **Culture:** Culture should be made on Sabouraud's agar to observe the characteristic conidial structures and arrangements necessary for identification of organisms.

Treatment

Amphotericin B injected directly into the lesions has proved curative. Local removal is the only other feasible treatment.

Epidemiology

Chromoblastomycosis is worldwide but occurs mainly in the tropics. The fungi are saprophytic in nature, probably occurring on vegetation and in the soil. The disease occurs chiefly on the legs of barefooted farm laborers, presumably following traumatic introduction of the fungus. It is not communicable. No animals have been found to be spontaneously infected. No control measures are known.

MADUROMYCOSIS

Maduromycosis is a slowly progressive infection of the subcutaneous tissue, usually of the foot; it is also called mycetoma and Madura foot. It can be caused by Nocardia and Streptomyces species, by *Monosporium apiospermum,* and by several filamentous fungi. It is principally a disease of the tropics, and is particularly prevalent in India.

Morphology & Identification

Monosporium apiospermum is found in tissues or exudates as a yellowish granule, composed of septate hyphae with many chlamydospores around the periphery. Grayish-white, cottony colonies are formed on Sabouraud's agar at room temperature; they have single ovoid conidia at the ends of conidiophores. Other species may produce black granules composed of dark septate hyphae. Each species has its own characteristic colonial morphology.

Pathogenesis & Clinical Findings

After the traumatic introduction of one of the causative fungi into the subcutaneous tissue of the foot, deep-seated nodules or abscesses form which increase in size and eventually drain, establishing chronic sinuses. The infection extends from the subcutaneous tissue to muscles and bones, causing deformity and loss of function.

Histologically, the lesions resemble actinomycosis, with prominent abscess formation, granulation tissue, necrotic foci, and fibrosis.

Diagnostic Laboratory Tests

Materials from sinuses or biopsy specimens should be examined for characteristic granules and should be cultured. Skin tests with a protein from *Nocardia brasiliensis* are positive in mycetoma patients, and precipitin tests in their sera can be performed with a polysaccharide from that organism.

Treatment

Antibiotics have been of no avail except to reduce secondary bacterial infection. Sulfonamides and sulfones have proved effective for some cases of nocardia and streptomyces infections.

Epidemiology & Control

The fungi producing maduromycosis occur free in nature, in the soil, or on vegetation. The disease is produced when they are introduced into tissues through trauma. Barefoot farm laborers are therefore most exposed. Wearing shoes is a reasonable control measure.

MUCORMYCOSIS & ASPERGILLOSIS

Saprophytic fungi of the genera Mucor, Rhizopus, and Aspergillus occasionally proliferate in debilitated hosts or injured tissues. *Aspergillus fumigatus* sometimes grows in external otitis, chronic sinusitis, or bronchiectasis, superimposed on other conditions. Aspergillus pneumonia occurs in leukemic or immunosuppressed patients.

In persons suffering from diabetes mellitus, extensive burns, tuberculosis, leukemia, and other severe chronic illnesses, *Rhizopus oryzae* or other species proliferate in the walls of blood vessels, producing thrombosis. Symptoms may be referable to many organs. The organism is rarely cultured during life but is seen in histologic preparations as nonseptate hyphae in thrombosed blood vessels or sinuses, with surrounding neutrophilic and giant cell response. The diagnosis of mucormycosis is usually made at autopsy, or in biopsy material. Occasional cure is accomplished by surgical removal of the lesion, eg, nephrectomy.

HYPERSENSITIVITY TO FUNGI

Several types of pneumonitis (eg, farmer's lung, maple bark disease) are caused by hypersensitivity reactions to inhaled antigens of a variety of fungi. These are discussed in Chapter 13.

MYCOTOXINS

Many fungi produce poisonous substances, called mycotoxins, which can cause acute or chronic damage in animals or man. Acute poisoning may occur, such as in acute mushroom poisoning caused by the ingestion of some types of mushrooms. Chronic damage to the liver or bone marrow may be produced, and neoplasms may be induced in animals (eg, aflatoxin from *Aspergillus flavus*). Derivatives of fungal products may cause profound mental derangement (eg, lysergic acid diethylamide).

•   •   •

General References

Campbell, C.C.: Use and interpretation of serologic and skin tests in the respiratory mycoses. Dis Chest 54:305–310, 1968.

Hart, P.D., & others: The compromised host and infection. 2. Deep fungal infection. J Infect Dis 120:169–191, 1969.

Littman, M.L., & J.E. Walter: Cryptococcosis. Am J Med 45:422–432, 1968.

Louria, D.B.: Deep-seated mycotic infections, allergy to fungi and mycotoxins. New England J Med 277:1065–1071, 1967.

23...

Normal Microbial Flora of the Human Body

The skin and mucous membranes always harbor a variety of microorganisms which can be arranged into 2 groups: (1) The resident flora consists of relatively fixed types of microorganisms regularly found in a given area at a given age; if disturbed, it promptly reestablishes itself. (2) The transient flora consists of nonpathogenic or potentially pathogenic microorganisms which inhabit the skin or mucous membranes for hours, days, or weeks; it is derived from the environment, does not produce disease, and does not establish itself permanently on the surface. Members of the transient flora are generally of little significance so long as the normal resident flora remains intact. However, if the resident flora is disturbed, transient microorganisms may proliferate and produce disease.

ROLE OF THE RESIDENT FLORA

The microorganisms that are constantly present on body surfaces are commensals. Their flourishing in a given area depends upon physiologic factors of temperature, moisture, and the presence of certain nutrients and inhibitory substances. Their presence is not essential to life because "germ-free" animals can be reared in the complete absence of a normal microbial flora. Yet the resident flora of certain areas plays a definite role in maintaining health and normal function. Members of the resident flora in the intestinal tract synthesize vitamin K and aid in the absorption of nutrients. On mucous membranes and skin, the resident flora may prevent colonization by pathogens and possible disease through "bacterial interference" (see Chapter 14).

On the other hand, members of the normal flora may themselves produce disease under certain circumstances. These organisms are adapted to the noninvasive mode of life defined by the limitations of the environment. If forcefully removed from the restrictions of that environment and introduced into the blood stream or tissues, these organisms may become pathogenic. For example, streptococci of the viridans group are the commonest resident organisms of the upper respiratory tract. If large numbers of them are introduced into the blood stream (eg, following tooth extraction or tonsillectomy), they may settle on abnormal heart valves and produce subacute bacterial endo-

carditis. Bacteroides are the commonest resident bacteria of the large intestine and are quite harmless in that location. If introduced into the free peritoneal cavity or into pelvic tissues along with other bacteria, as a result of trauma, they cause suppuration which may lead to sepsis. Spirochetes and fusiform bacilli are resident in every normal mouth. In the presence of tissue damage through trauma, nutritional deficiency, or infection they proliferate vastly in the necrotic tissue, producing "fusospirochetal" disease. There are many other examples, but the important point is that microbes of the normal resident flora are harmless and may be beneficial in their normal location in the host and in the absence of coincident abnormalities. They may produce disease if introduced into foreign locations and if predisposing factors are present. For these reasons, members of the resident flora that are found in disease are sometimes referred to as "opportunists."

NORMAL FLORA OF THE SKIN

Because of its constant exposure to and contact with the environment, the skin is particularly apt to contain transient microorganisms. Nevertheless there is a constant and well-defined resident flora, modified in different anatomic areas by secretions, habitual wearing of clothing, or proximity to mucous membranes (mouth, nose, and perineal areas).

The predominant resident microorganisms of the skin are aerobic and anaerobic diphtheroid bacilli (corynebacteria); nonhemolytic aerobic and anaerobic white staphylococci; gram-positive, aerobic, sporeforming bacilli which are ubiquitous in air, water, and soil; nonhemolytic or green streptococci (*S viridans*) and enterococci (*S faecalis*); and gram-negative coliform bacilli and mimeae. Fungi and yeasts are often present in skin folds; acid-fast, nonpathogenic mycobacteria occur in areas rich in sebaceous secretions (genitalia, external ear).

Among the factors that may be important in eliminating nonresident microorganisms from the skin are the low pH, the fatty acids in sebaceous secretions, and the presence of lysozyme. Neither profuse sweating nor washing and bathing can eliminate or significantly modify the normal resident flora. The number of superficial microorganisms may be diminished by vigorous surgical "scrubbing," but the flora is rapidly replenished from sebaceous and sweat glands even when contact with other skin areas or with the environment is completely excluded.

NORMAL FLORA OF THE MOUTH & UPPER RESPIRATORY TRACT

The mucous membranes of the mouth and pharynx are often sterile at birth but may be contaminated by passage through the birth canal. Within 4–12 hours after birth, alpha-hemolytic streptococci (*S viridans*) become established as the most prominent members of the resident flora and remain so for life. They probably originate in the respiratory tracts of the mother and attendants. Early in life aerobic and anaerobic staphylococci, gram-negative diplococci (neisseriae), diphtheroids, and occasional lactobacilli are added. When teeth begin to erupt, the anaerobic spirochetes and fusiform bacilli and some anaerobic vibrios and lactobacilli establish themselves. Actinomyces species are normally present in tonsillar tissue and on the gingivae in adults. Yeasts occur in the mouth.

In the pharynx and trachea, a similar flora establishes itself, whereas few bacteria are found in normal bronchi. Small bronchi and alveoli are normally sterile. The predominant organisms in the upper respiratory tract, particularly the pharynx, are nonhemolytic and alpha-hemolytic streptococci and neisseriae. Staphylococci, diphtheroids, hemophilus, pneumococci, mycoplasma, and bacteroides are also encountered.

The flora of the nose consists of prominent corynebacteria, white and yellow staphylococci, and streptococci.

The Role of the Normal Mouth Flora in Dental Caries

Caries is a disintegration of the teeth beginning at the surface and progressing inward. First the surface enamel, which is entirely noncellular, is demineralized. This has been attributed to the effect of acid products of bacterial fermentation. Subsequent decomposition of the dentin and cement involves bacterial digestion of the protein matrix.

An essential first step in caries production appears to be the formation of "plaque" on the hard smooth enamel surface. The "plaque" consists mainly of gelatinous deposits of high molecular weight dextrans in which acid-producing bacteria adhere to the enamel. The dextrans are formed mainly by certain anaerobic streptococci from sucrose as substrate. The essential second step in caries production appears to be the formation of large amounts of acid from carbohydrates by streptococci and lactobacilli in the plaque. High concentrations of acid demineralize the adjoining enamel and initiate caries.

In experimental "germ-free" animals, cariogenic streptococci can induce the formation of plaque and of caries. Certain diphtheroids can induce specific soft-tissue damage and bone resorption typical of periodontal disease. Proteolytic organisms, including actinomycetes and bacilli, play a role in the microbial action on dentin which follows damage to the enamel. The development of caries also depends on genetic, hormonal, nutritional, and many other factors. Control of caries involves physical removal of "plaque," limitation of sucrose intake, good nutrition with adequate protein intake, reduction of acid-production in the mouth by limitation of available carbohydrates and frequent cleansing. The application of fluoride to teeth or its ingestion in water results in enhancement of acid-resistance of the enamel.

NORMAL FLORA OF THE INTESTINAL TRACT

At birth the intestine is sterile, but organisms are soon introduced with food. In breast-fed children, the intestine contains large numbers of lactic acid streptococci and lactobacilli. These aerobic and anaerobic, gram-positive, nonmotile organisms (eg, bifidobacterium) produce acid from carbohydrates and tolerate pH 5.0. In bottle-fed children, a more mixed flora exists in the bowel, and lactobacilli are less prominent. As food habits develop toward the adult pattern, the bowel flora changes. Diet has a marked influence on the relative composition of the intestinal and fecal flora.

In the normal adult, the esophagus contains microorganisms arriving with saliva and food. The stomach's acidity keeps the number of microorganisms at a minimum (10^3-10^5/gm of contents) unless obstruction favors the proliferation of gram-positive cocci and bacilli. As the pH of intestinal contents becomes alkaline, the resident flora gradually increases. In the adult duodenum, there are 10^3-10^6 bacteria/gm; in the jejunum and proximal ileum 10^5-10^8 bacteria/gm; and in the lower ileum and cecum, 10^8-10^{10} bacteria/gm of contents. In the upper intestine, lactobacilli and enterococci predominate, but in the lower ileum and cecum the flora is fecal. In the colon and rectum, as in the feces, there are about 10^{11} bacteria/gm of content, constituting 10–20% of the fecal mass. In diarrhea, the bacterial content may diminish greatly.

In the adult normal colon, the resident bacterial flora consists of 96–99% anaerobes (bacteroides, anaerobic lactobacilli, eg, bifidobacterium, clostridia, anaerobic streptococci) and only 1–4% aerobes (gram-negative coliforms, enterococci, and small numbers of proteus, pseudomonas, lactobacilli, candida, and other organisms).

Intestinal bacteria are important in synthesis of vitamin K, conversion of bile pigments and bile acids, absorption of nutrients and breakdown products, and antagonism to microbial pathogens. The intestinal flora produces ammonia and other breakdown products which are reabsorbed and can contribute to hepatic coma.

Antimicrobial drugs taken orally can, in man, temporarily suppress the drug-susceptible components of the fecal flora. This is commonly done for the preoperative "sterilization" of the bowel by means of insoluble sulfonamides or antibiotics such as neomycin. For several days the count of fecal bacteria declines greatly, but at the end of 1–2 weeks the total count returns to normal or becomes higher than normal and the drug-susceptible microorganisms are replaced by drug-resistant ones, particularly staphylococci, aerobacter, enterococci, proteus, pseudomonas, and yeasts.

The feeding of large quantities of *Lactobacillus acidophilus* may result in the temporary establishment of this organism in the gut and the concomitant partial suppression of other gut microflora.

Growth of young chickens, turkeys, and pigs is greatly accelerated by admixture of antibiotics to the feed. The nature of this phenomenon is not clear; it probably does not occur in man or ruminants.

NORMAL FLORA OF THE VAGINA

Soon after birth, aerobic lactobacilli (Döderlein's bacilli) appear in the vagina and persist as long as the pH remains acid (several weeks). When the pH becomes neutral (remaining so until puberty), a mixed flora of cocci and bacilli is present. At puberty, lactobacilli reappear in large numbers and contribute to the maintenance of acid pH through the production of acid from carbohydrates, particularly glycogen. This appears to be an important mechanism in preventing the establishment of other, possibly harmful microorganisms in the vagina. If lactobacilli are suppressed by the administration of antimicrobial drugs, yeasts or various bacteria increase in numbers and cause irritation and inflammation. After the menopause, lactobacilli again diminish in numbers and a mixed flora returns. The normal vaginal flora often includes clostridia, anaerobic streptococci, listeriae, and others. The cervical mucus has antibacterial activity and contains lysozyme.

NORMAL FLORA OF THE EYE (CONJUNCTIVA)

The predominant organisms of the eye are diphtheroids (*Corynebacterium xerosis*), neisseriae, and small gram-negative bacilli resembling hemophilus (Morax-Axenfeld bacillus, Moraxella species). Staphylococci and nonhemolytic streptococci are also frequently present.

•   •   •

General References

Finegold, S.M.: Intestinal bacteria: Their role in physiology. California Med 110:455–459, 1969.

Morris, A.L., & R. Greulich: Dental caries. Science 160:1082–1083, 1968.

24...

Principles of Diagnostic Medical Microbiology

Diagnostic medical microbiology is concerned (1) with the etiologic diagnosis of infectious disease by means of the isolation and identification of infectious agents and the demonstration of immunologic responses (antibody, skin reactivity) in the patient; and (2) with the rational selection of antimicrobial therapy on the basis of laboratory tests.

In the field of infectious diseases, the results of laboratory tests are largely a function of the nature of the specimen, the timing of its collection, and the care with which it is collected; and the technical proficiency and experience of the laboratory personnel. Although any general physician should be competent to perform a few simple, crucial microbiologic tests (ie, should be able to make and stain a smear, examine it microscopically, and streak a culture plate), the technical details of the more involved procedures are usually left to the bacteriologist or virologist and the technicians working under him. Any physician who deals with infectious processes must know when and how to take a specimen, what laboratory examinations to request, and how to interpret the results.

COMMUNICATION BETWEEN PHYSICIAN & LABORATORY

When a physician sends a blood specimen to the laboratory and requests a chemical determination, the laboratory has no alternative but to employ a single chemical procedure and report the result to the physician. While that value may be reported higher or lower depending upon variations in the specimen, in the skill and experience of the technician, or in the equipment at hand in the laboratory, the physician generally accepts that value and takes it into account in making his clinical diagnosis. Little would be gained, in this situation, by further communication between the physician and the laboratory.

In microbiologic laboratory diagnosis the situation is different. No one method is available which will permit the isolation of all possible pathogenic organisms or differentiate them from nonpathogenic ones. Before the laboratory personnel can select the one technic best suited to the isolation of one or another organism, the physician must inform the laboratory of his tentative clinical diagnosis and of the type of infec-

tion he suspects. This forces the clinician to reason more closely than if he merely suspects "infection" and defers all attempts at etiologic diagnosis until the laboratory results are returned. Clinical information from the physician can often aid the laboratory in selecting the best methods available for the identification of an etiologic agent.

In contrast with chemical determinations, microbiologic laboratory procedures are often slow, requiring a series of sequential steps before the answer is reached. Many pathogenic microorganisms grow slowly, and days or even weeks may elapse before their identification. However, it is almost never possible to defer treatment until this laborious process is complete. It is therefore essential that the physician obtain proper specimens, inform the laboratory of his tentative clinical diagnosis, and then begin treatment with drugs aimed at the organism he supposes is responsible for the patient's illness. As the laboratory begins to derive information of clinical significance, it can feed it back to the physician so that he may reevaluate his diagnosis and perhaps make changes in the therapeutic program. This "feedback" information will consist of **preliminary reports** of the results of individual steps in the isolation and identification of the etiologic agent.

SPECIMENS

The results of many diagnostic tests in infectious diseases depend largely upon the selection, timing, and method of collection of specimens. These factors are often more crucial for microbiologic specimens than for those designed to yield chemical data. Microbial agents grow and die, are susceptible to many chemicals, and can be found at different anatomic sites and in different body fluids and tissues during the natural history of most infectious disorders. In general, the successful isolation of an infectious agent carries much more diagnostic weight in the formulation of a diagnosis than failure to do so. Therefore, the specimen must be obtained from the site most likely to yield the infectious agent at that particular stage of illness and must be handled in such a way as to favor survival and growth of the agent. For each type of specimen, suggestions for optimal handling are given in the following paragraphs.

Recovery of an infectious agent is most significant if the agent is isolated from a site normally devoid of microorganisms. Any type of microorganism cultured from blood, cerebrospinal fluid, or joint fluid or from the pleural cavity is a significant diagnostic finding. Conversely, many parts of the body have a normal microbial flora which may be altered by endogenous or exogenous influences. The recovery of potentially pathogenic microorganisms from the respiratory, gastrointestinal, or genitourinary tracts, from wounds, or from the skin must be considered in the context of the normal flora of each particular site. The situation is often further complicated by the presence of mixtures of different microorganisms each of which may or may not participate in a disease process of that particular tissue. Correlation of bacteriologic information with medical experience is then required to arrive at meaningful interpretation of results.

A few general rules apply to all specimens:

(1) A sufficient quantity of specimen must be provided to permit thorough study.

(2) The sample should be representative of the infectious process (eg, sputum, not saliva; pus from the underlying lesion, not from its sinus tract; a swab from the depth of the wound, not from its surface).

(3) Care must be taken to avoid contamination of the specimen by using only sterile equipment and aseptic precautions.

(4) The specimen must be taken to the laboratory and examined promptly.

(5) Meaningful specimens must be secured before antimicrobial drugs are administered. If antimicrobial drugs are given before specimens are taken for microbiologic study, drug therapy may have to be stopped and repeat specimens obtained several days later.

The above comments apply particularly to specimens intended for the isolation of bacterial or fungal agents. The isolation of viruses, rickettsiae, or chlamydiae is usually performed only in specialized laboratories. Specimens are often shipped to such laboratories in well stoppered containers packed in dry ice. All specimens must be accurately labeled and accompanied by adequate instructions, a clearly worded statement of the information desired, and background information.

The type of specimen to be examined is determined by the presenting clinical picture. If symptoms or signs point to involvement of one organ system, specimens are obtained from that source. In the absence of localizing signs or symptoms, repeated blood samples for culturing are taken first. Specimens from other sites are then considered in sequence, depending in part upon the likelihood of involvement of a given organ system in a given patient and in part upon the ease of obtaining the specimen.

SELECTION OF LABORATORY INVESTIGATIONS

Diagnostic tests in infectious diseases fall into 4 classes:

(1) The demonstration of an infectious agent (bacterial, mycotic, viral, protozoal, or helminthic) in specimens obtained from the patient.

(2) The demonstration of a meaningful antibody response in the patient. This frequently involves proof of a rise in specific antibody titer, and therefore requires 2 serum specimens obtained at an interval of 10–20 days.

(3) The demonstration of meaningful skin reactivity, as evidence of hypersensitivity to antigens of a particular infectious agent.

(4) The demonstration of deviations in a variety of clinical laboratory determinations which nonspecifically suggest or support a suspicion of infectious diseases.

In the following paragraphs, some important applications of these principal classes of tests will be described.

THE DEMONSTRATION OF AN INFECTIOUS AGENT

Laboratory examinations usually include microscopic study of fresh unstained and stained materials and preparation of cultures under environmental conditions which are suitable for growth of a wide variety of microorganisms, including the type of organism most suspect on clinical grounds. If a microorganism is seen or isolated, the physician is notified of its preliminary identification. Complete identification may then be pursued by bacteriologic, mycologic, or other technics. Antimicrobial sensitivity tests are not undertaken if the isolated organism is one whose response to chemotherapy is completely predictable (eg, pneumococci, group A streptococci). Other microorganisms may be tested for susceptibility to antimicrobial drugs or combinations of drugs. In certain types of diseases, assay of antibacterial activity in the patient's serum during treatment may be more informative than drug susceptibility tests (see Chapter 10). In all cases where significant pathogenic microorganisms are isolated before treatment, follow-up examinations during and after treatment are mandatory.

Blood

In the febrile ill patient, with or without localizing signs or symptoms, blood culture is the most useful and most frequently performed test for the presence of systemic infection. Proof of bacteremia is also essential in all persons suspected of having bacterial endocarditis even when they do not appear acutely or severely ill. In addition to its diagnostic significance, recovery of an infectious agent from the blood provides invaluable aid in guiding antimicrobial therapy. Every effort should therefore be made to isolate the etiologic organism in bacteremia.

In healthy persons, properly obtained blood cultures remain sterile. Although microorganisms from the normal respiratory and gastrointestinal flora enter the blood occasionally, they are rapidly removed by the reticuloendothelial system. These transients rarely affect the interpretation of blood culture results. If a blood culture yields microorganisms, this fact is of great clinical significance provided that technical error can be excluded. Proper technic in performing the procedure is therefore all-important.

Tissues, tissue fluids, or reducing substances must be used in such a way that the bottom part of the blood culture bottle will provide sufficiently low oxygen tension to permit growth of anaerobes while the top part permits growth of aerobes. Culture media often contain penicillinase to inactivate penicillin and PABA to overcome the inhibitory effect of sulfonamides.

The following rules, rigidly applied, yield reliable results:

(1) Use only sterile equipment and strict aseptic technic.

(2) Apply a tourniquet and locate a fixed vein by touch to minimize probing after insertion of the needle.

(3) Prepare the skin by applying 2% tincture of iodine in widening circles, beginning with the site of proposed skin puncture. Remove iodine with 70% alcohol. Do not touch the skin with the fingers after it has been prepared.

(4) Perform venipuncture and withdraw 12–15 ml blood.

(5) Detach the needle from the syringe with aseptic precautions (since the needle may have become contaminated with bacteria lodging within the skin). Add 1–2 ml of blood to a sterile tube containing 1 ml of 1.8% sodium citrate and mix well. Add the remainder of the blood to a flask containing 50–100 ml of a rich nutrient medium, which will permit the growth of fastidious organisms.

(6) Take the specimens to the laboratory promptly.

At the laboratory, a measured quantity of citrated blood is added to melted agar and poured into plates for quantitative cultures. The plates and the blood culture bottles are incubated at 37° C for up to 3 weeks. They are examined for bacterial growth every 2–3 days by inspection, smears, and subcultures. Colonies appearing on the poured plates are counted to give the number of bacteria per ml of blood in the original specimen.

In general, there is no significant advantage in arterial over the usual venous blood specimens.

If microorganisms grow from blood cultures, it then becomes necessary to determine their significance by ruling out technical error. Although it is not possible to state conclusively that any given positive blood culture does not reflect bacteremia, the following criteria may be helpful in differentiating "true" positives from contaminated specimens:

(1) Growth of the same type of organism in repeated cultures: bacteremia.

(2) Growth of large numbers of a single type of organism in quantitative cultures: bacteremia.

(3) Small numbers of several different organisms: suggestive of contamination.

(4) Common skin flora (white staphylococci [*Staphylococcus epidermidis; S albus*], diphtheroids) occurring in only one of several cultures: suggestive of contamination. (The presence of such organisms in more than one culture, or in bone marrow culture in addition to blood culture, enhances the likelihood of bacteremia.)

(5) "Expected" organisms (eg, viridans streptococci or enterococci) in suspected endocarditis are more apt to be etiologically significant than organisms commonly found as contaminants.

The number of blood specimens for cultures that should be drawn, and over what period, depends upon the severity of the clinical illness. In hyperacute sepsis, only 2 or 3 blood cultures can be taken in as many hours before antimicrobial therapy, based on the clinician's "best guess" regarding etiology, is begun. On the other hand, with a chronically ill patient who has suspected endocarditis, one or 2 cultures may be taken daily for 4 or 5 days before drugs are administered. In patients who eventually yield positive blood cultures, growth is usually obtained in the first few cultures taken, although there may be much delay until growth becomes evident. About 90–95% of positive blood cultures in proved cases of bacterial endocarditis are encountered among the first 5 cultures taken. Consequently, it is reasonable to begin treatment after 5–6 specimens have been obtained.

Virtually every microorganism other than viruses, rickettsiae, and chlamydiae has been grown in blood culture at some time. The following are most commonly found: Viridans streptococci, *Streptococcus faecalis,* staphylococci (*S aureus* and others), gram-negative enteric bacteria, including *Escherichia coli, Aerobacter aerogenes, Klebsiella pneumoniae,* Proteus species, Pseudomonas species, pneumococci, meningococci, bacteroides, Salmonella species, Brucella species, Pasteurella species, *Hemophilus influenzae,* spirilla, Leptospira species, and Candida species.

In most types of bacteremia listed above, examination of direct blood smears contributes little. However, in some spirochetal infections (eg, leptospirosis, relapsing fever) and parasitic infections (eg, malaria, trypanosomiasis), the etiologic organism can be detected in stained blood films. In some infections (eg, rickettsioses, leptospirosis, spirillosis, psittacosis), inoculation of blood into experimental animals may give positive results more readily than culture.

Urine

At present, bacteriologic examination of the urine is done mainly when signs or symptoms point to urinary tract infection, renal insufficiency, or hypertension. It should always be done in persons with suspected systemic infection or fever of unknown origin. It may some day become part of the routine periodic health examination.

Urine secreted in the kidney is sterile unless the kidney is infected. Uncontaminated bladder urine is also normally sterile. The urethra, however, contains a normal microbial flora which contaminates urine in passage, so that voided urine may contain small numbers of bacteria in the absence of urinary tract infection. Because it is necessary to distinguish contaminating from etiologically important organisms, only *quantitative* urine examination can yield meaningful results.

The following steps are essential in proper urine examination:

A. Proper Collection of Specimen: Because of the danger of introducing microorganisms into the bladder, catheterization is to be avoided whenever possible. Satisfactory specimens from males can usually be obtained by cleansing the meatus with soap and water and collecting midstream urine in a sterile container. Satisfactory midstream specimens from females can sometimes be obtained after cleansing the vulva and spreading the labia, but catheterization is sometimes unavoidable. Separate specimens from the right and left kidneys and ureters can be obtained by the urologist at cystoscopy using a catheter.

For most types of examinations, 0.5 ml of ureteral urine or 5 ml of voided urine is sufficient. Urine specimens must be delivered to the laboratory and examined within 1 hour, or refrigerated not longer than overnight. At room or body temperature, many types of microorganisms multiply rapidly in urine. To resolve diagnostic problems, urine can be aspirated directly from the bladder through suprapubic puncture of the abdominal wall.

B. Microscopic Examination: A great deal can be learned from the simple microscopic examination of urine. A drop of fresh uncentrifuged urine placed on a slide, covered with a coverglass, and examined with restricted light intensity under the high-dry objective of an ordinary clinical microscope reveals not only leukocytes and epithelial cells, but also bacteria if more than $10^4 - 10^5$ organisms per ml are present. This procedure informs the physician promptly that significant numbers of organisms are present and also indicates whether cocci (often *Streptococcus faecalis*) or motile rods (often gram-negative coliform organisms) are causing the infection. Similar semi-quantitative observations can be made with dried smears of urine stained with methylene blue or Gram's stain.

Bacteria are not sedimented by short (3–5 minutes) centrifugation at the usual speeds of the clinical centrifuge. However, brief centrifugation does readily sediment pus cells which may carry along bacteria and thus may help in rapid microscopic diagnosis of infection. The presence of other formed elements in the sediment—or the presence of proteinuria—is of little direct aid in the specific identification of active

urinary tract infection. Pus cells may be present without bacteria, and, conversely, bacteriuria may be present without pyuria.

C. Urine Cultures: As explained above, culture of the urine, to be meaningful, must be performed quantitatively. Properly collected urine is cultured in measured amounts on solid media, and the number of colonies appearing after incubation is counted to indicate the number of bacteria per ml. The usual procedure is to spread 0.1 ml of undiluted urine, 0.1 ml of 1:100 dilution, and 0.1 ml of 1:10,000 dilution on blood agar plates or to incorporate these amounts into agar pour plates for quantitative culture. If desired, a loopful of urine can be inoculated into thioglycollate medium (for anaerobes) and onto another blood agar plate for direct disk sensitivity tests. All media are incubated overnight at 37° C; colonies are then counted and the number of bacteria per ml of urine is estimated.

In active pyelonephritis, the number of bacteria in urine collected by ureteral catheter is relatively low. While accumulating in the bladder, bacteria multiply rapidly and soon reach numbers in excess of 10^5/ml, far more than could occur as a result of contamination by urethral or skin flora or from the air. Therefore, it is generally agreed that if more than 100,000 organisms per ml are cultivated from a properly collected and properly examined urine specimen, this constitutes strong evidence of active urinary tract infection. If fewer bacteria are cultivated, repeated examination of urine is indicated to establish the presence of infection.

If fewer than 1000–10,000 colonies per ml are present (especially if, as is often the case, there are several types), this suggests that the organisms come from normal flora or are contaminants. Intermediate counts (eg, 5000–50,000 colonies per ml) do not permit definitive interpretation from a single specimen and must be repeated with a fresh specimen. Such counts obtained repeatedly suggest persistent, chronic, or suppressed infection. If found only in a single specimen, they suggest contamination. If cultures are negative but clinical signs of urinary tract infection are present, tuberculosis, anaerobic infection, or ureteral obstruction must be considered.

Bacteria most commonly found in urinary tract infections are coliforms, other gram-negative rods, and enterococci.

Cerebrospinal Fluid (CSF)

The early, rapid, and precise diagnosis of meningitis ranks high among the medical emergencies. It depends upon maintaining a high index of suspicion; securing adequate specimens properly; and examining the specimens promptly. Because the risk of death or irreversible tissue damage is great unless treatment is started immediately, there is rarely a second chance to obtain pretreatment specimens—which are essential for specific etiologic diagnosis and optimal management.

The most urgent diagnostic issue is the differentiation of acute purulent bacterial meningitis from nonbacterial meningitis. The immediate decision is usually based on the results of cell count and glucose content of CSF, and of microscopic search for microorganisms. It is subsequently modified by the results of culture, CSF protein content, serologic tests, and other laboratory procedures. The table illustrates some typical findings. In evaluating the results of CSF glucose determinations, the simultaneous blood glucose level must be considered. In some CNS neoplasms the CSF glucose is low.

A. Specimens: As soon as infection of the CNS is suspected, blood cultures are taken and CSF is secured. Lumbar puncture is performed with strict aseptic technic, taking care not to risk compression of the medulla by too rapid withdrawal of fluid when the intracranial pressure is markedly elevated. CSF is usually collected in 3 or 4 portions (2–5 ml each) in sterile tubes. This permits the most convenient and most reliable examination for the several different values which determine the physician's course of action.

B. Microscopic Examination: Smears are made from fresh uncentrifuged CSF which appears cloudy; otherwise from the sediment of centrifuged CSF. Smears are stained with Gram's stain and occasionally with Ziehl-Neelsen stain. Ziehl-Neelsen stain is particularly indicated if a pellicle forms on the surface of the fluid, trapping acid-fast organisms. Study of stained smears under the oil immersion objective may reveal intracellular gram-negative diplococci (meningococci), intra- and extracellular lancet-shaped gram-positive

diplococci (pneumococci), or small gram-negative rods (*Hemophilus influenzae* or coliform organisms). In *H influenzae* meningitis, layering of CSF on specific type b antiserum may yield a precipitate at the interface, providing an etiologic diagnosis promptly even when no organisms are seen. Cryptococci are organisms best seen in India ink preparations. Common bacterial causes of meningitis can be rapidly identified by specific immunofluorescence. Initial treatment is usually aimed at the type of organism seen microscopically.

C. Culture: The culture methods used must be those which will favor the growth of microorganisms most commonly encountered in meningitis. Virus isolation can be attempted in aseptic meningitis or meningoencephalitis. It is often successful in infections caused by herpes simplex, mumps, and echo- or coxsackieviruses, but not usually so in the arthropod-borne encephalitides.

D. Follow-Up Examination of CSF: The return of CSF glucose to normal levels is the most reliable evidence of adequate initial therapy.

Respiratory Secretions

Symptoms or signs often point to involvement of a particular part of the respiratory tract, and specimens are chosen accordingly. In interpreting the laboratory results it is necessary to consider the normal microbial flora of the area from which the specimen was collected.

TABLE 24–1. Cerebrospinal fluid findings.

Diagnosis	Some Etiologic Microorganisms	Cells/ cu mm	Protein (mg/100 ml)	Glucose (mg/100 ml)	Remarks
Normal	. . .	0–5 lymphocytes	10–45	50–85	. . .
Acute purulent meningitis (bacterial)	Meningococci, pneumococci, *Hemophilus influenzae,* streptococci, staphylococci, coliform organisms, etc.	500–20,000 or more PMN's	Increased: 50–1000 or more	Low: 0–45	Organisms found in smear or culture
Viral meningo-encephalitis	Viruses of mumps, herpes simplex, lymphocytic choriomeningitis, poliomyelitis, coxsackievirus, echovirus, etc.	0–2000 or more, mostly lymphocytes	Normal or increased	Normal	Virus isolation or titer rise in paired serum specimen
Tuberculous or fungal meningitis	*Mycobacterium tuberculosis,* cryptococcus, coccidioides, histoplasma, etc.	10–1000 or more, mostly lymphocytes	Increased: 45–500 or more	Low: 0–45	Organisms found in smear or culture
Syphilitic or leptospiral meningitis	*Treponema pallidum,* Leptospira species.	25–2000 or more, mostly lymphocytes	Increased: 45–400 or more	15–75	Serologic tests positive
"Neighborhood reaction" to brain from extradural abscess, thrombosis, or intrathecal drug administration	. . .	Increased	Normal or increased	Normal	Cultures negative

A. Specimens:

1. Throat—Most "sore throats" are due to viral infection. Only 5–10% of such complaints in adults and 15–20% in children are associated with bacterial infections. The finding of a follicular yellowish exudate or a grayish membrane must arouse the suspicion of hemolytic streptococcal, diphtherial, fusospirochetal (Vincent's), or candidal infection; but such a membrane may also be present in infectious mononucleosis, adenovirus, and other virus infections.

Throat swabs must be taken from each tonsillar area before a swab is taken from the posterior pharyngeal wall. The normal throat flora includes an abundance of viridans streptococci, neisseriae, diphtheroids, staphylococci, small gram-negative rods, and many other organisms. Microscopic examination of smears from throat swabs is of no value in streptococcal infections because all throats harbor a predominance of streptococci, but it can rapidly identify fusospirochetal disease and may suggest diphtheria. By immunofluorescence, group A streptococci can sometimes be identified rapidly as the predominant organism.

Cultures of throat swabs are most reliable if inoculated promptly after collection, although special swabs are available which permit survival of important pathogens for several hours. When streaking culture plates (blood agar is used), it is essential to spread a small inoculum thoroughly and avoid overgrowth by normal flora. This can be done readily by touching the throat swab to one small area of the plate and using a second sterile applicator (or sterile bacteriologic loop) to streak the plate from that area. Incubation at 37° C must often be continued for 48 hours until hemolytic colonies can be clearly identified.

Reports on throat cultures should state the types of prevalent organisms. If potential pathogens (eg, beta-hemolytic streptococci) are cultured, their approximate number is important. A few colonies of beta-hemolytic streptococci may well represent only "transients" in the throat without pathogenic meaning. In "strep throat," the group A streptococci prevail. On a blood plate bearing massive growth, the "bacitracin disk" method most easily establishes the group A nature of the organisms. (See Levison & Frank reference at end of chapter.)

2. Nasopharynx—Specimens from the nasopharynx are studied infrequently because they must be obtained by special technics. (See Viral Diagnosis, below.)

3. Middle ear—Specimens are rarely obtained because puncture of the drum is necessary. In acute otitis media, 30–50% of aspirated fluids are bacteriologically sterile. The most frequently isolated bacteria are pneumococci, *Hemophilus influenzae,* and hemolytic streptococci.

4. Sputum—Bronchial and pulmonary secretions or exudates are usually studied by examining sputum. The most misleading aspect of sputum examination is the almost inevitable contamination with throat and saliva by flora. Thus, finding candida or *Staphylococ-cus aureus* in the sputum of a patient with pneumonitis has no etiologic significance unless supported by the clinical picture. Meaningful sputum specimens should be expectorated in the physician's presence from the lower respiratory tract and should be grossly distinct from saliva. The presence of many squamous epithelial cells suggests heavy contamination with saliva. Specimens can sometimes be obtained by catheter aspiration or bronchoscopy. In pneumonia accompanied by pleural fluid, examination of the latter may yield the etiologic organisms more reliably than sputum. Most bacterial pneumonias are caused by pneumococci. In suspected tuberculosis or fungal infection, gastric washings (swallowed sputum) may yield organisms when expectorated material fails to do so. Semiquantitative cultures are helpful.

5. Transtracheal aspiration—The flora in such specimens often reflects accurately the events in the lower respiratory tract.

B. Microscopic Examination: Smears of purulent flecks or granules from sputum stained by Gram's stain or by acid-fast methods may reveal etiologic organisms. Some mycotic organisms (eg, actinomyces) are best seen in unstained wet preparations.

C. Cultures: The media used must be suitable for the growth of bacteria (eg, pneumococci, klebsiella), fungi (eg, *Coccidioides immitis*), anaerobes (eg, bacteroides), mycobacteria (eg, *Mycobacterium tuberculosis*), mycoplasma (Eaton agent), and others. The relative prevalence of different organisms in the specimen must be estimated. Only a finding of one predominant organism or the simultaneous isolation of an organism from both sputum and blood can clearly establish its role in a pneumonic or suppurative process.

D. Viral Diagnosis: Most respiratory tract infections are caused by viruses. Throat swabs, throat washings, and sputum are fertile sources of virus if specialized laboratory facilities for virus isolation are available. Throat swabs immersed in broth, garglings with broth, or sputum must be brought to the virus laboratory promptly or kept frozen until they are inoculated into embryonated eggs, tissue cultures, or animals. To support the possible etiologic role of viral agents, a rise in specific antibody titer must be demonstrated. Serum specimens are obtained aseptically as early as possible in the disease and again 2–3 weeks later. The first serum specimen is stored in the refrigerator until the second specimen has been secured. Both serum samples are then submitted to the virus laboratory—with an adequate clinical description—for specific serologic diagnosis.

Gastrointestinal Tract Specimens

Acute symptoms referable to the gastrointestinal tract—particularly nausea, vomiting, and diarrhea—are commonly attributed to infection. In reality most such attacks are caused by food intolerance, intoxication, neurogenic impulses, or systemic illnesses. This is an important consideration if one is to avoid the error of administering antimicrobial drugs to everyone who has acute gastrointestinal symptoms. The objectives of management in such patients should be to restore water and electrolyte balance, restrict oral intake, and establish an etiologic diagnosis. The diagnosis must often be based on individual and community history.

Most cases of acute infectious diarrheas are due to viruses. On the other hand, many viruses (eg, adenoviruses, enteroviruses) can multiply in the gut without causing gastrointestinal symptoms. Similarly, some enteric bacterial pathogens may establish persistent residence in the gut following an acute infection. Thus, it is often difficult to assign significance to a microbial or viral agent cultured from the stool, especially in subacute or chronic illness.

These considerations should not discourage the physician from attempting laboratory isolation of enteric organisms, but should warn him of some common difficulties in interpreting the results.

The lower bowel has an exceedingly high normal bacterial flora. The most prevalent organisms are anaerobes (bacteroides, clostridia, and streptococci), coliform gram-negative rods, and *Streptococcus faecalis.* Any attempt to recover pathogenic bacteria from feces involves their separation from the normal flora, usually through the use of differential selective media and enrichment cultures. The most prominent bacterial pathogens are salmonellae, shigellae, enteropathogenic *Escherchia coli* of certain serotypes (O55, O111, O127, etc), and paracolon bacteria (see Chapter 18).

A. Specimens: Feces and rectal swabs are the most readily available specimens. Bile obtained by duodenal drainage may reveal infection of the biliary tract. The presence of blood, mucus, or helminths must be noted on gross inspection of the specimen. Special technics must be used in searching for ova and parasites. Stained smears may reveal a prevalence of certain abnormal organisms, eg, candida or staphylococci, but cannot differentiate enteric bacterial pathogens from normal flora.

B. Culture: Specimens are suspended in broth and cultured on ordinary as well as selective differential media (eg, SS agar, EMB agar) to permit separation of nonlactose-fermenting organisms from coliform bacteria. If salmonella infection (typhoid fever or paratyphoid fever) is suspected, the specimen is also placed in an enrichment medium (eg, selenite F broth) for 18 hours before plating. Identification of bacterial colonies proceeds by standard bacteriologic examination, and blood is drawn for serologic diagnosis. The agglutination of bacteria from suspected colonies by pooled specific antiserum is often the fastest way to establish the presence of salmonellae or shigellae in the intestinal tract. Elevation of the specific serum antibody titer often supports the diagnosis of salmonella infection.

Gastric washings represent swallowed sputum and may be cultured for tubercle bacilli and other mycobacteria on special media (eg, Dubos' medium). For virus isolation, frozen fecal specimens are submitted to special laboratories, accompanied by paired serum specimens.

Intestinal parasites and their ova are discovered by repeated microscopic study of fresh fecal specimens subjected to specialized handling in the laboratory. (See Appendix.)

Puncture Fluids

Exudates which have collected in the pleural, peritoneal, or synovial spaces must be aspirated with the most meticulous aseptic technic to avoid superinfection. If the material is frankly purulent, smears and cultures are made directly. If the fluid is clear, it should be centrifuged at high speed for 10 minutes and the sediment used for stained smears and cultures. The culture method used must be suitable for the growth of organisms suspected on clinical grounds—eg, Dubos' medium for mycobacteria, thioglycollate medium for anaerobic organisms, cooked blood agar in 10% CO_2 atmosphere for gonococci—as well as the commonly encountered pyogenic bacteria.

Although direct tests for etiologic microorganisms yield the most important answers, indirect supportive evidence of infection is also helpful. These include tests on oxalated puncture fluids. The following results are suggestive of infection: specific gravity over 1.018; protein content over 3 gm/100 ml, often resulting in clotting; and cell counts over 500–1000/cu mm. Polymorphonuclear leukocytes predominate in acute pyogenic infections; lymphocytes or monocytes predominate in chronic infections. Transudates resulting from neoplastic growth may grossly resemble infectious exudates in appearing bloody or purulent and in clotting on standing. Cytologic study of smears or of sections of centrifuged cells may prove the neoplastic nature of the process.

Genital Lesions

Prominent among the infections associated with local lesions of the external genitalia, discharge, and regional adenopathy are syphilis, gonorrhea, chancroid, lymphogranuloma venereum, granuloma inguinale, and herpes simplex. Each has a characteristic natural history and evolution of lesions, but one can mimic another. The laboratory diagnosis of most of these infections is covered elsewhere in the text. A few diagnostic tests are listed below.

A. Gonorrhea: Urethral or cervical exudate shows intracellular gram-negative diplococci in stained smear. Culture of freshly collected pus yields *Neisseria gonorrhoeae.* Serologic tests are not helpful.

B. Syphilis: Darkfield or immunofluorescence examination of tissue fluid expressed from the base of the chancre may reveal typical *Treponema pallidum.* Serologic tests for syphilis (STS) become positive 3–6 weeks after infection. A positive immunofluorescence treponemal antibody (FTA-ABS) test (see Chapter 29) proves syphilitic infection.

C. Chancroid: Smears and cultures from a suppurating ulcer usually show a mixed bacterial flora, including gram-negative rods in chains. Serologic tests are rarely done. The Ducrey skin test (*Hemophilus ducreyi* suspension) usually is positive within 3–5 weeks after infection. A positive skin test, however, cannot distinguish between old and recent infection.

D. Lymphogranuloma Venereum (LGV): While it is possible to grow the etiologic agent (a member of the psittacosis-LGV-trachoma group; see Chapter 26) by inoculating pus from suppurating lymph nodes into embryonated eggs, the procedure is difficult and infrequently tried. Serologic tests (usually complement fixation) can demonstrate a diagnostic rise in antibody titer of paired sera obtained 2 weeks apart. The Frei test is often employed to support the clinical diagnosis. This skin test employs as antigen (Lygranum) a suspension of egg-grown agent with proper controls. The delayed type of skin reaction may become positive within 2–3 weeks after infection and remain positive for life, but recently the test has been negative in a significant proportion of proved LGV infections. The skin test indicates reactivity to a group-specific antigen which is shared by all members of the group. Thus, past infection with psittacosis or trachoma may give rise to a positive Frei test as readily as past infection with lymphogranuloma venereum.

E. Granuloma Inguinale: The etiologic agent of this hard granulomatous proliferating lesion (*Calymmatobacterium [Donovania] granulomatis*) can be grown in complex bacteriologic media, but this is rarely attempted in practice. Histologic demonstration of intracellular "Donovan bodies" in biopsied material most frequently supports the clinical impression. Serologic tests are not helpful.

F. Herpes Progenitalis: Recurrent herpetic vesicles, evolving to ulcers and crusts and resembling the common "cold sores" on lips or skin, may occur on the genitalia. They may be mistaken for venereal lesions. A positive diagnosis depends upon finding typical multinucleated giant cells or positive immunofluorescence in scrapings from the ulcer base, or isolation and identification or herpes simplex virus from the aspirated contents of the vesicle. Specific antibodies are present (but do not rise), and the specific skin test is positive.

G. *Trichomonas Vaginalis* Vaginitis or Urethritis: Typical organisms can be seen or cultured from genital discharges.

H. Inclusion Conjunctivitis: This infection usually manifests itself as an acute conjunctivitis of the newborn, or as a venereal disease and eye infection of adults. Immunofluorescence or Giemsa-stained smears of scrapings from the eye, the cervix, or the male urethra may reveal typical crescent-shaped inclusion bodies in epithelial cells (see Chapter 26).

I. Abacterial Urethritis: From some cases of nongonococcal urethritis, T strain mycoplasmas can be grown on special media.

Wounds, Tissue Biopsies, Bone & Joint Infections, Abscesses

Microscopic study of smears and cultures of specimens from wounds or abscesses may often give early and important indications of the nature of the infecting organism and thus help in the choice of antimicrobial drugs. Specimens from diagnostic tissue biopsies should be submitted to bacteriologic as well as histologic examination. They are kept away from fixatives and disinfectants, minced and finely ground, and cultured by a variety of methods.

In closed undrained abscesses, the pus frequently contains only one organism as etiologic agent—most commonly staphylococci, streptococci, or coliforms. The same is true in acute osteomyelitis, where the organisms can often be cultured from the blood before the local lesion has become chronic. However, in open wounds, a multitude of microorganisms is frequently encountered, which makes it difficult to decide which are significant. When deep suppurating lesions drain onto exterior surfaces through a sinus or fistula, the flora of the surface drainage must not be mistaken for that of the deep lesion.

Only with reservations can organisms obtained from sinus tracts be used to guide therapy. Bacteriologic study of pus from closed or deep lesions must always include anaerobic methods. Anaerobic bacteria sometimes play an essential etiologic role, whereas aerobes may represent surface contaminants. The typical wound infections due to clostridia are readily suspected in gas gangrene. Pseudomonas in wounds gives rise to blue-green pus.

The methods employed must be suitable for the semiquantitative recovery of common bacteria and also for specialized microorganisms such as anaerobes, mycobacteria (eg, *Mycobacterium tuberculosis*), and fungi. Eroded skin and mucous membranes are frequently the sites of yeast or fungus infection. Candida, aspergillus, and others can be seen microscopically in smears or scrapings from suspicious areas and can be grown in cultures.

Viral antigens can sometimes be demonstrated directly in specimens from surface lesions by the fluorescent antibody method.

SEROLOGIC TESTS & THE DEMONSTRATION OF SPECIFIC ANTIBODY

In the course of many infections, serum antibodies are acquired relatively early, as microorganisms multiply, and these antibodies may persist for months or years. Thus, the serologic demonstration of antibody indicates effective exposure (by infection or vaccination) at some time in the past but may have no bearing on the current illness. For the diagnosis of a current infection it is often necessary to demonstrate an increase in antibody concentration, ie, a rise of antibody level in the second of 2 blood specimens obtained at an interval of 10–20 days. The 2 specimens of sera must be examined simultaneously in the same test for meaningful results. Blood specimens must be taken aseptically and the serum separated with sterile precautions.

Diagnostic antibody titers are sometimes obtained in the following infections:

Blastomycosis

Complement fixing antibodies appear principally in disseminated and progressive disease.

Brucellosis

During the acute infection, agglutinating antibodies appear; later, blocking and precipitating antibodies. Agglutinating antibodies persist for years in low titer without manifest activity of the disease, whereas precipitating antibodies disappear soon after the infection has subsided. Thus, the diagnosis of active chronic brucellosis may be suggested by the presence of precipitating antibodies or of high titer (over 1:160) agglutinating antibodies. Complement fixation tests are rarely employed.

Coccidioidomycosis

Soon after the initial infection, precipitating and complement fixing antibodies to *Coccidioides immitis* appear. In the absence of complications, these tend to subside to very low levels within months. Dissemination of the infection is accompanied by a rising titer of complement fixing antibodies (more than 1:32), which carries a grave prognosis.

Mycoplasmal (Eaton Agent) Pneumonia (Primary Atypical Pneumonia)

In some cases of pneumonitis not caused by common bacteria, cold agglutinins develop in the serum during the illness. These are substances which are capable of agglutinating human group O cells at 4° C but not at 20° or 37° C. Patients who develop cold agglutinins are usually infected with *Mycoplasma pneumoniae*. Antibodies to *M pneumoniae* can be detected by complement fixation, growth inhibition, or hemagglutination inhibition.

Histoplasmosis

Precipitating and complement fixing antibodies to antigens of *Histoplasma capsulatum* appear usually within 3–4 weeks of acute infection and, in the absence of complications, revert to negative after some months. If chronic lesions persist, complement fixation tests may remain positive (1:8 or higher) for years. If the infection disseminates and progresses, the complement fixation titer rises (more than 1:32). Thus, a complement fixation titer some time after the acute infection has serious prognostic as well as diagnostic implications.

Infectious Mononucleosis

It is probable, but has not been proved, that this disease is caused by a specific virus. Diagnosis of the clinically suggestive case rests on the identification of representative "atypical" lymphocytes in blood smears and on the "heterophil agglutination" test of Paul and Bunnel. This is a nonspecific reaction based on the accidental finding that persons suffering from infectious mononucleosis develop a high titer (usually more than 1:112) of antibodies which agglutinate fresh washed sheep cells. Similar agglutinating antibodies appear in a variety of hypersensitivity reactions but can be differentiated by absorption tests. The mononucleosis agglutinins cannot be absorbed by boiled guinea pig kidney, whereas agglutinins following other reactions are removed by this absorption.

In special laboratories, antibodies to EB (Epstein-Barr) virus can be demonstrated in sera of mononucleosis patients by several methods. (See Chapter 38.)

Leptospirosis

Agglutination, agglutination-lysis, and, occasionally, complement fixation tests give very high titers (often over 1:1000) following infection.

Parasitic Diseases

In cysticercosis, trichinosis, echinococcosis, and other parasitic infections, complement fixation, precipitin, or hemagglutination tests are occasionally employed for diagnosis.

Pasteurellosis (Plague, Tularemia)

Agglutination titers of 1:20 or higher, particularly with rising titers, can support the clinical diagnosis of acute infection. Low titers suggest cross-reactions (eg, with brucella or shigella organisms) or long-past infection. Complement fixation and precipitin tests are performed rarely.

Psittacosis, Ornithosis, Lymphogranuloma Venereum, Trachoma

Antibodies to the group antigen often become demonstrable by complement fixation tests within 2–4 weeks after symptoms appear. These antibodies cannot differentiate one infection of the group from another. The titer is usually low, rarely more than 1:16.

Rheumatoid Factor

In many disorders of possible "autoimmune" etiology, antibodies to the host's own antigens are encountered. Antithyroid antibodies are demonstrated in several thyroid disorders; antibodies which fix complement in the presence of nucleoproteins are found in disseminated lupus erythematosus. In rheumatoid arthritis, a macroglobulin (19 S, "rheumatoid factor") is present which resembles an antibody by reacting with human 7 S globulin. This can be demonstrated as a precipitin reaction or, more commonly, an agglutination of red cells or other particles coated with 7 S globulins by diluted sera from rheumatoid patients. It is of interest that more than half of individuals with bacterial endocarditis exhibit a very high titer of such "rheumatoid factor." These substances disappear when bacteriologic cure of endocarditis is established.

Rickettsioses

Complement fixation tests permit the demonstration of type-specific antibody rise; however, specific antigens often are not available. Various special strains of proteus organisms share antigens with the rickettsiae, and suspensions of these proteus organisms are agglutinated in high titer by the serum of infected persons (Weil-Felix test).

See Chapter 25 for further details about the diagnosis of viral infections.

Salmonellosis (Typhoid Fever, Paratyphoid Fever, Etc)

A rising agglutination titer to O antigens is particularly suggestive of active infection, whereas a rising titer to H antigens occurs commonly with vaccination and may persist for years. In carriers, antibody to Vi antigen may be more prominent than that to O or H. In previously vaccinated individuals with residual O or H titers, there may be no further titer rise with active infection.

Staphylococcal Infections

Persons with deep active suppurating staphylococcal infections frequently develop antibodies against a variety of staphylococcal antigens and extracellular products. In view of the ubiquity of many staphylococci, most such antibodies have little diagnostic meaning. However, a rise in antibody titer to staphylococcal leukocidin and staphylococcal alpha-hemolysin may indicate activity of a deep chronic lesion.

Streptococcal Infections & Poststreptococcal Disease

Persons infected with beta-hemolytic streptococci develop antibodies to a variety of streptococcal antigens and extracellular products. Most conveniently, antibodies to streptolysin O can be detected. If antistreptolysin O (ASO) is repeatedly found to be present in titers exceeding 125 units, this suggests recent or persistent infection with beta-hemolytic streptococci. Antistreptolysin formation is readily suppressed by early and adequate penicillin therapy. Type-specific bactericidal antibody may also be measured.

Syphilis

Most serologic tests for syphilis (STS) are based on the accidental relationship between lipid extracts of mammalian tissue and reagin, a substance developing in the serum of persons after treponemal infection. Flocculation tests (VDRL, Kahn, Kline, Hinton, Mazzini, etc) are simpler and more commonly employed than complement fixation tests (Kolmer, Wassermann). All of these tests estimate the presence of reagin, not specific antibody, and are therefore subject to biologic false-positive results. The latter are particularly frequent in various infectious and febrile disorders, in "collagen diseases," and after vaccinations. STS can be performed in a quantitative manner if desired. Most biologic false-positive results are of low titer.

The *Treponema pallidum* immobilization (TPI) test and the fluorescent treponemal antibody (FTA-ABS) test measure specific antibodies to the etiologic agent. The latter is cheaper to perform because it requires no living spirochetes. Positive TPI and FTA-ABS reactions occur only in syphilis or infections with closely related treponemes (yaws, bejel, pinta). Positive FTA-ABS reactions persist long after adequate therapy for syphilis whereas STS often revert to negative.

Toxoplasmosis

Toxoplasma gondii, a crescent-shaped protozoon, can be isolated with difficulty by inoculating lymph node material taken from patients with acute infection into mice. Three serologic tests can be applied. The dye test depends upon the ability of antibodies to prevent the uptake of methylene blue by living toxoplasma organisms. The test results become positive (frequently more than 1:1000) in 2–4 weeks after acquired toxoplasmosis, and may remain positive for years. In congenital toxoplasmosis, the dye test is often positive. The complement fixation test becomes positive (up to 1:100) in 4–8 weeks and declines to very low levels in a few months. Immunofluorescence antibody tests in low titer indicate only past infection, but high titers (1:10,000 or more) suggest recent infection. Positive tests in single samples of serum have little meaning because of the high frequency of asymptomatic infection.

Viral Infections

The diagnosis of viral infections is discussed in detail in Chapters 28 and 29.

SKIN TESTS

Under the antigenic stimulus of an infectious agent, the host may develop hypersensitivity, manifested by skin reactivity, to one or more antigens of that agent. The controlled application of known antigens can therefore give evidence of infection and serve as a valuable diagnostic aid. A positive skin reaction indicates only that the individual has, at some time in the past, been infected with the specific agent. It provides information about the relationship of a specific agent to a *current* illness only if conversion from a negative to a positive skin test occurs during or just preceding the current illness. The general skin reactivity declines markedly (anergy) during far-advanced stages of many infections and is a regular feature of sarcoidosis, Hodgkin's disease, and some childhood exanthematous diseases (eg, measles). Similarly, skin reactivity may be suppressed by the administration of large amounts of corticosteroids or corticotropin (ACTH).

Most skin test reagents are not pure antigens but a complex mixture of potentially reactive substances. For proper interpretation, it is essential to include suitable control materials in the test. Both immediate and delayed skin reactions may occur with some skin test preparations. In general, the delayed reaction is the only meaningful one for the diagnosis of specific infection.

In a properly performed test the entire test volume (usually 0.1 ml) of the standardized preparation must be injected intracutaneously. Unless the injection raises a well-circumscribed bleb, it is likely that part of the test volume has escaped into the subcutaneous tissue or onto the surface. This will diminish the reliability of the test. (Patch tests are occasionally used in small children, but they are not reliable.) In most instances the test should be read at 48 hours; additional readings at 24 and 72 hours are sometimes helpful.

The size of induration is the only important criterion of positive readings; erythema alone is not meaningful. When several strengths of test preparation are available, the smallest concentration of antigen must be injected initially, followed by increasingly higher concentrations if the previous test result was negative.

Diagnostic skin tests are frequently applied in the following clinical conditions.

Blastomycosis

Blastomycin is a filtered, concentrated broth in which *Blastomyces dermatitidis* has been grown for long periods. A test dilution of 1:100 gives 5 mm induration in persons with past infection. Interpretation is analogous to interpretation of the histoplasmin test (see below).

Brucellosis

Filtrates of old broth cultures of brucella (brucellin) or a brucella nucleoprotein extract (brucellergen) have been used for skin testing. Such preparations cannot be well standardized, and proper controls are not available. Therefore, the usefulness of the skin test is doubtful. Serologic tests are much to be preferred for diagnosis.

Candida

Candida antigens are used in skin tests to ascertain the individual's ability to respond with a delayed type hypersensitivity reaction. Virtually all normal adults react positively.

Cat Scratch Fever

Pus from active cases, diluted 1:5 and heated at 60° C for 10 hours, can be used as a skin test antigen. It gives a positive reaction in some individuals with a typical clinical picture. The nature of the etiologic agent and the significance of the test are not known.

Chancroid

A positive Ducrey test, a delayed skin reaction following the injection of a treated suspension of *Hemophilus ducreyi*, indicates past infection. A positive reaction may persist for years.

Coccidioidomycosis

Coccidioidin is a filtered, concentrated broth in which *Coccidioides immitis* has been grown for long periods. The usual test dilution is 1:100, and a positive reaction (more than 5 mm induration) occurs in 24–48 hours. In 1:10 dilution the material often gives cross-reactions with other fungal antigens. Positive skin tests commonly denote past subclinical infection and significant specific immunity to reinfection.

Echinococcosis

The injection of inactivated hydatid fluid (Casoni reaction) obtained from human or animal cases may give both immediate and delayed reactions in individuals with echinococcus infection.

Herpes Simplex

Injection of a soluble antigen obtained from growing virus gives a positive result in 18–24 hours in individuals who have had a primary infection with the virus and who are therefore usually not susceptible to systemic spread (encephalitis) but may develop local recurrences.

Histoplasmosis

Histoplasmin is a concentrated filtrate prepared from broth in which *Histoplasma capsulatum* has been grown for long periods. The usual test dilution is 1:100 and a positive reaction (more than 5 mm induration) occurs in 24–48 hours. Cross-reactions with other fungal products occurs relatively frequently. Positive skin tests commonly denote past subclinical infection and significant specific resistance to reinfection.

Lymphogranuloma Venereum

The Frei test antigen (Lygranum) is a chlamydial suspension prepared from infected chick embryo yolk sacs. A control injection with uninfected yolk sac material must be used as a control. A positive reaction consists of induration and erythema 8–20 mm in diameter, with a negative response at the control site. A positive Frei test may occur following infection with any member of the psittacosis-LGV-trachoma group at any time in the past.

Mumps

Intradermal injection of inactivated mumps vaccine gives a delayed positive skin test reaction in 18–36 hours provided the individual has had a past infection. The test has limited value in permitting identification of susceptibles (negative test) for epidemiologic control of virus spread.

Toxplasmosis

Toxoplasmin is prepared from a suspension of killed *Toxoplasma gondii* and evokes a delayed reaction in some individuals who also give positive serologic tests. Positive reactors are presumed to have been infected at some time in the past. The test has little diagnostic value, but has been employed in epidemiologic surveys.

Trichinosis

Antigens derived from trichinae (trichinella skin test) may give both immediate and delayed reactions in infected individuals, but most commercial antigens are too insensitive.

Tuberculosis

The tuberculin skin test can be performed with a concentrated filtrate of broth in which tubercle bacilli have been grown (old tuberculin, OT). However, the purified protein derivative (PPD) obtained by chemical fractionation of OT can be standardized accurately in terms of tuberculin units (TU) as well as weight and is almost universally preferred (see Chapter 17).

The initial test dose is usually 5 TU (intermediate strength PPD). Larger doses are injected when smaller doses have given negative results. The test is considered positive if induration 10 mm in diameter or more occurs in 48–72 hours following injection of 5 TU. In hypersensitive persons with erythema nodosum or phlyctenular conjunctivitis, not more than 1 TU should be injected to avoid serious general or local reactions.

PPD prepared from other mycobacteria are used in epidemiologic surveys. Many of them cross-react.

•   •   •

Toxin-Neutralization Tests

A. Schick Test: Although it is not designed for the diagnosis of infection, the Schick test is a valuable aid in the determination of probable susceptibility or resistance to diphtheria. The test consists of the intradermal injection of a standard skin test dose of active diphtheria toxin and of an identical amount of heated toxin as control. The test is usually read in 24 and 48 hours. A positive reaction consists of redness and swelling at the active toxin site which increases for 48 hours and then fades, leaving a brownish pigmented area. The control site shows no reaction. A positive reaction denotes the absence of an adequate amount of neutralizing circulating antitoxin and therefore susceptibility to diphtheria toxin. A negative reaction at both sites suggests the presence of adequate amounts of circulating neutralizing antitoxin and insusceptibility to diphtheria toxin.

The Schick test is at times complicated by individual hypersensitivity to constituents other than toxin contained in the injections.

Individuals who have positive Schick tests should be immunized with diphtheria toxoids. However, even if the Schick test is negative, diphtheria infection can sometimes occur.

B. Schultz-Charlton Reaction: If specific antitoxin to the erythrogenic toxin of beta-hemolytic group A streptococci is injected intradermally into a patient with scarlet fever, the rash will blanch and fade at the injection site because the antitoxin has neutralized the toxin. This test is rarely employed.

NONSPECIFIC CLINICAL LABORATORY TESTS

The usual laboratory procedures performed on most patients who undergo detailed medical examination frequently contain clues concerning possible infectious processes. Anemia and leukocytosis are suitable examples. Such abnormalities are compatible with a large variety of diagnoses and are helpful only if integrated with other findings into a meaningful pattern. No attempt is made here to list the many different laboratory findings which can thus aid in the diagnosis of infection. A few specific items will be discussed briefly for the sake of illustration.

Red Cell Count & Packed Cell Volume (PCV)

Anemia is a feature of many protracted infections, eg, bacterial endocarditis and malaria. Conversely, in acute gastrointestinal infections there may be dehydration with elevated PCV.

White Cell Count

In most suppurative infections the white count is elevated and the proportion of young polymorphonuclear cells is increased. A low white count in pneumococcal or staphylococcal pneumonia, especially in elderly patients, is an unfavorable prognostic sign.

In some infections caused by gram-negative bacilli there is a fall in the total white count and relative lymphocytosis. Similar findings occur in some viral infections (eg, myxoviruses). However, arbovirus infections with encephalitis commonly give rise to high white counts. In whooping cough, the white count is frequently high, with absolute lymphocytosis. Sudden widespread dissemination of any bacterial or fungal pathogen may be accompanied by a very rapid rise in the white count, at times to leukemoid levels. On the other hand, persons with depressed marrow activity do not develop white count elevations with infections.

These examples should indicate the complexity of interpreting white cell counts.

Erythrocyte Sedimentation Rate (ESR)

In many acute infections the ESR is normal; in prolonged infections it becomes accelerated. However, a rapid ESR can be associated with so many different processes which produce cell injury or derangements of blood proteins that it is rarely helpful in establishing the diagnosis of infection. It may be of use in evaluating therapeutic response.

C-Reactive Protein (CRP)

CRP is a substance in the serum of certain patients which reacts with the somatic C polysaccharide of pneumococci in vitro but is commonly measured by precipitation with a specific antiserum prepared in rabbits. It is a beta-globulin not found in normal sera but occurring frequently in sera of patients with inflammatory, neoplastic, or necrotizing processes. The laboratory test for the presence of CRP thus constitutes a nonspecific test for the presence of inflammation or tissue injury.

Tests for several mucoproteins in serum are likewise entirely nonspecific and so are of little help in diagnosis.

Transaminase & Similar Enzyme Tests

Glutamic oxaloacetic transaminase (SGOT), glutamic pyruvic transaminase (SGPT), lactate dehydrogenase (SLDH), and others are intracellular enzymes involved in amino acid or carbohydrate metabolism. In the course of many disease processes involving cellular injury, the enzyme concentration in blood serum increases markedly. Consequently, elevated enzyme levels are found in acute infections, neoplasms, infarctions, and many degenerative processes and are not necessarily due to hepatic insult or myocardial infarction, with which they are commonly associated.

Serum Bilirubin

The serum bilirubin may be elevated, indicating jaundice, particularly in infections of the newborn and in infections caused by gram-negative enteric organisms.

Biopsy

In many cases of protracted fever of unknown origin, all tests to establish the presence of infection fail to yield a definitive diagnosis. Surgical exploration and histologic examination of tissues may give the final answer. (See Petersdorf & Beeson reference.)

Nonspecific Organ System Response to Infections

Whenever an infectious process involves primarily one organ system, nonspecific laboratory tests may show abnormal values. For example, in renal infections, proteinuria and abnormal urinary sediment may be present even without bacteriuria. In CNS infections, abnormal values of CSF composition are of great help in diagnosis. In infections of the external eye, the cell picture of the conjunctival exudate assists in etiologic diagnosis. The roentgenographic appearance of bone or lung may not only support a diagnosis of infection but may even point to the etiologic agent.

LABORATORY AIDS IN THE SELECTION OF ANTIMICROBIAL THERAPY

The first drug used is chosen on the basis of clinical impression after the physician is convinced that a microbial infection exists and has made a tentative etiologic diagnosis on clinical grounds. On the basis of this "best guess," he can readily select a probable drug of choice (see Chapter 10). Before the probable drug of choice is administered, specimens are often obtained for laboratory isolation of the etiologic agent. The results of these examinations may necessitate selection of a different drug. The identification of certain microorganisms which are uniformly drug-susceptible eliminates the necessity for further testing and permits the selection of optimally effective drugs solely on the basis of experience. Under other circumstances, tests for drug susceptibility of isolated microorganisms may be helpful (see Chapter 10).

The commonly performed "disk test" must be used judiciously and interpreted with restraint. Only one member of each major class of drugs should be represented. For gram-negative rods, the following disks are used; ampicillin, cephalothin, streptomycin, chloramphenicol, tetracycline, kanamycin, gentamicin, and polymyxin (or colistin). For gram-positive organisms, penicillin G, cloxacillin, kanamycin, erythromycin, tetracycline, cephalothin, and lincomycin may be used. Vancomycin and methicillin may be tested against staphylococci; ampicillin against enterococci. Nitrofurantoin (Furadantin) disks are useful only against organisms isolated from the urine because the drug is only active in the urine—not systemically. Mandelamine disks are never used. Testing with sulfonamide disks is rarely indicated and is meaningless unless PABA-free media are employed.

The sizes of zones of growth inhibition vary with the molecular characteristics of different drugs. Thus zone size of one drug cannot be compared to the zone size of another drug acting on the same organism. However, for any one drug the zone size can be compared to a standard, provided media, inoculum size, and other conditions are carefully standardized. Then it is possible to list for each drug a minimum zone size which denotes "susceptibility."

The disk test measures the ability of drugs to *inhibit* the growth of microorganisms. Its results correlate reasonably well with therapeutic response in those disease processes where body defenses can frequently eliminate infectious microorganisms.

In a few types of human infections, the results of disk tests are of little assistance (and may be misleading) because a *bactericidal* drug effect is required for cure. Outstanding examples are bacterial endocarditis, acute osteomyelitis, and severe infections in a host whose antibacterial defenses are inadequate, eg, persons with neoplastic diseases which have been treated with radiation and antineoplastic chemotherapy, or persons who are being given corticosteroids in high dosage.

The selection of a bactericidal drug or drug combination for each patient can be guided by specialized laboratory tests. (See Jawetz, E., & others: Am J Clin Path 25:1016, 1955.)

Evaluation of the chemotherapeutic regimen in vivo can be performed by serum assay (see Chapter 10). This procedure consists of the following steps:

(1) An etiologic microorganism is isolated.

(2) Antimicrobial therapy is started.

TABLE 24–2. Bacteriologic diagnosis of specific microorganisms from clinical infections.

Organism	Principal Sources of Clinical Specimens	Preferred Culture Media	Special Conditions and Additional Tests Usually Required
Staphylococcus	Pus or exudate from site of infection; blood stream, spinal fluid, urine.	Blood agar plates; trypticase-soy broth; brain broth (3 weeks).	Aerobic or micro-aerophilic. Presence of hemolysis; coagulase reaction; mannitol fermentation.
Streptococcus			Aerobic or micro-aerophilic. Type of hemolysis; growth in 6.5% NaCl broth—enterococci.
Pneumococcus	Sputum, blood stream, spinal fluid, exudates, pus.	Blood agar plates; trypticase-soy broth; blood broth.	Hemolysis—alpha type; solubility in bile; typing with specific serum.
Gonococcus	Exudates from genitalia, eye, joints.	"Chocolate" agar plates incubated in 10% CO_2 (candle jar).	Intracellular diplococci on smear. Oxidase test.
Meningococcus	Blood stream, spinal fluid, nasopharynx, skin petechiae.		Intracellular diplococci on smear. Oxidase test; maltose fermented.
C diphtheriae	Nasopharynx, wounds, eye.	Löffler's slants; potassium tellurite medium; blood agar plates.	Typical morphology on smear. Virulence test; Schick skin test.
Clostridium	Wounds, exudates, pus, blood stream.	Blood agar plates; thioglycollate medium; chopped meat broth.	Strictly anaerobic. Type of hemolysis; milk coagulation.
M tuberculosis	Sputum, exudates, pus, spinal fluid, urine.	Petragnani's, Loewenstein's, or Dubos's media (2–4 weeks).	Guinea pig inoculation. Acid-fast stain; concentration.
Actinomyces	Sputum, exudates, pus.	Thioglycollate medium; blood agar plates.	Sulfur granules in specimen. Aerobic and anaerobic culture.
E coli–A aerogenes group	Urine, blood stream, spinal fluid, exudates, pus.	Blood agar plates, MacConkey's or eosin-methylene blue (EMB) agar.	Lactose fermented (paracolon bacilli ferment lactose slowly).
Salmonella	Feces, blood stream, urine, exudates.	MacConkey's or EMB agar plates; SS agar plates; tetrathionate broth; triple sugar iron agar.	Identified by slide agglutination with specific serum; patient's serum for agglutination test—H and O agglutination.
Shigella	Feces		Identified by slide agglutination with specific serum.
K pneumoniae (Friedländer's bacillus)	Sputum, blood stream, spinal fluid, exudates.	Blood agar plates; blood broth.	Typing with specific serum.
Proteus-Pseudomonas group	Urine, exudates, blood stream, spinal fluid.	Blood agar plates; nutrient agar plates.	Characteristic pigment, odor, "swarming"; lactose not fermented.
Pasteurella	Blood stream, sputum, exudates, pus.	Blood agar plates; cystine agar.	Patient's serum for agglutination test.
Brucella	Blood stream, exudates.	Trypticase-soy agar and broth, incubated in 10% CO_2 (candle jar).	Patient's serum for agglutination or precipitin tests.
Hemophilus species	Spinal fluid, blood stream, sputum, exudates.	"Chocolate" agar plates; blood agar plates.	Typing with specific serum. Precipitin test in spinal fluid.
Bacteroides	Exudates, blood stream.	Chopped meat broth; thioglycollate medium; blood agar plates.	Strictly anaerobic. Typical morphology.
T pallidum	Primary or secondary syphilitic lesion.	None.	Darkfield microscopy; serologic tests (STS, TPI, FTA).
Leptospira	Blood stream, urine.	Serum broth.	Darkfield microscopy.
B recurrentis	Blood stream.	Blood broth.	Stained blood film; serologic tests.
Yeasts and fungi	Skin, nails; exudates, pus; sputum, blood.	Blood agar plates; Sabouraud's medium.	Serologic tests on patient's serum.

TABLE 24–3. Diagnostic features of some acute exanthems.

Disease	Prodromal Signs and Symptoms	Nature of Eruption	Other Diagnostic Features	Laboratory Tests
Measles (rubeola)	3–4 days of fever, coryza, conjunctivitis and cough.	Maculopapular, reddish-brown; begins on head and neck, spreads downward. In 5–6 days rash brownish, desquamating.	Koplik's spots on buccal mucosa.	WBC low; specialized CF and virus neutralization in tissue culture.
German measles (rubella)	Little or no prodrome.	Maculopapular, pink; begins on head and neck, spreads downward, fades in 3 days. No desquamation.	Lymphadenopathy, postauricular or occipital.	WBC normal or low; specialized virus neutralization in tissue culture.
Chickenpox (varicella)	0–1 day of fever, anorexia, headache.	Rapid evolution of macules to papules, vesicles, crusts; all stages simultaneously present; lesions superficial, distribution centripetal.	Lesions on scalp and mucous membranes.	Specialized CF and virus neutralization in tissue culture.
Smallpox (variola)	3 days of fever, severe headache, malaise, chills.	Slow evolution of macules to papules, vesicles, pustules, crusts; all lesions in same stage; lesions deep-seated, distribution centrifugal.		Virus isolation on chorioallantoic membranes of chick embryos, CF.
Scarlet fever	½–2 days of malaise, sore throat, fever, vomiting.	Generalized, punctate, red; prominent on neck, in axilla, groin, skinfolds; circumoral pallor; fine desquamation involves hands and feet.	Strawberry tongue, exudative tonsillitis.	Group A hemolytic streptococci cultures from throat; antistreptolysin O titer rise.
Exanthem subitum (roseola infantum)	3–4 days of high fever.	As fever falls by crisis pink maculopapules appear on chest and trunk; fade in 1–3 days.		WBC low.
Fifth disease (erythema infectiosum)	None.	Red, flushed cheeks; circumoral pallor; maculopapules on extremities.	"Slapped face" appearance.	
Meningococcemia	Hours of fever, vomiting.	Maculopapules, petechiae.	Meningeal signs.	Cultures of blood, CSF.
Rocky Mt. spotted fever	3–4 days of fever, chills, severe headaches.	Maculopapules, petechiae, distribution centrifugal.	History of tick bite.	Agglutination (OX19, OX2), CF.
Typhus fevers	3–4 days of fever, chills, severe headaches.	Maculopapules, petechiae, distribution centripetal.	Endemic area, lice.	Agglutination (OX19), CF.
Infectious mononucleosis	Fever, adenopathy, sore throat.	Maculopapular rash resembling rubella, rarely papulovesicular.	Splenomegaly.	Atypical lymphs in blood smears; heterophil agglutination.
Enterovirus infections (echo, coxsackie)	1–2 days of fever, malaise.	Maculopapular rash resembling rubella, rarely papulovesicular.	Aseptic meningitis.	Virus isolation from stool or CSF; CF titer rise.
Drug eruptions	Occasional fever.	Maculopapular rash resembling rubella, rarely papulovesicular.		Eosinophilia.
Eczema herpeticum	None.	Vesiculopustular lesions in area of eczema.		Herpes simplex virus isolated in tissue culture; CF.

(3) Blood is drawn from the patient receiving treatment.

(4) Dilutions of the separated serum are tested for their ability to kill in vitro the microorganisms isolated from the patient.

This simple test can often help decide whether the patient is receiving the proper drug in adequate amounts or whether the regimen should be altered.

In urinary tract infections the antibacterial activity of *urine* is far more important than that of serum. The disappearance of infecting organisms from the urine during treatment can serve as a partial drug level assay.

Instead of the disk test, a semi-quantitative test tube procedure can be employed. This test measures more exactly the concentration of an antibiotic necessary to inhibit growth of a standardized inoculum under defined conditions. A series of broth tubes containing graduated amounts of an antibiotic is inoculated with a dilution of fresh broth culture of the test organism. After incubation, the tubes are examined for turbidity. The end point is considered to be that concentration of antibiotic contained in the last tube remaining clear. Upon this basis a rough estimate of the in vivo dose necessary to inhibit growth of the test organism can be arrived at. In addition, bactericidal effect may be determined by the tube dilution method, if tubes without growth are subcultured on drug-free media.

.   .   .

GRAM & ACID-FAST STAINING METHODS

Gram Stain (Hucker Modification)

(1) Fix smear by heat.

(2) Cover with crystal violet for 1 minute.

(3) Wash with water. Do not blot.

(4) Cover with Gram's iodine for 1 minute.

(5) Wash with water. Do not blot.

(6) Decolorize for 10–30 seconds with gentle agitation in acetone (30 ml) and alcohol (70 ml).

(7) Wash with water. Do not blot.

(8) Cover for 10–30 seconds with safranin (2.5% solution in 95% alcohol).

(9) Wash with water and let dry.

Ziehl-Neelsen Acid-Fast Stain

(1) Fix smear by heat.

(2) Cover with carbolfuchsin, steam gently for 5 minutes over direct flame (or for 20 minutes over a water bath).

(3) Wash with water.

(4) Decolorize in acid-alcohol until only a faint pink color remains.

(5) Wash with water.

(6) Counterstain for 10–30 seconds with Löffler's methylene blue.

(7) Wash with water and let dry.

Kinyoun Carbolfuchsin Acid-Fast Stain

(1) Formula: Basic fuchsin, 4; phenol crystals, 8; alcohol (95%), 20; distilled water, 100.

(2) Stain fixed smear for 3 minutes (no heat necessary) and continue as with Ziehl-Neelsen stain.

●   ●   ●

General References

Bauer, A.W., & others: Antibiotic susceptibility testing by a standardized single disc method. Am J Clin Path 45:493–496, 1966.

Fox, H.A.: Immunofluorescence in the diagnosis of acute bacterial meningitis. Pediatrics 43:44–79, 1969.

Kalinske, R.W., & others: Diagnostic usefulness and safety of transtracheal aspiration. New England J Med 276:604–608, 1967.

Levison, M.L., & P.F. Frank: Differentiation of group A from other beta hemolytic streptococci with bacitracin. J Bact 69:284, 1955.

Petersdorf, R.G., & P. Beeson: Fever of unexplained origin: Report of 100 cases. Medicine 40:1–30, 1961.

25...

Rickettsial Diseases

The rickettsiae were at one time considered closely related to the viruses because they are smaller than bacteria and because their growth, like that of viruses, occurs within cells. It is now clear that the rickettsiae are small, obligately parasitic, true bacteria, showing in thin sections all of the structural features of bacteria as well as possessing most of the enzymes of bacteria and a typical bacterial cell wall. The natural reservoir of these organisms is the arthropods, in which they propagate without, usually, producing any disease. When transmitted to an unnatural host such as man, they are likely to cause disease.

Except for Q fever organisms, the rickettsiae are transmitted by arthropods and produce infections in human beings characterized by fever and rash. The rickettsial diseases can be divided into groups on the basis of their clinical features, epidemiologic aspects, and immunologic characteristics.

Classification

A. **Typhus Group:**
  1. Epidemic typhus, louse-borne—*R prowazeki*.
  2. Endemic typhus, murine flea-borne—*R mooseri*.

B. **Spotted Fever Group:**
  1. Rocky Mountain spotted fever—*R rickettsi*.
  2. Mediterranean fever (boutonneuse fever), South African tick bite fever, Kenya tick typhus, Indian tick typhus—*R conori*.
  3. North Asian tick-borne rickettsiosis—*R siberica*.
  4. Queensland tick typhus—*R australis*.
  5. Rickettsialpox, Russian vesicular rickettsiosis—*R akari*.

C. **Scrub Typhus (Tsutsugamushi Fever):** *R tsutsugamushi*.

D. **Q Fever:** *Coxiella burneti*.

E. **Trench Fever:** *R quintana*.

Properties of Rickettsiae

The most extensively studied member of the group is *R prowazeki*. This organism may be found either as short rods, 600 × 300 μm in size, or as cocci. Rickettsiae are pleomorphic, being found singly, in pairs, in short chains, or in filaments. When stained with Giemsa's, Castaneda's, or Macchiavello's stain, they are readily visible under the optical microscope. With Giemsa's stain they stain blue; with Macchia-vello's stain they stain red and are in marked contrast to the blue-staining cytoplasm in which they appear.

A wide range of animals are susceptible to infection with rickettsial organisms. Rickettsiae grow readily in the yolk sac of the embryonated egg (yolk sac suspensions contain up to 10^9 rickettsial particles per ml). Pure preparations of rickettsiae can be obtained by differential centrifugation of yolk sac suspensions. Many rickettsial strains also grow in cell culture.

Purified rickettsiae contain both ribonucleic and deoxyribonucleic acids in a ratio of 3.5:1 (similar to the ratio reported for many bacteria). Rickettsiae have cell walls consisting of mucopeptides containing muramic acid, resembling cell walls of gram-negative bacteria. Rickettsiae divide like bacteria, and all forms similar to those present during the division of short bacterial rods can be seen.

Unlike true viruses, purified rickettsiae contain enzymes concerned with metabolism. Thus they oxidize intermediate metabolites like pyruvic, succinic, and glutamic acids and can convert glutamic acid into aspartic acid. Rickettsiae lose their biologic activities (toxicity, hemolytic activity, infectivity, and respiratory activity) when they are stored at $0°$ C; this is due to the progressive loss of diphosphopyridine nucleotide (DPN). All of these properties can be restored by subsequent incubation with DPN. They also may lose their biologic activity if they are starved by incubation for several hours at $36°$ C. This loss can be prevented by the addition of glutamate, pyruvate, or adenosinetriphosphate (ATP). Subsequent incubation of the starved organism with glutamate at $30°$ C leads to partial or complete recovery of activity. Analysis of the ATP content of the rickettsiae during the starvation and recovery process indicates that the ATP level falls to zero during starvation and rises again on addition of glutamate.

Rickettsiae may grow in different parts of the cell. Those of the typhus group are usually found in the cytoplasm; those of the spotted fever group, in the nucleus. Thus far, one of the rickettsiae, *R quintana*, has been grown on cell-free media. It has been suggested that rickettsiae grow best when the metabolism of the host cells is low. Thus, their growth is enhanced when the temperature of infected chick embryos is lowered to $32°$ C. If the embryos are held at $40°$ C, rickettsial multiplication is poor. Rickettsial growth can be inhibited by certain dyes which increase the oxidative processes of the host cells; it can be stimulated by metabolic inhibitors like cyanide. Conditions which influence the metabolism of the host can alter its susceptibility to rickettsial infection. Thus, if rats are maintained on a riboflavin-deficient diet, their susceptibility to rickettsial infection is increased.

Rickettsial growth is enhanced in the presence of sulfonamides, and rickettsial diseases are made more severe by these drugs. Para-aminobenzoic acid (PABA), the structural analogue of the sulfonamides, inhibits the growth of rickettsial organisms. This inhibition is reversed by parahydroxybenzoic acid, which may be the metabolite whose function is interfered with by PABA.

Chloramphenicol and the tetracycline drugs inhibit the growth of rickettsiae and are excellent therapeutic agents.

In general, rickettsiae are quickly destroyed by heat, drying, and bactericidal chemicals. Although usually killed by storage at room temperature, they can be stored frozen or lyophilized (although there is some loss in infectivity). However, dried feces of infected lice may remain infective for months at room temperature.

The organism of Q fever is the rickettsial agent most resistant to drying. This organism has also been found to survive pasteurization at 60° C for 30 minutes and has been recovered from the commercially pasteurized milk of infected herds.

Rickettsial Antigens & Antibodies

A variety of rickettsial antibodies are known; all of them participate in the reactions discussed below. The antibodies which develop in man after vaccination generally are more type-specific than the antibodies developing after natural infection.

A. Agglutination of *Proteus Vulgaris* **(Weil-Felix Reaction):** The Weil-Felix reaction is commonly used in diagnostic work. Rickettsiae and proteus organisms appear to share certain antigens. Thus during the course of rickettsial infections, patients develop antibodies which agglutinate certain strains of *Proteus vulgaris*. For example, the proteus strain OX19 is agglutinated strongly by sera from persons infected with epidemic or endemic typhus; weakly by sera from those infected with Rocky Mountain spotted fever; and not at all by those infected with Q fever. Convalescent sera from scrub typhus patients react most strongly with the proteus strain OXK (Table 25–1).

B. Agglutination of Rickettsiae: Rickettsiae are agglutinated by specific antibodies. This reaction is very sensitive and can be diagnostically useful when heavy rickettsial suspensions are available.

C. Neutralization of Infective Rickettsiae: Neutralizing antibodies are specific, but their measurement is too cumbersome for diagnostic work. The test requires the inoculation of chick embryos by the yolk sac route or of guinea pigs by the intraperitoneal route with serum-rickettsiae mixtures.

D. Complement Fixation With Rickettsial Antigens: Complement fixing antibodies are commonly used in diagnostic laboratories. The antigens found in the soluble substances of the organism are less type-specific than those found fixed to the rickettsiae. Washing purified rickettsiae removes most of the group antigens and leaves the type-specific antigens behind. A nucleoprotein has been extracted from *R prowazeki* which behaves as a type-specific antigen in complement fixation tests. Proteolytic enzymes alter this material so that it becomes group-specific, like the soluble antigen, and reacts almost to the same degree with epidemic and endemic antisera.

Persons immunized against epidemic typhus develop low titer complement fixing antibodies which are type-specific. If they later contract endemic typhus, their complement fixing antibodies against epidemic typhus antigen are boosted. This appears to be due to an anamnestic reaction to the common antigen shared by the 2 rickettsial species. A common soluble antigen has also been shown to exist for the rickettsiae of the spotted fever group.

E. Neutralization of Rickettsial Toxins: Rickettsiae contain toxins which produce death in animals within a few hours after inoculation. Toxin-neutralizing antibodies appear during infection, and these are specific for the toxins of the typhus group, the spotted fever group, and scrub typhus rickettsiae. Toxins exist only in viable rickettsiae and somewhat resemble bacterial endotoxins.

F. Hemagglutination-Inhibition: Rickettsiae and fractions derived from them by heating in dilute alkali have been shown to agglutinate erythrocytes. Antibodies which inhibit this reaction also appear in convalescence.

Pathology

Rickettsiae multiply in endothelial cells of small blood vessels. The cells become swollen and necrotic; there is thrombosis of the vessel, leading to rupture and necrosis. Vascular lesions are prominent in the skin. In the brain, aggregations of lymphocytes, polymorphonuclear leukocytes, and macrophages are associated with the blood vessels of the gray matter; these are called typhus nodules. The heart shows similar lesions of the small blood vessels. Other organs may also be involved.

Clinical Findings

Except for Q fever, in which there is no skin lesion, rickettsial infections are characterized by fever, headache, malaise, varying degrees of prostration, and skin rash.

A. Typhus Group:

1. Epidemic typhus—In epidemic typhus fever, the systemic infection and prostration are severe, and fever continues for about 2 weeks. The disease is more severe and is more often fatal in patients over 40 years of age. During typhus epidemics the case mortality has been 6–30%.

2. Endemic typhus—The clinical picture of endemic typhus has many features in common with that of epidemic typhus, but the disease is milder and is rarely fatal except in elderly patients.

B. Spotted Fever: The spotted fever group resembles typhus clinically; however, unlike the rash in other rickettsial diseases, the rash of the spotted fever group usually appears first on the extremities, moves centripetally, and involves the palms and soles. Some, like Brazilian spotted fever, may produce severe infections; others, like Mediterranean fever, are mild. The case mortality rate varies greatly; for Rocky Mountain spotted fever it may be as high as 20%. Rickettsialpox is a mild disease with a rash resembling that of varicella. About a week before onset of fever, a firm red papule appears at the site of the mite-bite and develops into a deep-seated vesicle which in turn forms a black eschar (see below).

C. Scrub Typhus: This disease resembles epidemic typhus clinically. One feature is the eschar, the punched-out ulcer covered with a blackened scab which indicates the location of the mite-bite. The eschar is usually present at the onset of symptoms. Localized eschars may also be present in the spotted fever group.

D. Q Fever: This disease resembles influenza and primary atypical pneumonia rather than typhus. There is no rash or local lesion. The Weil-Felix reaction is negative, and transmission appears to be air-borne rather than through the skin.

E. Trench Fever: The disease is characterized by headache, exhaustion, pain, sweating, coldness of the extremities, and fever associated with a roseolar rash. Relapses occur, and it may take over a year for the disease to run its course. Trench fever has been known only among armies during wars in central Europe.

Laboratory Findings

Isolation of rickettsiae is technically quite difficult and so is of only limited usefulness in diagnosis. Whole blood (or emulsified blood clot) is inoculated into guinea pigs, mice, or eggs. Rickettsiae are recovered most frequently from blood drawn soon after onset, but they have been found as late as the 12th day of the disease.

If the guinea pigs fail to show disease (fever, scrotal swellings, hemorrhagic necrosis, death), either "blind" passages to other animals are made or, more often, serum of the guinea pig is collected for antibody tests to determine if the animal has had an inapparent infection.

The agent of scrub typhus grows readily in the mouse. Regardless of the animal used for isolation of this agent, material should be passed through the mouse, for rickettsiae are readily seen in smears of peritoneal exudate.

Serologic tests of choice for the rickettsial diseases are indicated below. They are based on the discussion given above on Rickettsial Antigens and Antibodies. An antibody rise should be demonstrated during the course of illness.

TABLE 25–1. Serologic tests for rickettsial diseases.

Disease	Weil-Felix	Complement Fixation With Yolk Sac Antigen
Epidemic typhus	OX19	+
Endemic typhus	OX19	+
Scrub typhus	OXK	+
Rocky Mountain spotted fever	OX19 and OX2	+
Mediterranean (boutonneuse) fever	OX19 and OX2	+
South African tick fever	OX19 and OX2	+
Rickettsialpox	Negative	+
Q fever	Negative	+

Treatment

Chloramphenicol and the tetracyclines are effective. The initial loading dose, 2–3 gm for a 155 lb (70 kg) patient, is administered over a period of 2–4 hours. The total amount of antibiotic given in the first 24 hours of therapy is 4–6 gm. The daily dose thereafter is 2–3 gm divided into 4 doses. Response should be observed within 1–2 days, and the progression of the clinical disease is usually halted at the stage where treatment is started. To avoid relapses, continue treatment for 3–5 days after the temperature is normal.

Sulfonamides enhance the disease and are contraindicated.

The antibiotics do not free the body of rickettsiae, but they do suppress their growth. Recovery depends upon the immune mechanisms of the patient, which usually take 2 weeks to develop to the stage where they can control the parasite. If treatment is begun after the sixth day of illness, the immunity develops as in the untreated infection and relapses do not occur. If antibiotics are given earlier in the disease and a short course of treatment used, the immune mechanism is not properly stimulated, and relapses occur. Such relapses can be prevented in patients treated early in the infection by giving a second course of antibiotic 6 days after the first course of treatment has ended.

Epidemiology

A variety of arthropods, especially ticks and mites, harbor rickettsia-like organisms which do not harm the host. They are found in the cells which line the alimentary tract; from there they reach the genital tract and are transmitted from one generation to the next.

Rickettsiae, like other microorganisms, appear to be in a state of continuous evolution. They seem to be "bacteria" of arthropods which have become limited to an intracellular life cycle.

The life cycles of different rickettsiae vary according to the stage of their evolution:

(1) *R prowazeki* appears to have achieved a greater degree of parasitism for man than has any other member of the group. Its life cycle is limited to man and to the human louse (*Pediculus corporis* and *P capitis*). The louse obtains the organism by biting infected human beings and transmits the agent by fecal excretion on the surface of the skin of another person. Whenever a louse bites, it defecates at the same time. It is the scratching of the area of the bite which allows the rickettsiae excreted in the feces to penetrate the skin. As a result of the infection the louse dies, but the organisms remain viable for some time in the dried feces of the louse. Rickettsiae are not transmitted from one generation of lice to another. Typhus epidemics have been controlled by delousing large proportions of the population with insecticides like DDT.

Brill's disease is a recrudescence of an old typhus infection. The rickettsiae can persist for as long as 20 years in the body of an individual without any symptoms being manifest. The rickettsiae isolated from such cases behave like classical *R prowazeki;* this suggests that man himself is the reservoir of the rickettsiae of epidemic typhus. Epidemic typhus epidemics have been associated with war and the lowering of standards of personal hygiene, which in turn have increased the opportunities for human lice to flourish. If this occurs at the time of recrudescence of an old typhus infection, an epidemic may be set off. Brill's disease occurs in local populations of typhus areas as well as in persons who migrate from such areas to places where the disease does not exist. Serologic characteristics readily distinguish Brill's disease from primary epidemic typhus. Antibodies arise earlier, and are the 7 S recall type rather than the 19 S new type detected after primary infection. They reach a maximum by the tenth day of disease. The Weil-Felix reaction is usually negative. This early 7 S antibody response and the mild course of the disease suggest that partial immunity is still present from the primary infection.

(2) *R mooseri* has its reservoir in the rat, in which the infection is inapparent and long-lasting. The agent can be recovered from the rat for at least a year after exposure. Rat fleas carry the rickettsiae from rat to rat and sometimes from rat to man, who develops endemic typhus. In endemic typhus, the flea cannot transmit the rickettsiae through the egg.

(3) *R tsutsugamushi* has its true reservoir in the mites which infest rodents. Rickettsiae can persist in rats for over a year after infection. Mites transmit the infection transovarially. Occasionally infected mites or rat fleas bite man, and scrub typhus results. The rickettsiae persist in the mite-rat-mite cycle in the scrub or secondary jungle vegetation which has replaced the virgin jungle in areas of partial cultivation. Such areas may become infested with rats and trombiculid mites.

(4) *R rickettsi* may be found in healthy wood ticks (*Dermacentor andersoni*) and is passed transovarially. Vertebrate hosts such as deer and man are occasionally bitten by infected ticks in western USA. In order to be infectious, the tick carrying the rickettsiae must be engorged with blood, for this increases the number of rickettsiae in the tick. The dog is a natural host of the dog tick, but does not serve as a continuous source of infection with Rocky Mountain spotted fever rickettsiae in eastern USA.

(5) *R akari* has its vector in blood-sucking mites of the species *Allodermanyssus sanguineus.* These mites may be found on the mice (*Mus musculus*) trapped in apartment houses where rickettsialpox has occurred. Transovarial transmission of the rickettsiae occurs in the mite. Thus the mite may act as a true reservoir as well as a vector. *R akari* has also been isolated from a vole in Korea.

(6) *R quintana* is the etiologic agent of trench fever; it is found in lice and in man, and its life cycle is like that of *R prowazeki.* The disease has been limited to fighting armies. This organism can be grown on blood agar in 10% CO_2.

(7) *Coxiella burneti* is found in ticks, which transmit the agent to sheep, goats, and cattle. Workers in slaughterhouses and in plants which process wool and cattle hides have contracted the disease as a result of handling infected animal tissues. *C burneti* is transmitted by the respiratory pathway rather than through the skin. There may be a chronic infection of the udder of the cow. In such cases the rickettsiae are excreted in the milk, and may be transmitted to man. As many as 10,000 infective guinea pig doses for guinea pig or man may be contained in 1 ml of milk.

Infected sheep may excrete *C burneti* in the feces and urine. The placentas of infected cows and sheep contain the rickettsiae, and parturition creates infectious aerosols. The soil may be contaminated from one of the above sources and in turn becomes a continuous source of infectious rickettsiae. The high concentration of rickettsiae in the soil suggests that secondary aerosols (dust) lead to infection of man and livestock in the absence of active shedding of the organism by infected animal hosts. Coxiella can cause endocarditis.

Geographic Occurrence

A. Epidemic Typhus: Potentially worldwide, it has disappeared from the USA, Britain, and Scandinavia. It is still present in the Balkans, Asia, North Africa, Middle East, Mexico, and the Andes. In view of its long duration in man as a latent infection (Brill's disease), it can flourish quickly under proper environmental conditions, as it did in Europe during World War II as a result of the deterioration of community sanitation.

B. Endemic, Murine Typhus: Worldwide, especially in areas of high rat-infestation, such as seaports. It may exist in the same areas as—and may be confused with—epidemic typhus or scrub typhus.

C. Scrub Typhus: Far East, especially Burma, India, Ceylon, New Guinea, Japan, and Formosa. *Trombicula pallida,* the chigger most often found in Korea, maintains the infection among the wild rodents of Korea (*Apodemus agrarius*), but only infrequently does it transfer scrub typhus to man.

D. Spotted Fever Group: These infections occur around the globe, exhibiting as a rule some epidemiologic and immunologic difference in different areas. Transmission by a tick of the Ixodidae family is common to the group. The diseases which are grouped together include Rocky Mountain (Western and Eastern), Colombian, Brazilian, and Mexican spotted fevers; Mediterranean (boutonneuse), South African tick, and Kenya fevers; North Queensland tick typhus; and North Asian tick-borne rickettsiosis.

E. Rickettsialpox: The human disease has been found among inhabitants of apartment houses in northern USA. However, the infection also occurs in Russia, Africa, and Korea.

F. Q Fever: Since 1935, the disease is recognized around the world.

Seasonal Occurrence

Epidemic typhus is more common in cool climates, reaching its peak in winter and waning in the spring. This is probably a reflection of crowding, lack of fuel, and low standards of personal hygiene, which favor louse infestation.

Rickettsial infections which must be vector transmitted to the human host reach their peak incidence at the time the vector is most prevalent—the summer and fall months.

Control

Control is achieved by breaking the infection chain or by immunizing and treating with antibiotics.

A. Prevention of Transmission by Breaking the Chain of Infection:

1. **Epidemic typhus**—Delousing with DDT.

2. **Murine typhus**—Rat-proofing buildings and using rat poisons.

3. **Scrub typhus**—Clearing from camp sites the secondary jungle vegetation in which rats and mites live.

4. **Spotted fever**—Similar measures for the spotted fevers may be used: clearing of the infested land, and personal prophylaxis in the form of protective clothing such as high boots, socks worn over trousers; tick repellents, etc.

5. **Rickettsialpox**—Elimination of rodents and their parasites from human domiciles.

B. Prevention of Transmission of Q Fever by Adequate Pasteurization of Milk: Heating of *C burneti* in whole raw milk for 30 minutes at 143° F is not sufficient to destroy all the viable rickettsiae, but heating at 145° F does accomplish this. The presently recommended conditions of "high-temperature, short-time," 71.5° C (161° F) for 15 seconds are adequate.

C. Prevention by Vaccination: Active immunization may be carried out using formalinized antigens prepared from the yolk sacs of infected chick embryos. Such vaccines are available for epidemic typhus (*R prowazeki*), Rocky Mountain spotted fever (*R rickettsi*), and some others.

D. Chemoprophylaxis: Chloramphenicol has been used as a chemoprophylactic agent against scrub typhus in endemic areas. Oral administration of 3 gm doses at weekly intervals controls infection so that no disease occurs even though rickettsiae appear in the blood. The antibiotic must be continued for a month after the initiation of infection to keep the person well. Tetracyclines may be equally effective.

● ● ●

General Bibliography

Hazard, F., & others: Rocky Mountain spotted fever in USA. New England J Med 280:57–63, 1969.

Ormsbee, R.A.: Rickettsiae as organisms. Ann Rev Micro 23:275–292, 1969.

26...

Agents of the Psittacosis-LGV-Trachoma Group (Bedsoniae, Chlamydiae)

The agents of psittacosis, lymphogranuloma venereum (LGV), and trachoma are a large group of nonmotile, gram-negative, obligate intracellular parasites possessing a similar morphology and a common group antigen which multiply in the cytoplasm of their host cells by a distinctive developmental cycle. The group includes some important human and animal pathogens. In the interest of brevity, the generic term "chlamydiae" will be used here to denote agents of the psittacosis-LGV-trachoma group.

Because of their obligate intracellular parasitism, these organisms were once considered viruses. However, the chlamydiae differ from true viruses in the following important characteristics:

(1) They possess both RNA and DNA; viruses have only one nucleic acid.

(2) They multiply by binary fission; viruses never do.

(3) They possess bacterial type cell walls with mucopeptides containing muramic acid.

(4) They possess ribosomes; viruses never do.

(5) They have a variety of metabolically active enzymes, eg, they can liberate CO_2 from glucose. Some can synthesize folates.

(6) Their growth can be inhibited by many antimicrobial drugs.

It is probable that chlamydiae are derived from gram-negative bacteria. They can be viewed as bacteria which lack some important mechanisms for the production of metabolic energy. This defect restricts them to an intracellular existence.

Development Cycle

All chlamydiae share a general sequence of events in their reproduction. The infectious particle is a small cell ("elementary body") about 0.3 μm in diameter with an electron-dense nucleoid. It is taken into the host cell by phagocytosis. A vacuole, derived from host cell surface membranes, forms around the small particle. This small particle is reorganized into a large one ("initial body") measuring about 0.5–1 μm and devoid of an electron-dense nucleoid. Within the membrane-bound vacuole, the large particle grows in size and divides repeatedly by binary fission. Eventually the entire vacuole becomes filled with small particles derived by binary fission from large bodies to form an "inclusion" in the host cell cytoplasm. The newly formed small particles may be liberated from

the host cell to infect new cells. The developmental cycle takes 24–48 hours.

Structure & Chemical Composition

Examination of highly purified suspensions of chlamydiae, washed free of host cell materials, indicates the following: The outer **cell wall** resembles the cell wall of gram-negative bacteria. It has a relatively high lipid content, and the mucopeptide contains muramic acid. Cell wall formation is inhibited by penicillins and cycloserine, substances which inhibit mucopeptide synthesis in bacteria. **Both DNA and RNA** are present in both small and large particles. In small particles, most DNA is concentrated in the electron-dense central nucleoid. In large particles, the DNA is distributed irregularly throughout the cytoplasm. Most RNA probably exists in ribosomes, in the cytoplasm. The large particles contain about 4 times as much RNA as DNA, whereas the small, infective particles contain about equal amounts of RNA and DNA.

The protein content of small particles is about 60%, with at least 18 amino acids present. Chlamydiae contain large amounts of **lipids,** especially phospholipids, which are well characterized.

A toxic principle is intimately associated with infectious chlamydiae. It kills mice after the intravenous administration of more than 10^8 particles. Its chemical nature is not known.

Staining Properties

Chlamydiae have distinctive staining properties (similar to those of rickettsiae) which differ somewhat at different stages of development. Single mature particles (elementary bodies) stain purple with Giemsa's stain and red with Macchiavello's stain, in contrast to the blue of host cell cytoplasm. The larger, noninfective bodies (initial bodies) stain blue with Giemsa's stain. The gram reaction of chlamydiae is negative or variable, and Gram's stain is not useful in the identification of the agents.

Fully formed, mature intracellular inclusions are compact masses near the nucleus which are dark purple when stained with Giemsa's stain because of the densely packed mature particles. If stained with dilute Lugol's iodine solution, the inclusions formed by some chlamydiae (agents of mouse pneumonitis, LGV, trachoma-inclusion conjunctivitis [TRIC agents]) appear brown because of the glycogen-like matrix which surrounds the particles.

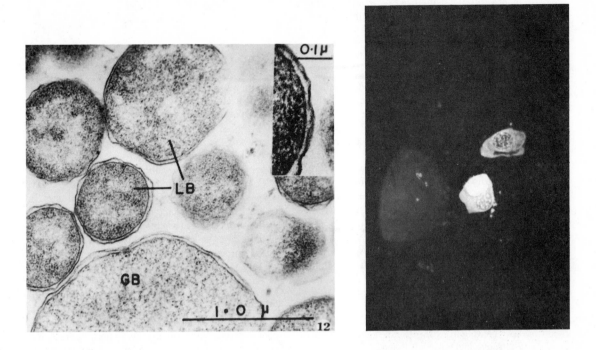

FIG 26–1. **Chlamydiae.** **Left**: Chlamydiae in various stages of intracellular development. LB, "elementary body" particles with cell walls. GB, "reticulate large body," "initial body." **Right**: Fluorescent inclusion body of TRIC agent in epithelial cell (conjunctival scraping) stained with specific fluorescein-labeled antiserum.

Staining with acridine orange or rhodamine permits an estimate of the relative content of RNA or DNA at different stages in the development of chlamydiae and correlates well with their relative infectivity.

Antigens

Chlamydiae possess 2 types of antigens. Both are probably located in the cell wall. *Group antigens* are shared by all members of the group of chlamydiae. They are resistant to heat, nucleases, and proteinases but are inactivated by periodate and lecithinase and removed in part by treatment with deoxycholate. They are probably lipopolysaccharides. *Specific antigens* remain attached to cell walls after group antigens have been largely removed by treatment with fluorocarbon or deoxycholate. Specific antigens can be detected by immunofluorescence and perhaps by gel diffusion reactions. Specific antigens are shared by only a limited number of chlamydiae, but a given organism may contain several specific antigens (perhaps up to a dozen). The toxic effects of infectious chlamydiae are associated with antigens. Specific neutralization of these toxic effects by antiserum permits limited antigenic grouping of organisms.

A hemagglutinin capable of clumping some chicken and mouse erythrocytes is present in chlamydiae. This hemagglutination is blocked by group antibody.

Growth & Metabolism

Chlamydiae require an intracellular habitat, presumably because they lack some essential feature of energy metabolism. All types of chlamydiae proliferate in embryonated eggs, particularly in the yolk sac. Some also proliferate in cell cultures and in various animal tissues.

Different chlamydiae differ somewhat in amino acid requirements, at times requiring fewer amino acids than their host cells. Chlamydiae appear to have an endogenous metabolism similar to that of some bacteria but participate only to a limited extent in potentially energy-yielding processes. They can liberate CO_2 from glucose, pyruvate, and glutamate; they also contain dehydrogenases. Nevertheless, they require assistance from the host cell in meeting their energy requirements for synthesis and have been called "energy parasites."

Reactions to Physical & Chemical Agents

Chlamydiae are rapidly inactivated by heat. They lose infectivity completely after 10 minutes at 60° C and partly after 3–12 hours at 37° C. They maintain infectivity for years at −50° C to −70° C. During the process of freeze-drying, much of the infectivity is lost, but successfully lyophilized preparations are stable for years. Some air-dried chlamydiae may also remain infective for long periods.

Chlamydiae are rapidly inactivated by ether (in 30 minutes), by formalin (0.1% for 24 hours), or by phenol (0.5% for 24 hours).

The replication of chlamydiae can be inhibited by many antibacterial antibiotics. Cell wall inhibitors such as penicillins and cycloserine result in the production of morphologically defective forms but are not very effective in clinical diseases. Inhibitors of protein synthesis (tetracyclines, erythromycins, chloramphenicol) are effective in laboratory models and at times in clinical infections. Some chlamydiae synthesize folates and are susceptible to inhibition by sulfonamides. Streptomycin, neomycins, and polymyxins have only minimal inhibitory activity for chlamydiae.

Characteristics of Host-Parasite Relationship

The outstanding biologic feature of infection by chlamydiae is the balance that is often reached between host and parasite, resulting in prolonged, often lifetime latency. Subclinical infection is the rule—and overt disease the exception—in the natural hosts of these agents. Spread from one species (eg, birds) to another (eg, man) more frequently leads to disease. Antibodies to several antigens of chlamydiae are regularly produced by the infected host. These antibodies have little protective effect. Commonly the infectious agent persists in the presence of high titers of antibodies. Treatment with effective antimicrobial drugs (eg, tetracyclines) for prolonged periods may eliminate the chlamydiae from the infected host. Very early, intensive treatment may suppress antibody formation. Late treatment with antimicrobial drugs in moderate doses may suppress disease but permit persistence of the infecting agent in tissues.

The immunization of susceptible animals with various inactivated or living vaccines tends to induce protection against death from the toxic effect of living challenge organisms. However, such immunization in animals or man has been singularly unsuccessful in protecting against infection. At best immunization, or prior infection, has induced some resistance which resulted in milder disease after challenge or reinfection.

Classification

Historically, chlamydiae have been arranged according to their pathogenic potential and their host range. Antigenic differences are beginning to emerge from studies employing toxin neutralization and specific antigen-antibody reactions. Chlamydiae can also be grouped according to the nature of the intracytoplasmic inclusion and the susceptibility to sulfonamides. TRIC agents, LGV, mouse pneumonitis, and other organisms of this group are inhibited by sulfonamides, and their intracellular inclusions are very compact and contain glycogen. These agents are sometimes called *Chlamydia trachomatis.* By contrast, the agents of psittacosis, meningopneumonitis, feline pneumonitis, and other organisms of this group are usually resistant to sulfonamides and their inclusions are diffuse and contain no glycogen. These agents are sometimes called *Chlamydia psittaci.* Rigid criteria for classification are not available.

PSITTACOSIS
(Ornithosis)

Psittacosis is a disease of birds which may be transferred to man. In man, the agent produces a spectrum of clinical manifestations ranging from severe pneumonia and sepsis with a high mortality rate to a mild inapparent infection.

Properties of the Agent

A. Size and Staining Properties: Similar to other members of the group (see above).

B. Animal Susceptibility and Growth of Agent: The agent can be propagated in embryonated eggs, in mice and other animals, and in cell cultures.

In all these host systems growth can be inhibited by tetracyclines and, to a limited extent, by penicillins. However, in intact animals and in man, antimicrobial drugs may not be able to eliminate the infectious agent or to terminate the carrier state.

C. Antigenic Properties: Complement-fixing antigens are associated with the agent. There is a heat-labile and a heat-stable component. The heat-labile antigen is also destroyed by phenol, acids, and proteolytic enzymes. The heat-stable antigen resists proteolytic enzymes but is destroyed by potassium periodate, which suggests that it may be a carbohydrate. The heat-stable antigen is shared by all the agents of the group whereas the heat-labile antigen is confined to relatively few.

Infected tissue contains a toxic principle, intimately associated with the agent, which rapidly kills mice upon intravenous or intraperitoneal infection. This toxic principle is active only in particles which are infective.

Specific serotypes characteristic for certain mammalian and avian species may be demonstrated by cross-neutralization tests of toxic effect. Neutralization of infectivity of the agent by specific antibody or cross-protection of immunized animals can also be used for serotyping.

D. Cell Wall Antigens: Walls of the infecting agent have been prepared by treatment with deoxycholate followed by trypsin. The deoxycholate extracts contained group-specific complement-fixing antigens, while the cell walls retained the species-specific antigens. The cell wall antigens were also associated with toxin neutralization and infectivity neutralization.

Pathogenesis & Pathology

The agent enters through the respiratory tract, is found in the blood during the first 2 weeks of the disease, and may be found in the sputum at the time the lung is involved.

Psittacosis causes a patchy inflammation of the lungs in which consolidated areas are sharply demarcated. The exudate is predominantly mononuclear. Only minor changes occur in the large bronchioles and bronchi. The lesions are similar to those found in pneumonitis caused by some viruses and mycoplasma.

Liver, spleen, heart, and kidney are often enlarged and congested.

Clinical Findings

A sudden onset of illness taking the form of influenza or atypical pneumonia in a person exposed to birds is suggestive of psittacosis. The incubation period averages 10 days. The onset is usually sudden, with malaise, fever, anorexia, sore throat, photophobia, and severe headache. The disease may progress no further and the patient may improve in a few days. In severe cases the signs and symptoms of bronchial pneumonia appear at the end of the first week of the disease. The clinical picture often resembles that of influenza, atypical pneumonia, or typhoid fever. The fatality rate may be as high as 20% in untreated cases, especially in the elderly.

Laboratory Diagnosis

A. Recovery of Agent: Laboratory diagnosis is dependent upon the recovery of psittacosis agent from blood and sputum, or, in fatal cases, from lung tissues. Specimens are inoculated intranasally, intra-abdominally, and intracerebrally into mice and into the yolk sacs of embryonated eggs. Infection in the test animals is confirmed by the finding of typical basophilic inclusion bodies and serologic identification of the recovered agent.

B. Serology: A variety of antibodies may develop in the course of infection. In humans, complement fixation with group antigen is the most meaningful diagnostic test. Acute and later phase sera should be run in the same test in order to establish an antibody rise. In birds the indirect complement fixation test may provide additional diagnostic information. Although antibodies usually develop within 10 days, the use of antibiotics may delay their development for 20–40 days, or suppress it altogether.

Sera of patients with LGV may fix complement in high titer with psittacosis antigen. In patients with psittacosis, the high titer persists for months and, in carriers, even for years. Infection of live birds is suggested by a positive complement fixation test and by the presence of an enlarged spleen or liver. This can be confirmed by demonstration of particles in smears or sections of organs and by passage of the agent in mice and eggs.

Immunity

Immunity in animals and man is incomplete. A carrier state in man has been known to occur for 10 years after recovery, even in the presence of antibodies. During this period the agent may continue to be excreted in the sputum.

Skin tests with group reactive antigen are positive soon after infection with any member of the group. Specific dermal reactions may be obtained by the use of some skin-testing antigens prepared by extracting suspensions of agent with dilute hydrochloric acid or with detergent.

Live or inactivated vaccines induce only partial resistance in animals.

Treatment

Tetracyclines are the drugs of choice. Psittacosis agents are not sensitive to streptomycin, and most strains are not susceptible to sulfonamides. While antibiotic treatment may control the clinical evidence of disease, it may not free the patient from the agent, ie, he may become a carrier. Intensive antibiotic treatment may also delay the normal course of antibody development. Strains may become drug-resistant.

With the introduction of antibiotic therapy, the case fatality rate has dropped from 20% to 2%. Death occurs most frequently in patients from 40–60 years of age.

Epidemiology

The term psittacosis is applied to the human disease acquired from contact with birds and also the infection of psittacine birds (parrots, parakeets, cockatoos, etc). The term ornithosis is applied to infection with similar agents in all types of domestic (pigeons, chickens, ducks, geese, turkeys, etc) and free-living birds (gulls, egrets, petrels, etc). Outbreaks of human disease can occur whenever there is close and continued contact between man and infected birds which excrete or shed large amounts of infectious agent. Birds often acquire infection as fledglings in the nest; may develop diarrheal illness or no illness; and often carry the infectious agent for their normal life span. When subjected to stress (eg, malnutrition, shipping), birds may become sick and die. The agent is present in tissues (eg, spleen) and is often excreted in feces by healthy birds. The inhalation of infected dried bird feces is a common method of human infection. Another source of infection is the handling of infected tissues (eg, in poultry rendering plants) and inhalation of an infected aerosol.

Birds kept as pets have been an important source of human infection. Foremost among these were the many psittacine birds imported from South America, Australia, and the Far East and kept in aviaries in the USA. Latent infections often flared up in these birds during transport and crowding, and sick birds excreted exceedingly large quantities of infectious agent. Control of bird shipment, quarantine, testing of imported birds for psittacosis infection, and prophylactic tetracyclines in bird feed help to control this source. Pigeons kept for racing or as pets or raised for squab meat have been important sources of infection. Pigeons populating civic buildings and thoroughfares in many cities are not infrequently infected but shed relatively small quantities of agent.

Among the personnel of poultry farms involved in the dressing, packing, and shipping of ducks, geese, turkeys, and chickens, subclinical or clinical infection is relatively frequent. Outbreaks of disease among birds have at times resulted in heavy economic losses and have been followed by outbreaks in humans.

Persons who develop psittacosis may become infectious for other persons if the evolving pneumonia results in expectoration of large quantities of infectious sputum. This has been an occupational risk to hospital personnel.

Control

Shipments of psittacine birds should be held in quarantine to ensure that there are no obviously sick birds in the lot. A proportion of each shipment should be tested for antibodies and examined for agent. An intradermal test has been recommended for detecting ornithosis in turkey flocks. The incorporation of tetracyclines into bird feed has been used to reduce the number of carriers. The source of human infection should be traced, if possible, and infected birds should be killed.

LYMPHOGRANULOMA VENEREUM (LGV)
(Lymphopathia Venereum)

LGV is a venereal disease, characterized by suppurative inguinal adenitis, which is common in tropical and temperate zones. The agent is related to that of psittacosis.

Properties of the Agent

A. Size and Staining Properties: Similar to other members of the group.

B. Animal Susceptibility and Growth of Agent: The agent can be transmitted to monkeys and mice, and can be propagated in tissue cultures in chick embryos. It does not infect birds readily. Only a few strains have been studied, and there are marked strain differences.

C. Antigenic Properties: The particles contain complement-fixing antigens and also serve as a skin-testing antigen (see Frei test, below). The agent possesses a heat-stable antigen (resistant to boiling) which it shares with other members of the psittacosis group. Infectious particles contain a toxic principle.

Clinical & Pathologic Findings

The progress of this disease is divided into 3 stages. The agent is disseminated widely in the blood, spinal fluid, and spleen during the early stages.

A. First Stage: The primary lesion is a small papule which develops 3–20 days after exposure to infection; it becomes vesicular and then bursts, leaving a shallow, grayish ulcer (lymphogranulomatous chancre). In the male the lesion may be on the glans penis, on the prepuce, or in the anterior urethra. In the female, it may occur either on the vulva or on the mucosa of the vagina or cervix. The initial lesion is painless and often is not noticed.

B. Second Stage: The disease then spreads through the lymphatics. Enlargement of regional lymph nodes usually is found about 2 weeks after the appearance of the primary lesion. The location of the initial lesion determines which glands will be involved. If the lesion is on the penis or vulva, the inguinal glands will be infected (inguinal bubo). In 60% of such cases the glands suppurate, adhere to the overlying skin, and drain pus. If the primary lesion is in the vagina or in the rectum, perirectal and para-aortic lymph nodes are involved. In addition to fever and general aches and pains, there may be rashes, arthritis, conjunctivitis, and meningoencephalitis.

C. Third Stage: The final stage is characterized by a genital and anorectal syndrome. The chronic inflammation of the lymphatics may last for years and induces fibrosis and strictures in the genital tract or rectum.

Elephantiasis of the labia and clitoris (esthiomene) or of the penis and scrotum may occur. Rectal strictures are common in women and in male homosexuals.

Laboratory Diagnosis

A. Smears: Pus, buboes, or biopsy material may be stained but particles are rarely recognized.

B. Isolation of Agent: Suspected material is inoculated into the yolk sacs of embryonated eggs or into the brains of mice. Streptomycin (but not penicillin or ether) may be incorporated into the inoculum to lessen the bacterial contamination. The agent is identified by its morphology and serologic tests. Few isolates have been obtained.

C. Complement Fixation Test: The complement fixation reaction is the simplest serologic test for the presence of antibodies. Antigen is prepared from infected yolk sac. The test becomes positive 2–4 weeks after onset of illness, at which time skin hypersensitivity can sometimes also be demonstrated. In a clinically compatible case, a rising antibody level during the course of the disease is good evidence of active infection. If treatment has eradicated the LGV infection, the complement fixation titer falls.

D. Frei Test (for Dermal Hypersensitivity): 0.1 ml of heat-inactivated agent is injected intradermally. The same amount of control material (prepared in the same way from normal yolk sac) is injected at a separate site. Readings are made after 48–96 hours. The control material should produce a mild reaction or none at all. An inflammatory nodule at the site of injection, reaching its maximum in 4 days and measuring at least 7 mm, constitutes a positive test (7–40 days after infection). The erythema accompanying the skin test has no significance.

Because the important antigen in the inactivated preparation is the heat-stable antigen which the agent shares with the other members of the group, the Frei test is not specific for LGV; a positive test will also be observed in persons infected with members of the group other than LGV. Treatment of the agent with dilute acid (0.02 N HCl) has been found to extract skin-testing antigen. The reactions evoked by such acid extracts appear to be specific for each member of the group.

The Frei test remains positive long after the acute infection has passed, perhaps for life. A positive test means only that infection has occurred; unless it is negative in the acute stage and becomes positive later, the test cannot be used to make a clinical diagnosis of LGV.

Immunity

Untreated infections tend to be chronic with persistence of the agent for many years. Little is known about active immunity. The coexistence of latent infection and antibodies is typical of all agents of the group.

Treatment

The sulfonamides and tetracyclines have been used with good results, especially in the early stages. In some drug-treated persons there is a marked decline in antibody level, which may indicate that the infective agent has been eliminated from the body.

Epidemiology

The disease is most often spread by venereal contact, but not exclusively so. The portal of entry may sometimes be the eye (conjunctivitis with an oculoglandular syndrome). The clinically cured patient may remain infective and continue to spread the disease.

LGV is global in distribution. The disease is reportable only in Alabama, California, Illinois, and Washington. A reservoir of infection may exist among Negroes in certain areas of the USA, as shown by 25–40% positive reactors to the Frei test or the complement fixation test. However, these tests cannot differentiate between LGV and inclusion conjunctivitis of adults, which may present similar clinical pictures.

Control

The measures used for the control of syphilis and gonorrhea apply also to the control of LGV. Case-finding and early medical care and control of infected persons are essential.

TRACHOMA & INCLUSION CONJUNCTIVITIS (TRIC AGENTS)

These 2 eye diseases differ somewhat in clinical and epidemiologic features but are caused by agents very closely related to each other and almost indistinguishable in the laboratory. The TRIC agents are typical members of the psittacosis-lymphogranuloma-trachoma group.

Trachoma is a chronic keratoconjunctivitis characterized by the development of follicles, papillary hypertrophy, and pannus, typically leading to scar formation and sometimes to blindness. Inclusion conjunctivitis is an acute purulent conjunctivitis of the newborn and a follicular conjunctivitis of the adult which does not produce major corneal involvement, scarring, or pannus formation. The usual habitat of the agent of inclusion conjunctivitis is the human genital tract, and in adults a venereal disease results.

Properties of TRIC Agents

A. **Size and Staining Properties**: Similar to other members of the group.

B. **Animal Susceptibility and Growth of TRIC Agents**: The natural host for the TRIC agents is man, and they produce disease only in the eye of man and other primates. All TRIC agents multiply in the yolk sacs of embryonated hen's eggs and result in death of the embryo when the titer is sufficient. TRIC agents can also be serially passaged in irradiated, nonmultiplying human cells in culture. A few isolates can proliferate in cell culture or in intracerebrally inoculated mice.

When TRIC agents multiply in cells they go through a well defined growth cycle. Elementary bodies enter the cell and soon cannot be visualized clearly. After some time, larger "initial bodies" appear near the nucleus of the cell, followed by the development of vacuoles, which gradually enlarge and fill with "elementary body" particles embedded in a matrix of carbohydrate resembling glycogen. This is the picture of the typical intracytoplasmic (Halberstaedter-Prowazek) inclusion which is diagnostic of TRIC infection in conjunctival epithelial cells. Occasional cells contain multiple inclusions. After disruption of cells, free elementary or initial bodies may be found in conjunctival exudates.

A toxic factor is associated with viable TRIC particles. After intravenous inoculation of 10^8 particles into mice, a shock-like state develops in 2–8 hours; this phase is followed by death. Vaccination of mice can specifically protect against this toxic death, and by this method several distinct antigenic types of TRIC agents have been delineated.

Clinical Findings

The incubation period in experimental TRIC infection is 2–9 days, depending upon the infectious dose. Inclusion conjunctivitis of the newborn begins between the fifth and twelfth days of life. The incubation period of naturally occurring trachoma is uncertain because the onset is often insidious.

A. **Trachoma**: The early symptoms of trachoma are lacrimation, mucopurulent discharge, and irritation. Early signs include conjunctival hyperemia and follicular hypertrophy. Biomicroscopic examination of the cornea reveals epithelial keratitis, subepithelial infiltration, and extension of limbal vessels into the cornea (pannus).

Progression of pannus across the cornea, scarring of subepithelial tissues, lid deformities, secondary bacterial infection, and blindness may occur over a period of months to years. There are no systemic symptoms or signs of infection.

B. **Inclusion Conjunctivitis**: Inclusion conjunctivitis is most commonly seen as an acute purulent conjunctivitis of the newborn, involving particularly the lower lids. After several weeks of intense inflammation, the disease gradually subsides and the conjunctiva becomes normal in several months. Pannus or scarring usually does not develop. In adults, eye infection ("swimming pool conjunctivitis") is manifested by follicular conjunctivitis with corneal subepithelial infiltration which usually resolves spontaneously. The genital infection in adults often produces no symptoms or signs. Rarely, spontaneous eye infection of adults with inclusion conjunctivitis agent produces a clinical picture indistinguishable from trachoma.

Laboratory Diagnosis

A. Recovery of TRIC Agents: Typical cytoplasmic inclusions are found in epithelial cells obtained in conjunctival scrapings stained by Giemsa's method or with fluorescent antibody. These are most frequent in early active disease. In trachoma they are most prevalent in the upper tarsal conjunctiva; in inclusion conjunctivitis, the lower lid conjunctiva is more intensively involved.

TRIC agents can be isolated in embryonated eggs inoculated by the yolk sac route. Often several passages are necessary to build up uniformly high titers. The susceptibility of embryonated eggs fluctuates intermittently, even when the eggs are derived from antibiotic-free poultry, perhaps as a result of some interference mechanism. X-irridated, nonmultiplying human cells can be used for isolating the agent and for supporting its growth through multiple passages. Sensitivity can be increased by centrifuging the agent into the cells.

The most sensitive method of establishing the diagnosis appears to be the finding of typical inclusions in conjunctival cells by use of the immunofluorescence technic. Specimens containing TRIC agents can also be centrifuged at high speed onto nonirradiated human cultured cells which can support 1–2 cycles of multiplication of the agent. Subsequent propagation of the isolate must take place in eggs because wild strains undergo only limited multiplication in cell culture.

B. Serology: TRIC agents share a common antigen with other members of the psittacosis-LGV-trachoma group. Individuals infected with TRIC agents often develop antibodies to the group antigen, but these antibodies do not appear to be protective against reinfection. As they are not species-specific, these antibodies have little diagnostic value. Species-specific antigens and antibodies are under study.

Treatment

A. Trachoma: In endemic areas trachoma must be diagnosed and treated in children because it can be affected by drugs before scarring occurs. The tetracyclines and sulfonamides have been most widely used, but the erythromycins may be equally effective. The tetracyclines are often applied topically and sulfonamides given orally. Treatment schedules are determined largely by convenience, cost, and feasibility. The most effective treatment of acute infections may be a combination of systemic sulfonamides for 3 weeks and ophthalmic tetracycline applied 4 times daily for 6 weeks. In chronic infection, full systemic doses of either sulfonamides or tetracyclines can suppress clinical signs but fail to eradicate the infection. Drug-resistant agents have thus far been encountered only in the laboratory. Topical application of corticosteroids is not indicated and can reactivate latent, persistent trachoma infection. The effect of antimicrobial drugs may partly be attributed to elimination of bacterial infections. TRIC agents may persist during and after drug treatment, and relapse is common.

B. Inclusion Conjunctivitis: Inclusion conjunctivitis is similarly susceptible to therapy, and often responds rapidly in the acute stage.

Epidemiology

A. Trachoma: It is believed that over 400 million people throughout the world are infected with trachoma and that 20 million have been blinded by it. Trachoma is spread mechanically from eye to eye by fingers and fomites, eg, shared cosmetics or towels. The disease is most prevalent in Africa and Asia, particularly where hygienic conditions are poor and water is scarce. In such endemic areas infection may be universally acquired in childhood. In the USA trachoma occurs sporadically in many areas, and endemic foci are found on many Indian reservations.

B. Inclusion Conjunctivitis: The epidemiology of inclusion conjunctivitis is quite different from that of trachoma. Inclusion conjunctivitis is fundamentally an infection of the adult human genital tract and is probably spread primarily by sexual contact. In the female the agent grows in the epithelium of the cervix; in the male, in the epithelium of the urethra. The agent enters the eye of the newborn during passage through the birth canal and produces acute conjunctivitis. Adults are occasionally infected by eye-to-eye transfer from the newborn, but most adult infections originate by sexual contact. Thus inclusion conjunctivitis is a typical venereal disease, occasionally manifest in the eye. In the past, infection may have occurred in swimming pools contaminated with genital secretions. However, chlorination has apparently limited this method of spread.

Control

A. Trachoma: Control of trachoma depends upon improvement of hygienic standards and drug treatment, and may be aided in the future by vaccination of children. Experimental vaccines have been prepared from egg-grown purified TRIC agents and can give significant protection to primates. Field studies with such vaccines have given variable and not often promising results. Experimental infection of volunteers and of subhuman primates with one strain of inclusion conjunctivitis agent resulted in resistance to reinfection with the same agent, but left the volunteers still fully susceptible to a second strain. This apparent partial strain-specific immunity may have important implications in the production of vaccines against TRIC agents.

B. Inclusion Conjunctivitis: Chlorination of swimming pools and drug treatment of the genital infection of adults are the principal control measures. Penicillin or silver nitrate instillation into the newborn's eye does not prevent inclusion conjunctivitis.

OTHER AGENTS OF THE GROUP

Many mammals carry infectious agents which are members of the psittacosis-LGV-trachoma group. Common animal disease entities are pneumonitis, arthritis, enteritis, and abortion, but infection is often latent. Some of these agents may also be communicated to man and cause disease in man.

Similar agents have been isolated from Reiter's disease in man, both from the involved joints and from the urethra. The etiologic role of these agents remains to be established.

●   ●   ●

General References

Christoffersen, G., & G.P. Manire: The toxicity of meningopneumonitis organisms (*Chlamydia psittaci*) at different stages of development. J Immunol 103:1085–1088, 1969.

Erskine, D.: Lymphogranuloma venereum. A review of 61 cases. Brit J Ven Dis 34:163–165, 1958.

Gordon, F.B. (editor): The biology of the trachoma agent. Ann New York Acad Sc 98:1–382, 1962.

Jawetz, E.: Chemotherapy of chlamydial infections. Advances Pharmacol Chemother 7:253–282, 1969.

Moulder, J.W.: *The Psittacosis Group as Bacteria*. CIBA Lectures in Microbial Biochemistry. Wiley, 1964.

27...

General Properties of Viruses

Viruses are the smallest infectious agents (20–300 nm in diameter), containing as their genome a molecule of either RNA or DNA which replicates within living cells. At one stage in their replication viruses undergo conversion into a noninfective form which is an essential process of their growth cycle. The viral genome causes the normal metabolic processes of the cell which it invades to be diverted into producing more viral nucleic acid and codes for a protein capable of forming an encasing shell (capsid). The total entity is called a virion, in which the capsid stabilizes the viral nucleic acid so that it survives extracellularly and facilitates its adsorption to, and perhaps penetration of, susceptible cells. Much information on virus-host relationships has been obtained from studies on bacteriophages, the viruses which attack bacteria. This subject is discussed in Chapter 9. Properties of individual viruses are discussed in Chapters 30–39.

Some useful definitions in virology are:

Capsid: The symmetric protein shell which encloses the nucleic acid genome.

Nucleocapsid: The capsid together with the enclosed nucleic acid.

Structure units: The basic building blocks of the capsid. These may be individual polypeptides.

Capsomeres: Morphologic units seen in the electron microscope on the surfaces of isometric virus particles (ie, those with cubic symmetry). They represent clusters of structure units.

Virion: The complete infective virus particle, which may be identical with the nucleocapsid. In more complex virions, this includes the nucleocapsid plus a surrounding envelope.

Primary nucleic acid structure: Primary structure refers to the sequence of bases in the nucleic acid chain.

Secondary structure: This refers to the spatial arrangement of the complete nucleic acid chain, ie, whether it is single- or double-stranded, circular or linear in conformation, branched or unidirectional.

Tertiary structure: Other elements of fine spatial detail in the helix, eg, presence of supercoiling, breakage points, deletions, gaps, catenation, regions of strand separation.

Transcription: The mechanism by which specific information encoded in a nucleic acid chain is transferred to messenger RNA.

Translation: The mechanism by which a particular base sequence in a nucleic acid results in production of a specific amino acid sequence in a protein.

CLASSIFICATION

Basis of Classification

The following properties, listed in the order of preference or importance, have been suggested as a basis for the classification of viruses. The amount of information available in these categories is not uniform for all viruses. For some agents knowledge is at hand about only a few of the properties listed.

(1) Nucleic acid type: RNA or DNA.

(2) Size and morphology, including type of symmetry, number of capsomeres, and presence of membranes.

(3) Susceptibility to physical and chemical agents, especially ether.

(4) Immunologic properties.

(5) Natural methods of transmission.

(6) Host, tissue, and cell tropisms.

(7) Pathology, including inclusion body formation.

(8) Symptomatology.

Classification by Symptomatology

A simple classification based on the human diseases produced by viruses offers certain conveniences for the clinician. However, this is not satisfactory for the biologist, inasmuch as the same virus may appear in several groups because it causes more than one disease depending upon the organ attacked.

A. Generalized Diseases: Diseases in which virus spread in the body is through the blood stream and which do not affect single organs only. Skin rashes may occur. These include smallpox, vaccinia, measles, rubella, chickenpox, yellow fever, dengue, Colorado tick fever, West Nile fever, sandfly fever, pleurodynia, and exanthem subitum; and rash due to enteroviruses, especially echoviruses 4, 9, 16, and 18, and coxsackieviruses A9, A19, B1, and B3.

B. Diseases Primarily Affecting Specific Organs: The virus may spread to the organ through the blood stream, along the peripheral nerves, or by other routes.

1. Diseases of the nervous system—Poliomyelitis, meningitis caused by the enteroviruses (polio-, coxsackie-, and echoviruses), rabies, encephalitis lethargica, arthropod-borne encephalitides, lymphocytic choriomeningitis, herpes simplex, herpes B; and meningoencephalitis of mumps, measles, vaccinia, and others.

2. Diseases of the respiratory tract—Influenza, bronchial pneumonia of children (RS virus, parainfluenza), bronchiolitis (RS virus, parainfluenza), laryngotracheobronchitis (parainfluenza), pharyngoconjunctival fever (adenovirus), common cold (caused by a number of different viruses, eg, rhinoviruses, parainfluenza viruses), and perhaps also primary atypical pneumonia.

3. Localized diseases of the skin or mucous membranes—Herpes simplex, molluscum contagiosum, warts, herpangina, and herpes zoster.

4. Diseases of the eye—Adenovirus conjunctivitis, Newcastle virus conjunctivitis.

5. Diseases of the liver—Infectious hepatitis and serum hepatitis.

6. Diseases of the salivary glands—Mumps and salivary gland virus disease (cytomegalovirus).

Classification by Biologic, Chemical, & Physical Properties (See Table 27–1.)

Viruses can be clearly separated into groups based on the type of nucleic acid and on the size, shape, and substructure of the particle. Within each group (genus) the species subgrouping is based on antigenic differences; such differences are expressed by type numbers. The properties of the main virus groups are discussed briefly below, and in greater detail in the chapters which follow.

A. Poxvirus Group: This group includes members which are chiefly pathogenic for the skin in many animal species. They are relatively large brick-shaped DNA viruses (230 X 300 nm) and have a complex structure (the DNA nucleoid and the entire virus are each enveloped by double membranes). Members of this group, some of which contain a common nucleoprotein antigen, include the viruses of smallpox, ectromelia of mice, fowlpox, molluscum contagiosum, myxoma of rabbits, and vaccinia.

B. Herpesvirus Group: These are medium-sized viruses containing DNA and with a lipid-containing envelope surrounding the viral capsid. The enveloped virion has a diameter of about 200 nm, but the naked virion is only about 110 nm in diameter. Latent infections may occur and last for the life-span of the host, even in the presence of circulating antibodies. Herpes simplex, varicella/zoster, EB, and cytomegaloviruses infect man. Related members occur in monkeys, rabbits, cattle, horses, pigs, dogs, and fowl.

C. Adenovirus Group: These are medium-sized, ether-resistant viruses containing DNA and exhibiting cubic symmetry. Thirty-one types pathogenic for man have been identified. Disease is rarely caused in labora-

tory animals, although certain types produce tumors in newborn hamsters. In man they have a predilection for mucous membranes, and may persist for years in lymphoid tissue.

D. Papovavirus Group: These are small, ether-resistant viruses containing circular DNA and exhibiting cubic symmetry. The human representative is the papilloma or wart virus. Other members are papilloma viruses of rabbits and cattle, polyoma and K viruses of mice, and vacuolating virus (SV40) of monkeys. They have relatively slow growth cycles characterized by replication within the nucleus. Papovaviruses produce latent and chronic infections in their natural hosts, and all are tumorigenic. The simian papovavirus has been injected or fed to millions of persons inadvertently as a contaminant of virus vaccines made in monkey tissue cultures.

E. Parvovirus (Picodnavirus) Group: This group of small DNA viruses includes the hamster osteolytic H viruses, the Kilham rat virus (RV), the X14 virus of rats, minute virus of mice (MVM), and the adeno-satellite viruses. These viruses are small (about 20 nm in diameter) and ether-resistant. They exhibit icosahedral symmetry, and contain DNA. The DNA liberated from adeno-satellites by conventional means acts as double-stranded, but the DNA within the virion stains with acridine orange and reacts with formaldehyde as single-stranded. The single-stranded DNA is present within satellite virions as plus and minus complementary strands in separate particles. Upon extraction of DNA the minus and plus strands unite to form a double-stranded Watson and Crick helix. Adeno-satellites are defective and cannot multiply in the absence of a helper adenovirus. The DNA of nondefective (autonomously replicating) parvoviruses appears to be single-stranded both before and after extraction, indicating that strands of similar polarity are present in all virions.

F. Myxovirus Group: Members are medium-sized viruses containing RNA and essential lipids and exhibiting helical symmetry. The diameter of the internal ribonucleoprotein helix is 6–9 nm. The RNA of the virus is made up of at least 3 components. The spherical viruses are about 100 nm in size, but vary from 80–200 nm. Many particles are pleomorphic; filamentous forms are common. Some contain an enzyme capable of splitting neuraminic acid from mucoproteins, which appears to be the reaction of the virus with cell receptors. The internal helix is synthesized in the nucleus while the hemagglutinin is formed in the cytoplasm. The virus matures at the cell membrane. Myxoviruses, which include the viruses of human and swine influenza and of fowl plague, are sensitive to dactinomycin during the early stages of their replicative cycle. Recently it has been shown that the internal helix of influenza A virus is 6 nm in diameter, whereas that of influenza C is 9 nm.

G. Paramyxovirus Group: Members are morphologically similar to but somewhat larger than the myxoviruses (100–300 nm). The diameter of the helix is 18 nm and the molecular weight of the nucleic acid is about 4 times greater than that of myxovirus RNA.

TABLE 27−1. Classification of viruses into groups based on chemical and physical properties.

Nucleic Acid Core	Capsid Symmetry	Virion: Enveloped or Naked	Ether Sensitivity	No. of Capsomeres	Virus Particle Size (nm)*	Molecular Weight of Nucleic Acid in Virion ($\times 10^6$)	No. of Genes (Approx.)	Virus Group
DNA	Icosahedral	Naked	Resistant	12 or 32	18−24	1.5	7	Parvovirus
				42 or 72	40−55	2−4	10	Papovavirus
				252	70−80	23	50	Adenovirus
		Enveloped	Sensitive	162	180−250 (110)†	40−84	150	Herpesvirus
	Unknown	(Complex)	Resistant		230 × 300	160−240	400	Poxvirus
RNA	Icosahedral	Naked	Resistant	32	18−30	2	10	Picornavirus
				92	70−75	10	50	Reovirus‡
	Unknown §	Enveloped	Sensitive	32§	50−60 (35)§	2	10	Togavirus §
					110**			Tacaribe-LCM**
					80−120			Coronavirus††
	Helical	Enveloped	Sensitive		80−200	2−5	10	Myxovirus
					100−300	7−10	40	Paramyxovirus
					60 × 225	3−4	10	Rhabdovirus
	Unknown	Enveloped	Sensitive		100	10−12	50	Leukovirus‡‡

*Diameter, or diameter × length.

†The naked virus, that is, the nucleocapsid, is 110 nm in diameter; however, the enveloped virion varies from 180−250 nm.

‡Recent evidence indicates that reovirus is one of a large group of viruses possessing double-stranded RNA (diplornaviruses).

§Included in the togavirus group are arboviruses of subgroups A and B. Rubella virus and lactic dehydrogenase (LDH) virus of mice have similar properties. One togavirus that has been studied in detail (Sindbis) has been shown to have a nucleocapsid 35 nm in diameter, containing 32 capsomeres in an icosahedral surface lattice with a triangulation number of T=3. The enveloped virion is about 50 to 60 nm in diameter.

**Lymphocytic choriomeningitis virus recently has been shown to be identical morphologically, and to cross-react serologically, with arboviruses of the Tacaribe complex, which includes the Junin and Machupo viruses of South American hemorrhagic fevers. A new taxonomic group of these RNA-containing, enveloped viruses has been proposed: the Tacaribe-LCM group.

††Included in this group of viruses with petal-shaped surface projections are a number of new human respiratory viruses, avian infectious bronchitis virus (IBV), and mouse hepatitis virus.

‡‡The leukovirus group refers to leukemia viruses of avian, feline, and murine species, since a human leukemia virus has not yet been described.

Both the nucleoprotein and the hemagglutinin antigens are made in the cytoplasm. The following viruses are included in this group: parainfluenza, respiratory syncytial, measles, and mumps of man; and Newcastle disease, distemper, and rinderpest of animals. The paramyxoviruses are resistant to the action of dactinomycin.

H. Rhabdovirus Group: This recently proposed group includes members that have an unusual morphology. Their structure is rod-shaped, resembling a bullet, flat at one end and rounded at the other (Fig 27−30). For animal members, the diameter of the cylinder is 65 nm and the length about 225 nm. An internal helix, resembling the nucleoprotein helix of the paramyxoviruses, has been observed for several members of this group. Members of this group include the following viruses: rabies virus, vesicular stomatitis virus of cattle, hemorrhagic septicemia virus of rainbow trout, Hart Park (Flanders) virus, cocal and sigma viruses of insects, and at least 3 viruses of plants (lettuce necrotic yellow, maize mosaic, and wheat striate mosaic).

I. Arbovirus Group: This is an ecologic grouping of over 150 viruses which survive through a complex cycle involving biting arthropods. They multiply in a variety of species, including man, horses, domestic and wild birds, bats, snakes, and insects (mosquitoes, ticks). On the basis of the antigenic overlap, they have been divided into several groups. Groups A and B, which have been most studied, are small (about 40 nm in diameter) and contain essential lipid. Those that

have been examined contain RNA. Common members pathogenic for man include the viruses of dengue, eastern and western equine encephalitis, Japanese encephalitis, St. Louis encephalitis, and yellow fever. Rubella virus has a similar size and morphology.

Included among arboviruses (an ecologic grouping) are members of other groups: rhabdovirus (vesicular stomatitis), reovirus (Colorado tick fever), and other diplornaviruses (bluetongue, African horse sickness), togaviruses, and the Tacaribe-LCM group.

J. Reovirus (Diplornavirus) Group: Reoviruses are medium-sized (75 nm in diameter), ether-resistant viruses containing double-stranded RNA and exhibiting cubic symmetry. Strains recovered from lower animals (chimpanzees, monkeys, cattle, mice) are indistinguishable from those of man. Antibodies occur in domestic animals.

Diplornaviruses form 2 subgroups based on the structure of the capsid. One group, with reovirus as its prototype and including Colorado tick fever and wound tumor viruses, possesses a double-layered capsid with 92 morphologic units in the outer layer. The other, represented by the bluetongue and horse sickness viruses as type species, has a smaller (40 nm) single-layered capsid consisting of 32 capsomeres.

K. Picornavirus Group: This group is subdivided into enteroviruses and rhinoviruses. At least 63 human enteroviruses are known; these include the polio-, coxsackie-, and echoviruses. Other types exist throughout the animal kingdom. More than 90 rhinoviruses have been isolated and are the most common cause of colds in man. Rhinoviruses are known to exist in other species; the most studied rhinovirus of animals is foot-and-mouth disease virus of cattle. Picornaviruses are small, ether-resistant viruses, containing RNA and exhibiting cubic symmetry. Unlike almost all other viruses, they are stabilized by $MgCl_2$ to thermal inactivation. The rhinoviruses are acid-labile and have a high density (1.4 gm/cu cm), and in these properties differ from the enteroviruses, which are acid-resistant and have a density of 1.34 gm/cu cm.

L. Leukoviruses: These include the avian leukosis complex and murine and feline leukemia viruses. They are characterized by RNA of high molecular weight. No leukoviruses of man have been identified as yet.

M. Coronavirus Group: Members of this newly defined group morphologically resemble the myxoviruses, with the exception that the surface projections are petal-shaped. The human strains of the virus group were isolated from patients with acute upper respiratory tract illness, primarily through the use of human embryonic tracheal and nasal organ cultures. Coronaviruses are known for lower animals: mouse hepatitis virus, rat pneumotropic virus, and avian infectious bronchitis virus.

N. Togavirus Group: Members of this group include most arboviruses of groups A and B, rubella virus and LDH (lactate dehydrogenase) virus of mice. Members of the group possess a lipid-containing envelope and are similar in size; the enveloped virion is 50–60 nm in diameter. They mature by budding from the cytoplasmic and plasma cell membranes. Although the capsid symmetry of most members is as yet unknown, recent studies of one member of the group, Sindbis virus, have revealed a nonhemagglutinating nucleocapsid 35 nm in diameter, with 32 capsomeres in an icosahedral surface lattice with a triangulation number of T=3. Within the nucleocapsid a further spherical structure (12–16 nm in diameter) was present as the central core component. Two proteins were found associated with the nucleocapsid, while a third viral protein was associated with the hemagglutinating surface envelope.

O. Tacaribe-LCM Group: This grouping of viruses has been proposed recently because of the morphologic and biologic similarity and serologic cross-reaction that have been found between arboviruses of the Tacaribe complex (including the Junin and Machupo viruses of South American hemorrhagic fevers) and lymphocytic choriomeningitis (LCM) virus. These RNA-containing, enveloped viruses have a mean diameter of 110 nm, with a range of 50–300 nm. The virions contain a number of electron-dense, RNA-containing granules about 20 nm in diameter which are indistinguishable in size, shape, and density from ribosomes. Antisera to all members of the Tacaribe complex react with LCM virus in the indirect fluorescent antibody test.

P. There are some viruses for which there are insufficient data to permit their inclusion in any of the above groups. These include viruses which cause infectious and serum hepatitis. However, they seem to belong to the "pico" viruses.

GENERAL PROPERTIES

Viruses are made up of nucleic acid contained within a protein coat. Animal and bacterial viruses contain either DNA or RNA, but not both, whereas plant viruses contain RNA. The usual procedure for isolating nucleic acid from the whole virion involves (1) lysis of the viral protein coat by a suitable detergent like sodium dodecyl sulfate, and (2) deproteinization of the nucleic acid by pronase and phenol.

Enteroviruses and arboviruses are among the animal viruses which have yielded an infectious RNA. Papovaviruses and bacteriophages have yielded infectious DNA. The infectious nucleic acid is inactivated by treatment with the respective nuclease (ribo- or deoxyribonuclease), whereas the intact virus is not affected by such nuclease treatment since it is protected by the protein coat. By contrast, antiserum against the virus will neutralize a virus because it reacts with the antigens of the protein coat, but the same antiserum is without effect when in contact with the free infectious viral nucleic acid.

Viruses call forth a different tissue response than do pathogenic bacteria, not only in the parenchymatous cells but also in cellular infiltration. Whereas polymorphonuclear leukocytes form the principal cellular response to the acute inflammation caused by pyogenic bacteria, infiltration with mononuclear cells and lymphocytes characterizes the inflammatory reaction of uncomplicated viral lesions.

A number of viruses are "toxic," ie, injection of concentrated suspensions will kill mice within a few hours. Pathologic examination of such animals reveals little except intense vascular congestion (the result of increased permeability of capillaries).

EVOLUTION OF VIRUSES

Three hypotheses have been brought forward to explain the origin of viruses.

(1) Viruses became parasites of the first cellular organisms, and present-day viruses are the direct descendants of these earliest subcellular structures. As new organisms and animals evolved, new viruses evolved with them. It is of interest in this connection that human beings may be harmlessly infected with latent herpes simplex virus for life and that monkeys may be infected in similar fashion with another type of herpesvirus. These viral species probably had a common origin; however, if man is accidentally infected with the monkey herpesvirus with which he has had no evolutionary experience, the infection is usually fatal.

(2) Viruses are not individual organisms but components of normal cells which sometimes get out of hand. Within the cell the virus might exert an auto-

catalytic property so that replicas of itself are formed from the materials within the cell. They might be said to resemble genes which have gotten out of control and continue to multiply as long as there is building material available. Cells of certain plant species, for example, contain what appear to be completely normal constituents of the species. However, when extracts of such cells are inoculated into other plants, the recipient host, if susceptible, behaves as if it has been inoculated with a true virus. If the second (susceptible) host were not known, the fact that the first host contained material of a viral nature would never have been recognized. This phenomenon has recently been shown to exist in rubella virus cultures derived from babies who acquired their infections in utero.

A corollary of this hypothesis is that viruses are derivatives of normal cellular genes (nucleic acids) which many eons ago became capable of autonomous replication and acquired the genetic information for coding for capsid protein. The capsid is essential in order to stabilize the nucleic acid of the subcellular organelle in its travel from cell to cell. Cancer viruses may exist in normal cells as repressed genes.

(3) Viruses have evolved from pathogenic bacteria through a retrograde evolutionary process. Certain bacteria have developed a highly specialized parasitic existence and grow with difficulty outside the host cells. They have given up some of the functions (mediated by enzymes) necessary for their independent existence, because these have been supplied by the parasitized cell. Rickettsiae and the agents of psittacosis and lymphogranuloma venereum appear to be good examples of intracellular organisms which have undergone parasitic degeneration. These are not viruses, however. There is at present no evidence to support the theory that true viruses have evolved from bacteria.

The recently discovered adeno-satellite virus is actually a defective virus and cannot replicate unless an adenovirus induces the cell to make the enzymes necessary for its replication. Such small viruses may have reached the very summit of parasitism.

Analysis of the patterns of nearest neighbor base sequences in the DNA of mammalian viruses suggests that small viruses (eg, papovaviruses) which contain very little information would conform closely in their frequency pattern to the doublet pattern of the host cells, which indeed they do. Doublet patterns of larger viruses (adeno-, pox-, herpesvirus) show only a limited resemblance to that of mammalian DNA. These results suggest that papovaviruses have evolved from cells of their hosts, whereas herpes-, pox-, and adenoviruses are probably of external origin.

BIOPHYSICAL PROPERTIES OF VIRUSES

Virus Particles & Electron Microscopy

Advances in x-ray diffraction technics and electron microscopy have made it possible to resolve fine differences in the basic morphology of viruses.

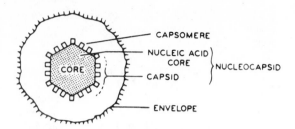

FIG 27–1. Schematic diagram illustrating the components of the complete virus particle or the virion.

The term "virion" is used for the complete infective virus particle, "capsid" for the protein coat, and "capsomere" for each of the protein morphologic subunits (Fig 27–1). The individual protein molecules that make up the capsomere are called the "structural units." More complicated virions may possess additional layers or envelopes which do not appear to be symmetric.

The capsids of animal viruses are arranged in 2 forms of symmetry: (1) helical symmetry (eg, myxoviruses) and (2) cubic symmetry (eg, picornaviruses). All cubic symmetry so far found in the animal viruses is of the icosahedral (5:3:2) pattern. The icosahedron is one of the 5 regular polyhedra of classical geometry. It has 20 faces, each an equilateral triangle, 12 vertices, and 5-fold, 3-fold, and 2-fold axes of rotational symmetry. The number of ways in which capsomeres can be arranged to comply with icosahedral symmetry is limited. In its simplest form this limitation may be expressed by the formula $N = 10(n-1)^2 + 2$, where N is the total number of capsomeres and n the number of capsomeres on one side of each equilateral triangle. Table 27–2 shows the number of capsomeres where n varies from 2–10, and the corresponding virus groups in this series.

Viruses exhibiting icosahedral symmetry can also be grouped according to their triangulation number, T, which for one class has values of 1, 4, 9, 16, and 25; for a second class, values of 3 and 12; and for a third

TABLE 27–2.

Virus	n	T	Capsomeres
Phage (ϕX-174)	2	1	12
Picorna group*	2	3	32
Papova group†	3	4	42
		7	72
Reo group	4	9	92
Herpes group	5	16	162
Adeno group	6	25	252
Iridescent group	10	81	812

*Picornaviruses are a special case and, for $n = 2$, fit the formula $N = 30 (n-1)^2 + 2$ (see below).

†At present the capsomere number (42 or 72) for this group of viruses is unsettled because of differences in the interpretation of electron micrographs. Recently examples of T = 1 and T = 3 structures have also been observed in papovavirus preparations.

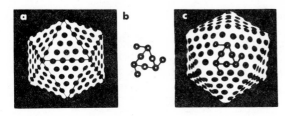

FIG 27–2. **(a)** Representation of the capsomere arrangement of an adenovirus particle, as viewed through the 2-fold axis of symmetry. **(b)** Arrangement of capsomere group of 9, obtained by treatment of an adenovirus with sodium lauryl sulfate. **(c)** Orientation of the capsomere group of 9 on the adenovirus particle.

class, values of 7, 13, 19, and 21. The number of morphologic units (capsomeres) is expressed by the formula M = 10T + 2. Table 27–2 shows the triangulation number for several virus groups.

An example of icosahedral symmetry is seen in Fig 27–2. The adenovirus ($n = 6$) model illustrated shows the 6 capsomeres along one edge (Fig 27–2[a]). Degradation of this virus with sodium lauryl sulfate releases the capsomeres in groups of 9 (Fig 27–2[b], [c]) and possibly groups of 6. The groups of 9 lie on the faces, plus one capsomere from each of the 3 edges of the face, and the groups of 6 would be from the vertices. The groups of 9 from the faces of the 20 triangular facets making the adenovirus icosahedron account for 180 subunits, and the groups of 6 which form the 12 vertices account for 72 capsomeres, thus totaling 252.

Viral Protein

The structural proteins of the viruses have several important functions. They serve to protect the viral genome against inactivation by nucleases, participate in the attachment of the virus particle to a susceptible cell, and are responsible for the structural symmetry of the virus particle. Also, the proteins determine the antigenicity of the virus, which is of importance in vaccine production and in viral diagnosis, particularly in distinguishing between closely related viruses. Thus far, the structural proteins of only a few viruses have been extensively examined. A good example of such a study was carried out with the picornaviruses. Electron microscopy has recently revealed that the capsids are composed of 32 morphologic subunits arranged to comply with the icosahedral form of cubic symmetry—but in the form of a rhombic triacontahedron (30 faces, each a rhombus) rather than a regular icosahedron. The results of x-ray crystallographic studies have also shown that the crystalline virus possesses icosahedral symmetry, and that the protein shell is composed of 60 structural units, or a multiple of 60 (a requirement for icosahedral symmetry). Now that the chemical subunits (ie, the individual polypeptide chains in the protein shell of the virus) have been studied, the most likely interpretation compatible with the x-ray and electron microscope results is that the structural

units are arranged in 12 groups of 5 identical polypeptide chains (around the 5-fold axis of symmetry) and 20 groups of 6 chains (around the 3-fold axis of symmetry), which corresponds to a total of 180 polypeptide chains in each virus particle. The molecular weight of these chains is approximately 25,000 for poliovirus. The protein shell forms a compact and highly stable structure which protects the infectious RNA; thus, the RNA does not contribute to the surface properties of the virus, such as electrophoretic mobility, serologic specificity, etc. The viral RNA has been isolated and shown to be infectious in the absence of protein. Each infective virion contains a single molecule of RNA with a molecular weight of 2 million. Little is known of the binding of the RNA to the protein.

The morphologic and x-ray studies of poliovirus have been extended, using polyacrylamide gel electrophoresis. By this technic, purified virus particles are disrupted to polypeptides by detergents and analyzed by electrophoresis on polyacrylamide gels. Such studies have shown that poliovirus contains 4 polypeptides: VP 1 (MW = 3.5×10^4 daltons) VP 2 (MW = 2.8×10^4 daltons), VP 3 (MW = 2.4×10^4 daltons), and VP 4 (MW = 6×10^3 daltons). While the exact location of these polypeptides in the virus particle has yet to be resolved, their molecular weight is close to that obtained by x-ray and electron microscopic studies. Polyacrylamide gel electrophoresis analysis has also been carried out on virus particles devoid of their RNA that have been separated from infectious virus by density gradient centrifugation. These particles were found to contain only VP 1 and VP 3 as well as a new polypeptide, VP 0. It is suggested that this RNA-free particle (or procapsid, as it has been termed) is a precursor of the infectious virus, and that, as the RNA becomes associated with the procapsid in some as yet unknown fashion, VP 0 is cleaved to yield VP 2 and VP 4. The mechanism of cleavage is unknown, but the possibility exists that one of the 3 procapsid polypeptides (VP 0, VP 1, or VP 3) may possess an appropriate enzyme activity.

In addition to the structural proteins, other virus-specific proteins are formed in an infected cell. For example, it has been shown that a new virus-specific enzyme, thymidine kinase, is found in herpes- and vaccinia-infected cells.

Viral Nucleic Acid

Virus particles contain either DNA or RNA (but not both), which carries the genetic information necessary for the replication of the virus. The molecular weight and type of nucleic acid are specific for each virus group (Table 27–1). The picornaviruses contain single-stranded RNA, whereas reoviruses contain double-stranded RNA. The molecular weight of biologically active viral RNA can range from as low as 1×10^6 daltons for bromegrass mosaic virus and 2×10^6 for polio- and influenza viruses to as large as 10×10^6 for reoviruses (Table 27–1). (One dalton equals the mass of one hydrogen atom.) The DNA animal viruses

TABLE 27–3. Identification of viral nucleic acids with acridine orange (AO).

Carnoy-Fixed Virus Smear	Color Reaction With 0.01% AO At pH 4.0	Enzyme Susceptibility	
		DNase	RNase
Double-stranded DNA virus	Yellow	+	−
Single-stranded DNA virus	Red	+	−
Single-stranded RNA virus	Red	−	+
Double-stranded RNA virus	Yellow	−	+

have a DNA molecular weight of the order of 2×10^6 daltons for the papovaviruses to 240×10^6 for the poxviruses.

The number of genes in a virus can be approximated (Table 27–1) if one assumes the following: (1) the genetic code is triplet and nonoverlapping; (2) nucleic acid of 10^6 daltons molecular weight in the form of a single strand (ie, the replicating form) contains 6000 nucleotides; and (3) the viral genes code for proteins, each containing about 200 amino acids.

The type of nucleic acid can be determined by a number of methods, using either the intact virus particle or the free nucleic acid. Both the type of nucleic acid and the strandedness can be determined by a simple fluorochrome procedure in the fluorescence microscope. After fixation with an alcoholic fixative, smears of purified virus preparations can be stained with acridine orange (pH 4.0, dye concentration 0.01%) and the nucleic acids identified by color reactions and enzyme digestion tests (Table 27–3).

Uranyl acetate has been shown to be a specific stain for DNA while having no affinity for RNA. The presence or absence of the stain in a virus can be determined in the electron microscope. Using the free nucleic acid, it is possible to determine the type by specific chemical reactions, ie, by treatment with specific nucleases or testing for the type of sugar (ribose or deoxyribose) present. Density gradient centrifugation in cesium salts can also be used to differentiate between DNA and RNA.

The quality of a virus preparation—ie, the ratio of complete particles with nucleic acid to empty viral capsids (protein shells)—can be determined in the electron microscope using heavy metal stains. Potassium phosphotungstate permeates the virus particle as a cloud and brings out the surface structure of viruses by virtue of "negative staining." It also enters into the center of coreless virus particles which do not contain nucleic acid and therefore are noninfectious. Thus the ratio of complete particles with nucleic acid to empty viral capsids (protein shells) can be determined at different stages of the growth cycle.

Although most viral genomes are physically quite fragile once they are removed from their protective protein capsid, it is now possible to examine many nucleic acid molecules in the electron microscope without disrupting them. The molecules are captured and spread in a special inert protein monofilm so that their complete contour lengths can be measured accurately. While most viral nucleic acids are linear, in some

instances (phage ϕX-174 and papovaviruses) the molecule takes the form of a circle—in the case of papovaviruses, a double-stranded circle. This circle is often hypercoiled (Fig 27–3). Using linear densities of approximately 2×10^6 daltons per micrometer for double-stranded nucleic acid and 1×10^6 daltons for single-stranded forms, molecular weights of viral genomes can be calculated from direct measurements (Table 27–1). The in vitro synthesis of small RNA and DNA viral genomes has been accomplished (see p 290).

The nucleic acid of reovirus is RNA; like other diplornaviruses, it fits a model of a double-helical polynucleotide with complementary strands running in opposite directions, similar to double-stranded DNA. However, the genome of reovirus may not be a single RNA helix, for the virus may contain several fragments of double-stranded RNA rather than a single RNA molecule. These fragments have been isolated both from intact viral particles and from cells in which reovirus is replicating, and this evidence, combined with the demonstration that these fragments are the intracellular templates for messenger RNA transcription, suggests that the reovirus genome is composed of a combination of different RNA molecules. Three dif-

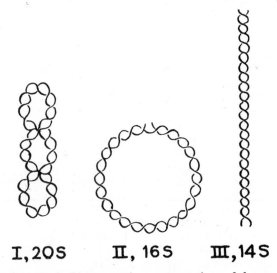

I, 20 S   II, 16 S   III, 14 S

FIG 27–3. Diagrammatic representation of hypercoiled (I), circular (II), and linear (III) forms of polyoma DNA. (After Vinograd.) Each morphologic form is associated with a specific sedimentation coefficient S. (The molecule probably exists in the virion in the hypercoiled formation.)

ferent fragments, with sedimentation coefficients of 14, 12, and 10.5 S (classes L, M, and S), can be isolated from reovirus virions, with a frequency in the complete virion of 2:2:3. The fragments are double-stranded as judged by the observations that they exhibit a sharp melting profile; they are resistant to ribonuclease; the sedimentation behavior is independent of ionic concentrations; and the base composition displays equality of A and U as well as G and C. An adenine-rich RNA fragment (82%) is also released from the reovirus virion. This RNA, which is of small size (2–3 S), makes up 20% of the viral genome and is synthesized at the same time as the double-stranded segments. It has been speculated that this adenine-rich material may serve to link together the double-stranded RNA fragments.

Viral Lipids

Relatively little information is available concerning viral lipids, primarily because of problems presented by the separation of lipids that are intimately associated with the virus from contaminating host cell lipids. The viruses that contain essential lipids as part of their structure have been shown to be ether-sensitive (Table 27–1). The lipids are generally added as the virus matures or buds through the membrane of the cell (Fig 27–4 and Fig 40–3). In this process, the host membranes are incorporated into the complete virus particle. However, there is some virus-specific change in the membranes of the infected cell, since differences do exist between the normal cell and the infected cell membranes. Thus, the limiting membrane of the myxoviruses contains enzyme activity (neuraminidase) that is not found in normal membranes.

This is further exemplified in a comparative study of the lipids of membranes of SV5, a simian parainfluenza virus, grown in primary rhesus monkey kidney (MK) and baby hamster kidney (BHK) cells. The lipid patterns of the membranes of these 2 cell types are significantly different from each other, especially with regard to the phospholipids. In MK membranes, phosphatidylethanolamine is the major phospholipid, and there is a relatively high content of phosphatidylserine, whereas in BHK membranes, phosphatidylcholine is present in highest amount, and there is relatively little phosphatidylethanolamine and phosphatidylserine. SV5 virions grown in MK or BHK cells have a lipid composition that is closely similar to that of the plasma membrane of the particular cell type in which the virus was grown. The data support the hypothesis that during the maturation of the virion by budding from the cell surface, lipids of the cell plasma membrane are incorporated into the viral envelope.

Herpesviruses are assembled into their nucleocapsid in the cell nucleus, and acquire envelopes from the nuclear rather than cytoplasmic membranes (Fig 27–5). The mechanisms seem to be: Virus is assembled in the nucleus and approaches the nuclear membrane (1). At the point of contact, the inner nuclear membrane becomes thicker and more electron dense. This membrane progressively envelops the virus particle

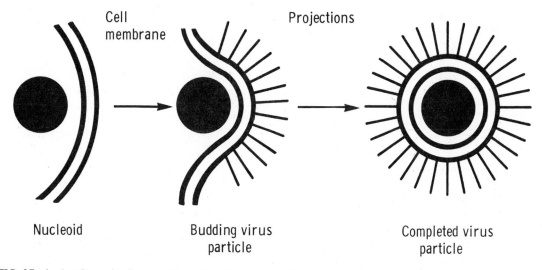

FIG 27–4. A schematic diagram illustrating the process of formation of a group A arbovirus particle. Left: A virus nucleoid, assembled elsewhere in the cytoplasmic matrix, approaches the plasma membrane, represented as a triple-layered unit membrane. **Center:** As the nucleoid buds through the membrane, a coating of projections is added to the outside of the membrane. **Right:** The virus particle, consisting of a nucleoid wrapped in a piece of membrane surrounded by projections, has been completed and lies free in the extracellular space. The diagram is drawn roughly to scale: the nucleoid is 28 nm in diameter, the unit membrane is 7.5 nm thick and separated from the nucleoid by a narrow (1–3 nm) space, and the projections are 11 nm long, making the whole virus particle approximately 70 nm in diameter. (From Acheson & Tamm.)

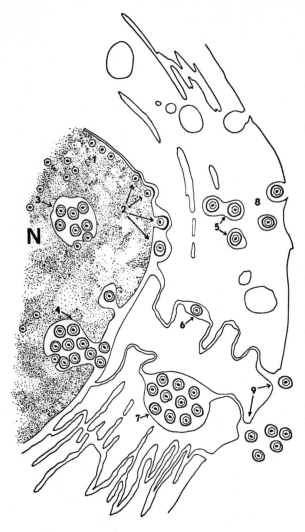

FIG 27–5. Envelopment and release of herpesvirus from infected cells. The numbers refer to specific steps in the process as discussed in text. (Darlington & Moss.)

(2) and finally pinches off, leaving the nuclear membrane intact and the enveloped particle free in the perinuclear cisterna. Nucleocapsids also may acquire envelopes by budding into nuclear vacuoles (3). These vacuoles seem to be indentations of the nuclear membrane cut in cross section, and are continuous with the perinuclear cisterna (4). The virus particle is now transported from the vicinity of the nucleus to an extracellular location. The outer lamella of the nuclear envelope wraps around the enveloped nucleocapsid and sequesters it from the cell cytoplasm (5). When the vacuole reaches the cytoplasmic membrane, the enveloped virion is released outside the cell (8). An additional route seems to be through the cistérnae of the endoplasmic reticulum (6, 7) to the exterior of the cell (9).

Later in the infection unenveloped particles may also appear in the cytoplasm where they may be enveloped, but breaks in the nuclear membrane are also present at this time. The envelopment process occurs whenever the nucleocapsid comes into contact with a cell membrane and may represent a cellular defense mechanism. Since the nuclear membrane is the first membrane encountered, it would be the primary site of envelopment.

MEASURING THE SIZE OF VIRUSES

Small size and ability to pass through filters which hold back bacteria are classical attributes of viruses. However, because some bacteria may be smaller than the largest viruses, filtrability is no longer regarded as a unique feature of viruses.

The following methods are used for determining the sizes of viruses, and of their components.

Filtration Through Collodion Membranes of Graded Porosity

The membranes with large pores allow the largest viruses to pass through readily; those with the smallest pores allow only small molecules like those of water and salt to pass through while small viruses and even protein molecules are held back. If the virus preparation is passed through a series of membranes of known pore size, the approximate size of any virus can be measured by determining which membranes allow the infective unit to pass and which hold it back. The size of the limiting APD (average pore diameter), multiplied by 0.64, yields the diameter of the virus particle. The limiting pore diameter is the diameter of the pores of a membrane which just allows the virus to pass or the average APD of the 2 membranes, one of which allows the virus to pass freely while the other holds it back completely.

Sedimentation in the Ultracentrifuge

If particles are suspended in a liquid and allowed to stand, they will settle to the bottom at a rate which is in proportion to their size. In an ultracentrifuge, forces of more than 100,000 times gravity may be used to drive the particles to the bottom of the tube. The relationship between the size of a particle and its rate of sedimentation permits determination of particle size.

Direct Observation in the Electron Microscope

As compared with the light microscope, the electron microscope uses electrons rather than light waves, and electromagnetic lenses rather than glass lenses. The electron beam obtained has a much shorter wavelength than that of light, so that objects much smaller than the wavelength of visible or ultraviolet light can be visualized. Viruses can be visualized not only in preparations made from tissue extracts but also in ultrathin sections of infected cells.

Ionizing Radiation

When a beam of charged particles such as high-energy electrons, alpha particles, or deuterons passes through a virus, it causes an energy loss in the form of primary ionization. The release of ionization within the virus particle inactivates certain biologic properties of the virus particle such as infectivity, antigenicity, and hemagglutination.

From the number of ionizations per unit volume or area which will destroy all but 37% of the biologic activity of the virus, the average sensitive volume or area per ionization can be determined. This is the point at which, according to the Poisson distribution, there has been an average of one hit per sensitive target, and so the volume or area per ionization is equivalent to the volume or area of the sensitive unit measured. Knowing the volume or area, one can readily calculate the diameter or area of the infective unit (or other biologic unit) in the virus particle. If the virus particle has properties other than infectivity, the rate of loss of each property will be proportionate to the size of the unit which governs the property in question. In this way the sizes of complement-fixing antigens and of hemagglutinins within the virus particle have been determined for certain viruses.

Comparative Measurements (See Table 27–1.)

For purposes of reference, it should be recalled that:

(1) Staphylococcus has a diameter of about 1000 nm.

(2) Bacterial viruses (bacteriophages) vary in size (10–100 nm). Some are spherical or hexagonal and have short or long tails.

(3) Representative protein molecules range in diameter from serum albumin (5 nm) and globulin (7 nm) to certain hemocyanins (23 nm).

It should be pointed out also that particles with a 2-fold difference in diameter have an 8-fold difference in volume. Thus, the mass of a poxvirus is about 1000 times greater than that of the poliovirus particle, and the mass of a small bacterium is 50,000 times greater.

Throughout this text, in accordance with modern terminology, the term **nanometer** (nm) is used to express a length of 10^{-9} meter, instead of the old term, millimicron (mμ), and the term micrometer (μm; 10^{-6} meter) instead of the old term, micron (μ).

PURIFICATION OF VIRUS PARTICLES

With the application of tissue culture methods to the growth and assay of virus infectivity, quantities of materials such as never existed before became available for purification studies. A variety of technics are avail-able, but the multistep procedure developed for the preparation of a very highly purified poliovirus suspension serves as a good illustration: (1) Precipitation of the virus from tissue culture fluid with 15% methyl alcohol at pH 4.0, and elution of the precipitate with 1/50 volume of molar NaCl solution at pH 9.0. (2) Two extractions with N-butanol. (3) Reprecipitation and elution of virus as in (1), but without methanol. (4) One cycle of high- and low-speed ultra-centrifugation. (5) Treatment with crystalline ribo- and deoxyribonucleases. (6) A final cycle of high- and low-speed ultracentrifugation.

Evidence for the high degree of homogeneity of the purified poliovirus preparations, which have been concentrated 50,000 times over the virus concentration of the original tissue culture fluid, is their ability to crystallize.

Equilibrium Density Gradient Centrifugation

Viruses can also be purified by high-speed centri-fugation in density gradients of cesium chloride (CsCl), potassium tartrate, potassium citrate, or sucrose. The gradient material of choice is the one that is least toxic to the virus. A density gradient is either preformed mechanically or in some cases (eg, CsCl) can be estab-lished during centrifugation. Virus particles migrate to an equilibrium position where the density of the solu-tion is equal to their buoyant density and the virus particles form a visible band. Virus bands may be harvested by puncture through the bottom of the plastic centrifuge tube and then assayed for infectivity. Viruses demonstrating cubic symmetry are banded in CsCl, since they are relatively stable in its presence. Relatively crude preparations of these viruses can be used, since they band at a density in the range of 1.3–1.4 gm/cu cm, whereas cell proteins float at 1.25 and free DNA bands at 1.7. Viruses exhibiting helical symmetry are generally unstable in the presence of CsCl, but have been successfully banded in potassium tartrate and citrate and in sucrose. In potassium citrate, murine leukemia viruses band at 1.16 and most myxoviruses at 1.20.

IDENTIFICATION OF A PARTICLE AS A VIRUS

When a characteristic physical particle has been obtained from various tissues, it should fulfill as many as possible of the following criteria before it is identi-fied as the virus particle. In brief, these are as follows: (1) The particle can be obtained only from infected cells or tissues. (2) Particles obtained from various sources are identical, regardless of the cellular species in which the virus is grown. (3) The degree of infective activity of the virus varies directly with the number of particles present. (4) The degree of destruction of the physical particle by chemical or physical means is asso-ciated with a corresponding loss of virus activity.

(5) Certain properties of the particles and virus must be shown to be identical, such as their sedimentation behavior in the ultracentrifuge and their pH stability curves. (6) The absorption spectrum of the purified physical particle in the ultraviolet range should coincide with the ultraviolet inactivation spectrum of the virus. (7) Antisera prepared against the infective virus should react with the characteristic particle and vice versa. (8) The particles should be able to induce the characteristic disease in vivo (if such experiments are feasible). (9) Passage of the particles in tissue culture should result in the production of progeny with biologic and serologic properties of the virus.

REACTION TO PHYSICAL & CHEMICAL AGENTS

Heat & Cold

Virus infectivity is generally destroyed by heating at 50–60° C for 30 minutes, although there are some notable exceptions (eg, serum hepatitis virus, adenosatellite virus).

Viruses can be preserved by storage at subfreezing temperatures, and some may withstand lyophilization and can thus be preserved in the dry state at 4° C or even at room temperature. Viruses which withstand lyophilization are more heat resistant when heated in the dry state.

Stabilization of Viruses by Salts

Many viruses can be stabilized by molar concentrations of salts. That is, they are not inactivated even by heating at 50° C for 1 hour. The mechanism by which the salts stabilize virus preparations is not known. Viruses are preferentially stabilized by certain salts (Table 27–4).

The stability of viruses is of particular importance in the preparation of poliovaccines, since the ordinary nonstabilized vaccine must be stored at freezing temperatures to preserve its potency. However, with the addition of salts for stabilization of the virus, potency can be maintained for weeks at the elevated ambient temperatures found in many parts of the world. In addition, heating of some virus preparations in the presence of high salt concentrations can be used to remove adventitious agents. For example, heating poliovirus suspensions in molar $MgCl_2$ will inactivate such simian contaminants as SV40, foamy virus, and herpes B virus, but have no deleterious effect on the infectivity of poliovirus.

pH

Viruses are usually stable between pH values of 5.0 and 9.0. However, because of the electrostatic forces in the hemagglutination reactions, variations of a few tenths of a pH unit may be the deciding factor in obtaining positive or negative results in this test.

Radiation

Ultraviolet, x-ray, and high-energy particles inactivate viruses. The dose varies for different viruses.

Vital Dyes

Viruses are penetrable to a varying degree by vital dyes such as toluidine blue, neutral red, and acridine orange. These dyes unite with the viral nucleic acid, and the virus then becomes susceptible to inactivation by visible light. A gradient of this photodynamic inactivation ranges from viruses which are impenetrable and therefore not inactivated (eg, polioviruses) through those which are moderately susceptible (adenovirus, reovirus) to those which are readily inactivated (herpesvirus, vaccinia). Impenetrable viruses like poliovirus, when grown in the dark in the presence of vital dyes, incorporate the dye into their nucleic acid and are then susceptible to photodynamic inactivation. The coat antigen is unaffected by the process.

Ether Susceptibility

Ether susceptibility has been useful for distinguishing viruses that possess a lipid-rich envelope from those that do not. The following viruses are inactivated by ether: herpes-, myxo-, paramyxo-, rhabdo-, corona-, leuko-, and most arboviruses. The following viruses are resistant to ether: parvo-, papova-, adeno-, pox-, picorna-, and reoviruses.

Virus-Lipid Interactions

Studies have been made of the lipophilic affinities of viruses, of the adsorption capacities of different lipids, and of the infectivity of lipid-virus suspensions. Lipophilic viruses include influenza, vaccinia, and herpes; hydrophilic viruses include polio-, echo-, and coxsackieviruses. The lipophilic nature of a virus appears to be correlated with its lipid content (25% for influenza, none for poliovirus).

Antibiotics

Antibacterial antibiotics and sulfonamides have no effect on the true viruses. Members of the psittacosis-LGV-trachoma group are susceptible to these agents, and are not true viruses. Rifampin, an antibiotic which markedly inactivates bacterial but not animal RNA polymerase, has been shown to be active against poxviruses. This is because these viruses carry their own RNA polymerase needed to transcribe the viral DNA to viral mRNA.

TABLE 27–4.

Molar $MgCl_2$	Molar $MgSO_4$	Molar Na_2SO_4
Picornaviruses	Myxoviruses	Herpesvirus
Polioviruses	Influenza virus	Herpes
Echoviruses	Paramyxoviruses	simplex virus
Coxsackie-	Parainfluenza	
viruses	virus	
Rhinoviruses	Measles virus	
Reoviruses	Rubella virus	

Metabolic analogues or antibiotics that interfere with synthesis of DNA or RNA will inhibit viral replication. These analogues also interfere with the metabolic processes of the host cell and are, therefore, too toxic to be of any chemotherapeutic value in the treatment of virus infections. However, a great deal of investigative work is continuing in this area (see p 295).

Antibacterial Agents

Bactericidal agents such as Lysol and Roccal are effective against only a few viruses, and larger concentrations of chlorine may be required to destroy viruses than to kill bacteria. For example, the chlorine treatment of stools recommended for typhoid carriers may be inadequate to destroy poliomyelitis virus present in feces. Dilute hydrochloric acid and formalin destroy resistant viruses like those of the poliomyelitis and coxsackie groups.

Organic iodine compounds also are relatively ineffective against viruses because tiny amounts of organic matter rapidly deplete the active iodine.

CULTIVATION OF VIRUSES

In the early years of virus work, the use of animals was mandatory for the recognition of viruses, and rapid, quantitative work was often difficult. For example, work in poliomyelitis was limited as long as the presence of the virus could be detected only by monkey inoculation. At present, many viruses can be grown in fertile eggs or in cell cultures under strictly controlled conditions. This has opened up many areas of investigation; for example, the nutritional requirements of virus synthesis now can be determined.

Chick Embryos

Virus growth in an embryonated chick egg may result in the death of the embryo (eg, encephalitis virus), the production of pocks or plaques on the chorioallantoic membrane (eg, herpes, smallpox, vaccinia), the development of hemagglutinins in embryonic fluids or tissues (eg, influenza), or merely the development of infective virus (eg, poliovirus, type 2).

Tissue Cultures

In tissue cultures, in which the host cells (chiefly of human or monkey origin) grow on the wall of the test tube and can readily be observed, the multiplication of the virus can be followed by determining the following:

(1) The cytopathic effect, or necrosis of the cells in the tissue culture (polio, herpes, measles, adenovirus, cytomegalovirus, etc).

(2) The inhibition of cellular metabolism, or failure of virus-infected cells to produce acid (eg, enteroviruses).

(3) The appearance of a hemagglutinin (eg, mumps, influenza) or complement-fixing antigen (eg, poliomyelitis, varicella, measles).

(4) The adsorption of erythrocytes to infected cells, called hemadsorption (parainfluenza, influenza). This reaction becomes positive before cytopathic changes are visible, and in some cases it is the only means of detecting the presence of the virus.

(5) Interference by a noncytopathogenic virus (eg, rubella) with replication and cytopathic effect of a second, indicator virus (eg, echovirus).

VIRAL HEMAGGLUTINATION

The red blood cells of man, chickens, and other animals can be agglutinated by a number of different viruses. These viruses can be separated into 3 different groups on the basis of hemagglutination.

The first group includes the myxoviruses. The hemagglutinin of these viruses is an integral part of their limiting membrane. Once these viruses have agglutinated with the cells, spontaneous dissociation of the virus from the cells can occur. The dissociated cells can no longer be agglutinated by the same virus species, but the recovered virus is able to agglutinate fresh cells. This is due to the destruction of specific mucopolysaccharide receptor sites on the surface of the erythrocyte by the enzyme neuraminidase of the virus particles. The hemagglutination reaction can be inhibited by mucopolysaccharides, since they compete with erythrocytes for the virus.

Hemagglutination can also be used as the basis of a method for purifying myxoviruses. After the virus has been adsorbed onto erythrocytes, it can then be eluted in a small volume of buffer and the erythrocytes removed by centrifugation. The reaction of red blood cells with virus can also be used as an indicator of the growth of paramyxoviruses in chick embryos or tissue cultures. The erythrocytes will hemadsorb to the infected cells, and this can be easily observed visually.

A second group of viruses also agglutinates red cells, but in this group (poxviruses) the hemagglutinin is separable from the intact, infective virus particle. The hemagglutinin, a phospholipid-protein complex, is smaller than the virus and is not so readily sedimented in the centrifuge.

A third group of viruses (arboviruses and others) have hemagglutinins in which there appears to be a reversible equilibrium:

Virus Particles + Free Erythrocytes ⇌
Agglutinated Cells-Virus Complex

The virus seems to be identical with the hemagglutinin.

Hemagglutination by viruses has led to rapid and inexpensive quantitative methods of virus assay. Since both noninfective and infective viruses give the reaction, the test measures the total number of virus particles present. In all 3 groups hemagglutination can be used for measurement of specific antibodies. When mixed with antibodies, the hemagglutinins lose their ability to clump erythrocytes; the degree of inhibition is a measure of the amount of hemagglutination-inhibiting antibodies present.

REPLICATION OF VIRUSES

The nutritional requirements of viruses are such that nutrients can be supplied only by the intact cell. The host cell must supply not only the energy and synthetic machinery, but also the low molecular weight precursors for the viral protein and nucleic acid. Virus particles do not respire, as do bacteria, nor do they have any of the enzymes associated with metabolic activity. However, they do have the necessary genetic information to convert the host into a virus factory. The number of new proteins (enzymes, structural antigens) synthesized in an infected cell is a function of the size of the viral genome (Table 27–1).

Virus multiplication was first studied successfully in the T-series of bacteriophages (which parasitize *E coli*) because of their short growth cycle (in terms of minutes, compared to hours or days for animal viruses) and their relative ease of quantification. These studies have resulted in a fairly complete picture of the mechanism of phage replication, in particular the T-even series of bacteriophages which is presented in Chapter 9. The studies of animal viruses have not been so fruitful, mainly because of the need for in vitro culture systems and technics for quantification. However, in the last several years these procedures have been devel-

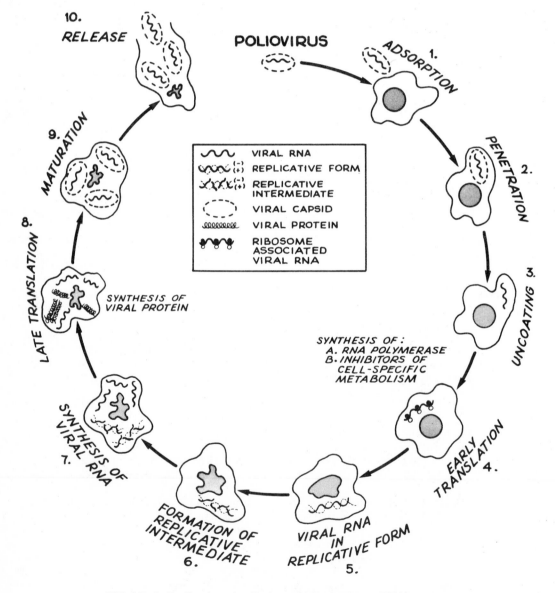

FIG 27–6. Replication of poliovirus which contains an RNA genome.

oped, and some of the steps of the interaction between the infecting virus and susceptible cells have been elucidated.

The specificity of receptor sites involved in the attachment of viruses to susceptible cells has been studied in some detail with myxoviruses. The receptor sites for these viruses are mucopolysaccharides on the cell surface. The adsorption can be prevented by pretreatment of the cells with an enzyme (receptor destroying enzyme, RDE) from *Vibrio cholerae* that destroys the mucopolysaccharide receptors. This system has been studied widely by means of the hemagglutination reaction.

Viruses released by a continuous process, in contrast to those released by cell lysis, have been found to contain lipid as an essential component, and they are inactivated by ether. It has been suggested that viruses containing lipids as essential components are assembled from viral subunits or from vegetative forms at or near the cell surface and are completed by obtaining a protective external lipid coat from the lipid structures at the cell periphery as the particles pass to the external cell surface (Fig 27–4). Viruses without essential lipid components seem to be completed within the cell and released in large numbers by a burst process. Specific

receptor sites have also been demonstrated for the picornaviruses.

The following 2 sections describe the replication of an RNA and a DNA virus that have been studied in some detail.

RNA Virus Replication (See Fig 27–6.)

The replication of poliovirus which contains a single-stranded RNA as its genome has been studied in some detail. All of the steps are independent of host DNA and occur in the host cell cytoplasm. Polioviruses adsorb to cells only through species-specific cell receptor sites (step 1). This is evidenced by the fact that intact poliovirus infects only primate cells in culture, while the isolated RNA will also infect nonprimate cells (rabbit, guinea pig, chick), and complete one cycle of multiplication. Only one cycle of infection is observed because the resulting progeny possess their protein coats, and will again only infect primate cells. The virus particles are then taken into the cell by pinocytosis (step 2) and the viral RNA is uncoated (step 3). The single-stranded RNA can then serve as its own messenger RNA. This messenger RNA is translated (step 4), resulting in the formation of an RNA polymerase necessary for the formation of a replicative

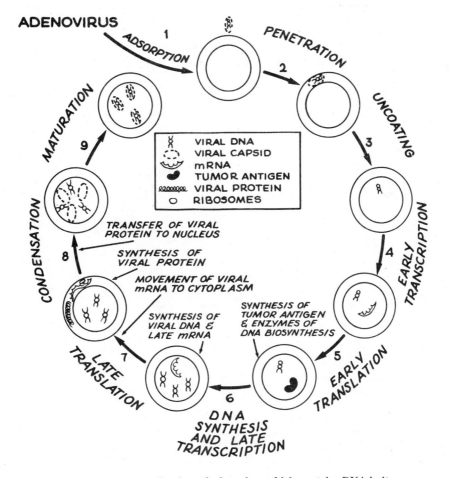

FIG 27–7. Steps in the replication of adenovirus which contains DNA in its genome.

form (step 5) and also in the formation of inhibitors that turn off the cellular RNA and protein synthesis. The number and nature of these inhibitors is unknown; however, a virus-induced stimulation of histone synthesis in the nucleus of infected cells has been described and is considered as the possible mechanism of inhibition of RNA synthesis. Single-stranded viral RNA molecules (+ strands) are then synthesized from the replicative form, first appearing as partially completed strands on the replicative intermediate (step 6). The synthesis of viral capsid proteins (step 7) is initiated at about the same time as RNA synthesis. Proteins condense to form the **procapsids** or empty protein shells. The viral genome, in some way, is then incorporated inside the procapsid, forming the mature virion (step 8). It has been shown by electrophoretic analysis that the protein capsid consists of at least 4 different subunits, each with a molecular weight of about 27,000. The virus particles are then released when the cell undergoes lysis (step 9).

DNA Virus Replication (See Fig 27–7.)

Of the DNA viruses, the replication of both the poxviruses and adenoviruses has been studied in detail. Many of the steps are similar for both viruses; poxvirus replication is described in detail in Chapter 36, and the following sequence depicts adenovirus replication. The adsorption (step 1) and penetration (step 2) of the virus into the cell are similar to steps described for poliovirus. After the virus enters the cell, the protein coat is removed (step 3), presumably by cellular enzymes, and the viral DNA reaches the nucleus. As in all DNA virus replication, a viral DNA strand is tran-

scribed (step 4) into specific mRNA, which in turn is translated (step 5) to synthesize virus-specific proteins such as tumor antigen and enzymes necessary for biosynthesis of virus DNA. This period involves the early virus function. Host-cell DNA synthesis is temporarily elevated and is then suppressed as the cell shifts over to the manufacture of viral DNA (step 6). As the viral DNA continues to be transcribed, late virus functions become apparent. Messenger RNA transcribed during the later phase of infection (step 6) migrates to the cytoplasm and is translated there (step 7). Proteins for virus capsids are synthesized during the late virus functions and are transported to the nucleus to be incorporated into the virus structure (step 8). Assembly of the protein subunits around the viral DNA results in the formation of complete virions (step 9), which are released after cell lysis.

IN VITRO SYNTHESIS OF INFECTIOUS VIRAL DNA

Infectious RNA and DNA have been synthesized for 2 small viruses. The recent work on DNA is of great importance since all living organisms have similar genomes. As shown in Fig 27–8, a DNA template molecule from the bacterial virus φX-174 is copied by purified DNA polymerase. The genome of this virus contains 5500 nucleotides and is in the form of a single strand in a covalently closed circle called the (+) strand. DNA polymerase copies the sequence of

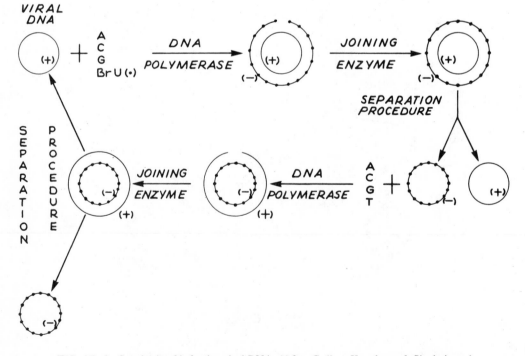

FIG 27–8. **Synthesis of infective viral DNA.** (After Gulian, Kornberg, & Sinsheimer.)

nucleotides of the (+) circle template and synthesizes a linear (−) strand complementary to the (+) circle, which the joining enzyme converts into a covalent duplex circle similar to that which occurs in vivo. The physical separation of the 2 DNA circles depends on the fact that the (−) circle synthesized in vitro is denser than the template (+) circle. The reason for this (Fig 27−8) is that 5-bromodeoxyuridylic acid (·) replaced thymidylic acid in the monomer mixture used for polymerization. The denser DNA produced can be separated from the lighter template by density gradient centrifugation. The dense synthetic (−) circles can be used as templates in an analogous system in which thymidine itself rather than BrU is present in the monomer mixture. The synthetic duplex now contains a light (+) circle which can be purified and shown to be identical with infectious DNA obtained from the whole virion.

VIRAL GENETICS & VIRAL INTERACTIONS

The genetic analysis of bacteriophage has been in progress for about 2 decades, but meaningful genetic studies with animal viruses have been possible in the past few years. Two primary factors have made these studies possible. The first was the development of the plaque assay for quantitation of virus infectivity. Since genetic interactions are relatively rare phenomena, it is necessary that a sensitive and accurate assay method be available. The second factor was the development of stable genetic **markers** (phenotypic expressions by a virus, such as a specific virus-induced enzyme). Such markers are prerequisite for meaningful genetic studies. They should be amenable to experimental study, should be easily recognized, and should result from single mutations. Some markers commonly used include specific virus-induced antigens, drug resistance, and inability to grow at elevated temperatures. Plaque size and pathogenicity have also been used as markers. Virus mutants that possess these markers are obtained either after spontaneous mutation or, more frequently, after treatment of the virus population with a mutagen.

Mutagens widely used for the induction of altered virus progeny fall into 3 classes: (1) base analogues which can replace the normal bases of DNA during replication; (2) substances which chemically alter the bases of resting DNA; and (3) those whose action is to remove DNA bases. An example of the first class of mutagens is 5-bromouracil, which replaces thymine quantitatively and which also binds with guanine. This substance can thus induce mutations by causing 2 types of base pair transitions depending upon whether the pairing error occurs during incorporation or during replication following incorporation, as shown in Fig 27−9(A). Nitrous acid is an example of the second class of mutagens. Its mutagenic action lies in its abil-

ity to oxidatively deaminate either adenine or cytosine, as illustrated in Fig 27−9(B). Representative of the third class of mutagens is ethyl ethanesulfonate, which is thought to act by removing guanine bases, as shown in Figure 27−9(C).

No genetic map is yet available for an animal virus, but studies have shown that when 2 different virus particles infect the same host cell they may interact in a variety of different ways. The types of interactions are summarized in Table 27−5 and presented diagrammatically in Table 27−6. Genetic interaction, one main division, results in some progeny which are **heritably** (genetically) different from either parent. Progeny produced as a consequence of nongenetic interaction, the other main division, are similar to the parental viruses.

The following terms are basic to the discussion of genetics which follows: **Genetics** is the study of heredity. By **genotype** is meant the genetic constitution of an organism. **Phenotype** refers to the observable properties of an organism which are produced by the genotype in cooperation with the environment. A **mutation** is an inheritable change in the genotype. The **genome** is the sum of the genes of an organism.

It should be realized that several types of interaction can occur simultaneously under the proper conditions.

Genetic Interactions

Recombination results in some progeny (recombinants) carrying traits not found together in either parent. This type of interaction is said to occur when both parental viruses are viable (active). It is postulated that the nucleic acid strands break, and part of the genome of one parent is recombined with part of the genome of the second parent. One important characteristic is that the recombinant virus is genetically stable, yielding progeny like itself upon replication. For example, a recombinant influenza virus was recognized because its hemagglutinin was antigenically identical with that of the type A parent while the antigenicity of its neuraminidase corresponded to that of the type A_2 parent.

Cross-reactivation occurs between the genome of an active virion and the genome of a virus particle which has been inactivated in some way. A portion of the genome of the inactivated virus recombines with that of the active parent, so that certain markers of the inactivated parent are rescued and appear in the viable progeny. None of the progeny produced are identical with the inactivated parent. The progeny carrying the rescued markers of the inactivated parent are genetically stable. Cross-reactivation was used to obtain an A_2 influenza virus suitable for vaccine production. Inactivated type A, which has the capacity to grow well in eggs, was mixed with active Asian (A_2) isolate. A recombinant was obtained with the desired A_2 antigenicity and the ability of the parental type A to grow in eggs.

Multiplicity reactivation occurs when an inactive virus particle is rendered active by interaction with

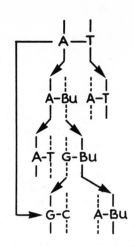

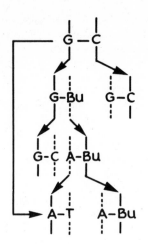

A

Erroneous pairing with guanine during
replication following incorporation.

Erroneous pairing with guanine
during incorporation.

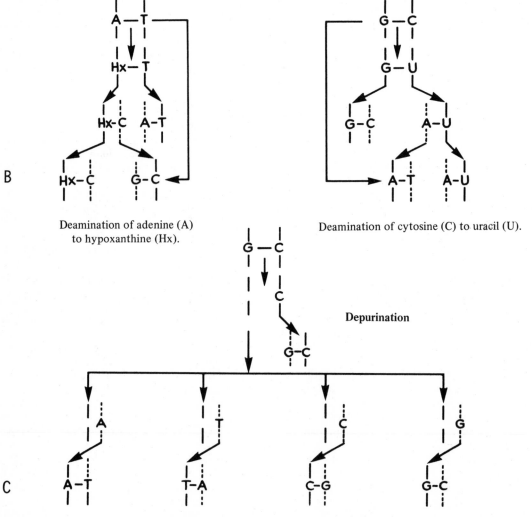

Deamination of adenine (A)
to hypoxanthine (Hx).

Deamination of cytosine (C) to uracil (U).

Depurination

B

C

Base pair substititution following removal of guanine by EES.

FIG 27–9. Mutagenesis. **A.** By 5-bromouracil (BU). **B.** By nitrous acid. **C.** By ethyl ethanesulfonate (EES).
(After Hayes.)

another inactive virus particle in the same cell. Recombination occurs between the damaged nucleic acids of the parents, producing a viable genome which can replicate. The greater the damage to the parental genomes, the larger the number of inactive particles required per cell to ensure the formation of such a viable genome. No progeny are produced that are identical with either parent.

Nongenetic Interactions

Phenotypic mixing is the association of a phenotype with a heterologous genotype. This occurs when the genome of one virus becomes randomly incorporated within the capsid of a different virus. It is not a stable genetic change because, upon replication, the phenotypically mixed parent will yield progeny encased in capsids homologous to the genotype, since protein synthesis is controlled by the virus genome. Phenotypic mixing was detected between 2 different picornaviruses in the following way: After a mixed infection, a virus population was obtained which could be neutralized by coxsackievirus antiserum. After replication, the progeny virus was neutralized only by poliovirus antiserum.

Genotypic mixing, or heterozygosis, is distinguished by a single virus particle which can give rise to progeny of 2 distinct parental types. This is not a stable genetic change and probably occurs when 2 complete genomes are accidentally incorporated within a single virus capsid.

Interference occurs when the multiplication of a superinfecting virus is inhibited because of the presence of the initially infecting virus. This phenomenon can be mediated either by interferon or by an alteration of cell receptor sites or metabolic pathways necessary for replication of the second virus. (For additional details, see p 297.)

Enhancement, in contrast to interference, is the increased production of one virus as the result of co-infection with a second virus. All the progeny will be like the parental viruses. Again, the basic mechanisms vary; one reported mechanism is the activity of the second virus in inhibiting the synthesis of interferon; for example, parainfluenza relieves autoinhibition by Newcastle disease virus, a potent interferon-producing virus.

Complementation is the functional interaction between 2 viruses, one or both of which may be defective, which results in the multiplication of one or both under conditions in which replication would not ordinarily occur. The progeny produced are like the parental viruses. Neither the genotype nor the phenotype of either virus is affected. A variety of different types of complementation may occur, as indicated in Table 27—5, and the mechanisms permitting complementation vary depending on the system. Examples include (a) the stimulation, by an active poxvirus (fibroma), of an uncoating enzyme necessary for the release of the genome of an inactive poxvirus (myxoma); and (b) the production, by active adenovirus, of coat protein utilized by defective SV40 (PARA). In the other examples cited, one or both of 2 defective viruses may act by inducing some essential gene product—as yet unidentified—which the other requires for replication but is unable to provide for itself.

TABLE 27—5. Types and characteristics of interactions between animal viruses.

Type of Interaction	Viability of Parental Viruses	Some Progeny Different From Parental	Progeny Genetically Stable	Example
I. Genetic				
A. Recombination	Active + active	Yes	Yes	Influenza, poliovirus
B. Cross-reactivation	Active + inactive	Yes	Yes	Influenza
C. Multiplicity reaction	Inactive + inactive	Yes	Yes	Vaccinia
II. Nongenetic				
A. Phenotypic mixing	Active + active	Yes	No	Picornaviruses
B. Genotypic mixing	Active + active	Yes	No	Myxoviruses
C. Interference	Active + active	No	Yes	Coxsackieviruses
	Defective + active	No	Yes	Satellite + adenovirus
D. Enhancement	Active + active	No	Yes	NDV + parainfluenza
E. Complementation	Active + inactive	No	Yes	Poxviruses
	Active + defective	No	Yes	(a) Rous-associated virus + Rous sarcoma virus
				(b) Murine leukemia + sarcoma
				(c) SV40 + adenovirus
				(d) Adenovirus + satellite
	Defective + defective	No	Yes	(a) PARA (SV40)-adeno + adenovirus
				(b) MAC-adeno + adenovirus

TABLE 27–6. Schematic representations of types of genetic and nongenetic interactions between animal viruses. (After Butel.)

Type of Interaction	Parental Types I	Parental Types II	Progeny Parental Types I	Progeny Parental Types II	Progeny Recombinants or Other	
I. GENETIC Recombination	(a₁b₁) active	+ (a₂b₂) active	(a₁b₁)	(a₂b₂)	(a₁b₂)	(a₂b₁)
Cross-reactivation	(a₁b₁) active	+ (a₂b₂) inactive ⟶	(a₁b₁)	none	(a₁b₂) or	(a₂b₁)
Multiplicity reactivation	(a₁b₁) inactive	+ (a₂b₂) inactive ⟶	none	none	(a₁b₂) or	(a₂b₁)
II. NONGENETIC Phenotypic mixing	(A) active	+ [B] active ⟶	(A)	[B]	Ⓐ or [Ⓐ] replication ↓ (A)	
Genotypic mixing	(A) active	+ [B] active ⟶	(A)	[B]	(A, B) replication (A) and [B]	
Interference 1.	(A) active	+ [B] active ⟶	(A) Less than usual	[B]	Possible	
2.	(A) active	+ [B] defective ⟶	(A) Less than usual	[B]	Possible	
Enhancement	(A) active	+ [B] active ⟶	(A) More than usual	[B]	Possible	
Complementation 1.	(A) active ↓ single infection (A)	+ [B] inactive ↓ no growth ⟶	(A)	[B]	Possible	
2.	(A) active ↓ single infection (A)	+ [B] defective ↓ no growth ⟶	(A)	[B]	Possible	
3.	(A) defective ↓ single infection no growth	+ [B] defective ↓ no growth ⟶	(A)	[B]	Possible	

EXPERIMENTAL CHEMOPROPHYLAXIS
OF VIRUS INFECTIONS

It is possible in the infected cell to inhibit some processes leading to the synthesis of viral constituents, or to inhibit adsorption, penetration, or release of infectious virus from the host cell. A number of different types of compounds have been described whose actions are directed toward metabolic reactions of the host cell. However, in order to be considered for chemoprophylaxis they must have a greater specificity for virus-directed reactions than for normal host cell reactions. The inhibitors which are used range from those which are highly virus specific to those which are only slightly virus specific. At this time there are no inhibitors available that can be used in the routine treatment of viral infections in man.

Very few inhibitors have been found which have a specific effect on virus penetration or release from the host cell. Amantadine (Symmetrel), a symmetrical amine, inhibits specifically certain members of the myxovirus group through blocking of viral penetration into the host cell. When administered prophylactically, amantadine is reported to have a significant protective effect in experimental animals and man against influenza A strains, but not against influenza B or other viruses. This protection consists mainly of a modification of the disease to a milder form.

Guanidine and 2-(a-hydroxybenzyl)-benzimidazole (HBB) specifically inhibit the replication of many picornaviruses in vitro by restricting the formation of virus specific RNA polymerase, which indirectly results in an inhibition of the synthesis of viral RNA and coat proteins. Once the RNA polymerase is formed, however, neither inhibitor can affect its activity. The action of the 2 compounds is similar but not identical since some viruses can be inhibited by one but not the other. The inhibitory action can be reversed by dilution with fresh medium. In some cases, HBB and guanidine have a synergistic effect. However, in experimentally infected animals, there is no protective effect by either of the inhibitors. This is probably due to rapid production of drug-resistant mutants.

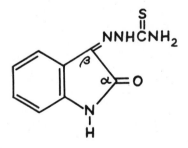

FIG 27–10. Methisazone (isatin-β-thiosemicarbazone, Marboran), an inhibitor of poxvirus reproduction.

Both drug-resistant and drug-dependent virus mutants have been isolated.

Methisazone (Marboran) is an inhibitor of many members of the poxvirus and adenovirus groups. Methisazone is highly virus specific and does not affect normal cell metabolism. In the presence of this inhibitor viral DNA synthesis occurs normally, but not all viral antigens are synthesized. The result is that immature, noninfectious virus particles are formed. The effect of methisazone cannot be reversed by dilution. Mutants resistant to this inhibitor have been found. Methisazone and an N-methyl derivative block poxvirus replication in the experimentally infected mouse. The N-methyl derivative is also an effective prophylactic for smallpox in man if given within 24–48 hours after exposure.

Many purine and pyrimidine analogues inhibit both RNA and DNA synthesis. By the incorporation of ribose or deoxyribose into the molecule to make the corresponding riboside or deoxyriboside, the activity of the analogue can be directed preferentially toward the inhibition of RNA or DNA. The significance of this structural specificity of the sugar component for the inhibition of virus synthesis is evident in the finding that the riboside of 5-fluorouracil is a much more effective inhibitor of the growth of tobacco mosaic virus, an RNA virus, than is its deoxyriboside. Ribosides of halogenated benzimidazoles are more selective inhibitors of influenza virus or poliovirus multiplication than the free benzimidazoles or their deoxyribosides.

Pyrimidine analogues may exert an action according to their structural similarities to either uracil or thymine (Fig 27–11). With halogenated pyrimidines, it has been found that the size of the particular halogen atom attached determines the character of the compound. The Van der Waals radii of fluorine and bromine resemble closely those of hydrogen and the methyl group, respectively; thus, the size and shape of 5-bromouracil is very similar to that of thymine, and that of 5-fluorouracil is similar to that of uracil. 5-Bromouracil is an effective inhibitor of the synthesis of DNA bacteriophage but is without effect on the synthesis of RNA tobacco mosaic virus. 5-Fluorouracil (FU), on the other hand, inhibits the growth of the RNA virus, and its action is reversed by uridine but not by thymidine.

5-Fluoro-2'-deoxyuridine (FUDR) inhibits DNA synthesis by inhibiting the enzymatic synthesis of thymidylic acid; 5-bromo-2'-deoxyuridine (BUDR) and 5-iodo-2'-deoxyuridine (IUDR) are incorporated into DNA, resulting in the production of a faulty nucleic acid which does not function normally. All 3 of these halogenated deoxyuridines inhibit replication of members of the major DNA virus groups: papova-, adeno-, herpes-, and poxviruses. Drug-resistant mutants of some viruses have been obtained, however, by growth in the presence of IUDR or BUDR. Topical administration of IUDR is being used in man in the treatment of corneal lesions due to herpes simplex virus. Systemic treatment of viral infections is not practicable because

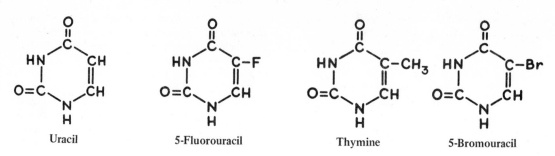

FIG 27–11. Structures of uracil, 5-fluorouracil, thymine, and 5-bromouracil.

of the toxicity of the drugs. However, in cases of herpesvirus encephalitis, massive near-lethal doses (400 mg/kg) of IUDR have been reported to lead to complete recovery.

The treatment of papovavirus- or herpesvirus-infected cells with IUDR arrests the synthesis of new infectious virus but not of viral components. Large amounts of viral antigen are found in IUDR-treated infected cells. In the electron microscope, structurally imperfect herpesvirus particles in large quantities are observed in the presence of IUDR, as many as 20,000 per cell. Perhaps the antiviral activity of IUDR is due to the faulty assembly of viral components which it induces.

In the presence of FU, herpesvirus-infected cells produce virus particles that are noninfectious because they lack DNA cores. With the papovavirus SV40, large amounts of viral antigen are produced in the nucleus but are not assembled into the capsid.

Mutations can be induced within host cells by purine and pyrimidine analogues such as 5-bromo-deoxyuridine and 2-aminopurine, indicating that specific changes in the viral genome can be brought about through the metabolism of the host cell. Nitrous acid is a mutagenic agent which has the added virtue that the virus or its nucleic acid can be treated directly, thus eliminating the complicating influence of the host cell. Experiments with tobacco mosaic virus have shown that nitrous acid deaminates the viral RNA, converting adenine to hypoxanthine, guanine to xanthine, and cytosine to uracil. It is considered that the transitions from cytosine to uracil, ie, from one natural base to another, have a mutagenic effect, whereas the transitions to xanthine and hypoxanthine, neither of which occurs naturally in RNA, cause inactivation.

Another pyrimidine analogue is 1-β-d-arabino-furanosylcytosine hydrochloride (cytosine arabino-side). It inhibits DNA synthesis, and thereby the replication of DNA viruses, primarily due to an inhibition of the reduction of the cytosine ribotide to the deoxy-ribotide. As with IUDR, cytosine arabinoside inhibits cellular DNA synthesis and viral DNA synthesis about equally and therefore exhibits little viral specificity. The compound has been found to have a differential inhibitory effect during the growth of certain viruses in tissue culture. In the presence of inhibitory concentrations of cytosine arabinoside, the tumor antigens of

both SV40 and adenoviruses are synthesized, but viral capsid proteins and infectious virus are not formed. The biochemical mechanism underlying this differential inhibition is not fully understood, but the difference is probably due to the fact that synthesis of the tumor antigens does not require replication of viral DNA, whereas formation of progeny viral DNA is a prerequisite for the formation of virus coat protein and new infectious virus.

Dactinomycin (actinomycin D) inhibits DNA-dependent RNA synthesis and thus inhibits the multiplication of DNA viruses, but not most RNA viruses. However, dactinomycin inhibits the multiplication of some RNA myxoviruses and of Rous sarcoma virus. The exact mechanism of this dactinomycin inhibition is not clear. The multiplication of some RNA viruses may be inhibited by dactinomycin through deleterious effects on the host cell, rather than by direct action on the replication of the RNA of the virus. Rifampin is an antibiotic whose action depends upon its preferential inhibition of bacterial RNA polymerase over animal cell RNA polymerase. Since poxviruses carry their own RNA polymerase for synthesizing viral mRNA (needed for transcription of the viral genome), rifampin was tried against this virus and found to be very effective in inhibiting its replication. Clinical trials against small-pox are now planned.

Although not practical as chemotherapeutic agents, protein inhibitors have been useful in the study of viral replication. For example, puromycin, cyclo-heximide, and p-fluorophenylalanine all inhibit synthesis of both viral and cell proteins. Thus they have proved useful in interrupting the cycle of virus replication at different stages.

With all specific inhibitors, it is necessary to demonstrate that inhibition is not merely due to direct cytotoxicity of the compound. Thus, the action of competitive inhibitors (cytosine arabinoside, IUDR, etc) can be reversed by the addition of the analogous normal metabolic compounds. Resumption of normal activity by the cell after reversal is indicative of the specificity of action of the drug employed.

Statolon, a penicillium mold product of *Penicillium stoloniferum,* shows inhibitory activity against several RNA viruses (eg, picornaviruses, arboviruses). After many years of work with this inhibitor, it has recently been found to be mycophage RNA which contaminates the penicillium cultures. It acts by stimulating interferon production.

INTERFERENCE PHENOMENON & INTERFERON

The term viral interference implies that superinfecting viral particles are in some way prevented from entering and multiplying in a cell already infected with virus of another kind. This phenomenon has been described using animal hosts or cells in culture. Interference in animals should be distinguished from specific immunity, ie, immunity resulting from antibody stimulation by the infecting virus. Also, interference has not been observed for all virus combinations; 2 viruses may infect and multiply within the same cell (eg, vaccinia and herpesviruses; measles and polioviruses).

Two mechanisms may be ascribed to the interference phenomenon: (1) the initial virus may alter either the host cell surface or its metabolic pathways, thus making them unavailable to the superinfecting virus; or (2) the first virus may stimulate the production of an inhibitor (interferon) which prevents the replication of the second virus. The first type of interference can occur between related as well as unrelated viruses; in some cases a virus will interfere with its own replication (autointerference).

Interference has been used as a basis for controlling outbreaks of infection with virulent strains of poliovirus by introducing into the population an attenuated poliovirus which interferes with the spread of the virulent virus. Theoretically, it would appear possible to use the interference phenomenon as a sort of immunization technic: Viruses of low virulence might be used to prevent subsequent infection with more virulent organisms. Infection with a mild respiratory virus produces a 2- to 6-week refractory period to infection by a related or unrelated respiratory virus. The development of suitable attenuated viruses which would produce a refractory response to subsequent infection, without themselves producing symptomatic illness, might be useful in preventing the more severe illness associated with influenza epidemics. Unfortunately, interference is generally short-lived and, when the first virus disappears from the cells, the cell receptors or other substances are rapidly regenerated, making the cell again susceptible to infection.

Interferon

Interferon is a virus inhibitor produced by intact animals or cultured cells when infected with viruses. Infection by virus in the animal host is associated with maximum virus production developing after an appropriate incubation period. Within 12–48 hours after virus titers reach a maximum, interferon is produced in large quantities and virus production rapidly decreases. Antibody does not appear in the blood of the animal until several days after virus production has abated. This temporal relationship of virus production to the appearance of interferon and then of antiviral antibody strongly suggests that interferon plays a major role in the defense of the animal against virus infections.

Interferon is characterized as protein which is acid-stable (pH 2.0), trypsin-sensitive, nondialyzable, and nonsedimentable by ultracentrifuge forces sufficient to pellet viruses. Interferon is effective as an antiviral substance on cells from the species of animal in which it was produced but is almost never effective on cells from other species. Thus, interferon produced by the intact mouse or by mouse cells in tissue culture will protect mouse cells from virus infection but has no protective effect for chicken cells. Although interferon is specific for the species of cells on which it is effective, it is not specific for the virus inhibited. Interferon production stimulated by one virus will effectively inhibit a wide variety of viruses.

Interferon is produced by cells in tissue culture when stimulated with viruses or synthetic double-stranded polynucleotides and by the intact animal when stimulated with viruses, rickettsiae, bacterial endotoxins, or synthetic anionic polymers or polynucleotides. Recent evidence indicates that many agents that are potent interferon stimulators have in common the presence of double-stranded RNA in the material inoculated, or the production of double-stranded RNA during the replication of the virus. The double-stranded RNA of reovirus extracted from the virion has been shown to have excellent ability to stimulate interferon. When stimulated, the host cell genome directs the synthesis of interferon, which is released from the infected cell.

When interferon is added to cells prior to infection, there is marked inhibition of virus replication. The presence of interferon in the cell stimulates the cell to produce another protein called the translational inhibitory protein (TIP). The TIP binds to cellular ribosomes and alters them in such a way that viral RNA is not translated. Cellular messenger RNA is translated normally. This permits normal cell functions to continue but prevents the synthesis of virus-directed protein. Without the production of necessary enzymes and coat protein for progeny virus, new virus is not formed. A schematic diagram of the mechanism of interferon action is presented in Fig 27–12.

All of the cells of the intact animal are probably capable of producing interferon; however, the elements of the reticuloendothelial system seem to provide the bulk of interferon during most virus infections.

Stimulation of animals with various substances has revealed at least 2 classes of interferons. One class appears to be preformed and is released into the blood stream within 2 hours after injection of statolon or endotoxins. This interferon has a higher molecular weight (ie, 8.5×10^4 daltons) than the interferon that is present in the serum 18 hours after stimulation. The late-appearing interferon has a molecular weight of $3–4 \times 10^4$ daltons, and is synthesized after a suitable stimulation. Interferons of still other molecular

HOW INTERFERON WORKS

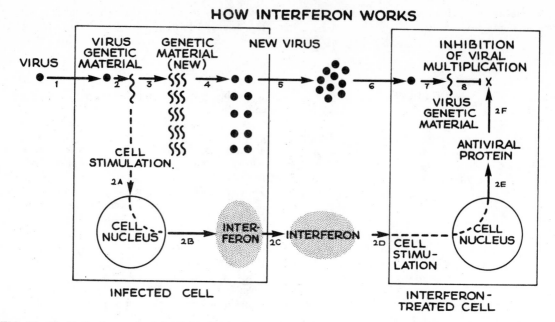

FIG 27–12. Beginning at the left of the figure (1), virus comes in contact with the cell and penetrates the cell membrane. The virus then releases its genetic material (2), which organizes the cell to make many copies of the genetic material (3). The new genetic material (4) is coated with viral protein to form completed new virus, and (5) the new virus is released into the fluid around the cells where it can now spread to other cells. During the early stages of infection the process of viral multiplication within the cell stimulates the cell (2a) to utilize the stored information for interferon synthesis. Through a series of complex procedures, the interferon protein is made (2b) and released rapidly (2c) into the extracellular fluid. In many instances the interferon precedes new virus to surrounding cells. The interferon stimulates the surrounding cells (2d) to utilize another set of stored information to produce an intracellular antiviral protein (2e). The antiviral protein (2f) acts to change the cell's protein-synthesizing machinery so that it cannot be used by viral genetic material subsequently encountered. Therefore, any infection by new virus of the interferon-protected cell (6) still leads to release of the viral genetic material (7), but that viral genetic material is discriminated against by the cell synthesizing machinery (8) and essential viral materials fail to be produced. Thus, viral multiplication is inhibited and the cell is protected. (Baron.)

weights have been found under various experimental conditions, and it is evident that interferon is a class of proteins that shares the biologic property of inhibiting virus replication by altering cell metabolism.

The low antigenicity and potent antiviral effect of interferon have created much interest in its possible application in controlling viral diseases of man. In experimental animals it has been possible to demonstrate the efficacy of exogenous interferon in preventing or decreasing the severity of virus infections. However, the difficulties in producing sufficient quantities of the material for human use have not been overcome. The substance has not been found effective in altering the course of viral diseases once the infection is well established. Present hope for the application of interferon to the control of human disease lies in the development of an interferon inducer; however, no such inducer is presently available for general use.

PATHOGENESIS OF VIRUS DISEASES

Virus implantation and multiplication occur in different tissues as the infectious agent travels to the target organ from the portal of entry. In the target organ, virus multiplication must reach critical levels before cell necrosis occurs and disease becomes manifest. In Fig 27–14 are shown examples of mousepox, a disease of the skin, and of human poliomyelitis, a disease of the CNS.

In mousepox, the virus enters the body through minute abrasions of the skin and multiplies in the epidermal cells. At the same time it is carried by the lymphatics to the regional lymph nodes, where multiplication also occurs. The few virus particles entering the blood by way of the efferent lymphatics are taken up by the macrophages of the liver and spleen. In both organs the virus multiplies rapidly. Following release of virus from the liver and spleen it passes by way of the blood stream and localizes in the basal epidermal layers of the skin, in the conjunctival cells, and near the

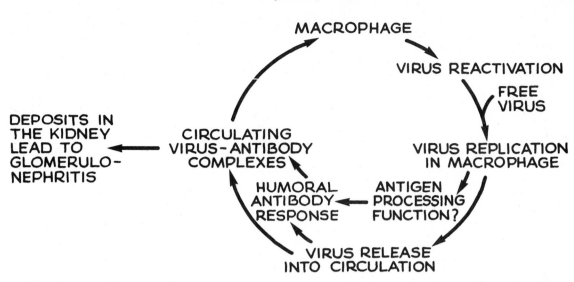

FIG 27–13. **Hypothetical mechanism leading to viral persistence and disease in Aleutian disease virus infection of mink.** Macrophages phagocytize virus-antibody complexes, reactivate the virus, and thus allow the virus to replicate in the phagocytic cell. This mechanism would negate any effect of antiviral antibody in terminating infection, and would promote viral persistence. The glomerulonephritis of Aleutian disease is largely due to deposition of virus-antibody complexes in the glomeruli.

lymph follicles in the intestine. The virus may occasionally also localize in the epithelial cells of the kidney, lung, submaxillary gland, and pancreas. A primary lesion occurs at the site of entry of the virus. It appears as a localized swelling which rapidly increases in size, becomes edematous, ulcerates, and goes on to scar formation. A generalized rash follows which is responsible for the release of large quantities of virus into the environment.

In poliomyelitis, virus enters by way of the alimentary tract and multiplies locally at the initial sites of viral implantation (tonsils, Peyer's patches) or the lymph nodes which drain these tissues, and begins to appear in the throat and in the feces. Secondary virus spread occurs by the blood stream to other susceptible tissues, namely, other lymph nodes, brown fat, and the CNS. Within the CNS the virus spreads by nerve fibers. If a high level of multiplication occurs as the virus spreads through the CNS, motor neurons are destroyed and paralysis occurs. The shedding of virus into the environment does not depend upon secondary virus spread to the CNS. Secondary spread to the CNS is readily interrupted by the presence of antibodies, induced by prior infection or vaccine.

Immunopathologic Virus Diseases

Certain viruses do not invariably kill the cells they infect. The immunologic response of the host to these viruses may be responsible for the observed pathologic changes and the clinical illness. This phenomenon is exemplified in lymphocytic choriomeningitis virus infection of mice. If adult mice are rendered immunologically incompetent by x-irradiation, immunosup-

pressive drugs, or antiserum directed against the lymphoid elements of the mouse, they do not become ill when infected with the virus. The virus replicates in the animal and establishes a chronic infection which persists until the competence of the immunologic response is restored, at which time the animal becomes ill. Infection of newborn mice before they develop immunologic competence results in a lifelong viral infection which is not associated with illness. Persistent infections occur with a number of animal viruses, and the persistence in certain instances depends upon the age of the host when infected. In human beings, rubella virus and cytomegalovirus infections acquired in utero characteristically result in viral persistence which is of limited duration, probably because of the development of the immunologic capacity to react to the infection as the infant matures.

Persistent viral infections may play a more far-reaching role in human disease than is now appreciated. In animals, persistent viral infections are associated with leukemias and sarcomas of chickens and mice (see Chapter 40) as well as progressive degenerative diseases of the CNS of man and animals (see Chapter 33). A persistent viral disease of Aleutian mink is associated with alterations of serum immunoglobulins very similar to the changes observed in human multiple myeloma. These alterations in immunoglobulins are thought to represent overreactivity of certain immunocytes in the host's response to the chronic presence of the viral agent. The infected minks also have pathologic alterations of their blood vessels and kidneys not unlike those seen in certain human connective tissue disorders. The role of the host response to the infecting virus does not appear to

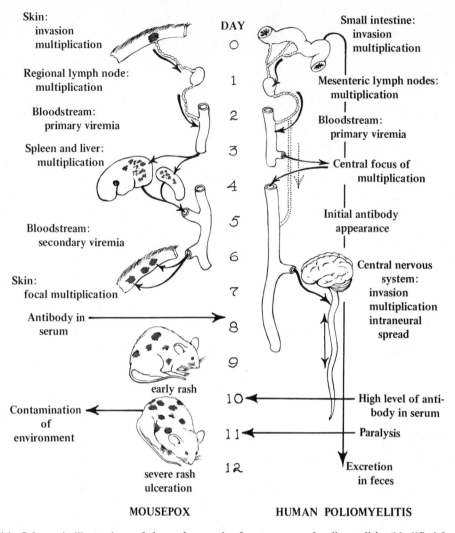

Skin:
invasion
multiplication

Regional lymph node:
multiplication

Bloodstream:
primary viremia

Spleen and liver:
multiplication

Bloodstream:
secondary viremia

Skin:
focal multiplication

Antibody in
serum

Contamination
of
environment

early rash

severe rash
ulceration

DAY
O
1
2
3
4
5
6
7
8
9
10
11
12

Small intestine:
invasion
multiplication

Mesenteric lymph nodes:
multiplication

Bloodstream:
primary viremia

Central focus of
multiplication

Initial antibody
appearance

Central nervous
system:
invasion
multiplication
intraneural
spread

High level of anti-
body in serum

Paralysis

Excretion
in feces

MOUSEPOX   HUMAN POLIOMYELITIS

FIG 27–14. Schematic illustrations of the pathogenesis of mousepox and poliomyelitis. (Modified from Fenner.)

be always beneficial to the host. Fig 27–13 illustrates the mechanism by which virus is believed to persist and to lead to glomerulonephritis in a slow virus infection.

INCLUSION BODY FORMATION

In the course of virus multiplication within cells, virus specific structures, called inclusion bodies, may be produced. They become far larger than the individual virus particle and often have an affinity for acid dyes such as eosin or acid fuchsin. They may be situated either in the nucleus or in the cytoplasm, or both (as in measles). In many virus infections the bodies are believed to be the site of development of the virions (the virus factories). In some infections (molluscum contagiosum) the inclusion body consists of masses of virus particles which can be seen in the electron microscope to ripen to maturity within the inclusion body.

In still others, as in the intranuclear inclusion body of herpes, the virus appears to have multiplied within the nucleus early in the infection before the typical eosinophilic inclusion forms. In the last instance the inclusion body appears to be a remnant of virus multiplication. Much remains to be learned about their significance.

Variations in the appearance of inclusion material depend upon the composition of the fixative used. When cells are fixed at a pH of 7.3, in formalin or osmium tetroxide, the inclusion material stains very faintly with acid dyes and generally occupies all of the chromatin-free areas of the nucleus. In contrast, when fixatives containing acetic acid are used, such as those of Zenker, Bouin, or Carnoy, the inclusion shrinks and a clear chromatin-free halo can be seen around the inclusion body, giving it its characteristic appearance. Inclusions may be very small, no larger than nucleoli. The cell nucleus may contain one or more of these inclusions. They may slowly grow and fuse until they occupy the whole nucleus, as in measles. The nucleolus may be forced by the inclusion mass against an apparently normal nuclear membrane.

The presence of inclusion bodies may be of considerable diagnostic aid. The intracytoplasmic inclusion in nerve cells, the Negri body, is pathognomonic for rabies. A mild case of smallpox may be difficult to differentiate clinically from a severe case of chickenpox. Histologic examination of the skin lesion permits a rapid diagnosis; with smallpox, intracytoplasmic inclusions will be present; with chickenpox, intranuclear inclusions will be found.

Correlated studies employing both cytochemical and immunofluorescent procedures are amassing a wealth of information on the intracellular development of viral nucleic acids and virus-specific antigens. For example, acridine orange staining of cells infected with reovirus has demonstrated the development in the cytoplasm of a viral inclusion containing double-stranded RNA within a protein matrix. Staining with fluorescein-labeled antibodies has shown that this matrix contains large quantities of reovirus antigen. In vaccinia virus-infected cells the use of 2 immune sera, each labeled with a different fluorescent dye, has shown that the cytoplasmic sites for synthesizing the LS protein antigen and the nucleoprotein NP antigen can be easily differentiated. The typical inclusion body seen in vaccinia-infected cells is composed mainly of the NP antigen; in companion cultures stained with acridine orange, the inclusion bodies are revealed to be centers of viral DNA synthesis.

CHROMOSOME DAMAGE

One of the consequences of infection of cells by viruses is derangement of the karyotype. Most of the changes observed are random in nature. Frequently, breakage, fragmentation, and rearrangement of the chromosomes occurs; abnormal chromosomes and changes in chromosome number have also been observed. Herpes zoster virus induces a colchicine-like effect in human cells; the mitotic cycle is interrupted at metaphase, the chromosomes overcontract, and micronuclei form. Some of the chromosomes undergo fragmentation. Chromosome breaks have also been observed in leukocytes from patients with chickenpox and from patients with measles. These viruses, as well as rubella virus, cause similar aberrations when inoculated into cultured cells. Cells infected with or transformed to malignancy by papovaviruses SV40 and polyoma, and cells exposed to adenovirus type 12, also exhibit random chromosomal abnormalities. Many of these findings are preliminary, and analysis of the effect of various viruses on chromosomes is continuing.

Special studies have been carried out with the Chinese hamster cell, which has the advantage for cytogenetic studies of a stable karyotype composed of only 22 chromosomes. Inoculation of these hamster cells with herpes simplex virus results in chromosome aberrations that are not random in distribution. Most of the breaks occur in region 7 of chromosome No. 1 and in region 3 of the X chromosome. The Y chromosome in region 3 of the X chromosome. The Y chromosome is unaffected. Replication of the virus is necessary for induction of the chromosome aberrations. To date, no pathognomonic chromosome alterations have been identified in either virus-infected or virus-transformed cells.

LATENT VIRUS INFECTIONS

Inapparent infection covers, at the host-parasite level, the whole field of infections which give no overt sign of their presence. "Subclinical" can be used as an alternative term, particularly in the discussion of human infections.

Latent infections are inapparent infections which are chronic and in which a certain virus-host equilibrium is established. "Occult virus" is the term used to describe those cases where virus particles cannot be detected and in which the actual state of the virus cannot as yet be ascertained.

Whenever it has been shown that viruses of animals or higher plants go through cycles as described for bacteriophage (see Chapter 9), the terms "provirus," "vegetative virus," and "infective virus" are appropriate for the corresponding stages. Infective virus is the fully formed virus particle.

A moderate virus (corresponding in some measure to a temperate phage) is one growing in a cell while still permitting the continued survival and multiplication of the cell. Some viruses may be moderate in one cell system and cytocidal in another. **Slow viral infections** are characterized by a prolonged incubation period lasting months or years, during which virus continues to multiply, producing increasing destruction of tissue.

Latency in tissue culture systems: The growth of cells in culture for many generations may be accompanied by a concomitant multiplication of virus. The number of cells supporting viral infection in such optimally growing cultures is usually only a small portion of the entire population.

Cells infected with some viruses can divide and grow into infected clones. In these respects, these infections resemble infections by moderate viruses, but there is no evidence that the viral nucleic acid has any real interaction with the host cell nucleic acid. In most of the cells of an actively growing virus-carrier culture, the virus seems to be under some control or repression, eg, local interferon. Culture manipulations that have been found to shift the virus-cell complex toward virus release (cell crowding, medium exhaustion, lowering of temperature) have been of the kind that also slow cell multiplication.

The examples in Fig 27–15 indicate (1) whether the infection is apparent or inapparent according to whether the threshold (dotted line) is passed; (2) whether the inapparent infection persists, ie, becomes truly latent; (3) whether it can be activated in the original host (shown by an arrow); and (4) whether the virus is occult (shown by shading).

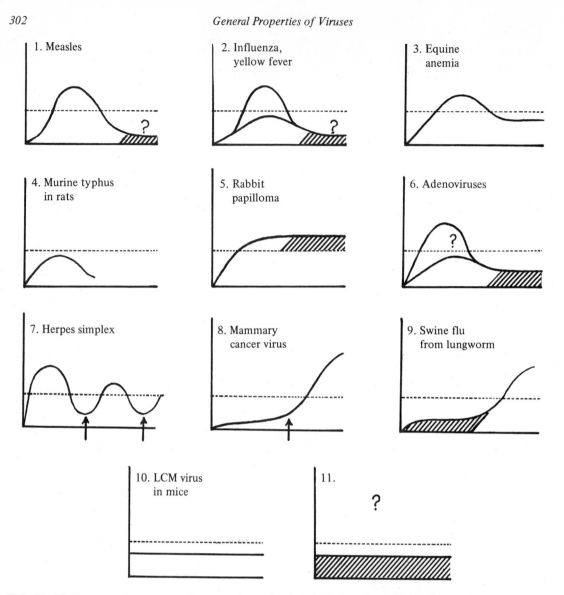

FIG 27–15. Inapparent, apparent, latent, and occult virus infections. (After Andrews.) **(1)** Measles runs an acute, almost always clinical, course. Long-lasting immunity may be associated with persistence of latent infection, possibly with occult virus. **(2)** Yellow fever and influenza show a similar pattern except that infection may be more often subclinical than clinical. **(3)** In equine infectious anemia and perhaps viral hepatitis in man, recovery from clinical disease is associated with latent infection in which fully active virus persists in the blood, sometimes in considerable amounts. **(4)** Some infections are, in a particular species, always subclinical. Examples are equine encephalitis in some species of birds and murine typhus in rats. **(5)** In rabbit papilloma, the course of the infection is chronic, and chronicity is associated with the virus becoming occult. **(6)** Infection of man with certain adenoviruses may be clinical or subclinical. There seems to be a long latent infection during which virus is present in small quantity and only detected by the sensitive technic of growing the infected cells in tissue culture. **(7)** The periodical activation of latent herpes simplex in man often follows an initial acute episode of stomatitis in childhood. **(8)** In many other instances infection is wholly latent for a long time before it is activated. Examples are afforded by mice carrying the mammary cancer virus and by sheep carrying scrapie virus. Kuru in man may be an example of a slow viral infection with a very long incubation period. **(9)** In pigs which have eaten virus-bearing lung worms, swine "flu" virus is occult until the appropriate stimulus induces the infection and simultaneously makes the virus readily demonstrable. **(10)** Lymphocytic choriomeningitis (LCM) virus may be established in mice by in utero infection. Antibodies fail to develop (immunologic tolerance), and the resulting latent infection almost never becomes active to the point of producing disease in the original host; its presence is readily revealed by transmission to an indicator host, eg, adult mice from a virus-free stock. **(11)** There is the theoretical possibility of a latent infection with an occult virus which cannot be activated. How to prove that such a virus is present at all remains a difficult task.

NATURAL HISTORY (ECOLOGY) & MODES OF TRANSMISSION OF VIRUSES & RICKETTSIAE

Viruses may be transmitted in the following ways: (1) Direct transmission from person to person by contact, in which droplet or aerosol infection may play the major role (eg, influenza, measles, smallpox). (2) Transmission by means of the alimentary tract (intimate association with carrier, food, and drink) (eg, enterovirus infections, infectious hepatitis). (3) Transmission by means of dust (eg, Q fever). (4) Transmission by bite (eg, rabies). (5) Transmission by means of an arthropod vector (eg, arboviruses).

Some of the viruses may be conveyed in several different ways and may therefore manifest a variable epidemiology.

The following cycles have been recognized among the arthropod-borne viruses:

1. Man-arthropod cycle—*Example:* Urban yellow fever.

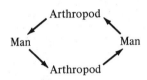

2. Lower vertebrate-arthropod cycle with tangential infection of man—*Examples:* Jungle yellow fever, equine encephalitis.

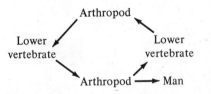

3. Arthropod-arthropod cycle with occasional infection of man and lower vertebrates—*Example:* Colorado tick fever.

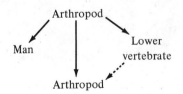

In (3) the virus may be transmitted from the adult arthropod to its offspring by means of the egg (transovarian passage); thus the cycle may continue with or without intervention of a vertebrate host.

In vertebrates the invasion of most viruses evokes a violent reaction, usually of short duration. The result is decisive. Either the host succumbs or it lives through the production of antibodies that neutralize or kill the virus. Regardless of the outcome, the sojourn of the active virus is usually short (although latent virus infec-

tions may occur, as in herpes, adenovirus, and cytomegalovirus infections). In arthropod vectors of the virus, the relationship is usually quite different. The viruses may produce little or no ill effect, and remain active in the arthropod throughout the latter's natural life. Thus arthropods, in contrast to vertebrates, act as permanent hosts and reservoirs.

SIMULTANEOUS ADMINISTRATION OF VIRUS VACCINES

The use of viral vaccines is detailed in the chapters dealing with specific diseases. However, there is one general point that needs to be made here. The USPHS Advisory Committee on Immunization Practices has recommended an interval of 1 month between inoculations of live virus vaccines. This was based on the theoretical consideration that adverse reactions might be more frequent or severe if the vaccines were given at closer intervals, and that antibody response might be diminished.

The above recommendation has sometimes been interpreted as being against administration of live virus vaccines at less than 1 month intervals **under any circumstances.** This misinterpretation has caused great inconvenience to travelers whose plans precluded waiting so long between inoculations. Immunization against yellow fever has sometimes been denied to persons recently vaccinated against smallpox when they presented themselves a few days before departure. However, the Advisory Committee recently stated that: "If the theoretically desirable 1 month interval is not feasible, as with the threat of concurrent exposures or disruption of immunization programs, the vaccines should preferably be given on the same day—at different sites for parenteral products. An interval of about 2 days to 2 weeks should be avoided because interference between the vaccine viruses is most likely then." The evidence upon which the Committee's latest recommendation is based is summarized below:

When vaccinia virus and attenuated yellow fever (YF) virus are given **simultaneously but at separate sites,** the dermal response to vaccinia and the YF antibody response are both satisfactory. In contrast, when vaccinia virus and YF virus are administered simultaneously and at the same site, the dermal response to vaccinia is normal but the antibody response to YF vaccine is suppressed. The vaccinia virus interferes with local replication of YF virus. Attenuated YF virus is sensitive to the antiviral effects of interferon in vitro and, when administered in combination with vaccinia virus, is inhibited by the interferon which is produced at the site of vaccinia virus inoculation.

Vaccinia takes may also be inhibited by interferon, and YF virus does induce circulating interferon, but only 4–6 days after vaccination. The dermal response to vaccinia virus is also known to be inhibited by measles virus vaccine but only if vaccinia virus is

[Cont'd on p 308.]

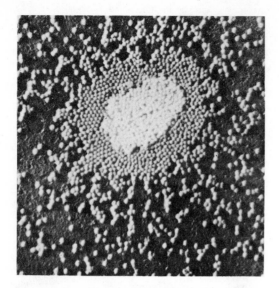

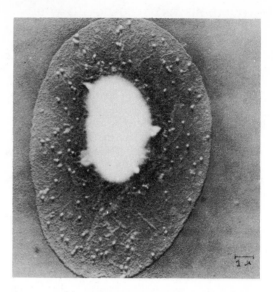

FIG 27—16. Electron micrograph typical of purified preparations of a spherical virus (20,000 ×). Shown are human wart virus particles (papovavirus group) having a diameter of 45 nm. (Melnick & Bunting.)

FIG 27—17. Influenza virus particles, PR8 strain, adsorbed on the membranes of a chicken erythrocyte. The particles are about 100 nm in diameter. (Werner & Schlesinger.)

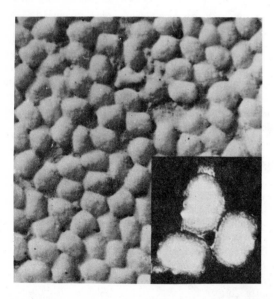

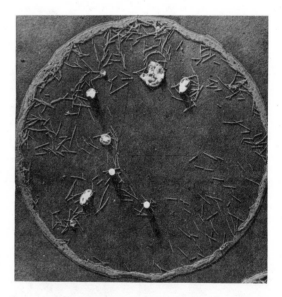

FIG 27—18. Electron micrograph of a purified sample of a brick-shaped poxvirus, molluscum contagiosum (20,000 ×). The virus particles, purified from human skin lesions by differential centrifugation, measure about 330 × 230 nm. (Melnick, Bunting, & Strauss.) Inset: Uranyl acetate stain of DNA-containing core of the virus (47,000 ×).

FIG 27—19. Meningopneumonitis virus ("nucleated" structures with diameters of about 400 nm) (2500 ×); standard latex particles (true spheres, 250 nm); and tobacco mosaic virus (rods, 15 × 280 nm). Purified preparations of the 2 viruses were mixed with standard latex particles, whose diameter is known, and sprayed to produce fine droplets. The contents of one droplet are shown. (Crocker.)

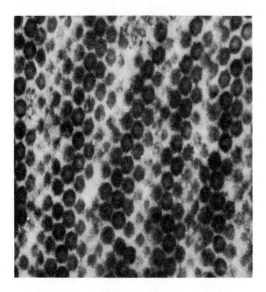

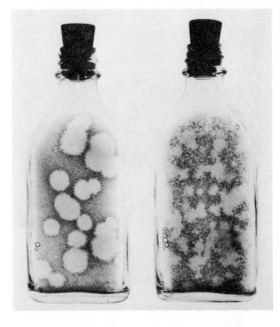

FIG 27−20. Adenovirus (60,000 X). Ultrathin section through the nucleus of a monkey kidney cell infected with type 3. Acrolein fixation, which also preserves viral antigen. Many virus particles are shown in hexagonal crystalline arrays. (Mayor & Jordan.)

FIG 27−21. **Plaques produced by poliovirus (left) and by an echovirus (right).** Both viruses are cultivated in bottle cultures of monkey kidney cells. After the viruses are seeded, the epithelial sheet is covered with an agar overlay containing a vital dye (neutral red). As the cytopathogenic effect of the virus becomes manifest, the cells lose their vital stain and clear areas appear in the culture. The progeny of a single virus particle are located in each clear area. The plaque morphology of each of the viruses shown is sufficiently clear so that the 2 virus groups can readily be distinguished from each other by this method. (Hsiung & Melnick.)

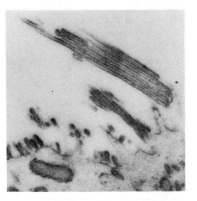

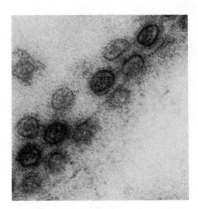

FIG 27−22. **Influenza virus at the cell surface (31,000 X).** Two bundles of filaments (one cut longitudinally, the other obliquely) extend into the extracellular space. At left, short filaments seem to be budding from the cell. (Morgan, Rose, & Moore.)

FIG 27−23. **Spherical forms of influenza virus (116,000 X).** The cell wall passes diagonally across the field, with host cell cytoplasm to the right. Several particles just beneath the cell membrane seem to be undergoing differentiation towards the mature extracellular form. (Morgan, Rose, & Moore.)

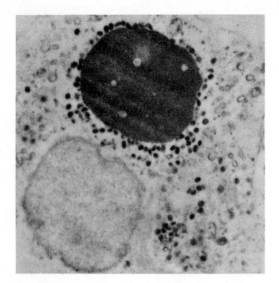

FIG 27—24. Mousepox virus within the infected cell (7400 X). Nucleus at lower left; above it can be seen a dark cytoplasmic inclusion body surrounded by virus particles. A colony of virus particles in the process of development is located to the right of the nucleus. (Gaylord & Melnick.)

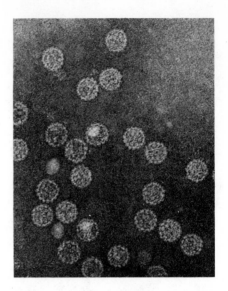

FIG 27—25. Papovavirus SV40. Purified preparation negatively stained with phosphotungstate (150,000 X). (McGregor & Mayor.)

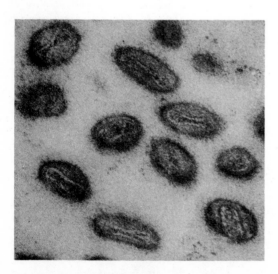

FIG 27—26. Ultrathin section of vaccinia virus particles within the cytoplasm of an infected cell (74,000 X). The internal structure of the mature virus is evident. (Morgan, Rose, & Moore.)

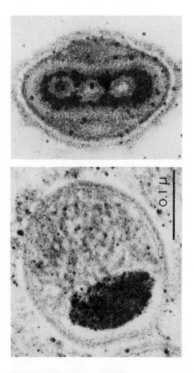

FIG 27—27. Localization of DNA in immature (bottom) and mature (top) vaccinia particles. After hydrolysis with HCl, a silver methenamine solution has been applied to Epon sections of the virus. Silver granules are specifically deposited at the sites of DNA. Other structures are made visible by counterstaining with uranyl acetate (170,000 X). (Peters.)

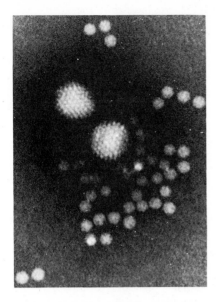

FIG 27–28. A group of satellite viruses and 2 adeno-virions which function as helpers for the defective satellites (250,000 X). (Mayor, Jordan, & Melnick.)

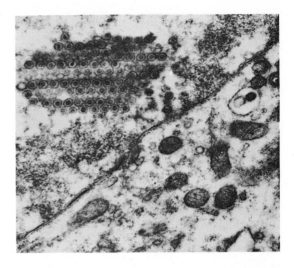

FIG 27–29. Herpesvirus in human amnion cell. The nuclear membrane runs from lower left to upper right. A regular array of virus particles, each possessing a dense central body and a single peripheral membrane, is present within the nucleus (27,000 X). (Morgan.)

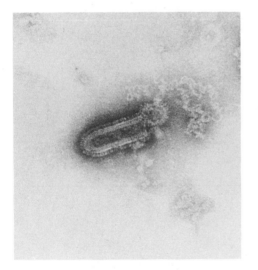

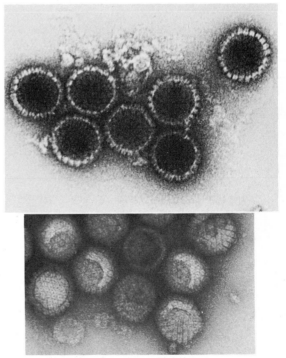

FIG 27–30. Electron micrograph of bullet-shaped particle typical of the rhabdovirus group (100,000 X). Shown here is vesicular stomatitis virus negatively stained with potassium phosphotungstate. (McCombs, Benyesh-Melnick, & Brunschwig.)

FIG 27–31. Top: Herpesvirus particles from human vesicle fluid, stained with uranyl acetate to show DNA core (140,000 X). Bottom: Virions stained to show protein capsomeres of the virus coat (140,000 X). (Smith & Melnick.)

TABLE 27–7. Principal vaccines used in prevention of virus diseases of man.

Disease	Source of Vaccine	Condition of Virus	Route of Administration
Recommended Immunization for General Public			
Poliomyelitis	Tissue cultures (formalinized, or treated with formalin and ultraviolet light) (monkey kidney)	Inactive	Intramuscular
	Tissue culture (monkey kidney)	Live attenuated	Oral
Measles	Tissue culture (chick embryo)	Live attenuated*	Intramuscular†
Smallpox and alastrim	Lymph from calf or sheep (glycerolated)	Active	Skin scarification or multiple pressure
	Chorioallantois, tissue cultures	Active	Subcutaneous or intradermal
Mumps	Tissue culture (chick embryo)	Live attenuated	Subcutaneous
Rubella	Tissue culture (duck embryo, rabbit, or dog kidney)	Live attenuated	Intramuscular
Immunization Recommended Only Under Certain Conditions (Epidemics, Exposure, Travel, Military)			
Yellow fever	Tissue cultures and eggs (17D strain)‡	Live attenuated	Subcutaneous or intradermal
Influenza	Allantoic fluid (formalinized, concentrated by various processes)	Inactive	Subcutaneous
Rabies	Duck embryo treated with phenol or ultraviolet light	Inactive	Subcutaneous
Adenovirus§	Monkey kidney tissue cultures (formalinized)	Inactive	Intramuscular
	Human diploid cell cultures	Live attenuated	Oral, by enteric-coated capsule
Japanese B encephalitis§	Mouse brain (formalinized), tissue culture	Inactive	Subcutaneous
Equine encephalo-myelitis§	Chick embryo (formalinized)	Inactive	Subcutaneous
Russian spring-summer encephalitis§	Mouse brain (formalinized)	Inactive	Subcutaneous

*Inactivated measles vaccine was available for a short period. However, a serious delayed hypersensitivity reaction often occurs when children who have received primary immunization with inactive measles vaccine are later exposed to live measles virus. Because of this complication, inactivated measles vaccine is no longer recommended.

†With less attenuated strains, gamma globulin is given in another limb at the time of vaccination.

‡A mouse-brain-grown neurotropic strain of virus (Dakar) is used in some parts of the world but is not recommended by the US Public Health Service.

§Not available in the USA except for the Armed Forces or for investigative purposes.

administered at the height of the measles virus-induced interferon response which occurs 10 days after vaccination. Therefore, it can be stated that inhibition of vaccinia virus replication by YF virus vaccine does not occur when the 2 viruses are administered **simultaneously**.

•　　•　　•

General References

Caspar, D.L.D., & A. Klug: Physical principles in the construction of regular viruses. Cold Spring Harbor Symposium 27:1–24, 1962.

Erikson, R.L.: Replication of RNA viruses. Ann Rev Microbiol 22:305–322, 1968.

Fenner, F., & J.F. Sambrook: The genetics of animal viruses. Ann Rev Microbiol 18:47–94, 1964.

Hilleman, M.R.: Toward control of viral infections in man. Science 164:506–514, 1969.

Joklik, W.K.: The molecular basis of the viral eclipse phase. Progr Med Virol 7:44–96, 1965.

Kaplan, A.S., & T. Ben-Porat: Metabolism of animal cells infected with nuclear DNA viruses. Ann Rev Microbiol 22:427–450, 1968.

Kit, S., & R. Dubbs: Enzyme induction by viruses. Monogr Virol 2:1–114, 1969.

Melnick, J.L.: Summary of classification of animal viruses, 1970. Progr Med Virol 12:337–341, 1970.

Mims, C.A.: Pathogenesis of viral infections of the fetus. Progr Med Virol 10:194–237, 1968.

Pagano, J.S.: Biologic activity of isolated viral nucleic acids. Progr Med Virol 12:1–48, 1970.

Rapp, F.: Defective DNA animal viruses. Ann Rev Microbiol 23:293–316, 1969.

Stich, H.F., & D.S. Yohn: Viruses and chromosomes. Progr Med Virol 12:78–127, 1970.

Wheelock, E.F., Larke, R.P.B., & N.L. Caroline: Interference in human viral infections: Present status and prospects for the future. Prog Med Virol 10:286–347, 1968.

28...

Isolation of Viruses From Clinical Specimens

Viruses can be isolated and identified during the course of many diseases, thus establishing the etiologic diagnosis. Generally, however, a specific diagnosis cannot be made in the first few days of the infection; the results of most diagnostic tests for viral diseases do not become available until the patient has recovered or died.

The time and cost entailed in isolating and identifying viruses necessitates careful selection of patients and proper collection and handling of specimens. As a general rule, the indications for attempting to isolate a virus from patients include the following: (1) Instances where the established diagnosis will directly affect the management of the patient, eg, laboratory-proved rubella in the first trimester of pregnancy would favor a decision to terminate pregnancy. (2) Instances where the diagnosis is vital to the health of the community, eg, laboratory confirmation of smallpox, poliomyelitis, influenza, or arbovirus encephalitis will provide the necessary information for instituting immunization programs or insect control measures. (3) Instances where the etiologic agent of a disease is being sought. Studies of patients for etiologic association require prior planning and cooperation between the physician, the public health worker, and the virologist, and must include the study of samples from control patients.

The laboratory procedures used in the diagnosis of viral diseases in human beings include the following:

(1) Isolation and identification of the agent.

(2) Measurement of antibodies developing during the course of the infection.

(3) Histologic examination of infected tissues. This should be performed on all fatal cases of virus infections and on animals suspected of infection with rabies virus (Negri inclusion bodies). Biopsy material is useful for distinguishing severe varicella (intranuclear inclusions present) from mild variola (cytoplasmic inclusions present).

(4) Detection of viral antigens in lesions. This method is useful today for detecting the antigen of variola in skin lesions and, using fluorescein-labeled antibodies, in the detection of rabies virus antigen. Myxovirus antigens (hemagglutinins) are detectable in respiratory secretions.

(5) Electron microscopic examination of vesicular fluids or tissue extracts treated with negative and positive stains to identify and count DNA and RNA virus particles (see Chapter 27). This procedure in the hands of trained personnel has provided diagnoses in a matter of hours in patients with vesicular diseases such as those produced by poxviruses or by herpesviruses, including chickenpox and myxoviruses in respiratory secretions.

CONSIDERATIONS IN THE DIAGNOSIS OF VIRAL DISEASES

Laboratory confirmation of a virus infection by serologic means is usually preferred, because antibody tests are more readily and quickly performed than isolation and typing of viruses. However, antibody tests can be carried out only for those illnesses for which the etiologic viruses have been grown in the laboratory. Virus isolation is required (1) when new epidemics occur, as with A_2 (Asian) influenza in 1957; (2) when serologic tests overlap and do not allow one to distinguish between 2 viruses, as with smallpox and vaccinia; (3) when it is necessary to confirm a diagnosis made by direct microscopic observation, eg, as detecting a herpesvirus in vesicle fluid; and (4) when the same clinical illness may be caused by many different agents.

In undertaking the diagnostic evaluation of a patient with a suspected viral disease one must bear in mind that the same clinical syndromes may be produced by a variety of agents. For example, aseptic (nonbacterial) meningitis may be caused by many different viruses as well as by spirochetes; similarly, respiratory disease syndromes may be caused by many viruses as well as mycoplasma and other agents.

The isolation of a virus is not necessarily equivalent to establishing the etiology of a given disease. A number of other factors have to be taken into consideration. Some viruses persist in human hosts for long periods of time, and therefore the isolation of herpes, poliomyelitis, echo, or coxsackie viruses from the secretions or cells of a patient with an obscure illness does not necessarily indicate that the virus is the cause of his disease. A consistent clinical and epidemiologic pattern must be established by repeated studies before one can be sure that a particular agent is responsible for a specific clinical picture.

Dual infections present still another problem in interpreting the result of virus isolation studies. Different viruses may have the same seasonal and geographic occurrence. Poliomyelitis and encephalitis viruses sometimes frequent the same area at the same time. Thus in one summer a patient may have inapparent infection with one virus and clinical infection with the other. If the clinical infection is mild, the syndrome (eg, aseptic meningitis) may be such that it could be produced by either virus. If antibody studies were made only for the virus which produced the inapparent infection, the diagnosis might be missed altogether. Isolation of 2 viral agents similarly confuses the etiologic significance of each agent unless their role in causation of the illness has been established by prior experience.

The same principle of identifying viral antigens using immunofluorescence has proved useful in rapid diagnosis of certain respiratory virus diseases by examining smeared epithelial cells from the nasopharynx. Buffy coat leukocytes obtained during the acute illness contain viral antigens (eg, enteroviruses), and this offers a rapid method for obtaining an accurate diagnosis of some viral diseases.

VIRUS ISOLATION TECHNIC

DIRECT EXAMINATION OF CLINICAL MATERIAL

The viral diseases for which direct microscopic examination of imprints or smears has been proved useful include rabies, herpes, varicella, and zoster. The procedure for staining viral antigens by immunofluorescence in a smear from a rabid animal has developed to such an extent that it has now become the method of choice for routine diagnosis of rabies. The procedure is carried out as outlined in Table 28–1.

The demonstration or isolation of active virus requires the proper collection of appropriate specimens, their preservation both en route to and in the laboratory, and the inoculation of susceptible animals, embryonated eggs, or suitable tissue cultures. Prior to the inoculation of the specimen, several preliminary procedures designed to eliminate bacteria from the specimen may be necessary (see below). The presence of a virus is demonstrated by the appearance of characteristic histologic lesions, inclusion bodies, or viral antigens (hemagglutinating and complement fixing) in the inoculated test system. Isolated viruses are specifically identified using known antibodies which inhibit

TABLE 28–1. Fluorescent rabies antibody test (direct method).

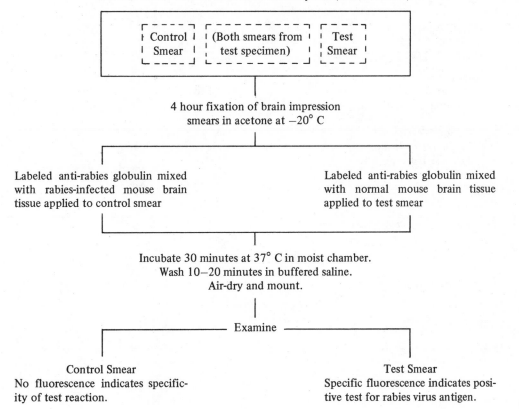

| Control Smear | (Both smears from test specimen) | Test Smear |

4 hour fixation of brain impression smears in acetone at −20° C

Labeled anti-rabies globulin mixed with rabies-infected mouse brain tissue applied to control smear

Labeled anti-rabies globulin mixed with normal mouse brain tissue applied to test smear

Incubate 30 minutes at 37° C in moist chamber.
Wash 10–20 minutes in buffered saline.
Air-dry and mount.

Examine

Control Smear
No fluorescence indicates specificity of test reaction.

Test Smear
Specific fluorescence indicates positive test for rabies virus antigen.

TABLE 28–3. Specimens for isolation of viruses.

Clinical Manifestations and Common Etiologic Agents	Source of Specimen for Virus Isolation	
	Clinical	Postmortem
Upper respiratory tract infections		
Rhinovirus Mycoplasma Parainfluenza	Throat swab or nasal secretions	. . .
Adenovirus Enterovirus Reovirus	Throat swab and feces	. . .
Lower respiratory tract infections Influenza Adenovirus Parainfluenza Mycoplasma	Throat swab and sputum	Lung
Pleurodynia Coxsackie virus	Throat swab and feces	. . .

Cutaneous and mucous membrane diseases
Vesicular
  Smallpox and vaccinia
  Herpes simplex
  Varicella-zoster
	Vesicle fluid	Liver, spleen, and lung

Enterovirus	Vesicle fluid, feces, and throat swab	. . .

Exanthematous
  Measles
  Rubella
	Throat swab and blood	. . .

Enterovirus	Throat swab and feces	. . .
CNS infections Enterovirus	Feces and CSF	Brain tissue and intestinal contents
Herpes simplex	Throat swab	Brain tissue
Mumps	Throat swab	Brain tissue
Lymphocytic choriomeningitis	Blood and CSF	Brain tissue

Arboviruses
  Western equine encephalitis
  Eastern equine encephalitis
  Venezuelan equine encephalitis
	Blood and CSF	Brain tissue

California encephalitis
  St. Louis encephalitis
  Japanese B encephalitis
	Usually not possible to isolate virus from clinical specimens	. . .

Rabies	Saliva	Brain tissue
Parotitis Mumps	Throat swab	. . .
Severe undifferentiated febrile illnesses Colorado tick fever Yellow fever Dengue	Blood	. . .
Congenital anomalies Cytomegalovirus	Urine and throat swab	Kidney, lung, and other tissues
Rubella	Throat swab and CSF	Lymph nodes, lung, spleen, other tissues

or neutralize the biologic effects of the virus or react with viral antigens (inhibiting hemagglutination or fixing complement).

SPECIMENS FOR STUDY

In the collection of material for virus identification studies it is well to remember that many viruses are most readily demonstrated in the early days of the disease. (See Table 28–2.)

Blood, sputum, nasal washings, stool, urine, pus, unfixed biopsy material, and spinal fluid all serve as sources of virus material from clinical cases (Tables 28–2 and 28–3). Tissues obtained at autopsy may also serve this purpose.

Owing to the variability of different viral types, care must be taken at the outset to prepare the inoculum in the proper manner and to determine which types of animals or culture media are to be inoculated (Table 29–10). There may be an unavoidable lapse of time between the collection of the material and its inoculation into a suitable animal or tissue culture; it is not enough, in such instances, to leave the material at the usual refrigerator temperature in the hope that the virus may survive for 1–2 days until it can be inoculated. This is particularly true if the material is left in a fluid state.

Material should, in general, be frozen at $-20°$ C or lower temperatures if there is a delay in bringing it to the laboratory. The principal exceptions to this rule are (1) whole blood drawn for antibody determination, which must have the serum separated before freezing, and (2) tissue for organ or cell culture (or urine for cytomegalovirus isolation), which should be placed at $4°$ C and taken to the laboratory as soon as possible for prompt processing.

The choice of specimens for viral study is of utmost importance. The specimens most likely to yield virus from common illnesses are listed in Table 28–3 along with the etiologic agents commonly associated with the diseases.

Generally, respiratory illnesses are associated with excretion of virus in the nasal or pharyngeal secretions. Virus can be demonstrated in the fluid of vesicular rashes. Illnesses manifested as meningoencephalitis are usually diagnosed more readily by serologic means. In such cases, if an enterovirus is the etiologic agent, it can be isolated readily. Arboviruses, herpes simplex virus, and mumps virus are not recovered from clinical specimens in most instances of CNS disease, although autopsy specimens of brain tissue from encephalitis patients who died early in the course of the disease often yield the etiologic virus. Other illnesses associated with enteroviruses, such as acute pericarditis, myocarditis, and fatal neonatal illness, are readily diagnosed by studying feces and throat swabs.

PRESERVATION OF VIRUSES

Freezing

A large, wide-mouthed thermos jar or insulated carton, half filled with pieces of solid CO_2 (dry ice), is useful for the transportation and temporary preservation of material containing viruses. The temperature within a dry ice storage cabinet can be maintained close to $-76°$ C. Electric deep-freeze cabinets can maintain temperatures of -50 to $-70°$ C.

Lyophilization

This procedure consists of rapid freezing at low temperature (in a bath containing alcohol and dry ice) and rapid dehydration from the frozen state at high vacuum; the containers are sealed under the original vacuum.

Ten to 50% of normal rabbit serum or other plasma or serum in the fluid menstruum protects the virus to be frozen and dried. The plasma or serum must not contain antibodies which might neutralize the virus. Skimmed milk is another "protective" menstruum in which virus-containing material may be suspended. If tissues are to be preserved by these methods, they may be ground to a paste and then desiccated in the same manner as are blood and other biologic suspensions.

Dried virus should be stored in the refrigerator. To reconstitute the virus, the sealed ampule containing the dried material is opened and a volume of distilled water equal to the original or desired volume is added.

Glycerol

This is the oldest and simplest method of preserving viruses. Small pieces of tissue or fecal material and suspensions of mucus can be preserved in 50% glycerol. The majority of pathogenic bacteria do not survive in glycerol after 5 or 6 days. Some viruses remain viable in glycerol longer than others.

TABLE 28–2. Relation of stage of illness to presence of virus in test materials and to appearance of specific antibody.

Stage or Period of Illness	Virus Detectable in Test Materials	Specific Antibody Demonstrable*
Incubation	Rarely	No
Prodrome	Rarely to occasionally	No
Onset	Frequently	Occasionally
Acute phase	Frequently	Frequently
Recovery	Rarely	Usually
Convalescent	Very rarely	Usually

*Antibody may be detected very early in vaccinated persons or in previously infected persons.

PREPARATION OF INOCULA

Bacteria-free fluid materials such as whole blood, plasma, serum, or CSF may be inoculated into animals, eggs, or tissue culture, directly or after dilution with buffered phosphate solution (pH 7.6).

Preparation of Tissues

The material is placed in a sterile Petri dish, washed in sterile water, drained, and weighed. Using sterile equipment and materials, it is cut into small pieces with scissors, placed in a mortar with sand (or particles of alundum), and ground to make a homogeneous paste. The diluent should be added in amounts sufficient to make up a concentration of 10–20%. This suspension can be centrifuged at low speed (not more than 2000 rpm) for 10 minutes to precipitate insoluble cellular debris. The supernatant fluid may be inoculated; if bacteria are present, they may be eliminated as discussed below.

Removal of Bacteria

If the material to be tested contains bacteria—as may be the case with oral washings or with suspensions of stools, infected tissue, or insects—these bacteria must be removed before inoculation.

A. Bactericidal Agents:

1. **Ether**—If it is not harmful to the virus in question (eg, poliomyelitis, vaccinia), ether may be added in concentrations of 10–15%.

2. **Antibiotics**—Antibiotics are used commonly as mixtures of penicillin and streptomycin, employed in combination with differential centrifugation (see below).

3. **Photodynamic inactivation**—The dye proflavine can irreversibly photosensitize microbial flora in stool and throat specimens. After incubation of dye-treated material in the dark at 37° C for 1 hour at pH 9.0 in 10^{-4} M proflavine, the dye is removed by cation resins and the photosensitized bacterial and fungal contaminants are inactivated by exposure to white light. With enteroviruses and rhinoviruses, little viral activity is lost.

B. Mechanical Methods:

1. **Filters**—Earthenware, porcelain, and asbestos filters reduce the virus concentration by adsorption, and are therefore used less frequently now.

2. **Differential centrifugation**—This is a convenient method of removing many bacteria from heavily contaminated preparations of the small viruses. It consists of sedimenting the bacteria at speeds which do not precipitate the virus: 18,000 rpm for 20 minutes in a 6-inch rotor has been recommended for viruses less than 100 μm in size. If the material is suspected of containing minimal quantities of infective virus, these may be concentrated by spinning the suspension in a vacuum ultracentrifuge at forces sufficient to sediment the virus into a small gelatinous pellet at the bottom of the tube. Centrifugation at 40,000 rpm (100,000 times gravity) for 60 minutes in a 6-inch rotor will throw down most viruses. The supernatant from such a run contains less than 1% of the original virus. The virus-containing sediment is then resuspended in a small volume.

ANIMAL INOCULATION

The laboratory animals employed for virus isolation include mice, hamsters, cotton rats, guinea pigs, rabbits, and monkeys. For certain viruses, infant mice (1 or 2 days old) are used. The animal of choice and the recommended route of inoculation for specific viruses are tabulated in Table 29–10. Only the intracerebral and intranasal routes will be discussed here.

Intracerebral Inoculation

This is the method of choice for many neurotropic viruses. The inoculum must be relatively free from pathogenic bacteria, for the brain is more susceptible to bacterial infection artificially introduced than are many other parts of the body. Mice are used in groups of at least 6; they should be anesthetized before inoculation. The technic consists of injecting 0.03 ml of inoculum above the orbital ridge into the brain.

Each day after inoculation all animals should be examined closely for signs of illness, and this daily observation should be pursued for an appropriate length of time (3–4 weeks). If the inoculated animal dies during the period of observation, bacterial cultures should be made of the brain and heart blood in order to rule out or confirm the possibility of supervening bacterial infection. If the animal survives without signs of illness until the end of the period of observation, it should be sacrificed and a careful autopsy performed.

Intranasal Inoculation or Instillation

Animals should be anesthetized and the material dropped on the nares with a capillary pipet.

Autopsies of inoculated animals should be performed with great care. Histologic sections are usually required to complete the examination.

CULTIVATION IN TISSUE CULTURE

Viruses do not multiply on inanimate culture media, but propagation may proceed in the presence of cells growing in vitro in tissue culture. Tissue culture technics are the most widely used methods for isolating viruses from clinical specimens. When viruses multiply in tissue culture, they produce biologic effects (cytopathic changes, viral interference, or hemadsorption) which permit identification of the agent.

Test tube cultures are prepared by adding cells suspended in 1–2 ml of nutrient fluid which contains balanced salt solutions and various growth factors (usually serum, glucose, amino acids, and vitamins). Cells of fibroblastic or epithelial nature attach and grow on the wall of the test tube where they may be examined with the aid of a low power microscope.

With many viruses, growth of the agent is paralleled by a degeneration of these cells. (See Fig 28–1.) Some viruses produce characteristic cytopathic effects in tissue culture, making a rapid presumptive diagnosis possible when the clinical syndrome is known. As examples, measles, mumps, parainfluenza, and respiratory syncytial viruses characteristically produce multinucleated giant cells, while adenoviruses produce grape-like clusters of large round cells, rhinoviruses produce focal areas of rounding and dendritic forms, and herpes simplex virus produces diffuse uniform rounding of cells.

Some viruses (eg, rubella virus) produce no direct cytopathic changes but rather can be detected by their interference with the cytopathic effect of a second challenge virus (viral interference).

Influenza virus as well as other myxoviruses may be detected within 24–48 hours if erythrocytes are added to infected cultures. Viruses maturing at the cell membrane produce a substance enabling the erythrocytes to adsorb at the cell surface (hemadsorption).

Recent work with organ cultures of ferret and human tracheal epithelium has shown that these cultures support the growth of a wide variety of viruses which cause upper respiratory tract disease, including some new viruses which do not grow in conventional tissue culture tubes. Viruses may cause general or focal necrosis of the ciliated epithelial cells or may be detected by a decline in ciliary activity.

Confirmation of the identity of a virus isolate requires use of type-specific antiserum, which inhibits both virus growth and the biologic (or cytopathic) effect. This inhibition has made possible relatively simple in vitro serologic tests for viruses.

CHICK EMBRYO TECHNIC

Embryonated eggs of varying age may be inoculated by several routes. After inoculation, the eggs are reincubated for several days at 36–38° C and examined daily.

Chorioallantoic Inoculation

This is performed in 10- to 12-day-old embryos. An area free of vessels is selected and marked at the greatest circumference of the egg. The air sac is also located. An artificial air sac is made by chipping the shell with a sharp-pointed instrument over the area

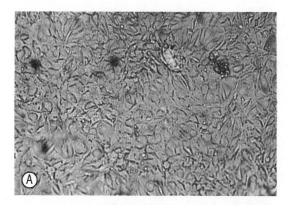

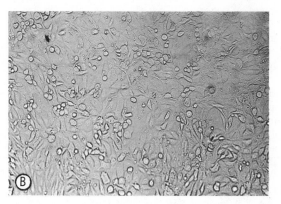

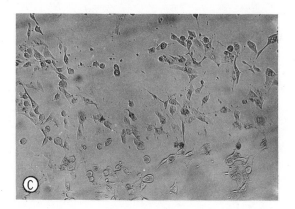

FIG 28–1. **A.** Monolayer of normal unstained monkey kidney cells in culture (120 X). **B.** Unstained monkey kidney cell culture showing early stage of cytopathic effects (CPE) typical of enterovirus infection (120 X). Approximately 25% of the cells in the culture show CPE indicative of virus multiplication (1+ CPE score). **C.** Unstained monkey kidney cell culture illustrating more advanced enteroviral cytopathic effect (3+ to 4+ CPE) (120 X). Almost 100% of the cells are affected, and most of the cell sheet has come loose from the wall of the culture tube.

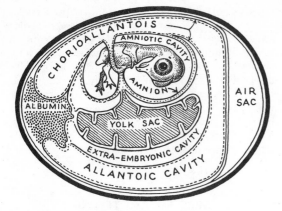

FIG 28—2. Schematic diagram showing developing chick embryo and indicating cavities and other structures used for various routes of inoculation.

marked on the side of the egg. The intact shell membrane is carefully exposed and slit by gentle pressure. The chorioallantois lying immediately beneath must not be ruptured in the process. A second hole is made in the air sac end of the egg. When gentle suction is applied through this opening the chorioallantois will drop away from the shell membrane beneath the first hole. The inoculum may be placed on top of the first hole and be drawn in when the membrane is dropped, or it may be placed later onto the membrane.

Amniotic Sac Inoculation

Embryos 7—14 days old have been used. After the chorioallantois is dropped the side opening is enlarged. A forceps is then thrust through the dropped chorioallantois and a small part of the amniotic membrane drawn through the chorioallantois, so that the inoculum can be introduced directly into the amniotic sac.

Allantoic Sac Inoculation

This procedure is perfomed in 10-day-old embryos through an opening made in the shell and underlying membranes over an avascular area of the chorioallantois. A hole is made in the air sac end to prevent back pressure of the inoculum.

Yolk Sac Inoculation

This is performed in 3- to 8-day-old embryos. At this age the yolk sac fills almost the entire egg. A hole is made in the air sac end, and the inoculum is introduced directly into the yolk sac.

Other Types of Inoculation

Intraembryonic, intravenous, and intracelomic inoculations may also be done in special instances.

EXAMINATION OF EMBRYOS

The shell over the artificial air space is chipped away and the shell membrane removed with sterile scissors and forceps. This exposes the ectodermal surface of the chorioallantois, on which lesions may have developed.

The membrane is removed, placed in sterile water, and examined for lesions against a dark background. If the virus is to be passed, the membrane is first ground to make a suspension. For some agents the whole embryo (minced and ground) may be used as a source of virus. Yolk sacs and the allantoic or amniotic fluid are also sometimes used as sources.

•   •   •

General References

Hoorn, B., & D.A.J. Tyrrell: Organ cultures in virology. Progr Med Virol 11:408—450, 1969.

Lennette, E.H., Melnick, J.L., & R.M. Chanock: Methods in clinical virology. Pages 489—497 in: *Manual of Clinical Microbiology.* Blair, J.E., Lennette, E.H., & J.P. Truant (editors). American Society for Microbiology, 1970.

Rapp, F., & J.L. Melnick: Applications of tissue culture methods in virus laboratories. Progr Med Virol 6:268—317, 1964.

Schmidt, N.J.: Tissue culture techniques for diagnostic virology. Pages 79—178 in: *Diagnostic Procedures for Viral and Rickettsial Infections,* 4th ed. American Public Health Association, 1969.

Sulkin, S.E., & R.M. Pike: Prevention of laboratory infections. Pages 66—78 in: *Diagnostic Procedures for Viral and Rickettsial Infections,* 4th ed. American Public Health Association, 1969.

29...
Serologic Diagnosis
of Virus Infections

Procedures Available

Procedures for the detection and measurement of antibody in virus diseases are based on ways in which the antibody reacts with the antigen. The reaction of the antibody with the virus may result in the neutralization of viral infectivity, the **neutralization** test; or prevention by antibody of the ability of the virus to agglutinate certain types of erythrocytes, the **hemagglutination inhibition** test. In other tests, the reaction may be visualized in the form of visible antigen-antibody complexes, the **precipitation** test, carried out either in liquid medium or in a semisolid medium. The virus-specific products in the infected tissue can also be demonstrated by reacting it with antibody conjugated with a fluorescent dye, the **fluorescent antibody** or **immunofluorescence** test. The **complement fixation** test utilizes the ability of the aggregates of virus and antibody to bind complement. For the correct diagnosis, it is necessary to have on hand the reference typing antisera and viruses.

The methods used in all of these tests are those of classical immunology (see Chapter 12), with certain modifications for certain viruses. This chapter will deal with methods chosen to illustrate some principles. A summary of the tests available is presented in Table 29–10.

Collection of Blood Specimens

Two or more serial samples of serum are essential for diagnostic purposes if antibodies are to be adequately tested and evaluated. In general, the first sample should be collected as soon as possible after the onset of the illness; the second, 2–3 weeks after onset. A third sample may be required later for special study. Antibodies seem to appear earlier in some viral infections than in others, and so the times of collecting specimens must be varied according to circumstances.

Blood specimens should be drawn with aseptic precautions and without anticoagulants and the serum separated and stored at 4° C or −20° C. Before performing serologic tests it may be necessary to heat the serum (56° C for 30 minutes) to remove nonspecific interfering or inhibiting substances. This is essential for complement fixation tests and also, with certain viruses, for neutralization tests.

NEUTRALIZATION TESTS

The principle of the neutralization test is that specific protective or virus-neutralizing antibodies can be measured by adding serum containing these antibodies to a suspension of virus and then injecting the mixture into a group of susceptible experimental animals. If the animals fail to develop the disease and control animals, who have received the virus plus a serum free of the antibody in question, do develop the disease, then the presence of neutralizing antibodies has been proved. In some infections, the virus-serum mixture may be inoculated into tissue culture (as in poliomyelitis) or embryonated eggs (as in mumps); failure of virus to grow indicates the presence of neutralizing antibodies.

It is possible to reactivate quantitatively neutralized poliovirus by treatment of the virus-antibody complex with hydrochloric acid (pH 2.0) or with fluorocarbon, which probably acts by dissociating the virus-antibody complex.

The level of such antibodies can be determined by using a constant amount of virus and falling concentrations of serum. In certain instances undiluted serum may be tested against falling concentrations of virus. In order to establish a diagnosis, one must be able to show a significant rise in antibody titer during the course of the infection.

A positive test in a single sample of serum is not of diagnostic value in acute recent infections. Neutralizing antibodies can persist for years, and their mere presence may indicate a past infection in a given individual. Thus, neutralization tests are useful in serologic epidemiology, where one is interested in knowing which viral agents have infected a given population in the past.

Although simple in principle, neutralization tests are expensive in time and in materials and may be difficult to interpret, chiefly because of the variability in the titration end-point and the possible nonspecificity of the neutralization. The technic of performing the test for neutralizing antibodies must be standardized for each viral agent. Among the variables which must be considered are (1) the selection of the experi-

mental animal, embryonated egg, or cell culture;
(2) the route of inoculation of the virus-serum mixture; (3) the age of the test animals; (4) the stability of
the test virus; (5) the reproducibility of the end-point;
(6) the relative heat-stability of the specific antibody
and of possible interfering substances in serum; (7) the
addition of an accessory factor found in fresh normal
serum of the homologous species; (8) the use of one
concentration of virus and varying dilutions of serum,
or vice versa (and the relationship between varying
concentrations of each); (9) the temperature of the
neutralizing mixture; and (10) the time of incubation
of the mixture.

QUANTITATIVE NEUTRALIZATION TESTS

Mouse Test

A stock of mice of known uniform susceptibility
and standard age is selected. The mice are inoculated
by a standard route with the virus-serum mixture.
They are observed daily for signs of illness, such as
weakness or paralysis, to establish specificity of the
deaths. Illness and deaths are recorded daily for 21
days. Deaths within 24 hours after inoculation are
attributed to traumatic or nonviral causes.

Titration of Virus

It is necessary to titrate the virus each time a test
is performed. The 50% end-points (ID_{50}, LD_{50}, or
TCD_{50}) are calculated according to the method of
Reed and Muench or the method of Kaerber. ID_{50}
indicates the dose which infects 50% of the inoculated
animals or eggs and LD_{50} the dose which kills 50% of
them. Variations of this expression include PD_{50}, the
dose which paralyzes 50% of the animals, and TCD_{50},
the dose which produces cytopathic changes in 50% of
the inoculated tissue cultures.

**A. Calculation of LD_{50} Titer by Reed-Muench
Method:**

The proportionate distance between the 2 dilu-
tions (in the example, between 10^{-3} and 10^{-4}), where-
in the 50% end-point lies, equals

$$\frac{\% \text{ mortality above } 50 - 50\%}{\% \text{ mortality above } 50\% - \% \text{ mortality below } 50\%} =$$

$$\frac{90 - 50}{90 - 22} = \frac{40}{68} = 0.6$$

Negative logarithm of LD_{50} titer =
negative log of dilution + proportionate
above 50% mortality   distance

Negative logarithm of LD_{50} titer =
3.0 + 0.6 = 3.6
LD_{50} titer = $10^{-3.6}$

TABLE 29-1. Animal mortality data.

Virus Dilution	Mortality Ratio	Died*	Survived*
10^{-1}	8/8	8	0
10^{-2}	8/8	8	0
10^{-3}	7/8	7	1
10^{-4}	2/8	2	6
10^{-5}	0/8	0	8

*Arrows indicate direction of addition for
accumulated values.

**TABLE 29-2. Accumulated values from mortal-
ity data.**

Virus Dilution	Died	Survived	Mortality	
			Ratio	Percent
10^{-1}	25	0	25/25	100
10^{-2}	17	0	17/17	100
10^{-3}	9	1	9/10	90
10^{-4}	2	7	2/9	22
10^{-5}	0	15	0/15	0

The same procedure is used for calculating
TCD_{50} titers. In the tissue culture calculations, the
mortality ratio (number of mice dead per number of
mice inoculated) is replaced by the cytopathogenic
ratio (number of cultures showing cytopathic changes
per number of cultures inoculated).

**B. Calculation of LD_{50} Titer by the Kaerber
Method:**

$$\text{Log } LD_{50} = 0.5 + \log \text{ of highest concentration}$$
of virus used
$$- \frac{\text{sum of \% of dead animals}}{100}$$

For the example shown above,

$$\text{Log } LD_{50} \text{ titer} = 0.5 + (-1.0) -$$
$$\frac{100 + 100 + 88 + 25}{100}$$

Log LD_{50} titer = 0.5 − 1.0 − 3.1
Log LD_{50} titer = −3.6
LD_{50} titer = $10^{-3.6}$

The same procedure is used for calculating
TCD_{50} titers. In the tissue culture titrations the "sum
of percent of dead animals" is replaced by "sum of
percent of cultures showing cytopathic changes."

Neutralization Index

The neutralization index is the expression of the
ratio of the virus control LD_{50} titer to the LD_{50} titer
of the serum-virus mixtures in which virus has been
added to undiluted serum. The logarithm of the LD_{50}

titer of the virus control minus the logarithm of the LD_{50} titer of the serum-virus mixture equals the logarithm of the neutralization index. The antilogarithm of this difference equals the neutralization index. A neutralization index of less than 10 is considered to indicate the absence of antibodies.

If the above virus titration had been that of the control, a positive serum might give the reaction shown in Table 29–3. (Each virus dilution is mixed with an equal volume of serum and the mixture incubated for 1 hour at room temperature before inoculation.)

A. Calculation of Neutralization Index by the Reed-Muench Method:

$$\text{Proportionate distance} = \frac{56 - 50}{56 - 8} = \frac{6}{48} = 0.1$$

$$\text{Negative logarithm of } LD_{50} \text{ titer} =$$
$$1.0 + 0.1 = 1.1$$
$$LD_{50} \text{ titer} = 10^{-1.1}$$

B. Calculation of Neutralization Index by the Kaerber Method:

$$\text{Logarithm of } LD_{50} \text{ titer} = 0.5 + (-1.0) - \frac{50 + 13}{100}$$
$$= 0.5 - 1.0 - 0.6 = -1.1$$
$$LD_{50} \text{ titer} = 10^{-1.1}$$

C. Logarithm of neutralization index =

$$\frac{\text{Neg log}}{\text{control titer}} - \frac{\text{Neg log of}}{\text{serum-virus mixture}}$$

$$\text{Neutralization index} = \text{Antilog of } 2.5 = 320$$

TABLE 29–3. Animal mortality data.

Virus Dilution Present in Each Virus-serum Mixture*	Mortality Ratio	Died	Survived
10^{-1}	4/8	4	4
10^{-2}	1/8	1	7
10^{-3}	0/8	0	8

*An equal volume of undiluted serum is added to each virus dilution 1 hour before inoculation of the mixture.

TABLE 29–4. Accumulated values from mortality data.

Virus Dilution	Died	Survived	Mortality Ratio	Mortality Percent
10^{-1}	5	4	5/9	56
10^{-2}	1	11	1/12	8
10^{-3}	0	19	0/19	0

Interpretation

As neutralizing antibodies for many viruses persist for a long time, it is essential to demonstrate a rise in titer in paired sera in order to establish recent infection by the virus. A positive test in a single specimen may be the result of an earlier and perhaps subclinical infection and is not useful for clinical diagnosis of the acute disease. For diagnostic purposes, the increase in neutralization index during convalescence should be at least 100. When antibodies are present in acute phase sera, their increase during the course of the disease is often more readily demonstrated by using a constant amount of virus and varying the dilutions of serum.

Soon after infection, the titer of 19S antibody, which is sensitive to 2-mercaptoethanol (2-ME), is much higher than that of 7S antibody, which is resistant to 2-ME. Long after infection, the 2-ME resistant antibody titer is much higher than that of the 2-ME susceptible antibody. If only a single serum specimen is available (usually acute or early convalescent), a 2-ME sensitivity test may be helpful. A significant fall in antibody titer after treatment with 2-ME in an acute phase serum is of presumptive diagnostic value.

THE NEUTRALIZATION TEST IN TISSUE CULTURE

The details of performing this test vary in different laboratories, but the same principle underlies all of them: The viral antibody specifically neutralizes the cytopathogenic action of the virus.

With each series of neutralization tests, control titrations of virus are made, the starting concentration being the highest dose (100 TCD_{50}) used in the serum-virus mixtures. It is also advisable to test the highest concentration of each serum in a tissue culture tube for possible nonspecific cell toxicity. A few tubes are left uninoculated to serve as tissue controls. A typical protocol of a patient infected with type 1 poliomyelitis virus is shown in Table 29–5. The cultures were incubated at 36° C for 3 days and then examined microscopically. At the end of that time the virus titration showed that 100 TCD_{50} doses had been added to each serum.

Suspensions of monkey kidney or continuous line cells may be used directly as cells in neutralization tests. The same basic principle which underlies any virus neutralization test, ie, that antibody specifically neutralizes the infectivity of the virus, also applies to the color (or metabolic inhibition) test. The color test employs known quantities of cell suspensions which are added to test tubes or plastic panel cups 1 hour after the serum-virus mixture. This eliminates the need for cultures in which cells have already grown out on glass. The color test utilizes the fact that, with continued cellular growth in control tubes or in the presence of an immune serum-virus mixture, acidic products of metabolism lower the pH of the medium.

TABLE 29–5. Tissue culture neutralization test with paired sera of patient infected with type 1 poliomyelitis virus.

Virus*	Serum (Day After Onset)	Cellular Degeneration (Cytopathic Effect) Final Serum Dilution					50% Serum Titer	
		1:2	1:10	1:50	1:250	1:1250	Logarithm	Antilog
Type 1	1	000	+++	+++	+++	+++	0.7	5
	20	000	000	000	00+	+++	2.5	320
Type 2	1	000	+++	+++	+++	+++	0.7	5
	20	000	000	0++	+++	+++	1.5	32
Type 3	1	+++	+++	+++	+++	+++	0	0
	20	+++	+++	+++	+++	+++	0	0
None	1	000						
	20	000						

*100 TCD_{50} doses of each virus used in test.

This effect is readily observed by incorporating the indicator dye phenol red into the medium. This dye is red at pH 7.4–7.8. It becomes salmon pink and finally yellow as the pH drops below 7.0. Conversely, cell necrosis induced by the virus leaves the medium red, for the dying cultures fail to reach the degree of acidity exhibited by the control cultures. The test can thus be read by color change alone rather than by the presence or absence of cellular degeneration as determined microscopically. Neutralizing antibodies are measured by determining the serum dilution which, in the presence of added virus, will allow the cells to metabolize normally and the pH to fall as in the controls.

The test described in the above paragraph is used with the enteroviruses. Because adenoviruses cause a stimulation of cellular metabolism and more rapid lowering of the pH than that of the control cultures, the color reaction is the opposite of that described above.

NEUTRALIZATION TESTS IN EGGS

The embryonated egg may also be used as an indicator system in virus neutralization tests. With influenza and mumps viruses, upon the inoculation of the virus-serum mixtures, the end-point is measured by determining whether viral hemagglutinins have developed in the allantoic fluid. For viruses such as herpes or vaccinia, which produce colonies or plaques on the chorioallantoic membrane, neutralization may be measured by comparing the number of plaques produced by the virus alone with the number produced in the presence of the serum. Such plaque reduction or plaque neutralization technics are available for many viruses grown in tissue culture.

COMPLEMENT FIXATION TESTS

Analogous to bacterial complement fixation, it has been shown that antiviral sera fix complement in the presence of their homologous antigens. Such tests are being employed for most viral diseases. The difficulty with viral complement fixation tests lies in the problem of preparing concentrated antigens free of nonspecific interfering substances. Infected tissue has often been employed in the past. At present, most antigens are derived from the allantoic fluid of the embryonated egg or from tissue culture fluids after infection with viruses. In some instances (eg, rubella), antigens are prepared from 10–20% suspensions of virus-infected cells which are disrupted by freezing and thawing or by sonication.

Preparation of Antigen

Various test procedures have been devised. A brief review of the Casals technic for the viral encephalitides follows; it illustrates principles common to many viral complement fixation tests. The antigens are often virulent, and caution should therefore be observed in handling them.

Antigen is prepared from mouse brains harvested at the first signs of infection. The weighed tissue is blended with 20 volumes of chilled acetone for 2 minutes. Following centrifugation, the sediment is re-extracted once with a mixture of equal parts of acetone and anhydrous ethyl ether and twice more with ether. After the last extraction, the ether is decanted and the residual material evaporated under vacuum. The ether-insoluble residue is resuspended in 3 volumes of physiologic saline solution and the suspension centrifuged. The supernatant constitutes the antigen.

Other methods have been advocated for the preparation of neurotropic virus antigens. These include the use of infected chick embroys as source material and the extraction with benzene of lyophilized chick

TABLE 29–6. An example of a complement fixation test response.

Time of Taking Serum	Serum Dilution						Titer
	1:5	1:10	1:20	1:40	1:80	1:160	
Acute phase	0	0	0	0	0	0	0
Recovery phase	4+	3+	0	0	0	0	1:10
Convalescent	4+	4+	4+	3+	2+	0	1:80

4+ indicates complement fixation (no hemolysis); 0 indicates complete hemolysis.

embryos or mouse brains followed by their resuspension in saline. For optimal reactivity, veronal buffer with added Mg^{++} and Ca^{++} may offer certain advantages over saline as a suspending medium for viral antigens.

Procedure

Complement should be titrated in the presence of each antigen under the same conditions as prevail in the test proper. A preliminary titration is made in saline. Another titration is set up at the same time with antigen and saline as control, and this is incubated along with the test for antibodies.

The test is run as follows: Inactivated sera (60° C for 20 minutes) are diluted 2-fold, beginning with the 1:2 dilution, and 0.25 ml is placed in a series of test tubes (13 × 100 mm). Then 0.25 ml of antigen is added plus 2 units of complement in 0.5 ml. The mixture of serum, antigen, and complement is incubated at 37° C for 1–2 hours or, for greater sensitivity, at 2–4° C for 18 hours. Following incubation the hemolytic system is added; this consists of 0.25 ml of a 3% suspension of packed sheep erythrocytes plus 0.25 ml of rabbit antisheep hemolysin diluted to provide 3 minimal hemolytic doses. The total volume of fluid in each tube is now 1.5 ml. The tubes are incubated at 37° C for 20 minutes and read visually: 4+ represents no hemolysis, which indicates complement fixation.

Interpretation

The titer is defined as the highest dilution of serum giving a 2+ or better fixation. Control tubes, in which 0.25 ml of saline replaces the serum or the antigen respectively, used in the test proper, are included for each antigen and for each serum as a measure of their anticomplementary power.

SOLUBLE & VIRAL ANTIGENS

Some viruses have been shown to possess 2 serologically distinct complement-fixing antigens, one being intimately associated with the virus and the other being much smaller ("soluble") and found in infected tissues. These observations have been of diagnostic value in mumps, particularly during the early stage of the disease. Antibodies against the soluble or S antigen appear earlier in the infection than do those against the virus-bound or V-antigen. Furthermore, anti-V bodies persist for much longer periods than anti-S bodies.

Thus, if the serum of an acutely ill patient has a high titer against the S-antigen and a negligible titer against the V-antigen of mumps virus, the illness is probably mumps. High levels of both antibodies indicate a recent infection or one of several days' duration. Negligible titers against V-antigen indicate long-past apparent or inapparent infection. With both S- and V-antigens, a presumptive diagnosis of infection with mumps virus often may be made in the first days of illness, for this is the only period when there occurs a high titer of anti-S and a low titer of anti-V. This has permitted the recognition of mumps meningoencephalitis in the absence of parotitis as early as 2 days after onset.

.   .   .

EPIDEMIOLOGIC INTERPRETATION

The interpretations of the various patterns of laboratory data obtainable on an individual are shown in Table 29–7 for a single infection of the enterovirus type. They are based on the duration of virus excretion and the different degrees of persistence of complement fixing and neutralizing antibody.

HEMAGGLUTINATION INHIBITION TESTS

There are a number of viruses which agglutinate erythrocytes, and this reaction may be specifically inhibited by immune or convalescent sera. As shown in Table 29–10, this reaction forms the basis of a number of diagnostic tests for viral infections.

TABLE 29–7. Interpretation of laboratory data in enterovirus infection.

Virus Isolation	Complement-fixing Antibody	Neutral-izing Antibody	Inter-pretation of Infection
−	−	−	None
+	−	−	Early
+	+	+	Current
−	+	+	Recent
−	−	+	Old

Diseases in Which an Antibody Response May Be Demonstrated by the Hemagglutination Inhibition Test

Influenza
Certain of the enterovirus infections
Mumps
Measles
Newcastle disease
Variola
Vaccinia
California virus encephalitis
St. Louis encephalitis
Western equine encephalitis
Japanese B encephalitis
West Nile fever
Dengue
Adenovirus infections
Rubella
Reovirus infections

As the same general principles apply for the hemagglutination inhibition tests used with different viral agents, the details will be presented only for influenza.

STANDARDS & TITRATION

Standard Erythrocyte Suspension

This suspension consists of 0.5% human type O erythrocytes in physiologic saline solution. The blood may be either freshly collected or preserved with sterile precautions in Alsever's solution for not longer than 1 month at 5° C. Formalinized chicken erythrocytes may also be used for measurement of influenza antibody. They may be stored for 3 months with no loss of hemagglutinating activity.

Standard Antigens

Standard influenza virus antigens types A, A_1, A_2, and B may be obtained from commercial sources. These consist of allantoic fluid from infected eggs and are distributed in lyophilized form.

Titration of Antigens

The hemagglutinating unit of antigen is defined as 0.5 ml of the highest dilution of antigen which completely agglutinates the 0.5 ml of standard human erythrocyte suspension. The virus-red cell mixture is read and recorded on the basis of the pattern of agglutination.

(1) Positive agglutination is indicated by a red, granular, diffused lining of the bowl of the tube.

(2) Absence of agglutination is indicated by the formation of a compact red button at the bottom of the tube.

(3) Partial agglutination is indicated by something in between a diffused lining of the bottom of the tube and a red button. This takes the form of a ring with a hollow center. The rings are of varying sizes, depending upon the extent of agglutination.

THE DIAGNOSTIC AGGLUTINATION INHIBITION TEST

Procedure

Two serum specimens from each patient must be tested with all types of antigen. The first of these (acute phase) is obtained within 2–3 days after the onset of illness; the second (convalescent phase) is obtained 10–14 days after the onset of illness. The tests are set up as follows:

(1) 0.3 ml amounts of the sera to be tested are inactivated at 53° C for 30 minutes; they are then diluted 1:8 by adding 2.1 ml of saline solution.

(2) For each serum to be tested set up 3 rows of tubes, preferably in a rack with 3 rows of 10 holes each. Saline solution in 0.75 ml amounts is added to the second to tenth tubes in the front row. The first tube on the far left in the front row and all the tubes in the middle and back rows are left empty. The

TABLE 29–8. An example of a hemagglutination inhibition test response.

Time of Taking Serum	Serum Dilution						Titer
	1:8	1:16	1:32	1:64	1:128	1:256	
Acute phase	0	+	+	+	+	+	1:8
Recovery phase	0	0	0	+	+	+	1:32
Convalescent	0	0	0	0	0	+	1:128

+ = Agglutination. 0 = No agglutination.

inactivated 1:8 dilution of serum in 0.25 ml amounts is transferred to the first tube of each of the 3 rows and 0.75 ml of the same solution of the serum is placed in the second tube of the front row. This is mixed thoroughly, and 0.25 ml is transferred to the second tube of the middle and back rows and 0.75 ml is placed in the third tube of the front row. The operation is repeated in this manner until 3 identical series of 2-fold dilutions have been prepared. Each tube contains 0.25 ml and the serum dilutions range from 1:8 through 1:4096.

(3) After the serum dilutions have been prepared, 0.25 ml amounts containing 4 hemagglutinating units of the 3 test antigens are added to the tubes in the first, second, and third rows respectively.

(4) Shake well and then add 0.5 ml of the 0.5% erythrocyte suspension to the serum-antigen mixtures.

(5) Shake well and incubate at room temperature for 60 minutes. Be careful not to bump or move the racks.

(6) The tests are read and recorded in terms of degree of inhibition of agglutination by each serum using each antigen. The titer of a given serum using a given antigen is defined as the highest dilution of serum which effects complete inhibition of agglutination.

Controls

Known antisera to A, A_1, A_2, and B influenza are set up in the same manner as are the unknown sera, except that a 1:100 initial dilution of the standard titrated serum is used instead of the 1:8 dilution in the human sera described.

The test antigens must be re-titrated at the same time that the agglutination inhibition tests are performed.

Interpretation

Results are reported in terms of the titers of each of the paired sera obtained with each antigen. An example is shown in Table 29–8. A 4-fold or greater increase in titer during convalescence is considered of diagnostic significance.

MIXED HEMADSORPTION TEST

This test has been used to detect and identify viral antigens at the cell surface of monolayer cultures infected with a variety of viruses. The principle of the test is similar to the indirect immunofluorescence test except that specially prepared erthrocytes are used as an indicator instead of fluorescence. Erythrocytes are coated with red cell antibody made in the same animal species used to prepare antibodies against the virus. To the coated erythrocytes, antiglobulin antibody is added. Now viral antibody is added to the infected cells and coats the cell surface if virus antigens are present. The erythrocytes with their external coat of

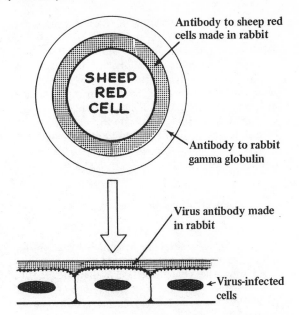

FIG 29–1. Espmark's schematic representation of the postulated principles underlying the mixed hemadsorption reaction. In the given example the test antibody is of rabbit origin and the indicator red cells are prepared accordingly.

gamma globulin are added, and attach to those cells coated with viral antibody.

The test can be used to quantitate antigen or viral antibody. There is a good correlation between the mixed hemadsorption and the neutralization and complement fixation tests. Although the mixed hemadsorption titers are about 100- to 1000-fold higher than in the corresponding CF and neutralization test, the test is not yet widely used in the diagnosis of human disease.

PRECIPITATION REACTIONS

Immunodiffusion Test

In immunodiffusion tests, the antigen and antibody are allowed to diffuse toward each other in a semisolid medium, such as agar. A precipitate is formed at the zone of optimal proportions which acts as a specific barrier to the further diffusion of antigen or antibody past the precipitation line. The number of precipitation lines formed will depend upon the number of distinct antigen-antibody reactions taking place; each line represents one antigen-antibody system. The technic is well suited for the analysis of soluble antigens associated with viruses. The test, commonly performed with the Ouchterlony technic, provided the basis for demonstrating the antigen of serum hepatitis (SH or Australia antigen). Microscopic slides are covered with 1% agarose containing 0.1 M NaCl,

0.01 M tris buffer, 0.0001 M EDTA and 1 mg protamine sulfate. After hardening, wells are cut in the agarose. The center well is filled with a rabbit serum or a human serum containing antibodies to the antigens. Opposite wells are filled with serum from persons with acute or chronic hepatitis. The slides are incubated in a moist chamber for 24–48 hours. The appearance of a precipitation line indicates the presence of the antigen. Similar technics have been used to detect antigens or antibodies to a number of viruses.

MICROFLOCCULATION TEST

A simple procedure for determining viral precipitating antibodies has been developed for poliomyelitis. Pyrex spot plates containing 9 depressions are used. To each is added 0.02 ml of virus and the same volume of serum by means of a dropping pipet (blunt needle attached to a glass barrel fitted with a rubber bulb). The plates are placed in a deep pan containing a wet paper towel to prevent drying of the drops; the lid of the pan is sealed with masking tape; and the plates are incubated overnight at 37° C. The drops in each depression are then examined for flocculates, using a microscope with a low-power objective and reduced light. The serum end point titer is the highest dilution of serum giving a 2+ or greater flocculation reaction with the standard dilution (2 units) of antigen.

IMMUNOFLUORESCENCE TEST

The indirect immunofluorescence technic has been effectively applied for quantitating antibodies to certain viruses (eg, rubella). Tissue culture cells on coverslips are infected with the virus and the culture incubated to allow virus replication. The coverslips are washed, fixed in acetone, and covered with 2-fold dilutions of the test serum along with known positive and negative control sera. The excess antibody is removed after 30 minutes by washing with salt solution, and the coverslips are covered with fluorescent antibody against human globulin. (Before use, this indicator antibody is labeled with fluorescein isothiocyanate.) The excess labeled antibody is removed after 30 minutes by washing; the coverslips are then dried, mounted, and examined in the darkfield microscope under ultraviolet light. The presence of viral antibody in the test serum produces a distinct fluorescence in the infected cells.

A presumptive diagnosis can be made by detecting virus specific IgM antibodies in a single serum sample obtained within 3 weeks after a viral illness by using fluorescent-labeled antibody against immunoglobulin M. This technic has the advantage of being rapid and requiring small quantities of serum. The technic, however, is usually less sensitive than other methods of quantitating antibody and requires a higher degree of technical proficiency to obtain reproducible results.

With the direct immunofluorescence test, the virus antibody is labeled. The diagnosis of influenza can be established within 2 hours by direct staining of sputum. Diagnosis can also be made in 36 hours by culturing infected cells (monkey kidney or human trachea).

DIAGNOSIS OF INFECTIOUS MONONUCLEOSIS

In patients with infectious mononucleosis, the development of antibodies against a herpes-type virus has been demonstrated by an indirect immunofluorescence test in which the antigen is a virus-bearing cell line derived from a Burkitt lymphoma. Similar cell lines have been obtained from peripheral blood and bone marrow of patients with infectious mononucleosis or leukemia, as well as from some normal individuals. The antibodies, absent in pre-illness serum specimens, usually appear very early in the acute disease, rise to peak levels within a few weeks, and remain at relatively high levels during convalescence. They are distinctive from heterophil antibodies and, unlike the latter, they persist for years (probably for life).

Complement-fixing antibodies also develop, quickly against the virus-associated antigen but slowly against the soluble nonviral antigen present in infected cell lines.

Infectious mononucleosis is accompanied by the appearance of unique sheep cell hemagglutinins. The serologic procedure for detecting the hemagglutinins of infectious mononucleosis has long been used for diagnosis and is described below.

HETEROPHIL AGGLUTINATION TEST

Collection of Specimen

It is desirable to have matched specimens of serum, the first taken as soon as infectious mononucleosis is suspected, the second taken in the second week of the disease, and the third taken during the third or fourth week after the onset of the disease. If only one specimen is available it may yield more valuable information if obtained in the second or third week of the disease than if obtained in the first week.

Procedure

Blood is drawn and serum is separated from the clot by centrifugation, removed, and inactivated at 56° C for 30 minutes. Inactivation is necessary because some normal sera possess a relatively high lytic titer for sheep cells.

For the antigen a 1% suspension of sheep erythrocytes, washed with physiologic saline 3 times, is used. Freshly washed cells are used or citrated blood (10 volumes of blood plus 2 volumes of sterile 3.8% sodium citrate solution) up to 1 week old. For serial tests, blood from the same sheep should be used.

Two-fold serial dilutions (1:2.5–1:1280) of inactivated serum in amounts of 0.5 ml each with an equal volume of 1% sheep red blood cell suspension yield a final serum dilution of 1:5–1:2560, and all titers should be reported on this basis. For a control, 0.5 ml of the cell suspension is added to 0.5 ml of saline. The tubes are incubated at 37° C in the water bath for 2 hours and then placed in the refrigerator overnight. Readings are made the following morning, after shaking, and the highest final serum dilution showing agglutination is taken as the titer. It is essential that the tests be read after the times specified.

Interpretation

There is some disagreement concerning the diagnostic titer of sheep cell agglutinins in infectious mononucleosis serum; this can be explained, in part at least, by the fact that variable technics have been used. Titers which range from 1:10–1:40 should be considered negative; titers from 1:80–1:160 are suspicious; and agglutination titers of 1:160 or more are considered as definitely elevated and may be regarded as positive. The best criterion in the early stages is that of a rising titer, especially after the adsorption tests described below are performed.

ADSORPTION TEST FOR INCREASED SPECIFICITY

Sheep cell agglutinins in infectious mononucleosis are adsorbed by bovine erythrocytes but are not reduced significantly by adsorption with guinea pig kidney. Sheep cell agglutinins in serum sickness are completely adsorbed by both guinea pig kidney and bovine erythrocytes. Sheep cell agglutinins in normal human serum are almost completely adsorbed by guinea pig kidney (Table 29–9).

Procedure

One ml of guinea pig kidney suspension is added to 1 ml of a 1:2.5 dilution of the serum to be tested. The mixture is incubated at 37° C for 30 minutes and then centrifuged at 4000 rpm for 15 minutes. The supernatant is tested in serial dilutions for sheep cell agglutinins, as described above. If agglutinins remain, a second adsorption with bovine red cells may be done.

TABLE 29–9. Adsorption reactions of agglutinins in human serum.

	Agglutinins Adsorbed By	
Type of serum	Guinea Pig Kidney	Bovine Erythrocytes
Normal	Yes	No
Infectious mononucleosis	No	Yes
Serum sickness	Yes	Yes

To 1 ml of the serum dilution adsorbed with guinea pig kidney, 0.5 ml of packed bovine red cells is added, mixed, and incubated at 37° C for 30 minutes. After centrifugation the supernatant is tested for sheep cell agglutinins as before.

Interpretation

The relationships of the different types of sheep cell agglutinins in human serum are shown in Table 29–9. Agglutinins, which may be present in normal serum to a titer of 1:160 and in serum sickness to a titer of 1:20,000, are removed by adsorption with guinea pig kidney. The failure of guinea pig kidney to affect the sheep cell agglutinin titer of the patient's serum is adequate evidence of infectious mononucleosis in most cases; adsorption with bovine red cells is rarely required for confirmation.

TESTS FOR DERMAL HYPERSENSITIVITY (SKIN TESTS)

When available, tests for dermal hypersensitivity offer certain advantages in determining, easily and quickly, prior exposure to infectious agents. Tests are available for mumps, herpes simplex, cat scratch fever, Western equine encephalomyelitis, and variola (or vaccinia). The skin test may lead to increase in antibodies.

Technic of Inoculation

The test for dermal hypersensitivity to virus is carried out by injecting 0.1 ml of the skin test antigen intradermally into the flexor surface of the right arm, and 0.1 ml of the control material into the same area of the left arm. The sites of injection are examined after 12–48 hours. The width of erythematous reaction and induration is measured and compared to the control.

Character of the Reaction

If the individual is hypersensitive to the skin test antigen, an area of induration and erythema varying from about 10 mm to 60 or 80 mm may be observed.

TABLE 29–10. Laboratory diagnosis of viral diseases.

(TC, tissue culture. Nt, neutralization. CF, complement fixation. HI, hemagglutination inhibition. CAM, chorioallantoic membrane. ID, immunodiffusion. IF, immunofluorescence.)

Disease	Human Specimens to be Tested	Primary Isolation of Virus				Diagnostic Serologic Tests	
		Material or Animals to Be Inoculated	Route	Tissue to Be Harvested for Passage	Positive Result in Test System: Signs and Pathology	Type of Test	Source of Virus or Antigen
ARTHROPOD-BORNE							
Encephalitides California St. Louis Japanese B Western equine Eastern equine Venezuelan Russian spring-summer West Nile fever Bwamba, etc	Brain, blood	Mice	Intracerebral	Brain	Encephalitis	Nt in Mice or TC CF HI	Mouse brain or TC Mouse brain or TC Infant mouse brain
Yellow fever	Blood, viscera	Monkeys	Intraperitoneal	Viscera	Hepatic necrosis	Nt	Mouse brain
		Mice	Intracerebral	Brain	Encephalitis		
Rift Valley fever	Blood	Mice	Intraperitoneal	Liver	Hepatitis	Nt, CF	Mouse liver
Dengue	Blood	Mice (difficult)	Intracerebral	Brain	Encephalomyelitis	Nt, CF	Mouse brain
Sandfly fever	Blood	Infant mice	Intracerebral	Brain	Encephalomyelitis	Nt, CF	Mouse brain
Colorado tick fever	Blood	Hamsters	Intraperitoneal	Brain	Encephalitis	Nt	Mouse brain
		Mice	Intracerebral	Brain	Encephalitis	CF	Mouse brain
NEUROTROPIC, NONARTHROPOD-BORNE							
Poliomyelitis	Spinal cord, feces, throat swabbings	TC		Fluid of infected culture	Cytopathic effect	Nt, CF	TC
Rabies	Brain	Mice	Intracerebral	Brain	Encephalitis, Negri inclusion bodies in cytoplasm	IF	
Lymphocytic choriomeningitis	Brain, blood, spinal fluid	Mice	Intracerebral	Brain	Encephalitis and choroiditis	Nt	Mouse brain
		Guinea pig	Intraperitoneal	Spleen	Death with pneumonia, focal infiltration in liver	CF	Guinea pig spleen
B virus infection	Brain, spleen	Rabbit	Intracutaneous	Spinal cord	Necrosis of skin, myelitis, intranuclear inclusion bodies	CF, Nt	Rabbit kidney TC
		Rabbit kidney TC		TC fluid		CF, Nt	Rabbit kidney TC

DERMOTROPIC

Disease	Source of virus	Host	Site of inoculation	Material examined	Recognition of virus	Serologic tests	Rapid diagnosis
Variola (smallpox)	Skin lesions, vesicle fluid, blood	Embryonated egg	CAM	CAM	Pocks on membrane, cytoplasmic inclusion bodies	CF, HI	Vesicle fluid or crusts from patient against standard serum for rapid results
Vaccinia	Skin lesions, vesicle fluid	Embryonated egg; Rabbit	CAM; Intracutaneous	CAM; Skin	Pocks on membrane; Skin lesion, cytoplasmic inclusion bodies	CF	CAM, rabbit skin or testicle, or mouse brain
Varicella (chickenpox)	Vesicle fluid	TC		Cells of infected culture	Intranuclear inclusions in skin lesions and in TC	CF, Nt†	TC
Zoster	Vesicle fluid	TC		Cells of infected culture	Intranuclear inclusions	CF	TC
Measles	Nasopharyngeal secretions, blood	TC		TC fluid	Multinucleate giant cells and intranuclear inclusions	CF, Nt	TC
Rubella (German measles)	Nasopharyngeal secretions, blood	TC		TC fluid	Interference, or cytopathic effect	Nt, CF, HI, IF	TC
Congenital rubella syndrome	Throat swab, urine, feces, spinal fluid, blood, bone marrow, conjunctival swab	TC		TC fluid	Interference, or cytopathic effect	Nt, CF, HI, IF	TC
Exanthem subitum	Blood	Monkeys	Intravenous	Blood	Experimental exanthem		
Herpes simplex	Skin lesions, brain	Mouse (newborn); Embryonated egg; TC	Intracerebral; CAM	Brain; Allantoic fluid; Fluid	Encephalitis; Pocks; Cytopathic effect, intranuclear inclusion bodies	Nt in mice or eggs; CF; CF	Mouse brain, allantoic fluid; Allantoic fluid; TC

RESPIRATORY AND PAROTID

Disease	Source of virus	Host	Site of inoculation	Material examined	Recognition of virus	Serologic tests	Rapid diagnosis
Influenza A, Influenza B, Influenza C	Nasal washings, lung	Eggs	Amniotic and allantoic sacs	Embryonic fluids	Hemagglutinin produced	HI	Allantoic fluid
		Ferrets, mice	Intranasal	Lung	Pneumonitis	CF	Allantoic fluid
		TC		Fluid phase	Cytopathic effect, hemadsorption	Nt in eggs, mice or TC	Allantoic fluid, mouse lung, TC
Para-influenza		TC			Hemadsorption	Nt, CF	TC
Respiratory syncytial, RS		TC			Multinucleate giant cells with cytoplasmic inclusions	Nt, CF	TC
Common cold (rhinovirus group)	Nasopharyngeal washings, swabs	TC		TC fluid	Cytopathic effect	Nt	TC
Mumps	Saliva, spinal fluid, urine	Monkeys; Eggs; TC	Parotid gland; Amniotic and yolk sacs	Parotid gland; Amniotic fluid, yolk sac; Fluid phase	Parotitis; Hemagglutinin produced; Cytopathic effect	CF; HI; Nt in TC	Amniotic fluid; Monkey parotid gland; TC

TABLE 29–10 (cont'd). Laboratory diagnosis of viral diseases.

(TC, tissue culture. Nt, neutralization. CF, complement fixation. HI, hemagglutination inhibition. CAM, chorioallantoic membrane. ID, immunodiffusion. IF, immunofluorescence.)

Disease	Human Specimens to Be Tested	Primary Isolation of Virus				Diagnostic Serologic Tests	
		Material or Animals to Be Inoculated	Route	Tissue to Be Harvested for Passage	Positive Result in Test System: Signs and Pathology	Type of Test	Source of Virus or Antigen
Adenovirus group	Pharyngeal washings, stool	TC		TC fluid and cells	Cytopathic effect	CF, Nt	TC
HEPATIC							
Infectious hepatitis	Blood, feces	(No satisfactory experimental animal. Preliminary indications of success in TC with D6 cells.)					
Serum hepatitis	Blood					CF, ID	Serum
MISCELLANEOUS							
Coxsackie infection	Feces, throat washings, spinal fluid	Infant mice	Subcutaneous	Muscle	Paralysis with myositis and, with certain types, encephalitis, steatitis; pancreatitis	Nt in infant mice or TC	Mouse muscle
Echovirus infection	Feces, throat swabbings, spinal fluid	TC		TC fluid	Cytopathic effect	Nt, CF, HI	TC
		TC		TC fluid	Cytopathic effect	Nt, CF, HI	TC
Reovirus infection	Feces, throat swabbings	TC		TC fluid	Cytopathic effect	Nt, CF, HI	TC
Molluscum contagiosum	Skin lesions	(No satisfactory experimental animal. Characteristic cytoplasmic inclusion bodies. Elementary bodies can be seen in the electron microscope.)					
Verrucae (warts)	Skin lesions	(No satisfactory experimental animal. Electron microscopic examination of warts shows elementary bodies.)					
Encephalomyocarditis (Col. SK-Mengo)	Blood	Mice	Intracerebral	Brain	Encephalitis	Nt in mice	Mouse brain
Epidemic kerato-conjunctivitis	Conjunctivas	TC		TC cells and fluid	Cytopathic effect	Nt test for adenovirus 8	TC
Foot-and-mouth disease	Skin lesions	Guinea pigs Newborn mice	Intracutaneous, foot pads	Foot pads Muscle	Hyperkeratosis with vesicle formation, paralysis with myositis	CF	Guinea pig foot pad Mouse muscle
Cytomegalic (inclusion) disease	Oral swabs, urine, various organs	TC		TC fluid and cells	Cytopathic effect, inclusion bodies	Nt, CF	TC

Its maximum intensity is usually attained between 24 and 48 hours after injection. After 48 hours, the erythema rapidly fades.

Interpretation

In mumps, persons exhibiting dermal reactions exceeding 10 mm in mean diameter 48 hours after the inoculation of inactivated virus (positive reaction) may be regarded as resistant.

In Western equine encephalomyelitis, as in mumps, children have less dermal sensitivity than do adults.

Inoculation of skin test antigens may result in an increase in complement-fixing antibody. This must be taken into account when the complement fixation test is employed as a diagnostic aid after a skin test.

●　　●　　●

General References

Lennette, E.H.: General principles underlying laboratory diagnosis of viral and rickettsial infections. Pages 1–65 in: *Diagnostic Procedures for Viral and Rickettsial Infections,* 4th ed. American Public Health Association, 1969.

Liu, C.: Fluorescent-antibody techniques. Pages 179–204 in: *Diagnostic Procedures for Viral and Rickettsial Infections,* 4th ed. American Public Health Association, 1969.

Svehag, S.E.: Formation and dissociation of virus-antibody complexes with special reference to the neutralization process. Progr Med Virol 10:1–63, 1968.

30 . . .

Arthropod-Borne (Arbo)
Viral Diseases

The **arthropod-borne viruses**, or **arboviruses**, are functionally classified as a group of infectious agents which are biologically transmitted between susceptible vertebrate hosts through the bite of a hemophagous arthropod. These viruses have the capacity to multiply in the tissues of susceptible arthropods without producing any apparent disease or damage. A vertebrate → arthropod → vertebrate cycle in nature is maintained by the vector, which develops a lifelong infection through ingestion of vertebrate blood from a viremic host.

Names of the individual viruses were originally those of the diseases produced since recognition of the disease complex preceded the isolation of the infectious agent (yellow fever, dengue, the equine encephalitides). After that, a combination of the geographic location of the isolate with the disease produced was favored (St. Louis encephalitis, Colorado tick fever, West Nile fever, Russian spring-summer encephalitis). More recently, the convention has been to name newly isolated viruses after the geographic area where the original isolation was made (Hart Park, Kern Canyon, Cache Valley).

Although arboviruses are found on all temperate and tropical continental land masses and on some islands, they are most prevalent in the tropical rain forest areas of the earth. This is understandable in view of the favorable climatic conditions and of the abundance in kind as well as in number of animal and insect species. As the arboviruses are maintained by cycles involving arthropods as well as vertebrates, the tropics offer the most favorable conditions for these complex biologic cycles.

It is now becoming possible to classify arboviruses in terms of their chemical and physical properties. Most of the arboviruses of group A and B belong to a newly proposed group called **togaviruses**; this group also includes rubella virus and the lactic dehydrogenase (LDH) virus of mice. A grouping of the **Tacaribe-LCM viruses** has been proposed for the Tacaribe group of arboviruses (which includes the Junin and Machupo viruses of South American hemorrhagic fevers together with the lymphocytic choriomeningitis [LCM] virus).

All arboviruses that have been studied have been found to contain RNA. All but 5 of 154 arboviruses tested are inactivated by ether or sodium deoxycholate (exceptions are Nodamura, African horse sickness, bluetongue, Tribec, and epizootic hemorrhagic disease of deer). Recent experimental evidence would link the viruses of African horse sickness and bluetongue to a newly recognized group, the diplornaviruses (containing double-stranded RNA), members of which include the reoviruses and apparently Colorado tick fever virus. Size estimates have ranged from 20 to > 150 nm in diameter, but most seem to be between 20 and 60 nm.

The arbovirus group consists of about 220 different viruses which are at present classified into several groups according to their antigenic relationships. Each group is composed of members sharing to varying degree complement fixing (CF), hemagglutination inhibiting (HI), and—less frequently—neutralizing (Nt) antigens. About 59% of these viruses fall into 7 major groups (10 or more per group); 17% are in 16 small groups (2–7 members per group); and 24% remain ungrouped.

(1) **Group A:** These viruses are significantly larger (40–60 nm) than group B arboviruses (20–40 nm). Sulfhydryl reagents do not inactivate group A viruses, and they appear resistant to proteases, whereas group B viruses are sensitive to proteases. Western equine, eastern equine, and Venezuelan equine encephalitis viruses have received most study. Other viruses of group A include Mayaro (Trinidad, Brazil, Bolivia), Semliki (Africa), Chikungunya (Africa, Southeast Asia), Sindbis (Africa and India), Aura and Una (Brazil), Getah (Malaya), Ross River (Australia), Whataroa (New Zealand), Middelburg (South Africa), and O'nyong-nyong (Uganda). This group is responsible primarily for fevers of an undifferentiated type ("dengue-like") or encephalitis.

(2) **Group B:** This group can be divided into 4 antigenic subgroups of closely related viruses. These include the following: (1) Japanese B, St. Louis, and Murray Valley encephalitis viruses; West Nile fever, Ilheus, and Kunjin viruses; (2) the dengue viruses; (3) yellow fever, Uganda S, and Zika viruses; and (4) the tick-borne complex. The latter subgroup is composed of viruses capable of causing hemorrhagic fever (Omsk hemorrhagic fever, Kyasanur Forest disease viruses) or encephalitis (Russian spring-summer encephalitis, biphasic meningoencephalitis, or Powassan viruses). Other members of group B are Modoc, Spondweni, Israel turkey meningoencephalitis, Wesselsbron, louping ill, Bussuquara, Rio Bravo (U.S. bat salivary gland), Ntaya, and Langat viruses.

(3) **Group C:** A group of arboviruses isolated from man, "sentinel" monkeys, and mosquitoes in Trinidad, Panama, the Florida everglades, and the

Amazon forest near Belem. These viruses, which cause acute undifferentiated febrile illnesses with headache in man, can be placed in 3 subgroups on the basis of close interrelationships by hemagglutination inhibition and neutralization tests: Maritiba, Murutucu, Restan, Nepuyo, and Gumbo Limbo; Caraparu, Ossa, Apeu, and Madrid; and Oriboca and Itaqui.

(4) **Bunyamwera group**: A group of arboviruses isolated from mosquitoes in different parts of the globe: Bunyamwera from Aedes in Africa; Wyeomyia from *Wyeomia melanocephala* in Colombia; Kairi from *Aedes scapularis* in Trinidad; and Cache Valley virus from *Culiseta inornata* in Utah and from *A scapularis* in Belem, Brazil, and Trinidad. Other viruses in this group are Batai (India, Malaya), Germiston (South Africa), Guaroa (Colombia, Brazil), and Ilesha (West Africa).

(5) **Phlebotomus (sandfly) fever group**: There are 10 members of this group, 4 of which have been implicated in an undifferentiated febrile syndrome in man. The Sicilian and Neapolitan phlebotomus fever viruses (Italy, Egypt, Iran, and Pakistan) are transmitted by *Phlebotomus papatasii* females, whereas no vector has yet been demonstrated for the Candiru (Brazil) or Chagres (Panama) viruses.

(6) **California group**: There are 11 members of this group, 8 isolated within the USA (see California Encephalitis).

(7) **Miscellaneous groups**: These represent 16 small groups. The most important associated with disease in man or animals are (a) the Tacaribe-LCM group: Argentinian hemorrhagic fever (Junin) and Bolivian hemorrhagic fever (Machupo); and (b) the diplornaviruses: bluetongue and African horse sickness. The latter has spread from its enzootic area in Africa through the Eastern Mediterranean to Pakistan and India, causing in 1960 alone over 50,000 equine deaths and unknown numbers of cases in these new areas of distribution. Its pathogenicity for man is as yet unknown.

(8) There are about 50 viruses unrelated to each other or to any agent with which they have been compared. Included are the viruses causing Colorado tick fever, Crimean hemorrhagic fever, Rift Valley fever, and Nairobi sheep disease. Colorado tick fever and Chenuda viruses have recently been shown to have the same size and morphology as the diplornaviruses (eg, reovirus).

Although most groups are antigenically distinct, subtle interrelationships between groups through some of their members by cross-reactions in hemagglutination inhibition, complement fixation, or neutralization tests have been seen. For example, Guaroa reacts with the Bunyamwera group by the complement fixation test and weakly to the California group by the hemagglutination inhibition and neutralization tests; Ťahyňa (California group) is neutralized by Bunyamwera antiserum; and low titer hemagglutination inhibition reactions occur between the Bunyamwera-California-Bwamba-Simbu and group C-Guama-Capim-unassigned complexes. This has led to the tentative establishment

of the Bunyamwera supergroup under which the above 8 groups are listed.

About 75 of the arboviruses are capable of infecting man, although only about 60% of these are known to cause overt disease. Those infecting man are all believed to be zoonotic, with man usually the accidental host who plays no important role in the maintenance or transmission cycle of the virus. Exceptions to this are urban yellow fever and dengue. Some of the natural cycles are simple and involve a nonhuman vertebrate host (mammal or bird) with a species of mosquito or tick (jungle yellow fever, the equine encephalitis viruses, and the viruses of Japanese B, St. Louis encephalitis, and Colorado tick fever). Others, however, are quite complex. For example, many cases of central European biphasic meningoencephalitis occur following ingestion of raw milk from infected goats and cows. These animals become infected by grazing in tick-infested pastures where a tick-rodent cycle is occurring.

Diseases produced by the arboviruses may be divided into 3 clinical syndromes: (1) fevers of an undifferentiated type, frequently called "dengue-like," with or without the presence of a maculopapular rash and usually relatively benign; (2) encephalitis, often with a high case fatality rate; and (3) hemorrhagic fevers, also frequently severe and fatal. These categories are somewhat arbitrary.

The intensity of viral multiplication in the organism and its predominant site of localization within the tissues or organs will determine the clinical syndrome finally observed. Thus, individual arboviruses can produce a minor febrile illness in some patients and encephalitis or a hemorrhagic diathesis in others. However, in an epidemic situation one of the above syndromes will predominate, permitting a tentative differential diagnosis to be entertained. A final diagnosis is based on further epidemiologic and serologic data.

The initial stage of infection by an arbovirus is asymptomatic and corresponds to the intrinsic incubation period of viral multiplication. This is followed by the abrupt onset of clinical manifestations which are closely related to viral dissemination. General signs of malaise, headache, nausea, vomiting, and myalgia accompany fever, which is an invariable clinical symptom and sometimes the only one observed. The symptom complex could terminate at this stage, recur with or without a rash, or reveal hemorrhagic manifestations secondary to vascular abnormalities. Not infrequently, the period of viremia is asymptomatic, with the acute onset of encephalitis following localization of the virus in the CNS.

The above clinical categories are utilized in the following sections in discussing some of the most important diseases caused by the arboviruses.

ARBOVIRUS ENCEPHALITIDES

Encephalitis may be produced by a number of neurotropic viruses. Such agents produce an infection, often in epidemic form, in which the primary clinical findings are produced by involvement of the brain and spinal cord. A number of these diseases of similar epidemiology have been grouped together as the arthropod-borne encephalitides. Although they have much in common, their geographic distribution is often quite distinct (Table 30–1). Thus, **western equine encephalitis (WEE)** occurs primarily in the western USA and Canada; **eastern equine encephalitis (EEE)** occurs in the eastern and southern USA; **Venezuelan equine encephalitis (VEE)** occurs in South America and Panama; **St. Louis encephalitis (SLE)** in almost all of the USA (but its distribution in the country varies widely from one year to the next); **Japanese B encephalitis (JBE)** in the Far East (Japan, Korea, China, Malaya, India); and **Murray Valley encephalitis (MVE)** in Australia. A more recently recognized group of arboviruses that produce encephalitis, the California complex, will be discussed in a separate section.

One of the reasons epidemics of viral encephalitis have not been recorded in the Middle East may be the prevalence of West Nile virus in this area. This virus, which produces a mild, self-limiting disease in man, shares some antigens and other properties with JBE, SLE, and MVE viruses. The widespread occurrence of West Nile fever in the Middle East may result in an increase of the resistance of the population to encephalitis caused by the related Japanese type; that is to say, a population immune to West Nile fever may not be able to support an epidemic caused by a virus like that of Japanese encephalitis.

Practically all of the arboviruses show encephalitogenic properties in suckling mice. Fortunately, only a few produce this disease in man, at least when acquired normally by the peripheral route. Individual host susceptibility, the immune status of the patient, the development of a viral mutant, or the dosage inoculated may be important in the occasional production of encephalitis by such viruses as West Nile fever, yellow fever, or dengue.

Encephalitis (or meningoencephalitis) may also occur as a complication of a variety of diseases (measles, mumps, infectious hepatitis, variola, varicella, herpes zoster, herpes simplex, and others), which are caused by viruses other than the arboviruses. In many cases, a delayed hypersensitivity reaction occurs, and for this reason they have been called "postinfectious" encephalitides.

Properties of the Viruses

A. **Nucleic Acid**: RNA.

B. **Size**: The arthropod-borne encephalitis producing viruses are small, between 20 and 60 nm. Certain of the viruses have been purified and were found to contain phospholipids, fatty acid, and cholesterol in addition to nucleoprotein.

C. **Reaction to Physical and Chemical Agents**: New isolates are unstable at room temperature. They may be preserved by freezing at $-70°$ C, particularly in the presence of 25% rabbit serum or 4% bovine albumin. Arboviruses are inactivated by ether or by 1:1000 sodium deoxycholate. In this way new isolates may

readily be distinguished from the deoxycholate-resistant enteroviruses.

D. **Animal Susceptibility and Growth of Viruses**: The viruses are infectious for a variety of animals, and the WEE and EEE viruses are responsible for much illness in horses and mules. The chief experimental animal is the mouse, which can be infected most easily by inoculation into the brain. Infant mice are especially susceptible to infection. In the susceptible vertebrate host, primary virus multiplication occurs either in myeloid and lymphoid tissues or in the vascular endothelium. Multiplication in the CNS seems to depend upon the ability of the virus to pass the blood-brain barrier and to infect nerve cells. After the parenteral administration of small amounts of virus into chickens, doves, ducks, bats, guinea pigs, rabbits, and monkeys, a silent, inapparent infection often develops during which the virus circulates in the blood for several days. In nature this type of infection serves as a source of virus for the insect vectors of the disease.

The viruses multiply in chick embryos when inoculated by the yolk sac or chorioallantoic routes. They readily grow in tissue cultures of chick or mouse embryo, baby hamster kidney, duck embryo, or in cultures of mammalian cell lines. In addition, *Aedes albopictus* and *A aegypti* cell lines have recently shown selective susceptibility to infection with mosquito-borne viruses, especially from group B. All arboviruses so far investigated have been shown to be formed in the cytoplasm and acquire their membrane at the cell surface by budding (Fig 27–4). Viral multiplication can be measured by direct observation of cytopathic changes and of virus-specific immunofluorescence, or by production of viral hemagglutinin as measured directly in the tissue culture by the hemadsorption test. By means of the plaque method, more consistent and more sensitive endpoints have been described with group A, B, and C viruses in cultures of chick embryo, duck kidney, hamster BHK-21, and Vero monkey cells. Homotypic and heterotypic interference, as well as susceptibility to interferon, has been demonstrated for some of the arboviruses studied.

E. **Antigenic Properties**: Complement fixing antigens and viral hemagglutinins may be prepared; infected brains of newborn mice, because of their low fat content, are the starting materials of choice for both preparations. The hemagglutinins of these viruses are part of the infectious virus particle. The union between hemagglutinin and red cell is irreversible. The erythrocyte-virus complex is still infective, but it can be neutralized by the addition of antibody which results in large lattice formations. This phenomenon, plus the fact that infectivity is lost at alkaline pH whereas hemagglutinin is lost at acid pH, indicates that the sites on the virus responsible for infectivity and for hemagglutination are separate.

Some of these viruses have an overlapping antigenicity which is most readily demonstrated by cross-reactions in hemagglutination-inhibition tests. The overlapping is due to the presence of one or more cross-reactive antigens in addition to the strain-specific antigen. Thus immune sera prepared for one strain will contain strain-specific as well as group-specific antibodies.

A considerable degree of specificity can be obtained by adsorption of the immune serum with a heterologous virus belonging to the same group. The resulting serum, when tested for hemagglutination-inhibiting activity, reacts only with the homologous but not with the heterologous strain. Such adsorbed sera have facilitated the analysis of the complex antigenic structure of many arboviruses within a major group as well as the identification of newly isolated strains.

Pathogenesis & Pathology

The pathogenesis of the disease in man has not been well studied, but in certain instances the disease in experimental animals may afford a model for the human disease. Thus the equine encephalitides in horses are diphasic. In the first phase (minor illness) the virus multiplies in nonneural tissue and is present in the blood 3 days before the first signs of involvement of the CNS. In the second phase (major illness) the virus multiplies in the brain, cells are injured and destroyed, and encephalitis becomes apparent at the clinical level. The 2 phases may be distinct or may overlap. It has not been established in man whether or not there is a period of primary viral multiplication in the viscera with a secondary liberation of virus into the blood before its entry into the CNS. The viruses have been found to multiply in nonneural tissues of experimentally infected monkeys.

Certain concentrations of virus in brain tissue are necessary before the clinical disease becomes manifest. In mice the level to which the virus multiplies in the brain is influenced by genetic (a mendelian trait) as well as other factors.

The primary encephalitides are characterized by lesions in all parts of the CNS, particularly in the basal structures of the brain and in the cerebral cortex, and to a lesser degree in the spinal cord. Small hemorrhages with perivascular cuffing and meningeal infiltration—chiefly with mononuclear cells—are common. Nerve cell degeneration associated with neuronophagia occurs in the cerebral cortex, cerebellar cortex, basal ganglia, pons, medulla, and upper spinal cord. Purkinje's cells of the cerebellum may be destroyed. There are also patches of encephalomalacia; acellular plaques of spongy appearance in which medullary fibers, dendrites, and axons are destroyed; and focal microglial proliferation. Thus not only the neurons but also the cells of the supporting structure of the CNS are attacked.

Although widespread neuronal degeneration is observed with all arboviruses producing encephalitis, predominant characteristics are noted. Lesions due to EEE tend to be localized in the cortex while the basal nuclei are involved in WEE. Pathologic changes seen in SLE are most marked in the brain stem and midbrain, especially the substantia nigra. The production of severe diffuse lesions with focal necrosis in WEE, EEE, and could account for the occurrence of permanent sequelae in these infections. Many of the tick-borne encephalitides produce lesions in the anterior horn cells indistinguishable from those of poliomyelitis.

Clinical Findings

Incubation periods of the encephalitides are between 4 and 21 days. There is a sudden onset with severe headache, chills and fever, nausea and vomiting, generalized pains, and malaise. Within 24–48 hours, marked drowsiness develops and the patient may become stuporous. Nuchal rigidity is common. Mental confusion, dysarthria, tremors, convulsions, and coma develop in severe cases. Fever lasts 4–10 days. The mortality rate in most encephalitides is 5–25% or even 40% (see Table 30–1). With JBE, the mortality rate in older age groups may be as high as 80%. Sequelae may occur and include mental deterioration, personality changes, paralysis, aphasia, and cerebellar signs.

Abortive infections simulate aseptic meningitis and are difficult to distinguish from nonparalytic poliomyelitis. In addition, inapparent infections are common in certain areas.

In California, where both WEE and SLE are prevalent, WEE has a predilection for children and infants. In the same area SLE rarely occurs in infants, even though both viruses are transmitted by the same arthropod vector (*Culex tarsalis*).

Laboratory Diagnosis

A. Recovery of Virus: The virus occurs in the blood only early in the infection, usually before the onset of symptoms. The virus is most often recovered from the brains of fatal cases. Samples should be taken under aseptic conditions as soon as possible after death. A 20% suspension in 0.75% bovalbumin phosphate-buffered saline is prepared, and 0.02 ml is injected intracerebrally into newborn mice. Embryonated eggs have also been employed.

If a transmissible agent free from bacteria is recovered in the brains of the inoculated mice (or in the embryo), it should be identified by suitable neutralization, complement fixation, or hemagglutination inhibition tests with known antisera. The hemagglutinin of arboviruses has been demonstrated through the use of 1-day-old chick cells or adult goose erythrocytes. A modified Ouchterlony agar gel precipitation method, employing the principle of double diffusion (crude brain antigen against known antibody) has been used for rapid identification of some encephalitis agents, especially group B and the California complex.

B. Serology: Neutralizing and hemagglutination inhibiting (HI) antibodies are detectable within a few days after the onset of illness. Complement fixing (CF) antibodies appear later. The neutralizing antibody and probably the HI antibody endure for years, if not for life. The complement fixing antibody is less persistent and may be lost within 1–2 years.

The HI test is the simplest diagnostic test, but it primarily identifies the group rather than the specific etiologic virus. If adult goose rather than newly hatched chick erythrocytes are used, the serum must first be adsorbed with goose erythrocytes in order to remove the nonspecific hemagglutinin found in human and other sera.

It is necessary to establish a rise in specific antibodies during infection in order to make the diagnosis. The first sample of serum should be taken as soon after the onset as possible and the second sample about 2–3 weeks later. The matched specimens must be run in the same serologic test.

The cross-reactivity that takes place among the group A or B arboviruses must be considered in making the diagnosis. Thus, following a single infection by one member of the group, antibodies to other members may also appear. These group-specific antibodies are usually of lower titer than the type-specific antibody and are easy to interpret. Serologic diagnosis becomes difficult when epidemics occur in endemic areas or when the individual has been infected previously by a closely related arbovirus. Under these circumstances, a definite etiologic diagnosis may not be possible. Neutralizing, CF, and HI antibodies have a decreasing degree of specificity for the etiologic viral type (in the order listed).

Immunity

Immunity is believed to be permanent after a single infection. In endemic areas the population may build up immunity as a result of inapparent infections; the proportion of persons with antibodies to the local arthropod-borne virus increases with age.

Attempts at the production of artificial immunity with killed vaccines prepared from mouse brain or chick embryo have not yielded striking results in man. Effective vaccines have been developed to protect horses against eastern (and western) equine encephalitis. No effective vaccines for these diseases are at present available for man.

An attenuated vaccine for Venezuelan equine encephalitis is available to laboratory workers engaged in research with this agent. Recent serologic trials with a new attenuated Japanese B encephalitis vaccine hold promise for future prevention of this disease.

Because of antigens common to several members within a group, the response to immunization or to infection with one of the viruses of a group may be modified by prior exposure to another member of the same group. In general, the homologous response is greater than a cross-reacting one. Repeated inoculation of a virus in group A or group B confers protection on animals against another virus of the same group, particularly when the challenge is given by peripheral inoculation. This mechanism may be important in conferring protection on a community from an epidemic against another related agent. This theory has been postulated for the reduced number of typical cases of St. Louis encephalitis among persons previously infected with dengue, another group B arbovirus.

Treatment

There is no proved specific treatment. In experimental animals, hyperimmune serum is ineffective if given after the onset of disease. However, if given 1–2 days after the invasion of the virus but before the signs of encephalitis are obvious, serum can prevent lethal infection.

Epidemiology

In severe epidemics caused by the encephalitis viruses, the case rate is about 1–3/1000. In the large urban epidemic of St. Louis encephalitis that occurred in 1966 in Dallas (population 1 million), there were 545 reported cases, 145 (27%) laboratory-confirmed cases, and 15 deaths. The overall attack rate was 15 cases per 100,000, with a case fatality rate of 10%. All deaths were in persons 45 years of age or older.

Most infections with the arboviruses occur in mammals or birds, with man serving as an accidental host. Viruses have been isolated from mosquitoes and ticks, which serve as reservoirs of infection.

The epidemiology of the arthropod-borne encephalitides must account for the maintenance and dissemination of the viruses in nature in the absence of man. The virus is transmitted from the animal through the bites of arthropod vectors. In ticks, the viruses may pass from generation to generation by the transovarian route, and in such instances the tick acts as a true reservoir of the virus as well as its vector.

The mechanism for the maintenance of arboviruses in certain geographic areas has not yet been elucidated. It is not known, for example, whether the virus is reintroduced each year from the outside, presumably by birds migrating from southern or tropical areas, or whether it somehow survives the winter in the local area. A relatively simple overwintering mechanism would be that of hibernating mosquitoes, which could reinfect birds at the time of their emergence and thus reestablish each year a simple bird-mosquito-bird cycle. Or it may be that the virus remains latent during this period in birds, mammals, and arthropods. Certain arboviruses have been recovered from birds and bats several months after infection and after the development of serum antibodies. However, the true role of cold-blooded vertebrates (snakes, turtles, lizards, alligators, and frogs) in the ecology of certain arboviruses has not been satisfactorily explained.

Garter snakes experimentally injected with western equine encephalitis virus can hibernate overwinter and circulate virus in high titers and for long periods the following spring. Normal mosquitoes can be infected by feeding on the emerged snakes, and then can transmit the virus to chicks. This is a possible mechanism of overwintering of arboviruses, since the virus can be found in the blood of wild gopher snakes, garter snakes, and blue racers and in their offspring.

A. Serologic Epidemiology: In highly endemic areas, almost the entire population may become infected, and most infections are asymptomatic. This is true for Japanese encephalitis infection in Japan, Korea, and Okinawa. In Korea, no large-scale epidemics have been reported among the natives, although at times the disease has broken out among Americans stationed there. A high rate of inapparent infection may also be found among domestic animals (pigs, cows, and horses). It has been estimated that in a single epidemic (Murray Valley encephalitis) one clinical case of encephalitis occurred for every 700 minor or inapparent infections. Similar high infection-to-case ratios exist among specified age groups for other arbovirus infections (Table 30–1).

In the 1964 Houston SLE epidemic (712 reported cases), there was an inapparent infection rate of 8% in a random city survey, but in the epidemic area of the city the inapparent infection rate was 34%. The infection-to-case ratio remained about the same, however. It is obvious that the presence of infected mosquitoes is required before human infections can occur, although socioeconomic and cultural factors (air conditioning, screens, sitting outside) affect the degree of exposure of the population to these virus-carrying vectors. In areas of the city where intensive, weekly mosquito control programs had been carried on from early spring to late fall for pest control, there was no evidence of infection. Antibodies were found in many chickens and wild birds, especially sparrows, tested in the Houston area.

In endemic areas of California, 11% of infants are born with maternal antibody to WEE and 27% have SLE antibody. A direct relationship exists between the length of residence of the mother in the endemic area and the acquisition of antibody.

B. Mosquito-Borne Encephalitis: Infection of man occurs when a mosquito like *Culex tarsalis, C quinquefasciatus, C pipiens,* or *C tritaeniorhynchus* (Japan), or another arthropod, bites first an infected animal and later man.

The equine encephalitides, EEE and WEE, are transmitted by culicine mosquitoes to horses or man, from a mosquito-wild bird-mosquito cycle. Equines, like man, are tangential and unessential hosts for the maintenance of the virus. Human encephalitis cases occurring in conjunction with an epizootic of encephalitis in horses should alert physicians and the community to the possibility that an arbovirus epidemic may be developing. Horse cases often occur as long as 2 weeks before the first human cases. EEE in horses is severe, with up to 90% of the affected animals dying within the first day or two. In contrast, epizootic WEE is less frequently fatal for horses. In addition, EEE produces severe epizootics in certain domestic game birds such as pheasants, Pekin ducks, and partridges. A mosquito-wild bird-mosquito cycle is also observed in SLE and JBE, although swine are also an important host of the latter virus. Mosquitoes remain infected for life (several weeks to months). Only the female feeds on blood in response to oviposition and therefore can feed and transmit the virus more than once. The growth cycle in the mosquito has been established for several of the arboviruses. The cells of the midgut are the site of primary virus multiplication. This is followed by viremia and consequently by invasion of several organs—chiefly salivary glands and nerve tissue, where secondary virus multiplication occurs. The arthropod remains healthy.

Infection of insectivorous bats with arboviruses produces a viremia lasting 6–12 days without any illness or pathologic changes in the bat. While the virus concentration is high, the infected bat may infect mosquitoes which then are able to transmit the infection to chickens as well as to other bats.

In nature, mosquitoes have a close association with bats, not only in summer daytime resting places but also during the winter, in hibernation sites. Under experimental conditions simulating the bat's winter environment, mosquitoes were capable of transmitting virus to the bat provided they had passed through an adequate extrinsic incubation period at 27° C before low-temperature exposure. Bats thus infected were capable of maintaining a latent virus infection, with no detectable viremia, for over 3 months at 10° C under simulated hibernation conditions. When the bats were returned to room temperature, no virus could be detected immediately; but after 3 days a viremia appeared. The titers following hibernation were above the minimal level required to infect mosquitoes. The mosquito-bat-mosquito cycle has been suggested as a possible overwintering mechanism for some arboviruses.

Coldblooded animals (snakes, turtles, lizards, alligators, and frogs) have been shown to harbor arboviruses and may play a role in the overwintering of these viruses.

C. Tick-borne Encephalitis Complex:

1. Russian spring-summer encephalitis—This disease occurs chiefly in the early summer, particularly in adult males exposed to the ticks *Ixodes persulcatus* and *I ricinus* in the uncleared forest. Ticks can become infected at any stage in their metamorphosis, and experimental studies have shown trans-stadial and transovarial transmission. The virus is believed to persist throughout the winter in hibernating ticks or vertebrate hosts such as hedgehogs, dormice, or bats. Virus is secreted in the milk of infected goats for long periods, and infection may be transmitted to those who drink unpasteurized milk. Characteristic of this disease is its involvement of the bulbar or cervical cord areas and the development of ascending paralysis or hemiparesis. Residual paralysis is not uncommon.

2. Louping ill—This disease of sheep in Scotland and northern England is spread by the tick *Ixodes ricinus.* Man is occasionally infected.

3. Tick-borne encephalitis (Central European or biphasic meningoencephalitis)—This virus (or closely related strains) is antigenically related to Russian spring-summer encephalitis virus and louping ill virus. Typical cases have a biphasic course, the first phase being influenza-like and the second a meningoencephalitis with or without paralysis.

4. Kyasanur Forest disease—An Indian hemorrhagic disease similar to Omsk hemorrhagic fever, both of which are caused by viruses of the Russian spring-summer encephalitis complex. Langur (*Presbytis entellus*) and bonnet (*Macaca radiata*) monkeys are found naturally infected in southern India. Experimentally infected lactating monkeys were found to excrete the virus in the milk during the period of viremia. The infection can be transmitted through the milk to the suckling infant.

5. Powassan encephalitis—This tick-borne virus is the first member of the Russian spring-summer com-

TABLE 30–1. Summary of 5 major human arbovirus infections which occur in the USA.

Diseases	Exposure	Distribution	Vectors	Infection: Case Ratio (Age Incidence)	Sequelae	Mortality Rate (%)
WEE	Rural	Pacific, Mountain, West Central, Southwest	*Culex tarsalis*	50:1 (under 5) 1000:1 (over 15)	+	2–3
EEE	Rural	Atlantic, Southern Coastal	*Aedes sollicitans* *A vexans*	10:1 (infants) 50:1 (middle aged) 20:1 (elderly)	+	50–70
SLE	Urban-rural	Widespread	*C pipiens* *C quinquefasciatus* *C tarsalis* *C nigripalpus*	>400:1 (young) 64:1 (elderly)	±	5–10
California encephalitis	Rural	North Central, Atlantic, South	(Aedes sp?)	Unknown ratio (most cases under 20)	±	Fatalities rare
Colorado tick fever	Rural	Pacific, Mountain	*Dermacentor andersoni*	Unknown ratio (all ages affected)	Rare	Fatalities rare

plex to have been isolated in North America (Canada, 1958). Only the initial case has been reported. Serologic surveys in humans have been unrewarding.

Each virus is limited to definite areas. It has been postulated that the viruses may have a common ancestor and have become adapted to different parts of the globe, each with its special arthropod vectors and animal reservoirs. On the other hand, a virus may be kept out of an area because the local established virus has built up an immunity in the population which, because of the overlapping serologic response, protects against a virus from another area. In this way, perhaps, the Middle East, where West Nile fever is prevalent, may be spared from the more serious Japanese encephalitis.

Similarly, in the Caribbean area, where dengue is a common infection, antibodies against dengue virus may offer a degree of protection against yellow fever virus or SLE. This might also account for the fact that yellow fever has never gained a foothold in India. However, dengue and yellow fever can and have occurred in the same geographic area. Since the same mosquito vector is often involved in these diseases, it is possible that interference prevents the insect from transmitting both viruses at once.

Control

Biologic control of the natural vertebrate host is generally impractical, especially against wild birds. The most effective control, therefore, is through arthropod control. Since the period of viremia in the vertebrate is of short duration (3–6 days for SLE infections of birds), any suppression of the vector for this period should break the transmission cycle. During the 1966 Dallas SLE epidemic, low-volume, high-concentration malathion mist was sprayed aerially over most of Dallas County. A striking decrease in the number and infectivity rate of the mosquito vectors occurred, demonstrating the effectiveness of the treatment.

Inactivated vaccines have not met with success, although preliminary encouraging results had been obtained in Japanese children. A new attenuated strain of Japanese B virus is undergoing extensive field trials at this time. The development of other attenuated strains by serial passages in cultures of various types of cells is still in its experimental stages, and, except for Venezuelan equine encephalitis, no attenuated vaccines against the encephalitides are available for use in man. A live attenuated variant of WEE virus has produced high antibody levels in horses and may be safe. However, these attenuated strains have yielded virulent mutants on further passages in animals.

CALIFORNIA ENCEPHALITIS

The California complex comprises 11 closely related but antigenically distinct members. Eight are found within continental USA and include California encephalitis, La Crosse, trivittatus, Jamestown Canyon, Keystone, Snowshoe Hare, Jerry Slough, and San Angelo viruses. Strains from other areas are Melao (Trinidad and Brazil), Ťahyňa (Czechoslovakia and Yugoslavia), and Lumbo (Mozambique). This group has recently been recognized to be part of a larger complex, the Bunyamwera supergroup, through cross-reactions in HI, CF, or Nt tests.

Properties of the California Group

The virions are spherical, 50–80 nm in diameter, and are inactivated by sodium deoxycholate and ether. Hemagglutinins are difficult to demonstrate. Success has been achieved with most members through the use of spinner cultures, sonication, or trypsin treatment (alone or in combination) of mouse brain antigen. All members are pathogenic for suckling mice and hamsters and for a variety of cell culture preparations.

Clinical Findings & Diagnosis

The onset of California encephalitis virus infection is abrupt, typically with a severe bifrontal headache preceding a fever which ranges between 38.3 and 40.6° C. Vomiting, lethargy, and local or generalized convulsions may occur. Less frequently, aseptic meningitis with nuchal rigidity alone is noted.

Polymorphonuclear leukocytosis is frequent, with the peripheral white count above 10,000/cu mm and occasionally as high as 29,000. CSF pleocytosis, predominantly lymphocytic, is present at some stage of the illness with a range of 30–1000/cu mm, with the majority below 250. Serum protein is slightly elevated, but serum glucose is within normal limits. The EEG reveals generalized cerebral dysfunction with high-amplitude slow activity.

Histopathologic changes include neuronal degeneration and patchy inflammatory response with some perivascular cuffing and edema in the cerebral cortex and meninges. Inclusion bodies are not seen.

The prognosis is usually excellent, although convalescence may be prolonged, and fatalities have been reported. Although gross evidence of residual neurologic abnormalities have not been observed, abnormal EEG patterns have occasionally persisted in the more severe cases for at least 1–2 years.

Serologic confirmation by hemagglutination inhibition, complement fixation, or neutralization tests is necessary in all suspected cases with appropriately spaced acute and convalescent specimens.

Epidemiology

The first member of the group, **California encephalitis virus,** was isolated from mosquitoes in California in 1943. It was not until 1964, however, that major outbreaks were recognized and studied. A significant occurrence at this time was a new isolation from the brain of a 4-year-old child from La Crosse, Wisconsin, who had died in 1960 following acute meningo-encephalitis. Laboratory tests with this antigen (La Crosse) appear to be more sensitive in detecting antibody in human infections than the other members of the group. This suggests either a greater avidity of this antigen for humoral antibody or that this strain is the principal human pathogen in the parts of the USA where outbreaks have occurred.

Cases occur primarily in late July through early September in rural communities and have been most common in the upper Mississippi and Ohio River valleys, particularly in Indiana, Wisconsin, and Ohio. Scattered cases have been reported from North Carolina, Minnesota, Iowa, New York, Florida, Louisiana, Mississippi, and California. Clinical infections have occurred only in persons less than 21 years of age, with the majority between 4 and 14 years.

The ecologic information available suggests that these viruses are transmitted between various woodland mosquitoes and small mammals such as squirrels and rabbits. Human infection is tangential and is usually acquired in rural areas in association with the natural cycle.

WEST NILE FEVER

West Nile fever is an acute, mild, febrile disease with lymphadenopathy and rash that occurs in the Middle East, tropical or subtropical Africa, and southwest Asia.

Properties of the Virus

The virus has the properties of the other group B arboviruses. It propagates in chick embryo and tissue culture, producing plaques on cell monolayers under agar.

Clinical Findings

The virus is introduced through the bite of a Culex mosquito, and produces viremia and a generalized systemic infection characterized by lymphadenopathy, sometimes with an accompanying maculopapular rash. Although not common, transitory meningeal involvement may occur during the acute stage. The virus may produce fatal encephalitis in older people, who have a delayed (and low) antibody response.

Laboratory Diagnosis

To recover the virus, blood is taken in the acute stage of the infection. In serologic tests the first sample should be taken early in the disease; the second, about 2–3 weeks later. CF, HI, and Nt tests may be used. Complement fixing titers of 32–128 are commonly found in the convalescent specimen, remain at this level for about 3 months, and then fall slowly. Neutralizing antibodies rise somewhat more slowly, reach maximum height at about 4 months, and persist almost at the same level for over 2 years. During convalescence, heterologous complement fixing and neutralizing antibodies develop to JBE and SLE, which are members of this same group. The heterologous response is shorter and lower than the homologous response.

Immunity

Only one antigenic type exists, and immunity is presumably permanent. Maternal antibodies are transferred from mother to offspring, and disappear during the first 6 months of life.

When volunteers were first sensitized by a mild West Nile virus infection and then given the killed Japanese virus vaccine, they formed neutralizing antibodies of high titer to Japanese encephalitis and of lower titers to the related group B arboviruses.

Epidemiology

West Nile fever appears to be limited to the Middle East, endemic in Egypt, and epidemic in Israel. However, antibodies have been found in normal adults in Africa, India, and Korea. In nonimmune populations, the attack rate is high, and abortive and inapparent infections also occur. In Cairo, over 70% of the inhabitants aged 4 years and above have both neutralizing and complement fixing antibodies.

This summer disease is more prevalent in rural than in urban areas. The virus has been isolated on several occasions from Culex mosquitoes during epidemics, and also from the blood of febrile children. Experimentally infected mosquitoes can transmit the virus after an extrinsic incubation period of 1–3 weeks.

Ticks may play a role as reservoir vectors of West Nile virus. Nymphs of the tick *Ornithodoros moubata* can be infected by gorging on viremic mice. The virus multiplies in the nymph and persists into the adult stage for at least 224 days. The ticks in turn can pass the virus on to chicks and mice.

Control

Mosquito abatement is a logical control measure but has not yet been proved to be effective.

YELLOW FEVER

Yellow fever (YF) is an acute, febrile, mosquito-borne illness. Severe cases are characterized by jaundice, proteinuria, and hemorrhage.

Properties of the Virus

A. Size: YF virus is about 22–38 nm in diameter.

B. Reaction to Physical and Chemical Agents: The virus may be preserved for a month in blood at 4° C, for 3 months in 50% glycerol at 0° C, and for years at −70° C. After lyophilization, it survives for years at 0° C. The virus is killed by heating at 60° C for 10 minutes and also by contact with 0.1% formalin for 48 hours at 0° C. The virus is rapidly inactivated by diluting it in physiologic saline solution, unless 5% normal serum or 0.75% bovalbumin is added to the diluent.

C. Animal Susceptibility and Growth of Virus: YF virus multiplies in a variety of animals (monkeys, mice, guinea pigs) and in mosquitoes. It is readily cultivated in the developing chick embryo and in tissue cultures made from chick or mouse embryos. All strains of the virus produce encephalitis in mice following direct inoculation into the brain. Infant mice also develop encephalitis after subcutaneous and intraperitoneal inoculations.

When freshly isolated from nature (from man, monkey, or mosquito), the virus is pantropic, ie, it invades all 3 embryonal layers. Fresh strains usually produce a severe (often fatal) infection with marked damage to the livers of monkeys after parenteral inoculation. After serial passage in the brains of monkeys or mice, such strains lose much of their viscerotropism; they cause encephalitis after intracerebral injection but only asymptomatic infection after subcutaneous injection. Cross-immunity exists between the pantropic and neurotropic strains of the virus.

During the serial passage of a pantropic strain of YF through tissue cultures, the relatively avirulent 17D strain was recovered. This strain lost its capacity to induce a viscerotropic or neurotropic disease in monkeys and in man and is now used as a vaccine. The virus in the vaccine may be diluted 10,000 times and still produce encephalitis and death in mice inoculated intracerebrally.

D. Antigenic Properties: Hemagglutinins and complement fixing antigens may be prepared from infected mouse brain or from infected monkey liver or serum. Each antigen has 2 separable components, one of which is associated with the infectious particle. The other is probably not the virus, and may be a product of the action of YF virus on the tissues which it infects. By serologic tests, YF virus is classifed as a member of the group B arboviruses.

Pathogenesis & Pathology

Our understanding of the pathogenesis of YF is based on work with the experimental infection in monkeys. The virus enters through the skin and then spreads to the local lymph nodes, where it multiplies. From the lymph nodes it enters the circulating blood and becomes localized in the liver, spleen, kidney, bone marrow, and lymph glands. Even after the virus has been cleared from the blood, it may still be present for days in the lymph nodes, spleen, and bone marrow. With highly virulent strains (Asibi), the virus is found in highest concentration in the liver. With an attenuated strain (17D), it is found only in the spleen, lymph nodes, and bone marrow.

The lesions of YF are due to the localization and propagation of the virus in a particular organ. Death follows upon the severe necrosis produced by these lesions in the liver and kidney. In severe cases, there may be almost complete destruction of the parenchymatous cells of the liver. In fatal cases, the most frequent site of hemorrhage is the mucosa at the pyloric end of the stomach.

The distribution of the necrotic cells in the liver may be spotty, but is most evident in the midzones of the lobules. The necrosis is hyaline in nature and may be restricted to the cytoplasm. These irregular hyaline masses are eosinophilic and are called Councilman bodies. Intranuclear eosinophilic inclusion bodies are also present and are of diagnostic value. Hemorrhage is rare in the liver. During the recovery period, the parenchymatous cells are replaced and the liver may be completely restored.

In the kidney there is fatty degeneration of the tubular epithelium which may be secondary to the hemorrhagic diathesis. Degenerative changes also occur in the spleen, lymph nodes, and heart. Intranuclear, acidophilic inclusion bodies may be present in the nerve and glial cells of the brain. Perivascular infiltrations with mononuclear cells also occur in the brain.

Clinical Findings

The incubation period is from 3–6 days. At the onset, the patient has fever, chills, headache, and backache. This is soon followed by nausea and vomiting. A short period of remission often follows the prodrome.

On about the fourth day, the period of intoxication begins. Faget's sign—a slow pulse rate (90–100) relative to a high fever—is observed, and moderate jaundice becomes apparent. In severe cases, marked proteinuria and hemorrhagic manifestations appear. The vomitus may be black in nature due to altered blood. Lymphopenia is present. When the disease progresses to the severe stage (black vomitus and jaundice), the mortality rate is high. On the other hand, the infection may also be so mild as to go unrecognized. Regardless of severity, there are no sequelae; patients either die or recover completely.

Laboratory Diagnosis

A. Recovery of Virus: The virus may be recovered from the blood up to the fifth day of the disease. Mice inoculated intracerebrally with serum of a suspected case develop encephalitis if the virus is present. If virus is isolated, it should be identified by neutralization with specific antiserum.

Some strains of the virus act paradoxically when first isolated from patients. Undiluted serum may produce no disease in inoculated mice, whereas the same serum diluted 10 or 100 times may cause encephalitis in the inoculated mice. The explanation of this paradoxic behavior might be (1) that antibody is present in the serum in only small amounts, and that the virus may be reactivated by simple dilution, which dissociates, in part, the virus-antibody complex; or (2) that a relatively large amount of inactive virus is also present in the specimen, which interferes with the growth of the active virus unless it is diluted out. For this reason, the serum should be inoculated undiluted into one group and in various dilutions into other groups of mice.

B. Serology: Neutralization antibodies develop early (by the fifth day) even in severe and fatal cases. In patients who survive the infection, circulating antibodies endure for life. Neutralization tests are carried out by mixing varying dilutions of virus with undiluted serum and injecting the mixture intracerebrally into adult mice or intraperitoneally into infant mice. An accessory factor in the form of fresh human or monkey serum is used as a diluent to enhance the neutralization of the virus by specific antibody.

Complement fixing antibodies are rarely found after mild infection or vaccination with the attenuated, live 17D strain. In severe infections they appear later than the neutralizing antibodies and disappear more rapidly.

The serologic response in YF may be of 2 types. In **primary infections** of yellow fever, specific HI antibodies appear first, followed rapidly by antibodies to other group B viruses. The titers of homologous HI antibodies are usually higher than those of heterologous antibodies. CF antibodies rise slowly and are usually specific, as are neutralizing antibodies in primary infections especially.

In secondary infections where YF occurs in a patient previously infected with a group B arbovirus, HI and CF antibodies appear rapidly and to high titers.

There is no suggestion of specificity. The highest HI and CF antibodies are usually heterologous. The heterologous response may be so great that accurate diagnosis by Nt test may be impossible.

Histopathologic examination of the liver in fatal cases is useful in those regions where the disease is endemic.

Immunity

Subtle antigenic differences are observed between YF strains isolated in Africa and South America. The pantropic prototype strain, Asibi, is antigenically somewhat different from the 17D vaccine strain.

An infant born of an immune mother will have antibodies at birth which are gradually lost during the first 6 months of life. Reacquisition of these antibodies is dependent upon the individual's exposure to the virus under natural conditions or by vaccination.

Epidemiology

Two major epidemiologic cycles of YF are recognized: (1) classic (or urban) epidemic YF and (2) sylvan (or jungle) YF. Urban YF involves person-to-person transmission by domestic or peridomestic Aedes mosquitoes. In the western hemisphere and West Africa, this species is primarily *A aegypti,* which breeds in the accumulations of water that accompany human settlement. Most adult mosquitoes remain within 100 yards of their point of origin, and rest during the daytime in the houses. They become infected by biting a viremic individual. Urban YF is perpetuated in areas where there exists a constant influx of susceptible persons, cases of YF, and *A aegypti.* With the use of intensive measures for mosquito abatement, urban YF has been practically eliminated in South America.

Jungle YF is primarily a disease of monkeys. In South America, it is transmitted from monkey to monkey by arboreal mosquitoes such as members of the Haemagogus family which inhabit the moist forest canopy. In Africa, reservoirs of infection include certain monkeys, with Aedes mosquitoes acting as vectors. The infection in animals may be severe or inapparent. Persons such as woodcutters, nut-pickers, or road-builders come in contact with these mosquitoes in the forest and become infected. Jungle YF may also occur when an infected monkey visits a human habitation and is bitten by *A aegypti,* which then transmits the virus to man.

The virus multiplies in mosquitoes, which remain infectious for life. After the mosquito ingests a virus-containing blood meal, an interval of 12–14 days is required for it to become infectious. This interval is called the extrinsic incubation period.

All age groups are susceptible, but the disease in infants is milder than that in older groups. Large numbers of inapparent infections occur. The disease usually is milder in Negroes. Yellow fever has never been reported in India or the Orient, even though the vector, *A aegypti,* is widely distributed there.

Large-scale epidemics occurred in Ethiopia in 1961 and in Senegal in 1965–1966.

Control

Vigorous mosquito abatement programs have virtually eliminated urban YF. The last reported outbreak of YF in the USA occurred in 1905. However, with the speed of modern air travel, health officers must be on the alert in areas where infections, once brought in, might take hold. Most countries insist upon proper mosquito control of airplanes and vaccination of all persons at least 10 days before arrival in or from an endemic zone. Until complete eradication of *A aegypti* is accomplished, the threat of a YF outbreak will be always present.

An excellent attenuated, live vaccine is available in the 17D strain. Vaccine is prepared in eggs and then dispensed as a dried powder in small vials. Because it is a live virus, it must be kept cold. It is rehydrated just before use and injected subcutaneously. The vaccine contains egg proteins, and vaccinees should be questioned about allergic reactions to such proteins. The vaccine can also be administered by the skin scarification technic. A single dose produces a good antibody response in more than 95% of vaccinated persons. Persistence of antibody levels have resulted in lengthening the recommended interval for revaccination from 6 years to 10 years, although most individuals maintain significant neutralizing titers for even longer periods of time. An avian leukosis-free YF vaccine seed has recently been developed and should be available for distribution soon. After vaccination, the virus multiplies and may be isolated from the blood before antibodies develop. With viremia, a circulating virus inhibitor with properties similar to interferon has been detected. It may limit the duration of viremia, and may provide early resistance.

See Table 27–7 for USPHS recommendations about simultaneous administration of YF and smallpox vaccines.

DENGUE
(Breakbone Fever)

Dengue is a mosquito-borne infection characterized by fever, muscle and joint pain, lymphadenopathy, and rash.

Properties of the Dengue Viruses

A. Size: The diameter of these viruses is about 25 nm.

B. Reaction to Physical and Chemical Agents: The viruses are stable for at least 5 years in the frozen state at $-70°$ C and in the lyophilized state at $5°$ C. Human blood may be infectious if kept at $5°$ C for several weeks.

C. Animal Susceptibility: Human serum containing dengue virus produces only inapparent infection in chimpanzees and monkeys. The infection is followed by the appearance of CF and NE antibodies, which persist for many months.

Mice inoculated with human serum containing dengue virus rarely show signs of disease. Several strains of virus have been adapted to mice. After intracerebral inoculation, mice exhibit flaccid paralysis with the histologic lesion chiefly in the neurons. Mouse-adapted dengue virus may produce a fatal paralytic disease in monkeys, which is similar, both clinically and pathologically, to experimental poliomyelitis.

Dengue virus grows to high levels in cultures of monkey kidney (LLC-MK$_2$), hamster kidney, and HeLa cells, producing cytopathic changes which may be used for titrating virus and for measuring neutralizing antibodies. Recent successful primary isolation of dengue virus has been reported using *A albopictus* cell cultures.

D. Antigenic Properties: At least 4 distinct serotypes exist, designated types 1–4. In addition, 2 other agents, dengue TH-36 (closely related to type 2) and dengue TH-Sman (closely related to type 1) may represent new serotypes—dengue 5 and 6, respectively.

Complement fixing and hemagglutinating antigens can be prepared from the brains of infected newborn mice. Although dengue and YF viruses show group relationships, this is not associated with any significant cross-immunity. Human volunteers immunized against YF are fully susceptible to small doses of dengue virus.

Pathogenesis & Pathology

Viremia is present at the onset of fever and may persist for 3 days. The histopathologic lesion is in and about the small blood vessels, producing endothelial swelling, perivascular edema, and infiltration with mononuclear cells.

Dermal inoculation with small doses of virus may produce typical attacks of dengue, mild attacks without rash, or no evidence of disease. Immunity is achieved in all 3 instances. A laboratory worker developed dengue 9 days after serum from a patient had been accidentally squirted in his eye.

Clinical Findings

The incubation period is 5–8 days. The onset of fever may be sudden or there may be prodromal symptoms of malaise, chills, and headache. Pains soon develop, especially in the back, joints, muscles, and eyeballs. A flushed face and injected conjunctivas are common. The temperature returns to normal after 5–6 days or may subside on about the third day and rise again about 5–8 days after onset ("saddle-back" form). A rash (maculopapular or scarlatiniform) may appear on the third or fourth day and lasts for 24–72 hours, terminating without desquamation. Lymph nodes are frequently enlarged. Leukopenia with a relative lymphocytosis is a regular occurrence. Convalescence may take weeks, although complications and death are rare.

Dengue may also occur as a mild febrile illness lasting 1–3 days. Dengue should be suspected if the patient has fallen ill in or has recently arrived from an area where the specific mosquito vectors are present.

Hemorrhagic fever, a syndrome consisting of a bleeding diathesis, profound shock, and a mortality rate of 5–10%, has been observed, often in epidemic form, in the Philippines, Southeast Asia, and India associated with the dengue viruses. The factors responsible are poorly understood, but may be related to a delayed hypersensitivity reaction. The presence of more than one dengue serotype in an area of high endemicity has frequently been observed, suggesting that this syndrome is the result of secondary rather than primary infection. Other contributory factors of a genetic and nutritional nature have not been entirely excluded.

Laboratory Diagnosis

Isolation of the virus is difficult. Until the use of Aedes cell cultures for primary isolation is fully evaluated, the following diagnostic tests may be done.

A. Presumptive Test: One group of mice is inoculated with fresh acute-phase serum and another group with heated serum (56° C for 30 minutes). One month later, both groups of mice are challenged with 100 LD_{50} doses of the known mouse-adapted dengue viruses. If the mice which received the fresh serum resist the challenge and the mice which received the heated serum succumb, then the serum contained dengue virus.

B. Serology: Following infection, Nt and HI antibodies appear within 7 days of onset, and CF antibodies appear 7–14 days later.

Antigens representing the local serotypes present must be used in testing for antibodies. Although patients develop heterotypic as well as homotypic dengue antibodies, the homotypic antibodies reach higher titers.

1. Neutralizing antibodies–Homotypic antibodies have a higher titer than heterotypic antibodies in primary infections.

2. Complement fixing antibodies–The response may be the same to both homotypic and heterotypic antigens, but often the heterotypic response is lower and does not persist as long.

3. Hemagglutination inhibiting antibodies–Homotypic antibodies may appear 1 week before, may be of higher titer, and may persist for longer periods than heterotypic antibodies. Antibodies to other members of group B also appear after primary infection.

Immunity

At least 4 antigenic types of the virus exist, as established by the following: (1) active cross-immunity tests in human volunteers; (2) dermal Nt tests with convalescent sera in human volunteers; (3) neutralization tests in mice with convalescent sera from patients and from monkeys; and (4) CF and HI tests with serum from patients and monkeys.

Reinfection with a virus of a different serotype, 2–3 months after the primary attack, may give rise to a short, mild illness without a rash. If mosquitoes are allowed to feed on these reinfected patients, they can transmit the disease. Dengue type 1 and 2 infections are associated with the highest antibody levels. Sufficient cross-reacting antibody may be present in these situations to prevent infection with type 3 or 4.

The mouse-adapted and tissue culture-adapted strains have become attenuated; strains free of monkey paralytogenic properties are recommended for use as vaccines. They no longer produce disease in man. Persons inoculated with the attenuated virus have a solid immunity to unmodified virus transmitted by infected mosquitoes or by inoculation of large doses of highly infectious human serum.

Persons previously vaccinated against yellow fever give a broad anamnestic antibody response to immunization with attenuated dengue virus; the same is true of persons previously infected with other members of group B.

Epidemiology

The known geographic distribution of the dengue viruses today is India, the Far East, and the Hawaiian and Caribbean Islands. Dengue has occurred in the southern USA and in Australia. In addition, most subtropical and tropical regions around the world where Aedes vectors exist are endemic areas (or potential ones).

Dengue virus is transmitted only by certain species of Aedes mosquitoes, particularly *A aegypti*.

The infectious cycle is as follows:

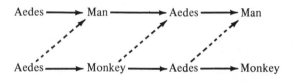

A aegypti is a domestic mosquito; *A albopictus* exists in the bush or jungle and may be responsible for maintaining the infection among monkeys (jungle dengue). In an epidemic, large numbers of people usually become infected within a short period, as would be expected where there are many infected vectors as well as susceptible persons.

Mosquitoes can become infected if they feed on infected hosts from 12 hours before to 72 hours after onset of symptoms. An extrinsic incubation of 11–14 days is required before the mosquitoes can transmit the virus. They can then act as vectors for the remainder of their lives (1–3 months or more).

The virus is not passed from one generation of mosquitoes to the next. The disease is maintained constantly in the tropics, where mosquitoes are present throughout the year. Outbreaks in colder areas are terminated with the advent of cold weather.

Epidemics of dengue are usually observed when the virus is newly introduced into an area or if susceptibles, such as troops, move into an endemic area. If there is a year-round maintenance of the virus cycle, the disease becomes endemic, as has happened in the Caribbean area. If the infection is introduced into a more temperate region where the vector disappears during the winter, the epidemic promptly comes to an end and does not reappear the next year. Thus the endemic dengue in the Caribbean is a constant threat to the USA, where *A aegypti* mosquitoes are prevalent in the summer months. A large epidemic of dengue involving several thousand persons occurred in the southern USA in 1934. The epidemic ceased with the coming of winter.

In 1963, epidemic dengue occurred in Puerto Rico, with over 20,000 cases. In some towns the attack rate was over 30%, with the highest rate among the 20–30 year old age group. More than 20 known cases were imported into the USA from these epidemic areas.

Control

Control depends upon antimosquito measures, eg, elimination of breeding places and the use of insecticides such as DDT. An experimental attenuated virus vaccine has been produced, but it has not had a large-scale field test.

HEMORRHAGIC FEVER

Hemorrhagic fever has been reported from Siberia, Soviet Central Asia, Eastern and Northern Europe, Southeast Asia, and South America. It first received widespread attention in the USA during the early 1950's when American troops fighting in Korea experienced an outbreak of Korean hemorrhagic fever.

Three categories have recently been suggested for classifying the hemorrhagic fevers: (1) tick-borne, which includes some members of the Russian spring-summer encephalitis complex (Omsk hemorrhagic fever and Kyasanur Forest disease), and the Crimean hemorrhagic fever group; (2) mosquito-borne, which includes the dengue viruses (see above) and probably Chikungunya virus; (3) zoonotic, which includes the viruses of Korean hemorrhagic nephroso-nephritis, Argentinian hemorrhagic fever (Junin), and Bolivian hemorrhagic fever (Machupo). Junin, Machupo, Tacaribe (isolated from bats in Trinidad), and Tamiami viruses (isolated in the Florida Everglades) are closely related antigenically. With the exception of the Korean virus, all of the viruses listed in the zoonotic category now can be classified in the Tacaribe-LCM group on the basis of morphologic and biologic similarities and serologic cross-reactions.

Common clinical features of the epidemic hemorrhagic fevers include fever, petechiae or purpura, gastrointestinal, nasal, and uterine bleeding, hypotension, prostration, CNS signs, and thrombocytopenia. Leukopenia occurs in all except hemorrhagic nephroso-nephritis, and gross proteinuria occurs in all except the mosquito-borne hemorrhagic fevers.

Argentine hemorrhagic fever was first noted near the town of Junin in 1955. Virus was isolated from patients' blood and from local rodents and their mites. No evidence has been produced to suggest that these arthropods (mites) serve as biologic vectors for this disease. Cases have continued to occur in increasing numbers, and the virus is gradually spreading. From

300 to 1000 cases per year have been reported, with case fatality rates as high as 20%.

Machupo virus was recovered from the spleen of a patient in Bolivia who died of hemorrhagic fever in 1963. The virus has been isolated from the small pastoral mouse, *Calomys callosus,* but not yet from any arthropods. Experimental and epidemiologic investigations have suggested that these rodents are chronically infected and directly contaminate their environment through infected excreta. A similar hypothesis is advanced for the spread of Junin virus. The systematic extermination of this field mouse has been successful in controlling the spread of the disease in Bolivia.

Recently the isolation of the virus of Crimean hemorrhagic fever has been accomplished. It is immunologically similar to Congo virus, an agent recovered in Africa from cattle ticks, hedgehogs, mosquitoes, and humans.

SANDFLY FEVER
(Pappataci Fever, Phlebotomus Fever)

Sandfly fever is a mild, insect-borne disease which occurs commonly in countries bordering the Mediterranean Sea and in Russia, Iran, Pakistan, and India. The sandfly, *Phlebotomus papatasii,* is present in endemic areas between 20 and 45° latitude.

Properties of the Virus

The virus has a diameter of about 25 nm.

Although at least 10 separate antigenic types exist, only 2 are responsible for sandfly fever (Neapolitan and Sicilian types). Members of the group are antigenically distinct from other arbovirus groups, can be grown in tissue culture, and have been adapted to infant mice and hamsters, in which they produce encephalitis. They are stable to freezing and lyophilization.

Clinical Findings

In man the bite of the sandfly results in small itching papules on the skin which persist for up to 5 days. The disease begins abruptly after an incubation period of 3–6 days. For 24 hours before and 24 hours after the onset of fever, the virus is found in the blood. The clinical features consist of headache, malaise, nausea, fever, conjunctival infection, photophobia, stiffness of the neck and back, abdominal pain, and leukopenia. All patients recover. There is no specific treatment. The pathology in man is not known.

Laboratory Diagnosis

The diagnosis is made usually on clinical grounds. It may be confirmed by demonstrating a rise in antibody titer in paired serum specimens, either through Nt tests with mouse-adapted virus or HI tests utilizing a hemagglutinin associated with the virus.

Immunity

The immunity is specific for each antigenic type of virus and persists for at least 2 years.

Epidemiology

The disease is transmitted by the female sandfly, a midge only a few mm in size. In the tropics the sandfly is prevalent all year; in cooler climates only during the warm seasons. It is not definitely known how the virus remains viable during the winter although transovarial transmission may occur.

The extrinsic incubation period in the sandfly is about 1 week. The insect feeds at night; during the day, it may be found in dark places (cracks in walls, caves, houses, and tree trunks). Eggs are laid a few days after a blood meal. About 5 weeks are required for the eggs to develop into winged insects. The adult lives only a few weeks in hot weather.

In endemic areas infection and immunity occur commonly in childhood. When nonimmune adults (eg, troops) enter the area, large outbreaks can occur among the new arrivals and are occasionally mistaken for malaria.

Control

Sandflies are commonest just above the ground. Because of their small size they can pass through ordinary screens and mosquito nets. Their flight range is up to 200 yards. Prevention of disease in endemic areas rests on application of insect repellents during the night and the use of residual insecticides in and around living quarters.

COLORADO TICK FEVER
(Mountain Fever, Tick Fever)

Colorado tick fever (CTF) is a mild febrile disease, without rash, which is transmitted by a tick.

Properties of the Virus

Electron microscopic studies have demonstrated close ultrastructural and morphologic similarities to reovirus (diplornavirus group). However, the biophysical and biochemical properties are different, and its RNA strandedness has not yet been elucidated. Since it fulfills the functional classification of an arbovirus, it will be considered here. The differences in properties between reovirus and CTF virus may be due to a functional lipid-containing envelope of the latter virus.

The diameter of the virus is 80 nm with an inner capsid of 50 nm. The virus is stable to freezing and also to lyophilization. The virus is pathogenic for hamsters and mice. Upon intracerebral inoculation, mice develop paralysis. The virus multiplies in human tissue cultures and in the chick embryo when inoculated into the yolk sac, and highest concentrations are found in the CNS of the embryo. The virus is antigenically distinct from all other agents.

Pathogenesis & Pathology

The virus is transmitted through the bite of an infected tick. Virus is present in the blood during the acute stage of the illness. The pathology in man is not known.

Clinical Findings

The incubation period is 4–6 days. The disease has a sudden onset with chilly sensations and myalgia. Symptoms include headache, deep ocular pain, muscle and joint pains, lumbar backache, and nausea and vomiting. The temperature is usually diphasic. After the first bout of 2 days, the patient may feel well. Symptoms and fever then reappear and last 3–4 more days. The white count falls to 2000–3000. No complications are known. No fatal cases have been reported.

Laboratory Diagnosis

The virus may be isolated from whole blood by the intracerebral or intraperitoneal inoculation of baby hamsters or suckling mice. Viremia in man persists for at least 2 weeks. Experimentally injected monkeys fail to show any signs of illness, but viremia may persist for as long as 50 days.

Specific complement fixing antigens are available from infected mouse brain. Complement fixing and neutralizing antibodies appear during the second week of disease and persist for at least 3 years.

Immunity

Only one antigenic type is known. A single infection is believed to produce a lasting immunity.

Epidemiology

Colorado tick fever is limited to areas where the wood tick, *Dermacentor andersoni,* is distributed, primarily Colorado, Oregon, Utah, Idaho, Montana, and Wyoming. Patients have been in a tick-infested area 4–5 days before onset of symptoms, and in many cases ticks are found attached to their bodies. One is often unaware of the ticks' presence since their bite is painless. Cases occur chiefly in adult males, because this group is subject to greater exposure to ticks.

D andersoni collected in nature has been found to be infected with the virus. This tick is a true reservoir of the virus, for the agent is transmitted transovarially by the adult female. Natural infection occurs in rodents, which act as hosts for immature stages of the tick.

Control

The disease can be prevented by avoiding tick-infested areas. If this is not possible, suitable clothing is recommended (high boots, socks worn outside of trouser legs). In tick-infested areas, the body should be examined for ticks that might become attached, and these should be removed as soon as found. A strain adapted to chick embryo culture has had limited trials as a modified, live vaccine.

RIFT VALLEY FEVER
(Enzootic Hepatitis)

The virus of this disease is primarily pathogenic for sheep and other domestic animals. Man is secondarily infected during the course of epizootics in domesticated animals in Africa. Infection among laboratory workers is common.

The clinical features are similar to those of dengue: acute onset, fever, prostration, pain in the extremities and joints, and gastrointestinal distress. The temperature curve is like that of dengue and yellow fever (saddle-back type). There is a marked leukopenia. The disease is shortlived, and recovery almost always is complete.

The virus has a diameter of about 30 nm. It may be propagated in a number of animals, but mice are the laboratory animals of choice. The virus can be isolated from human blood during the first 3 days of the disease. Complement fixing, neutralizing, and hemagglutination inhibiting antibodies develop during convalescence and persist for many years.

The disease is not contagious but is transmitted by a bloodsucking insect active at night, presumably the mosquito. Sheep can be protected if they can be screened at night.

LASSA FEVER

The first recognized cases of this disease occurred in 1969, among Americans stationed in the Nigerian village of Lassa. The causative virus, which appears to be an arbovirus, is extremely virulent for persons not native to the area. Of 5 Americans who have been infected, 3 died. Lassa fever can involve almost all of the organ systems, although symptoms may vary in the individual patient. The disease is characterized by very high fever, mouth ulcers, skin rash with minute hemorrhages, pneumonia, infection of the heart, kidney damage, and severe muscle aches. The virus can be isolated from the blood of the patient and can be grown in Vero cell cultures, a continuous line from African green monkey kidney. The virus has been shown to be antigenically unrelated to known arboviruses, but little is known about its properties.

•   •   •

General References

Arboviruses and Human Disease. Report of a WHO scientific group. WHO Technical Report Series No. 369, 1967.

Hammon, W.M., & G.E. Sather: Arboviruses. Pages 227–280 in: *Diagnostic Procedures for Viral and Rickettsial Infections,* 4th ed. American Public Health Association, 1969.

Luby, J.P., Sulkin, S.E., & J.P. Sanford: The epidemiology of St. Louis encephalitis: A review. Ann Rev Med 20:329–350, 1969.

Spence, L., Jonkers, A.H., & L.S. Grant: Arboviruses in the Caribbean islands. Progr Med Virol 10:415–486, 1968.

Work, T.H.: Arthropod-borne viral encephalitides. Pages 90–102 in: *Textbook of Medicine,* 12th ed. Beeson, P.B., & W. McDermott (editors). Saunders, 1967.

31...

Picornavirus Group
(Enterovirus & Rhinovirus Subgroups)

The picornavirus group is made up of the small, ether-insensitive RNA viruses. The following biologic subgroups are recognized:

Picornaviruses of Human Origin
  A. Enteroviruses:
   1. Polioviruses, types 1–3.
   2. Coxsackieviruses A, more than 24 types.
   3. Coxsackieviruses B, types 1–6.
   4. Echoviruses, more than 30 types.
   5. Enterovirus type 68. Starting in 1969, new types are assigned *enterovirus* type numbers rather than attempting to subclassify them as coxsackie or echoviruses.
  B. Rhinoviruses: More than 90 types.

Picornaviruses of Lower Animals
   An example is bovine foot-and-mouth disease (a rhinovirus).

Plant Viruses
   Certain plant viruses (tomato bushy stunt, turnip yellow mosaic) have properties similar to those of the picornaviruses. Some of the recently discovered RNA-containing bacteriophages have similar properties.
   Enteroviruses include over 60 members, all transient inhabitants of the human alimentary tract. They may be isolated from the throat or lower intestine, or from both sites. They have the following properties: (1) Particle size, 17–28 nm. (2) Architecture, capsid of the virus particle composed of 32 morphologic subunits arranged to comply with the icosahedral form of cubic symmetry, but in the form of a rhombic triacontahedron rather than a regular icosahedron. (3) RNA core, molecular weight 2×10^6 daltons, making up about 25% of the virus particle. (4) Resistance to ether due to lack of essential lipids. (5) Protection by magnesium chloride against inactivation by heat.
   Rhinoviruses differ from the enteroviruses in several properties: (1) Whereas the cytopathogenic enteroviruses grow in primary cultures of human and monkey kidney cells, and certain strains even in continuous human heteroploid cell lines (such as HeLa), rhinoviruses are more readily isolated in embryonic human kidney or human diploid cell strains than in monkey kidney cells. Most strains can only be recovered in cells of human origin. (2) Rhinoviruses are isolated from the nose and throat rather than from

feces. (3) Their initial growth in primary fetal cell cultures is favored when cultures are rolled at 33° C, whereas enteroviruses grow readily in stationary cultures at 36–37° C. (4) Unlike enteroviruses, the rhinoviruses are unstable when held at pH 3.0–5.0 for 1–3 hours. (5) The density in cesium chloride has been shown to be 1.4 gm/ml, whereas enteroviruses have a density of 1.34 gm/ml. (6) Rhinoviruses can further be differentiated from enteroviruses by their binding to $Al(OH)_3$ and $AlPO_4$ precipitates; enteroviruses bind to $Al(OH)_3$ but not to $AlPO_4$.
   The host range of the picornaviruses varies greatly from one type to the next, and even among strains of the same type. They may readily be induced, by laboratory manipulation, to yield variants which have host ranges and tissue tropisms different from those of certain wild strains; this has led to the development of attenuated poliovaccine strains.
   Many picornaviruses cause diseases in man ranging from severe paralysis to aseptic meningitis, pleurodynia, myocarditis, skin rashes, and common colds. However, subclinical infection is far more common than clinically manifest disease. Different viruses may produce the same syndrome; on the other hand, the same picornavirus may cause more than a single syndrome. For these reasons, clinical disease is not a satisfactory basis of classification.

POLIOMYELITIS

Poliomyelitis is an acute infectious disease which in its serious form affects the CNS. The destruction of motor neurons in the spinal cord results in flaccid paralysis. However, only a small number of infections are clinically recognizable.

Properties of the Virus
   A. Size: Poliovirus particles are 28 nm in diameter, and have the properties of enteroviruses as listed above.
   B. Reactions to Physical and Chemical Agents:
   1. Ultraviolet light, drying–Poliomyelitis virus is inactivated by ultraviolet light and usually by drying. It may be preserved by freezing.
   2. Reactions to heat–Poliovirus (as found in fecal material) is destroyed in aqueous suspension when

heated at 50–55° C for 30 minutes, but in the presence of molar divalent cations (Mg⁺⁺) no loss of virus occurs. Milk, cream, and ice cream exert a protective effect; the virus is able to withstand temperatures about 5° C higher when suspended in these materials than when suspended in water. Adequate pasteurization of milk destroys the agent.

3. Chemicals—In the absence of extraneous organic matter, the virus may be inactivated by low concentrations of chlorine (0.1 ppm). However, much higher concentrations are required if the virus is to be destroyed in the feces of a virus carrier. Many common disinfectants are poor inactivating agents. The virus is destroyed only slowly by alcohol and not at all by ether or deoxycholate. This distinguishes it from the arboviruses.

C. Animal Susceptibility and Growth of Virus: Polioviruses have a very restricted host range. Most strains will infect only monkeys and chimpanzees. Infection is initiated most readily by direct inoculation into the brain or spinal cord. Chimpanzees and cynomolgus monkeys can also be infected by the oral route; in chimpanzees the infection thus produced is usually asymptomatic. The animals become intestinal carriers of the virus; they also develop a viremia that is quenched by the appearance of antibodies in the circulating blood. Unusual strains have been transmitted to mice or chick embryos.

Most strains can be grown in primary or continuous cell line cultures derived from a variety of human tissues or from monkey kidney, testis, and muscle.

In poliovirus synthesis, the viral RNA serves as its own messenger RNA. Polysomes held together by host messenger RNA break down early during infection and later are built up again, now held together by viral RNA. Viral protein is synthesized on the polysomes. For a detailed description of poliovirus replication, see Fig 27–5.

Guanidine in concentrations greater than 1 mM and 2-(alpha-hydroxybenzyl)-benzimidazole inhibit poliovirus multiplication in tissue culture. Guanidine inhibits synthesis of RNA polymerase. On the basis of this guanidine effect, it is believed that 12–14 electrophoretically distinct virus-specific proteins are formed in poliovirus-infected cells.

The limited virus progeny which grow in the presence of the guanidine become 10,000 times more resistant to the drug. Further passage in the presence of guanidine results in the selection of strains which become dependent upon the drug for virus growth. These dependent strains are no longer neurovirulent for monkeys in vivo. When guanidine dependence is reversed in vitro, there is a return of the neurovirulence in vivo.

D. Antigenic Properties: There are 3 antigenic types. Complement fixing antigens are known for each. They may be prepared from tissue culture or infected CNS. Inactivation of the virus by formalin, heat, or ultraviolet light liberates a soluble complement fixing antigen. This antigen is cross-reactive and fixes comple-

ment with heterotypic poliomyelitis antibodies. A type-specific precipitin reaction occurs when virus in sufficient concentration is used with immune animal or convalescent human sera. Two type-specific antigens are contained in poliovirus preparations, and can be detected by precipitin and complement fixation tests. They are called D and C, or N and H. The D antigen is observed as a band in the lower or more dense regions of a sucrose density gradient and comprises most of the virus infectivity. The upper band containing the C antigen has little infectivity. The virus in the D zone appears intact in electron micrographs, and contains 20–25% RNA, whereas that in the C zone is damaged and contains little or no RNA. There is a direct relationship between the amount of D antigen, measured by complement fixation, and the number of intact physical particles of poliovirus as counted by electron microscopy. The 2 antigens are also known as N and H (native and heated). Heat changes N (or D) preparations from complete virus particles to empty particles when viewed in the electron microscope.

Pathogenesis & Pathology

The mouth is the portal of entry of the virus, and primary multiplication takes place at the sites of viral implantation in the oropharynx or intestines. The virus is regularly present in the throat and in the stools before the onset of illness. One week after onset there is little virus in the throat, but virus continues to be excreted in the stools for several weeks, even though high antibody levels are present in the blood.

The virus may be found in the blood of patients with abortive and nonparalytic poliomyelitis, and in orally infected monkeys and chimpanzees in the preparalytic phase of the disease. Antibodies to the virus appear early in the natural disease and also early in the experimental disease after oral infection. They are usually present before paralysis is noted.

Viremia is also associated regularly with type 2 oral vaccination. Free virus is usually present between days 2 and 5 after vaccination, and virus is bound to antibody for an additional few days. Bound virus is detected by acid treatment, which inactivates the antibody and liberates active virus.

These findings have led to the view that the virus first multiplies in the tonsils, the lymph nodes of the neck, Peyer's patches, and the small intestine. The CNS may then be invaded by way of the circulating blood. In monkeys infected by the oral route, small amounts of antibody prevent the paralytic disease, whereas large amounts are necessary to prevent the passage of the virus along nerve fibers. In man also, antibody in low titer in the form of gamma globulin may prevent paralysis if given before exposure to the virus.

Poliovirus can spread along axons of peripheral nerves to the CNS, and there it continues to progress along the fibers of the lower motor neurons to the spinal cord or brain. This may occur in children after tonsillectomy. Poliovirus present in their oropharynges may enter nerve fibers exposed during tonsillectomy, and spread to the brain. A similar mechanism of virus spread may be responsible for the rare instances of paralysis in a limb recently injected with an irritating material during a period of high poliovirus prevalence. Perhaps traces of virus are inadvertently introduced with the injection into peripheral nerve fibers.

Poliovirus invades certain types of nerve cells, and in the process of its intracellular multiplication it may damage or completely destroy these cells. The anterior horn cells of the spinal cord are most prominently involved, but in severe cases the intermediate gray ganglia and even the posterior horn and dorsal root ganglia are often involved. Lesions are found as far forward as the hypothalamus and thalamus. In the brain, the reticular formation, the vestibular nuclei, the cerebellar vermis, and the deep cerebellar nuclei are most often affected. The cortex is virtually spared, with the exception of the motor cortex along the precentral gyrus.

Poliovirus does not multiply in muscle in vivo. Its chief site of action is in the neuron, and the changes which occur in peripheral nerves and voluntary muscles are secondary to the destruction of the nerve cell. Changes occur rapidly in nerve cells, from mild chromatolysis to neuronophagia and complete destruction. Cells which lose their function may recover completely. Inflammation occurs secondary to the attack on the nerve cells; the focal and perivascular infiltrations are chiefly lymphocytes with some polymorphonuclear cells, plasma cells, and microglia.

In addition to pathologic changes in the nervous system, there may be myocarditis, lymphatic hyperplasia, ulceration of Peyer's patches, prominence of follicles, and enlargement of lymph glands.

Clinical Findings

When an individual susceptible to infection is exposed to the virus, one of the following responses may occur: (1) inapparent infection without symptoms, (2) mild illness, (3) aseptic meningitis, (4) paralytic poliomyelitis. As the disease progresses, one response may merge with a more severe form, often resulting in a biphasic course: a minor illness, followed first by a few days free of symptoms and then by the major, severe illness. Only about 1% of infections are recognized clinically.

The incubation period is usually between 7 and 14 days, but it may be as short as 3 days or as long as 35 days. The incubation period is defined as the time from exposure to onset of any symptoms.

A. Abortive Poliomyelitis: This is the commonest form of the disease. The patient has only the minor illness, characterized by fever, malaise, drowsiness, headache, nausea, vomiting, constipation, or sore throat in various combinations. The patient recovers in a few days. The diagnosis of abortive poliomyelitis cannot be made with assurance, even during an epidemic, except when the virus is isolated or antibody development is measured.

B. Nonparalytic Poliomyelitis (Aseptic Meningitis): In addition to the above symptoms and signs, the patient with the nonparalytic form presents stiffness and pain in the back and neck. The disease lasts 2–10 days, and recovery is rapid and complete. In a small percentage of cases the disease advances to paralysis. Poliovirus is only one of many viruses which produce aseptic meningitis. In the absence of virologic diagnosis, poliovirus must be suspected if the disease occurs in persons associated with paralytic patients.

C. Paralytic Poliomyelitis: The major illness usually follows the minor illness described above, but it may occur without the antecedent first phase. The predominating complaint is flaccid paralysis resulting from lower motor neuron damage. However, incoordination secondary to brain stem invasion and painful spasms of nonparalyzed muscles may also occur. The amount of damage and destruction varies from case to case. Muscle involvement is usually maximal within a few days after the paralytic phase begins. The maximal recovery usually occurs within 6 months, but it may take longer.

Laboratory Diagnosis

A. Cerebrospinal Fluid: The CSF contains an increased number of leukocytes—usually 10–200/cu mm, seldom more than 500/cu mm. In the early stage of the disease, the ratio of polymorphonuclear cells to lymphocytes is high, but within a few days the ratio is reversed. The total cell count slowly subsides to normal levels. The protein content of the CSF is mildly elevated (average about 40–50 mg/100 ml), although high levels may occur and persist for several weeks after the cell count declines. The glucose content is normal.

B. Recovery of Virus: In vitro cultures of human or monkey tissues may be used.

In nonfatal cases, the virus may be recovered from throat swabs taken within a few days of the onset of illness and from rectal swabs or feces collected for longer periods. The chance of recovering the virus decreases as the disease runs its course. The virus has been found in about 80% of patients during the first 2 weeks of illness, but in only 25% during the third 2-week period. No permanent carriers are known. Recovery of poliovirus from the CSF is uncommon, unlike that of the coxsackie or echoviruses.

In fatal cases, the virus should be looked for in the cervical and lumbar enlargements of the spinal cord, in the medulla, and in the colon contents. Histologic examination of the spinal cord and parts of the brain should be made. If paralysis has lasted 4–5 days, it is difficult to recover the virus from the cord.

Material collected from patients should be frozen as soon as possible after collection and, if possible, kept stored in the frozen state during transit to the diagnostic laboratory.

In the laboratory, the specimens are treated with penicillin, streptomycin, and sometimes ether, to destroy bacteria before inoculation of tissue cultures. If the specimen contains an agent which destroys the cells in the culture, it must be shown to be neutralized by specific antipoliomyelitis serum before the agent can be identified as poliovirus. Usually 3–6 days are required to isolate and type a strain of virus.

C. Serology: Paired serum specimens are required; the first sample must be taken as soon after the onset of illness as possible; the second, about 3—4 weeks later.

N and H complement fixing antigens of poliovirus are described above. In the course of poliomyelitis infection, H antibodies form before N antibodies, and subsequently the level of H antibodies declines first. Early acute stage sera thus contain H antibodies only; 1—2 weeks later, both N and H antibodies are present; in late convalescent sera, only N antibodies are present. Only first infection with poliovirus produces strictly type-specific complement fixation responses. Subsequent infections with heterotypic polioviruses recall or produce antibodies, mostly against the heat-stable antigenic components shared by all 3 types of poliovirus, ie, against the poliovirus group antigen.

Neutralizing antibodies which can be measured quantitatively and rapidly by tissue culture methods also appear early and are usually already detectable at the time of hospitalization. However, if the first specimen is taken sufficiently early, a rise in titer can be demonstrated during the course of the disease. In addition to the homologous antibody which persists at high levels for years, if not for life, antibodies to other virus types may appear transiently and at low levels. Neutralizing antibody also occurs in the urine.

Type-specific viral precipitating antibodies develop in convalescence. By the microprecipitation test, only 50% of poliomyelitis patients show a 4-fold or greater rise in antibody titer (due to the early appearance and early decline of the precipitating antibody). Therefore, the microprecipitation test appears to be less useful than the complement fixation and neutralization tests.

Immunity

Immunity is permanent to the type causing the infection. There may be a low degree of heterotypic resistance induced by infection, especially between type 1 and type 2 polioviruses. This may account for the observation that second attacks of polio have most often involved types 1 and 3.

Passive immunity is transferred from mother to offspring. The maternal antibodies gradually disappear during the first 6 months of life. Passively administered antibody lasts only 3—5 weeks.

Virus neutralizing antibody forms within a few days after exposure to the virus, often before the onset of illness, and persists, apparently, for life. Its formation early in the disease implies that viral multiplication occurs in the body before the invasion of the nervous system. As the virus in the brain and spinal cord is not influenced by high titers of antibodies in the blood (which are found in the preparalytic stage of the disease), immunization is of value only if it precedes the onset of symptoms referable to the nervous system.

Treatment

Patients with paralysis when admitted to hospitals already have antibodies in their blood. An increase in antibody is not beneficial. Neither gamma globulin from normal adults nor convalescent serum was of value in controlled trials. Antibiotics obviously have no effect.

Epidemiology

Poliomyelitis occurs all over the world, throughout the year in the tropics and during the summer and fall in the temperate zones. Winter outbreaks have rarely been recorded. Epidemics have been rare in tropical and subtropical countries, but the virus in those areas is widely prevalent.

The disease occurs in all age groups, but children are usually more susceptible than adults because of the acquired immunity of the adult population. In isolated populations (Arctic Eskimos), poliomyelitis attacks all ages equally. In crowded primitive areas, where conditions favor the wide dissemination of virus, poliomyelitis continues to be a disease of infancy, with all children over 4 years of age already immune. In many areas of the temperate zones (USA, England, Denmark, Sweden, and Australia), the age incidence of poliomyelitis had shifted into the older age groups during recent decades. For example, in the USA, just before the development of poliovaccines, 25% of the patients were over 15 years old and most were between 5 and 15.

The case fatality rate is not easily determined, because of the difficulties in diagnosing nonparalytic infections. In years of high prevalence, the case fatality rate may appear lower than in years of low prevalence, because nonparalytic poliomyelitis may be diagnosed more readily at times of epidemic prevalence. The usual rate varies between 5 and 10%, and is highest in the older age groups. In recent epidemics, in which a third of the cases occurred in patients over 15, two-thirds of the deaths were in this age group.

The only known reservoir of infection is man. Under conditions of poor hygiene and sanitation in warm areas, where almost all children become immune early in life, polioviruses maintain themselves in the human population by continuously infecting a small part of the total population. In countries which have high levels of hygiene, in temperate zones, epidemics have been followed by periods of low spread of virus, until sufficient numbers of susceptible children have grown up to provide a mechanism for continuous cycles of transmission in the area. Epidemics are caused when the high degree of virus spread is accompanied by strains of high virulence. Warm weather favors the spread of virus by increasing human contacts, the susceptibility of the host or the dissemination of virus by extra-human sources. The virus is spread by human contact. Virus can be recovered from the pharynges and intestines of both patients and healthy carriers. The prevalence of infection among family associates is higher than among nonhousehold contacts. When the first case is recognized in a family, all susceptibles in the family are already infected, the result of rapid dissemination of virus.

During periods of epidemic prevalence, in both rural and urban areas, house flies (*Musca domestica*) and filth flies (*Phormia regina, Phaenicia sericata,* Sarcophaga species) may be found contaminated with poliomyelitis virus. The importance of flies in the transmission of the disease is not easily evaluated, although it is important to note that virus has been found in food naturally contaminated by flies. The virus is also present in urban sewage during periods when subclinical or clinical disease is prevalent. Although no epidemiologic evidence suggests that sewage is a common source of infection, it may serve as a source of contamination of flies or of water supplies used for drinking or bathing, or through its use as fertilizer.

In temperate zones infection with poliovirus (and other enteroviruses) and the acquisition of antibodies is almost limited to the summer months. Regardless of geographic location, antibodies are acquired at an early age by those populations which live under primitive sanitary conditions, and particularly if crowding also exists. Even in the same city, there is a direct correlation between unfavorable socioeconomic status and the early development of antibodies. Neutralizing (but not complement fixing) antibodies to each of the 3 antigenic types of poliomyelitis virus persist for several decades, even in the absence of reinfection.

Prevention & Control

Both live and killed virus vaccines are available. Formalinized vaccine (Salk) is prepared from virus grown in monkey kidney cultures. Because of the varying levels of potency of commercial vaccine, a series of at least 4 inoculations over a period of 1–2 years is recommended in the primary series. A booster immunization is necessary every 2–3 years to maintain immunity.

Until 1956, the epidemic pattern was one of wide and rather uniform attack rates over large areas irrespective of race or socioeconomic class. After the widespread use of killed vaccine, several localized epidemics occurred with the cases concentrated in slum areas among unvaccinated preschool children. However, the killed vaccine is not perfect; in a study of several thousand paralytic cases, 17% were in triply vaccinated children. In 1959, about 6000 paralytic cases were still reported in the USA.

Oral vaccines containing live attenuated virus have been prepared from virulent strains manipulated in the laboratory by genetic procedures, or from naturally attenuated strains isolated from healthy children in nonepidemic periods. The vaccine can be stabilized by molar $MgCl_2$ so that it can be kept without losing potency for over a year at 4° C and for about a month at room temperature.

The live poliovaccine multiplies, infects, and thus immunizes. In the process, infectious progeny of the vaccine virus are disseminated in the community. Although the viruses, particularly type 3, mutate in the course of their multiplication in vaccinated children, only rare cases of paralytic poliomyelitis have occurred in recipients of oral poliovaccine (OPV) or their close contacts. To minimize the contact problem (ie,

infecting a contact with reverted virus progeny of greater neurovirulence than the licensed vaccine), whole communities can be given the vaccine at one time. Repeat vaccinations seem to be important to establish permanent immunity.

Another potential limiting factor on the use of the oral vaccine is that of interference. The alimentary tract of the child may be infected with another enterovirus at the time the vaccine is fed. This interferes with, and blocks, the establishment of infection and immunity, and is an important problem in areas (particularly in tropical and subtropical regions) where enterovirus infections are common. Interference with immunity can be minimized if the immunization schedule recommended is followed, thereby allowing immunization to begin in any season.

To simplify record keeping and scheduling, trivalent OPV has largely replaced the monovalent forms. The vaccine has failed to take in about half of the newborns to whom it was administered as a single dose. Therefore, primary immunization for infants should begin at 6–12 weeks of age simultaneously with the first DPT inoculation. The second dose should be given 2 months later with a third dose 8–12 months after the second. A trivalent OPV booster is recommended for all children entering elementary school. No further boosters are presently recommended. The primary immunization schedule for children and adolescents is similar to that for infants. Routine immunization for adults residing in the continental USA is not felt to be necessary because of the small risk of exposure. However, adults who are at increased risk because of contact with a patient or who are anticipating travel to an endemic or epidemic area can be immunized according to the schedule outlined above. Pregnancy is not an indication nor a contraindication for required immunization.

Alternatively to the above, separate monovalent OPV types may be administered at least 6–8 weeks apart. The recommended sequence of types is 2, 1, 3. Trivalent OPV vaccine should be given as a booster 8–12 months after the third dose of monovalent OPV. Type 3 oral vaccine is not recommended for adults unless there is some special risk involved, such as foreign travel to an area where poliovirus may be present. The reason is the possibility of disease in adults from type 3 vaccine strains, although the risk is very low indeed.

Since the introduction of live poliovirus vaccine, the number of paralytic cases in the USA has decreased to less than 50 a year by 1968.

Both killed and live virus vaccines produce antibodies and protect the CNS from subsequent invasion by wild virus. Low levels of antibody resulting from killed vaccine have little effect in preventing intestinal carriage of virus. However, the alimentary tract develops a far greater degree of resistance after live virus vaccine, which seems to be dependent on the extent of initial vaccine virus multiplication in the alimentary tract rather than on serum antibody level. In some cases the alimentary tract has been completely resistant after a single feeding. In others, particularly with type 3, each subsequent feeding of vaccine (about a year apart) has produced a shorter period of virus excretion.

Gamma globulin can provide protection for a few weeks against the paralytic disease, but does not prevent subclinical infection. The dose is about 0.14 ml/lb IM. Gamma globulin is effective only if given shortly before infection; it is of no value after clinical symptoms of the disease are apparent.

It is not possible to list rules for the prevention of poliomyelitis other than vaccination. Quarantine either of patients or of exposed family or intimate contacts is ineffective in controlling the spread of the disease. This is understandable in view of the large number of inapparent and therefore unrecognized infections during an epidemic.

During epidemic periods (defined now as 2 or more local cases caused by the same type in any 4-week period), children with fever should be given bed rest. Undue exercise or fatigue should be avoided, especially if there is any suspicion of involvement of the nervous system. Elective nose and throat operations and dental extractions should be avoided. Children should not travel unnecessarily to or from epidemic areas. Food and human excrement should be protected from flies. Once the poliovirus type responsible for the epidemic is determined, type-specific monovalent oral poliovaccine should be administered to susceptible persons in the population.

Patients with poliomyelitis should be admitted to general hospitals, provided appropriate isolation precautions are employed. All pharyngeal and bowel discharges are considered infectious and should be disposed of quickly and safely. Patients may be cared for at home if facilities and medically supervised care are adequate; or they may be discharged to home care when there is no medical indication for further observation or treatment in the hospital. Admission to or care in a hospital solely for isolation purposes is not indicated. When suspected cases are admitted to a hospital, they should be segregated from known cases until the diagnosis has been established.

COXSACKIEVIRUS GROUP

The coxsackieviruses comprise a large group of the enterovirus family. They produce a variety of illnesses in human beings, including aseptic meningitis, herpangina, pleurodynia, myo- and pericarditis, and common colds. Coxsackieviruses have been divided into 2 groups, A and B, having different pathogenic potentials for the mouse.

Properties of the Viruses

A. Size: 28 nm in diameter. Density: 1.34 gm/ml.

B. Reactions to Physical and Chemical Agents: Commonly used antiseptics, including ethanol (70%),

Lysol (5%), Roccal (1%), and ether, fail to inactivate coxsackieviruses. Treatment with 0.1 N HCl or 0.3% formaldehyde, however, effects rapid inactivation. Unlike the arboviruses, they are resistant to deoxycholate.

C. Animal Susceptibility and Growth of Virus: Coxsackieviruses are highly infective for newborn mice. Strains of certain types (B 1–6, A-9) also grow preferentially in monkey kidney tissue culture. Some group A strains grow in human amnion cells. Chimpanzees and cynomolgus monkeys can be infected subclinically; virus appears in the blood and throat for short periods and is excreted in the feces for 2–5 weeks. Type A-14 produces poliomyelitis-like lesions in adult mice and in monkeys, but upon inoculation into suckling mice this type produces only myositis. Type A-7 strains produce paralysis and severe CNS lesions in monkeys.

On histologic as well as clinical grounds, these viruses have been divided broadly into 2 groups. Group A viruses produce widespread myositis in the skeletal muscles of newborn mice, resulting in flaccid paralysis without other observable lesions. Group B viruses can produce a myositis which is more focal in distribution than that produced by viruses of group A but also give rise to a necrotizing steatitis, involving principally the maturing fetal fat lobules (interscapular pads, cervical and cephalic pads, etc). Encephalitis is found at times, the animals dying with paralysis of the spastic type. Some B strains also produce pancreatitis, myocarditis, endocarditis, and hepatitis in both suckling and adult mice. The corticosteroids may enhance the susceptibility of older mice to infection of the pancreas.

D. Antigenic Properties: At least 29 different immunologic types of coxsackieviruses are now recognized; 23 are listed as group A and 6 as group B types. Evidence for the existence of multiple distinct immunologic types has been obtained by means of (1) cross-neutralization tests in infant mice, (2) cross-complement fixation tests, (3) cross-protection tests in infant mice born of immunized mothers, and (4) cross-protection tests in chimpanzees (production of subclinical infection). Antigenic variants occur within each of the group B virus types and some of the group A types.

Occasionally, 2 types of coxsackieviruses are isolated in the same mice from injections of specimens of sewage, flies, or pooled human feces. Rarely have 2 types been isolated from a single human patient.

Several of the coxsackieviruses hemagglutinate the human type O erythrocytes, a method which can be used to differentiate these strains.

Pathogenesis & Pathology

Virus has been recovered from the blood in the early stages of infection in man and in chimpanzees. Virus is also found for a few days early in the infection in the throat and for longer periods, up to 5–6 weeks, in the stools. The situation as far as distribution of virus is concerned is similar to that found in the other enteroviruses (poliomyelitis, echo).

Characteristic lesions of herpangina are caused by types A-2, 4, 5, 6, 8, and 10. Deaths attributable to the group B coxsackieviruses have been reported in infants, in whom acute interstitial myocarditis may be produced. Lesions may also be present in the CNS and liver, indicating that myocarditis of the newborn is a generalized systemic disease analogous to that produced by group B viruses in newborn mice. The potential of a virus to cause myocarditis appears to correlate with its ability to produce myositis.

Clinical Findings

The incubation period of coxsackievirus infection ranges from 2–9 days. The clinical manifestations of infection with various coxsackieviruses are diverse and may present as distinct disease entities.

Infection with a coxsackievirus is suggested by the clinical manifestations of herpangina, pleurodynia, aseptic meningitis, summer minor illnesses of nonbacterial origin, or neonatal disease, particularly myocarditis. Evidence is accumulating that the coxsackievirus B group may be responsible for some cases of myocarditis or pericarditis in persons over the age of 12. In some series, up to 39% of the persons infected with coxsackie B5 will have cardiac abnormalities. Confirmation must be obtained by isolation of the virus from feces or oropharyngeal swabs and demonstration of an antibody titer rise. Virus is present in the CNS and heart muscle of fatal cases in the newborn.

A. Herpangina: This disease is caused by certain group A viruses; it is characterized by an abrupt onset of fever and sore throat. There may be anorexia, dysphagia, vomiting, and abdominal pain. The pharynx is usually hyperemic, and characteristic discrete vesicular lesions may be seen on the anterior pillars of the fauces and, less frequently, on the palate, uvula, tonsils, or tongue. The illness is self-limited, and most frequent in small children.

B. Summer Minor Illnesses: Coxsackieviruses are often isolated from patients with acute febrile illnesses of short duration and without distinctive features, occurring during the summer or fall. Information is lacking on the frequency of oropharyngeal lesions in these patients, whose illnesses in other respects resemble herpangina.

C. Pleurodynia (Epidemic Myalgia, Bornholm Disease): This disease is caused by certain group B viruses. Fever and chest pain are almost invariably present together; they are usually abrupt in onset, although they may be preceded by malaise, headache, anorexia, and other vague prodromal symptoms. The chest pain may be located on either side or substernally, is intensified by movement, and may last from 2 days to almost 2 weeks. Abdominal pain occurs in approximately half the cases and in children may be the chief complaint. The illness is self-limited, and recovery is complete although relapses are common.

D. Aseptic Meningitis and Mild Paresis: This syndrome is caused by all types of group B; certain coxsackie A types (A-7, A-9) also have been clearly implicated in several epidemics. Signs of meningeal irritation with stiffness of the neck or back and vomiting may appear 1–2 days later. Fever, malaise, headache, nausea, and abdominal pain are common early symptoms. The disease sometimes progresses to mild muscle weakness which is often confused clinically with paralytic poliomyelitis. Patients almost always recover completely from nonpoliovirus paresis with no residual disability. Examination of the CSF early in the acute phase of the illness reveals an increase in the number of leukocytes which, in most instances, does not exceed 100/cu mm. The percentage of polymorphonuclear cells ranges from 10–50.

E. Neonatal Disease: Neonatal disease caused by group B coxsackieviruses may be more common than has generally been recognized. The clinical syndrome may consist merely of lethargy, feeding difficulty, and vomiting with or without fever. In severe cases, myocarditis or pericarditis with or without severe generalized disease can occur within the first 8 days of life; it may be preceded by a brief episode of diarrhea and anorexia. Cardiac and respiratory embarrassment are indicated by tachycardia, dyspnea, cyanosis, and changes in the electrocardiogram. The clinical course may be rapidly fatal, or the patient may progress to complete recovery. The disease may sometimes be acquired transplacentally. Myocarditis has also been caused by some of the group A coxsackieviruses.

F. Colds: It has become apparent that the common cold may be caused by many different viruses. A number of the enteroviruses have been associated with common colds; among these are coxsackieviruses A-10, A-21, A-24, and B-3.

G. Other Syndromes: The sudden death syndrome, which accounts for a conspicuous percentage of deaths among children, particularly infants 2–3 months of age, has been associated with coxsackie B viruses. Hand, foot, and mouth disease has been associated with coxsackievirus A-16. Immunofluorescence results on heart tissue obtained at autopsy have suggested that coxsackie B viruses might play a role in myocarditis of children and adults.

Laboratory Diagnosis

A. Recovery of Virus: Although the virus has been isolated from the blood early during infection, it can more readily be found in the throat washings during the first few days of illness and in the stools during the first few weeks. In general, virus isolated from the throat will also be found in the stool, although the corollary is not necessarily true. In coxsackievirus A-21 infections, the largest amount of virus is found in nasal secretions. In cases of aseptic meningitis, strains have been recovered from the CSF as well as from the alimentary tract. The procedures are similar to those employed for isolating poliomyelitis virus from clinical specimens. The specimen is inoculated into tissue cultures and also into suckling mice if these animals are available. In tissue culture a cytopathic effect appears within 5–14 days. In suckling mice, signs of illness appear usually within 3–8 days with group A strains and 5–14 days with group B strains. The virus is identified by the pathologic lesions it produces and also by immunologic means.

B. Serology: Neutralizing antibodies appear early during the course of the infection. The first sample of serum should be taken as soon as possible and the second about 2 weeks later, when the antibodies are already at their peak level. They persist for years.

After a coxsackievirus infection, patients may develop complement fixing antibodies to a number of both group A and group B agents, but the neutralizing response appears to be specific for the infecting type of virus. Complement fixing antibodies may disappear or drop to a low level within 6 months. The large number of possible etiologic agents associated with the clinical syndromes discussed makes it impractical to perform serologic tests on adequately collected acute and convalescent specimens unless an isolate is obtained from the patient. During an epidemic, however, the prevalent pathogen can be used.

It is possible to detect and titrate serum antibody using the immunofluorescence technic. Infected coverslip cultures for use as a source of antigen may be prepared and kept frozen at $-20°$ C for at least 1 year, making this test readily available for rapid diagnosis.

Immunity

Because mice early in life acquire a natural resistance to infections by coxsackieviruses, it is not possible to vaccinate newborn mice and later to test for immunity by direct challenge; however, by challenging infant mice less than 48 hours old and born of mothers previously vaccinated, cross-protection tests can be carried out. Strains of virus studied in this way showed the same type-specificity as that observed in neutralization and complement fixation tests. The immunity conferred by the milk of the mother or foster mother is type-specific, and there is a simultaneous transfer of complement fixing antibodies from the mother to her young. In humans a passive transfer of neutralizing and complement fixing antibodies from the mother to the offspring also occurs.

Adults have antibodies against more types of coxsackieviruses than do children, which suggests that multiple experience with these viruses is common and increases with age.

Epidemiology

Viruses of the coxsackie group have been encountered around the globe. Isolations have been made mainly from human feces, pharyngeal swabbings, sewage, and flies. That coxsackieviruses are widely distributed is also indicated by the detection of antibodies in serum collected from individuals in different parts of the world and by the capacity of gamma globulin prepared from pooled human serum to neutralize all of the coxsackieviruses identified and tested.

Coxsackieviruses are recovered much more frequently during the summer and early fall. Also, children develop neutralizing and complement fixing antibodies during the summer, indicating infection by these agents during this period; such children have much higher incidence rates for acute, febrile minor illnesses during the summer than children who fail to develop coxsackievirus antibodies.

Familial or household exposure is important in the acquisition of infections with coxsackieviruses. Once the virus is introduced into a household all susceptible persons usually become infected, although all do not develop clinically apparent disease.

In herpangina only about 30% of infected persons within households develop faucial lesions. Others may present a mild febrile illness without the throat lesions. In a community study virus was found most often in patients with herpangina (85%), next most often in their neighborhood (65%) and family contacts (40%), and least often in all persons in the community (4%).

The coxsackieviruses share many properties with the echo- and polioviruses. Because of their epidemiologic similarities, enteroviruses may occur together in nature, even in the same human host or the same specimens of sewage or of flies.

ECHOVIRUS GROUP

The echoviruses (enteric cytopathogenic human orphan viruses) are grouped together because they infect the human enteric tract and because they can be recovered from man only by inoculation of certain tissue cultures. Over 30 serotypes are known, but only certain of these have been known to cause human illness. Aseptic meningitis, febrile illnesses with or without rash, and common colds are some of the diseases caused by certain echoviruses.

Properties of the Viruses

A. Size: Variable, mostly 24–48 nm in diameter. The complement fixing antigen (which may be part of the total virus particle) has a diameter of about 10 nm. Their general properties are like those of the other enteroviruses: RNA core, ether-resistant, stabilized by magnesium ions. Density: 1.34 gm/ml.

B. Growth of Virus: Monkey kidney tissue culture is the medium of choice for the isolation and propagation of these agents. However, they also multiply in human amnion cells. They have been adapted to cell lines such as HeLa. Cultures from the African green and tantalus monkeys seem to be as susceptible as rhesus and cynomolgus monkey cells. New types have been discovered which grow in HeLa and other human cells but not in monkey kidney cultures.

Certain echoviruses agglutinate human group O erythrocytes. The hemagglutinins are associated with the infectious virus particle; they are sedimented together in the ultracentrifuge and are adsorbed together by erythrocytes during the process of agglutination. The virus and hemagglutinin may be eluted, and in the process the red cells become exhausted. The hemagglutinin is not affected by neuraminidase.

The echoviruses came to be distinguished from the coxsackieviruses by their failure to produce pathologic changes in newborn mice. Classification problems have arisen because echovirus-9, responsible for tens of thousands of cases of aseptic meningitis (many with rash) during 1956–1957, frequently produced paralysis in newborn mice. These mice developed a widespread myositis like that produced by coxsackie A viruses. However, unlike the coxsackieviruses, the original material collected from echo-9 patients failed to produce disease in newborn mice. Passage in tissue culture was required in order to select out mouse-pathogenic virus particles. Even after tissue culture passage, only a certain proportion of recently isolated strains proved pathogenic for mice. Conversely, strains of some coxsackievirus types (especially A-9) lack mouse pathogenicity, and thus resemble echoviruses. This variability in biologic properties is the chief reason why new enteroviruses are no longer being subclassified as echo or coxsackieviruses.

C. Antigenic Properties: Over 30 different antigenic types have already been identified. The different types may be separated on the basis of cross-neutralization or cross-complement fixation testing. Cross-neutralization tests are necessary not only to guard against mixtures of virus types, but also because of the frequent occurrence of the so-called "prime" strains. A "prime" strain is neutralized to very low titer or not at all by the existing prototype antiserum, whereas an antiserum against the prime strain neutralizes the prototype virus as well as homologous virus. Types 1 and 8 overlap antigenically.

Neutralizing antibodies are determined by measuring the dilution of serum capable of preventing the cytopathogenic effect of the virus or by plaque reduction tests. Culture fluids to be used in neutralization tests must be harvested early, before heat-inactivated particles accumulate, because such inactivated virus may bind antibody and give apparent low serum titers. Complement fixing antigens may be prepared from a harvest of infected tissue culture fluids. Treatment with fluorocarbon may remove anticomplementary activity, as it does for the other enteroviruses (coxsackie- and polioviruses). Neutralizing antibodies persist much longer after infection than complement fixing antibodies.

D. Animal Susceptibility: In order to be included in the echo group, prototype strains must not produce disease in suckling mice, in rabbits, or in monkeys. However, different strains related to the prototypes have been found to produce certain variants which may exhibit animal pathogenicity. A number of the echoviruses have produced inapparent infections in monkeys, as evidenced by the occurrence of antibodies after inoculation and the appearance of lesions within the CNS even though the lesions have not been severe enough to produce obvious disease. The pattern of infection of the echoviruses in the chimpanzee is the same as that for the other enteroviruses. No apparent illness is produced, but infection is readily demonstrable by the presence and persistence of virus in the throat and in the feces, and by the type-specific antibody responses.

Pathogenesis & Pathology

The pathogenesis of the alimentary infection is similar to that of the other enteroviruses. Virus may be recovered from the throat and stools; in a number of types (4, 5, 6, 9, and 14) which have been associated with aseptic meningitis, the virus has been recovered from the CSF.

Clinical Findings

In order to establish etiologic association of echovirus with disease, the following criteria are used: (1) A much higher recovery rate of the virus must be obtained from patients with the disease than from healthy individuals of the same age and socioeconomic level living in the same area at the same time as the patient. (2) Antibodies against the virus develop during the course of the disease. If the clinical syndrome can be caused by other known agents, then virologic or serologic evidence must be negative for concurrent infection with such agents. (3) The virus is isolated in significant concentration from body fluids or tissues manifesting lesions, for example, from the CSF in cases of aseptic meningitis.

Echoviruses 4, 6, 9, 11, 14, 16, and 30 have been repeatedly associated with aseptic meningitis. Other types (2, 3, 5) have been associated with aseptic meningitis only in sporadic cases. With echo-6, muscle weakness and mild paralysis have been observed. However, recovery was usually complete. A rash appears to be a common manifestation of infection with type 9 and, less frequently, with type 4.

Echovirus 9 may produce aseptic meningitis or undifferentiated febrile illness, either of which may be accompanied by a rash. (In rare instances echo-9 may cause a more extensive involvement of the CNS.) The incidence of rash, high in young children, decreases with age. Conjunctivitis may also be present. The virus may occur in spinal fluid even in the absence of pleocytosis. Muscle weakness and spasm may occur and may persist for weeks. The virus has been recovered in high titer from the medulla of a fatal case.

Echo-16 can produce aseptic meningitis and also "Boston exanthem disease." Type 20 has been associated with a febrile disease involving both the respiratory and enteric tracts. Echo-28, associated with upper respiratory illness, has produced colds in volunteers and has been reclassified as rhinovirus type 1. Type 18 and others have been associated with infant diarrhea. Echo-4 has recently been associated with vaginitis and cervicitis. For many of the echoviruses, as for many of the coxsackieviruses, no disease entities are yet known.

Laboratory Diagnosis

It is impossible in an individual case to diagnose an echovirus infection on clinical grounds. However, in the following epidemic situations, echoviruses must be considered: (1) summer outbreaks of aseptic meningitis; (2) summer epidemics, especially in young children, of a febrile illness with rash; and (3) outbreaks of diarrheal disease in young infants from whom no pathogenic enterobacteria can be recovered.

The diagnosis is dependent upon laboratory tests. The procedure of choice is isolation of virus from throat swabs, stools, rectal swabs, and, in aseptic meningitis, CSF. Echoviruses 9 and 16 have been recovered from the blood when specimens were collected very early in the disease. Serologic tests by themselves are impractical because without some clue as to the predominating virus too many enterovirus tests would be necessary. As with other enteroviruses, neutralizing and hemagglutination inhibiting (HI) antibodies are type-specific, but heterotypic responses are common with the complement fixation (CF) test. To illustrate the situation for these agents, the development and persistence of different antibodies in patients from whom type 6 was isolated may be cited. Neutralizing antibodies developed in 96% of patients, reached peak levels 2 weeks after the onset of illness, and persisted with virtually no decline for at least 3 years. HI antibody developed in 67%, reached peak levels at 2 weeks, declined rapidly, and persisted at significant levels for 3 years. CF antibody developed in 67% and also reached peak levels at 2 weeks, but was undetectable at 3 years.

After an agent is isolated in tissue culture it is tested against a variety of pools of antisera against the enteroviruses. In order to determine the type of virus present, it must be neutralized by a single serum; infection with 2 or more enteroviruses may occur simultaneously. Tests on progeny from different types of plaques produced by the specimen on monkey kidney cell monolayer cultures under agar are useful for detecting mixed infections.

Epidemiology

The epidemiology of the echoviruses is similar to that of other members of the enterovirus family. They occur in all parts of the globe. Unlike the enterobacteria, which are constantly present in the intestinal tract, the enteroviruses produce only transitory infections. They are more apt to be found in the young than in the old. In the temperate zone they occur chiefly during summer and autumn, and are about 5 times more prevalent in children of the lower socioeconomic groups than in those living in more favorable circumstances. In southern USA, they are prevalent over a greater part of the year than they are in the north.

In one longitudinal study conducted over a 3-year period, 1540 specimens were tested from the lower economic districts. Of these, 11.4% were positive, whereas in the upper districts, of 1427 specimens tested, only 2.6% yielded virus. Studies of families into which enteroviruses were introduced demonstrated the ease with which these agents spread and the high frequency of infection in persons who had formed no antibodies from earlier exposures. This is the case no matter which enterovirus is considered.

The rapid and usually silent dissemination of the agent in households is a property shared by all enteroviruses. Hospitalized patients may not give a true picture of the extent of illness caused by an entero-

virus in a community. Thus, a survey during an echo-4 outbreak in which 27 cases of aseptic meningitis were reported in a town of 20,000 revealed that 16% of the population had a compatible illness. Similarly, during a period when 149 inhabitants of a city of 740,000 were hospitalized with echo-9 disease, it was estimated that approximately 6%, or 45,000 persons, had a compatible illness.

Control

No specific control measures are known. Avoidance of contacts with patients exhibiting acute febrile illness, especially those with a rash, is advisable for premature babies and very young infants. Members of institutional staffs responsible for caring for young or premature infants should be tested to determine whether they are carriers of enteroviruses. This is particularly important during outbreaks of diarrheal disease among infants.

RHINOVIRUS GROUP

The rhinoviruses are isolated from the nose and throat, but very rarely from the feces. These viruses, as well as a number of other viruses including certain enteroviruses, influenza, parainfluenza, RS (respiratory syncytial), adenoviruses, and reoviruses, cause common colds in adults and children.

Properties of the Virus

A. Nucleic Acid: RNA, with a molecular weight of 2.1×10^6 daltons, similar to that of the enteroviruses.

Size of virion: 17–30 nm in diameter.

B. Density: Rhinoviruses banded by gradient centrifugation in CsCl have a density of 1.40 gm/ml compared to enteroviruses, which have a density of 1.32–1.34. In density gradient studies, complement fixing activity is noted in 2 distinct bands. One peak of activity is associated with the virion at a density of 1.40 and is found to be type-specific whereas the other peak, with a density of 1.30, is group-specific and possibly represents empty virions. This is analogous to the D and C (or N and H) antigens of poliovirus.

C. Reactions to Physical and Chemical Agents: All strains thus far studied have been shown to be acid-labile at pH 3.0–5.0. They are ether-stable and are generally more stable at 50° C than are enteroviruses. Some have been shown to be stabilized by 1 M $MgCl_2$ or 1 M $MgSO_4$. These viruses may be stored for short periods at −4° C and indefinitely at −70° C, without significant titer loss.

D. Animal Susceptibility and Growth of Virus: These viruses have a limited host range which has made it necessary to perform all animal experiments in man or in chimpanzees. They have been propagated in cultures of human embryonic lung, diploid human fibroblast tissue (WI 38), human aortic tissue, and in organ cultures of ferret and human tracheal epithelium. They are grown best at 33° C under slightly acidic conditions in rolled cultures. Certain of these viruses (M strains) can be isolated in, or adapted to, monkey kidney cells, while others grow only in cultures of human origin (H strains). However, some viruses grown only in human cell cultures have been shown by neutralization test to be M strain viruses.

E. Antigenic Properties: There are 89 recognized distinct serotypes and a number of new candidates identified by neutralization tests, using type-specific guinea pig, calf, baboon, and goat antisera.

Pathogenesis & Pathology

The virus enters via the upper respiratory tract. It may be present in nasal secretions as early as 2–4 days after infection and is associated with maximal illness. Thereafter, viral titers fall, although illness persists.

Histopathologic changes are limited to the submucosa and surface epithelium. These include engorgement of blood vessels, edema, mild cellular infiltration, and desquamation of surface epithelium which is complete by the third day. Nasal secretion increases in quantity and in protein concentration.

Experiments under controlled conditions have not shown that chilling, including the wearing of wet socks, produces the cold itself or increases susceptibility to the virus. Chilliness is an early symptom of the common cold.

Clinical Findings

The incubation period is brief, from 2–4 days, and the acute illness usually lasts for 7 days although a nonproductive cough may persist for 2–3 weeks. The average individual has 1–2 attacks each year, usually during fall, winter, and spring. Usual symptoms in adults include sensations of irritation or fullness in the upper respiratory tract, nasal discharge, headache, mild cough, malaise, and a chilly sensation. Fever, if present, is mild, or the temperature may be subnormal. There is injection and swelling of the nasal and nasopharyngeal mucosa, and the sense of smell becomes less keen. Mild hoarseness may be present. While small cervical nodes may be palpable, prominent adenopathy does not occur. There may be a secondary bacterial infection of the respiratory tract. Acute otitis media or sinusitis, in addition to more serious lower respiratory disease, may complicate the later stages of the illness, especially in children. Type-specific antibodies appear or rise with each infection.

Immunity

Natural immunity is brief indeed, yet some exists. Only 30–50% of volunteers can be infected with infectious material; yet the "resistant" volunteers may catch cold at other times. Furthermore, people in isolated areas have more severe colds and a higher incidence of infection when a cold is introduced than people in areas regularly exposed to small doses of the virus.

Recent work with human volunteers has shown that resistance to the common cold is independent of measurable serum antibody, but perhaps related to specific antibody in the nasal secretions. These secretory antibodies are primarily 11 S IgA immunoglobulins, related to the 7 S serum IgA but containing additional determinants. Furthermore, secretory antibody appears to be made locally in the mucosal lining and is not a transudate from the serum. These 11 S IgA antibodies do not persist as long as those in serum, and could explain the paradox of reinfection in a person with adequate serum antibodies. Since antibody production does not appear until the illness subsides, recovery may be more temporally related to the production of interferon. Results regarding the role of interferon are inconclusive to date.

In addition, volunteers infected with one rhinovirus serotype resist challenge with both homologous and heterologous virus for 2–16 weeks after initial infection. Resistance to homologous challenge is complete during this period, while resistance to heterologous challenge is already incomplete by 5 weeks and apparently gone by 16 weeks. This nonspecific resistance may be a factor in the control of naturally occurring colds.

Epidemiology

The disease occurs throughout the world. In the temperate zones, the attack rates are highest in early fall and winter, declining in the late spring. Members of isolated communities form highly susceptible groups. The virus is believed to be transmitted through close contact, by large droplets. Colds in children spread more easily to others than do colds in adults. Adults in households with a child in school have twice as many colds as adults without this contact.

In a single community, many rhinovirus serotypes have been found to be responsible for outbreaks of disease in a single season. Different serotypes predominate during different respiratory disease seasons and during different outbreaks in a single season.

Treatment & Control

No specific treatment is available. Problems hindering the development of a potent rhinovirus vaccine are the inability to grow rhinoviruses in high titer in tissue culture and the fleeting immunity. Even if a potent and safe monovalent vaccine were developed, it would be of little value in controlling rhinovirus infections in view of the many serotypes already recognized. In addition, many rhinovirus serotypes are present during single respiratory disease outbreaks, and may recur only rarely in the same area. Recent experiments using highly purified vaccines have shown that the high serologic responses obtained are frequently not associated with similar elevations of local secretory antibody.

FOOT-AND-MOUTH DISEASE
(Rhinovirus of Cattle)

This highly infectious disease of cattle, sheep, pigs, and goats is of great economic importance. It is rare in the USA but has become endemic in Mexico and Canada. The disease may be transmitted to man by contact with infected animals or by ingestion of infective materials. In man the disease is characterized by fever, salivation, and vesiculation of the mucous membranes of the oropharynx and of the skin of the palms, soles, fingers, and toes.

The disease in animals is highly contagious in the early stages of infection when viremia is present and when vesicles in the mouth and on the feet rupture and liberate large amounts of virus. Excreted material remains infectious for long periods. Mortality in animals is usually low, although severe epizootics have been known in which the mortality rate was as high as 70%. Even though the disease does not always kill, infected animals become poor producers of milk and meat. In addition, many cattle become carriers for long periods, and can serve as foci for infections up to 8 months.

The infective particle contains RNA and has a diameter of 23 ± 2 nm; a noninfective 12 S particle which is associated with it has a diameter of 7–8 nm. Both particles can function as complement fixing antigens. The virus is acid-labile (at pH 3.0) and has a density of 1.43 gm/ml. The properties of RNA content, size, morphology, density, and ether resistance place foot-and-mouth disease virus in the rhinovirus subgroup of the picornaviruses. The virus survives freezing and is not affected by drying at ordinary temperatures.

Immunity is adequate, but of short duration. Passive antibody is transferred in the colostrum. At least 7 antigenic types are known with approximately 53 subtypes.

A variety of animals is susceptible to infection. The typical disease can be reproduced by inoculating the virus into the pads of the foot. The reaction in infant mice inoculated with the virus of foot-and-mouth disease is similar to their reaction to inoculation with coxsackieviruses: Paralysis results due to myositis. The virus grows readily in tissue cultures of cattle tongue or hamster BHK-21 cells. Formalin-treated vaccines have been prepared from virus grown in such tissue cultures. However, such vaccines do not produce a long-lasting immunity, and frequent booster inoculations are necessary. Recent experience with vaccines inactivated with acetylethyleneimine and containing an oil adjuvant have been shown to be more efficient. Attenuated virus vaccines have recently been developed and used in the field with reported success.

The methods of control of the disease are based on its high degree of contagiousness and on the resistance of the virus to inactivation. When foci of infection occur in the USA, all exposed animals are slaughtered and their carcasses destroyed. Strict quarantine is established, and the area is not presumed to be safe until susceptible animals fail to develop symptoms within 30 days. Another method which has been attempted in enzootic areas is to quarantine the herd and vaccinate all unaffected animals. Other countries have successfully employed systematic vaccination schedules. Some nations (eg, USA and Australia) forbid the importation of potentially infective materials such as fresh meat, and the disease has been eliminated in these areas. Even so, migrating birds may play a role in carrying the virus from one country to another, as from France and Holland to England.

• • •

General References

Evidence on the safety and efficacy of live poliomyelitis vaccines currently in use, with special reference to type 3 poliovirus. Report of a WHO scientific group. Bull WHO 40:925–945, 1969.

Hamre, D.: Rhinoviruses. Monogr Virol 1:1–85, 1968.

Melnick, J.L.: Enteroviruses: Vaccines, epidemiology, diagnosis, classification. CRC Critical Reviews in Clinical Laboratory Sciences 1:87–118, 1970.

Melnick, J.L., & H.A. Wenner: Enteroviruses. Pages 529–602 in: *Diagnostic Procedures for Viral and Rickettsial Infections,* 4th ed. American Public Health Association, 1969.

32...

Hepatitis Viruses

Acute viral hepatitis remains a major worldwide public health problem. Epidemiologic and laboratory investigations have strongly implied that 2 specific viruses are involved in this disease. These agents have been designated (1) **infectious hepatitis virus** (IH, viral hepatitis A, epidemic jaundice, short-incubation hepatitis) and (2) **serum hepatitis virus** (SH, viral hepatitis B, homologous serum jaundice, long-incubation hepatitis). Both agents produce acute inflammation of the liver, resulting in a clinical illness characterized by fever, gastrointestinal symptoms such as nausea and vomiting, and jaundice. Identical histopathologic lesions are observed in the liver.

The epidemiologic distinctiveness of these 2 viruses has recently been challenged. Infectious hepatitis, transmitted primarily by the fecal-oral route, is also transmitted by the parenteral route. Serum hepatitis occurs sporadically following parenteral inoculation of virus-infected blood products, although recent studies have demonstrated that oral transmission can also occur.

Appreciation of the existence of these lesser known transmission patterns is important when attempting to correlate presently established clinical classifications of viral hepatitis with the presence or absence of a recently discovered hepatitis associated antigen. This antigen was originally detected in 1963 in the serum of an Australian aborigine following its reaction in immunodiffusion tests with sera from multiply transfused hemophiliacs. Although the association of this Australia (Au) antigen with viral hepatitis was not recognized until 1967, it represents a major breakthrough in the field of hepatitis research. The relationship of Au antigen to long-incubation (serum or MS-2) hepatitis is now well established. In the discussion that follows, infectious hepatitis will designate the highly contagious short-incubation type (also designated MS-1), and serum hepatitis the long-incubation type in which Au antigen is found.

Properties of the Viruses

The physical and chemical properties of hepatitis viruses have been studied with human volunteers, the only experimental host. Recent work suggests that the virus of infectious hepatitis may have been isolated in Detroit 6 (D6) cells. The agent isolated in D6 cells has a diameter of 18–20 nm, in the same size range as the hepatitis associated Au antigen.

Infectious hepatitis virus is remarkably resistant to heating (56° C for 30 minutes), acid, and disinfecting chemicals. It contains no essential lipids, as indicated by its resistance to ether. The resistance of infectious hepatitis to disinfection procedures emphasizes the need for extra precautions in dealing with hepatitis patients and their products. The virus can be destroyed by autoclaving (121° C at 15 lb per square inch for 20 minutes), boiling in water for at least 15 minutes, or with dry heat (180°C for 1 hour). It withstands freezing for prolonged periods.

Serum hepatitis virus has been shown by ultrafiltration experiments to be about 25 nm in diameter. It is also resistant to heat (60° C for 20 hours) and stable in acid; it also survives a wide variety of chemical treatments, repeated freezing and thawing, and storage at room temperature for at least 6 months or at −20° C for more than 20 years. Peak Au antigen reactivity after sedimentation has been observed at densities of 1.20–1.25 in CsCl and between 1.16 and 1.18 in sucrose. The virus may persist following ultraviolet irradiation of plasma or other blood products. The stability of serum hepatitis virus has resulted in numerous warnings against the indiscriminate use of blood products in therapy.

Electron microscopy of serum from patients who possess the Au antigen has revealed virus-like particles, 20 nm in diameter. Tubular and filamentous forms are occasionally observed. Ether treatment reduces the size of the particles, suggesting the removal of a 2 nm lipid coat.

Pathology

Microscopically, there is necrosis of hepatocytes with inequality in cell size and lobular disarray. These parenchymal changes are accompanied by hyperplasia of the reticuloendothelial (Kupffer) cells, periportal infiltration by mononuclear cells, and localized areas of necrosis with acidophilic degeneration. Later in the course of the disease, there is an accumulation of lipofuscin in Kupffer cells due to the breakdown of hepatocytes. As liver cells enlarge, they block biliary excretion, resulting in bile stasis. Preservation of the reticulum framework allows hepatocyte regeneration so that the highly ordered architecture of the liver lobule can be ultimately resumed. The damaged hepatic tissue is usually restored in 8–12 weeks.

More extensive damage may prevent orderly regeneration; fibrosis occurs in some areas, and large regenerating nodules in others. This state may lead to postnecrotic cirrhosis. Electron microscopic studies reveal little specific alteration, and virus particles have not been detected.

Clinical Findings (See Table 32–1.)

In individual cases it is not possible to make a reliable clinical distinction between infectious hepatitis and serum hepatitis. Other viral diseases which may present as hepatitis are infectious mononucleosis, yellow fever, cytomegalovirus infection, herpes simplex, and some enterovirus infections. Hepatitis may occasionally be caused by infectious diseases such as leptospirosis, syphilis, tuberculosis, toxoplasmosis, and amebiasis, all of which are susceptible to specific drug therapy. Other important differential diagnoses are biliary obstruction, drug toxicity, and drug hypersensitivity reactions.

In viral hepatitis, the onset of jaundice is often preceded by gastrointestinal symptoms such as nausea, vomiting, severe anorexia, and fever which may mimic influenza. Jaundice may appear within a few days of the prodromal period, but anicteric hepatitis is common. Complete recovery occurs in the majority of cases. However, hepatocellular damage may be so severe as to cause massive hepatic necrosis with a fatal outcome, ie, fulminant hepatitis. Extensive involvement of the liver may also lead to clinical recovery but with the development of fibrosis, ie, postnecrotic cirrhosis. Another complication is the development of chronic hepatitis.

Infectious hepatitis is more severe in adults than in children, in whom it often goes unnoticed. The mortality rate is low in the young (0.1–0.3%), but increases with the age of the patient. The more severe course and higher mortality rates often observed in serum hepatitis may reflect the underlying condition for which transfusion was given rather than any increased inherent pathogenicity of the specific etiologic agent. Relapses may be manifested by abnormalities in liver function, or jaundice may appear. The posthepatitis syndrome may occur, especially in postmenopausal women. It is characterized by repeated episodes of anorexia, irritability, lethargy, weakness, headaches, and right upper quadrant pain. This syndrome is due to interference with normal estrogen metabolism in the liver and can be successfully treated in women with estrogens and progesterone.

As shown in Table 32–1, virus persists in the blood and stools of patients with infectious hepatitis for variable times, and virus may be found in the stools even a year after recovery. Serum hepatitis virus and Au antigen may persist in the blood of a healthy person for years after infection and consequently represents a continual potential source of infection.

Laboratory Diagnosis

Liver biopsy permits a tissue diagnosis of hepatitis. Tests for abnormal liver function, such as serum transaminase and thymol turbidity, supplement the clinical, pathologic, and epidemiologic findings, especially in cases of hepatitis without jaundice. Transaminase values range between 500 and 2000 units and are almost never below 100 units. SGPT values are usually higher than SGOT. A spiking rise in the SGOT with a short duration (3–19 days) is more indicative of IH, whereas a gradual rise with prolongation (35–200 days) appears to characterize SH. In addition, the thymol turbidity is often abnormal in IH but relatively normal in SH. Sulfobromophthalein (BSP) excretion is the most sensitive measure of liver function and may be of diagnostic value early in the preicteric phase of the disease. Leukopenia is typical in the pre-icteric

TABLE 32–1. Epidemiologic and clinical features of human hepatitis virus infections.

	Short-Incubation (Infectious) Hepatitis	Long-Incubation (Serum) Hepatitis
Incubation period	15–50 days	43–180 days
Age distribution	Children and young adults	All ages
Seasonal incidence	Autum and winter	All year
Route of infection	Predominantly fecal-oral	Predominantly parenteral
Duration of infectivity of patient		
Blood	Days	Months-years
Stool	Weeks-months	?
Clinical and laboratory features		
Fever > 38° C (100.4° F)	Common	Less common
Duration of transaminase elevation	1–3 weeks	1–3 months
Thymol turbidity	Abnormal	Usually normal
Immunoglobulins (IgM levels)	Elevated	Usually normal
Australia antigen	Not present	Present
Immunity		
Homologous	Yes	Yes
Heterologous	No	No
Duration	?	?
Gamma globulin prophylaxis	Prevents jaundice	Variable response

phase and may be followed by a relative lymphocytosis. Large atypical lymphocytes such as are found in infectious mononucleosis may occasionally be seen. Further evidence of liver dysfunction and host response are reflected in a decreased serum albumin and increased serum globulin.

Immunodiffusion technics—and the more sensitive complement fixation method—have been employed in the detection of Au antigen in the serum or plasma of patients with viral hepatitis. About 80% of patients clinically diagnosed as having serum hepatitis are positive for Au antigen, compared with only 20% of patients clinically diagnosed as infectious hepatitis. This discrepancy may reflect difficulties in their classification, as discussed above. The absence of Au antigen in sera from well documented cases of common source epidemics of infectious hepatitis or sera from volunteers who had received short-incubation (MS-1 or IH) virus is noteworthy in this regard.

Au antigen usually appears in advance of clinical and biochemical evidence of hepatitis. It is detectable for varying periods of time from a few days or weeks up to several years. Not infrequently it will disappear, only to reappear at another time.

Except in multiply transfused patients, such as those with hemophilia, antibody detection has not proved fruitful for diagnostic application. Attempts to grow hepatitis virus in laboratory animals or in tissue culture were not successful. A number of strains from patients with short-incubation infectious hepatitis were recently grown in D6 cells, but the work has not yet progressed to the point where the agent can be classified as hepatitis virus. Patients yielding the virus in D6 tissue culture were negative for Au antigen.

Immunity

There is evidence for only 2 types of hepatitis virus—short-incubation infectious hepatitis virus and long-incubation serum hepatitis virus. A single infection with either confers homologous but not heterologous protection against reinfection. The nature and duration of immunity are not known, since there are no methods of measuring them at the present time. Factors such as impaired immunity and virus dose must be considered in analyzing the incidence of reinfections.

Most cases of infectious hepatitis presumably occur without jaundice during childhood, and by late adulthood there is a widespread resistance to reinfection. Evidence for this comes from the relatively higher incidence of infectious hepatitis in children and young adults as well as the protective effect of normal adult gamma globulin given during the incubation period of hepatitis.

The virus-host relationship in serum hepatitis may be more complex than in infectious hepatitis for it may often involve the persistence of the virus in the blood stream for long periods. The failure of or delay in virus and Au antigen clearance in a healthy individual is not understood.

Various host factors, immunologic or genetic, have been proposed to account for the long-term presence of Au antigen in a significant proportion of patients with leukemia (acute leukemia and chronic lymphocytic leukemia), lepromatous leprosy, thalassemia, or Down's syndrome, and in persons without obvious disease living in Oceania, Japan, or Southeast Asia. The relationship of Au antigen to blood transfusions is obvious in many of these disorders, but its presence cannot be explained so easily in others.

Some long-term carriers continue to exhibit biochemical and histologic evidence of chronic liver disease. About 25% of patients with chronic active hepatitis have detectable Au antigen in their serum.

Immunoglobulin levels during acute viral hepatitis have been studied. Patients with infectious hepatitis have an abnormally high level of IgM which appears 3—4 days after the SGOT begins to rise. Serum hepatitis patients have slightly elevated to normal IgM levels.

Treatment

Treatment of the patient with hepatitis is directed at allowing hepatocellular damage to resolve and repair itself under optimal conditions. This requires adequate bed rest and a nutritious diet. Patients should be advised to avoid hepatotoxins such as alcohol during convalescence.

Epidemiology

As shown in Table 32—1, there are marked differences in the epidemiologic features of infectious and serum hepatitis.

A. **Short-Incubation (Infectious) Hepatitis:** Outbreaks of infectious hepatitis are common in families and institutions, summer camps, and especially among troops. The most likely mode of transmission under these conditions is by the fecal-oral route through close personal contact. The clinical disease is most often manifest in children and young adults. The ratio of anicteric to icteric cases in adults is about 1:1; in children, it may be as high as 12:1.

Sharp, explosive epidemics usually result from contamination of a single source (eg, drinking water, food, milk, or nonhuman primates). Infectious hepatitis virus may also be transmitted by the use of contaminated needles and syringes or through the administration of blood. Under these conditions, the shortened incubation period may be of epidemiologic significance. Using the incubation period as the criterion for IH, as many as 1/3 of cases of posttransfusion hepatitis may be due to this agent. Water-borne epidemics of infectious hepatitis have resulted from sewage contamination of a water supply. The largest such epidemic occurred in New Delhi in 1955—1956, resulting in an estimated 1100 cases among 250,000 people in a single week. The consumption of raw oysters or clams obtained from water polluted with sewage has also resulted in several outbreaks of hepatitis.

Other recently identified sources of potential infection are nonhuman primates. Since 1961 there have been over 20 outbreaks in which primates, usually chimpanzees, have infected humans in close personal contact with them. Most of the primates responsible were recent arrivals in the United States, less than 3 months having elapsed from their entry to the appearance of the index case. These animals probably acquire the infection after arrival, and transmit the virus to their caretakers. A persistent carrier state is unlikely since the number of new cases diminishes with residence.

B. Long-Incubation (Serum) Hepatitis: The virus of serum hepatitis is also believed to be worldwide in distribution. There is no seasonal trend and no particular predilection for any age group, although there are definite high risk groups such as narcotic addicts and individuals who have recently received blood transfusions. The incidence of SH following blood transfusions is 0.3–4% for the recipients. Case fatality rates increase with age and are 11% overall (5.5% in persons less than 40 years of age). Cases appear sporadically and are often associated with the parenteral inoculation of infective human blood (or its products), usually obtained from an apparently healthy carrier with virus in his blood. Thousands of cases have been produced by injecting human serum, vaccines containing human serum, plasma, and whole blood. Many others have been infected by improperly sterilized syringes or needles, lancets, or even in tattooing. Serum hepatitis virus is also infectious by the oral route, but this mechanism of spread at present does not seem the major one. The estimated ratio of anicteric to icteric infections is reported to be greater than 100:1.

The incubation period for serum hepatitis is 43–180 days, with a mean between 60–90 days. It appears to vary with the type of blood product injected. The mean incubation period was significantly shorter in a group of patients receiving whole blood (69 days) than in a group receiving blood products only (102 days).

Gamma globulin and albumin are 2 blood products which appear free from the risk of serum hepatitis. Their method of preparation includes cold-ethanol fractionation (gamma globulin) and heating to 60° C for 10 hours (albumin).

Prevention & Control

Until vaccines are available, prevention and control of hepatitis must be directed toward interrupting the chain of transmission and the use of passive immunization.

A. Infectious Hepatitis: Sanitation procedures which prevent fecal contamination are recommended. An attempt should be made to avoid employing food handlers who may be carriers of the virus and to keep other food handlers free of infection. The appearance of the disease in camps or institutions is often an indication of poor sanitation and poor personal hygiene. In special instances, asymptomatic carriers can be found by determining SGOT levels. All needles, syringes, blood-counting pipets, and lancets which have come in

contact with the blood of hepatitis patients should be sterilized by heating. (See Properties of the Viruses.)

Gamma globulin prepared from large pools of normal adult plasma confers passive protection when injected intramuscularly during the incubation period up to 6 days before the onset of disease. A dose of 0.06–0.12 ml/kg (0.02–0.03 ml/lb) is recommended. Passive immunity probably lasts 3–6 months, depending on the dose administered. Continued exposure of persons receiving gamma globulin to carriers of the virus produces an active immunity superimposed on the passive immunity. Gamma globulin does not prevent infection, but it modifies the illness so that clinical symptoms and jaundice do not usually develop. Gamma globulin is recommended for the interruption of epidemics in institutions or camps. Prophylactic administration of gamma globulin (0.12 ml/kg every 5–6 months) to persons at high risk (missionaries, Peace Corps volunteers, military personnel, or travelers to endemic areas) has been practiced. Recent evidence suggests that protection against IH is afforded by this regimen, but that a further reduction in cases might be obtained if the interval between injections were shortened to every 4 months.

B. Serum Hepatitis: Persons who have had hepatitis should not be used as blood donors. However, even persons without a history of hepatitis and with normal liver function tests may be carriers of the virus. The duration of the carrier state is not known. With the recent introduction of the Au antigen test, it is recommended that test be routinely employed to avoid using blood from Au-positive donors.

The resistance of the virus to physical and chemical agents makes it difficult to treat human blood and its products to render them safe for human inoculation. Neither ultraviolet irradiation nor nitrogen mustard treatment is entirely reliable. The combined use of ultraviolet irradiation and 0.35% propiolactone may be successful. Prolonged storage of plasma (for several months at room or body temperature) may reduce the hazard of producing hepatitis but may alter plasma proteins. Little is known of the virucidal action of chemical disinfectants used on surgical and dental instruments.

Since as little as 0.004 ml of plasma can transmit the disease, a single carrier of virus might infect a large batch of pooled plasma. It has been recommended, therefore, that pooled plasma should not be used. If pools must be used, they should be made from no more than 5 donors. Plasma should be used only in cases of emergency, because of the possibility of transmitting serum hepatitis to a patient already ill.

The use of disposable needles and syringes is recommended to reduce the possibility of viral contamination. Cases have also been traced to tattooing.

Prevention of transfusion associated hepatitis by the administration of immune globulin has not been adequately demonstrated in carefully conducted trials. Therefore, its routine administration to recipients of blood transfusions is not recommended. Proper donor selection and the development of a central registry for identification of carriers can lower the incidence of transfusion associated hepatitis. In addition, blood or its products should be used only when necessary, since the risk of hepatitis appears to increase with the number of units administered.

• • •

General References

Giles, J.P., & others: Relation of Australia/SH antigen to the Willowbrook MS-2 strain. New England J Med 281:119–122, 1969.

Havens, W.P., Jr., & J.R. Paul: Infectious hepatitis and serum hepatitis. Pages 965–993 in: *Viral and Rickettsial Infections of Man,* 4th ed. Horsfall, F.L., Jr., & I. Tamm (editors). Lippincott, 1965.

Hirschman, R.J., & others: Virus-like particles in sera of patients with infectious and serum hepatitis. JAMA 208:1667–1670, 1969.

London, W.T., Sutnick, A.J., & B.S. Blumberg: Australia antigen and acute viral hepatitis. Ann Int Med 70:55–59, 1969.

Prince, A.M.: An antigen detected in the blood during the incubation period of serum hepatitis. Proc Nat Acad Sc 60:814–821, 1968.

33...

Rabies & Certain Other Viral Diseases of the Nervous System; Slow Viruses

RABIES

Rabies is an acute infection of the CNS which is almost always fatal. The virus is usually transmitted to man from the bite of a rabid animal.

Properties of the Virus

A. Size: Rabies virus is a member of the rhabdovirus group (see Chapter 27 and Fig 27–26). The virion is enveloped and is covered with projections; it contains an internal filamentous structure. The virus particle is bullet-shaped, with a cylinder diameter of about 70 nm and a length of about 210 nm (similar to vesicular stomatitis virus of cattle and certain viruses of fish, insects, and plants). The nucleic acid is RNA. Its density in CsCl solution is about 1.2 gm/ml.

B. Reaction to Physical and Chemical Agents: The virus survives storage at 4° C for weeks; it can survive subzero temperatures for much longer periods, but only in the absence of CO_2. On dry ice, therefore, it must be stored in glass-sealed ampules. In glycerol it may be kept alive for weeks at room temperature. After desiccation from the frozen state, rabies virus is stable for years at 4° C. The virus deteriorates in dilute suspension in the absence of protein. For this reason, normal serum or 0.75% bovalbumin fraction V is added to the diluent when the virus is titrated.

The rabies virus is killed rapidly by ultraviolet irradiation or sunlight. Thermal inactivation occurs in 1 hour at 50° C and in 5 minutes at 60° C. Lyophilized virus is more thermostable and resists temperatures of 55° C even after an exposure period of 24 hours.

The virus is rapidly inactivated by strong acids and alkali and by bichloride of mercury. Viral infectivity is destroyed by 0.1% sodium deoxycholate, by ether, and by trypsin.

C. Animal Susceptibility and Growth of Virus: Rabies virus has a wide host range. All warm-blooded animals, including man, are susceptible. The virus is widely distributed in infected animals, having been detected (in order of decreasing frequency) in the nervous system, saliva, urine, lymph, milk, and blood. Recovery from infection is rare except in the vampire bats, where the virus has become peculiarly adapted to the salivary glands. Vampire bats may transmit the virus for months without themselves ever showing any signs of disease. Latent rabies virus has been reac-

tivated in a laboratory animal 5 months after infection by inoculation of corticotropin.

When freshly isolated in the laboratory, the strains are referred to as street virus. Such strains show long and variable incubation periods (usually 21–60 days in dogs) and regularly produce intracytoplasmic inclusion bodies. The inoculated animals may exhibit long periods of excitement and viciousness. The virus may invade the salivary glands as well as the CNS.

Serial brain-to-brain passage in rabbits yields a "fixed" virus which no longer multiplies in extraneural tissues. This fixed virus multiplies rapidly, and the incubation period is shortened to 4–6 days. At this stage, inclusion bodies are found only with difficulty.

The virus may be propagated in chick embryos. Baby hamster kidney cells are especially susceptible to rabies virus. The virus also multiplies in human diploid cell cultures, even though it cannot be passaged in such cultures by transfer of tissue culture fluid. However, virus can be propagated by transfer of infected cells to uninfected human diploid cultures.

One strain (Flury), after serial passage in chick embryos, has been modified so that it fails to produce disease in animals injected extraneurally. The attenuated virus is used for vaccination of animals.

D. Antigenic Properties: Neutralizing and complement fixing antibodies develop during the course of the disease; they may develop following vaccination. A soluble complement fixing antigen, about 12 nm in size, is produced in infected cells but is unassociated with infectious virus.

Pathogenesis & Pathology

Rabies virus infects and multiplies in the muscle or connective tissue and is propagated through the endoneurium of the Schwann cells or associated tissue spaces of the sensory nerves to the CNS. It multiplies there and may then spread through peripheral nerves to the salivary glands and other tissues. Rabies virus has not been isolated from the blood of infected persons.

It has been suggested that the incubation period depends on the distance the virus has to move from its point of entry to the brain. Support for this view lies in the higher attack rate and shorter incubation period in persons suffering from wounds about the face. In experimental infection, on the other hand, there is no relationship between incubation period and area of inoculation, and some feel that the higher attack rates and shorter incubation periods associated with face wounds are due to the more severe lacerations and the greater degree of penetration of infecting virus. Even after direct introduction of the virus into the brains of animals, the incubation period is sometimes 12 weeks. The long incubation periods in rabies appear, therefore, to result from a transitory failure of the virus to multiply.

There is a general hyperemia and pronounced nerve cell destruction in the cerebral and cerebellar cortex, midbrain, basal ganglia, pons, and especially in the medulla. Demyelinization occurs in the white matter, and degeneration of axons and myelin sheaths is common. In the spinal cord, the posterior horns are most severely involved. If the bite has occurred on an arm or leg, the corresponding posterior horn shows extensive destruction (neuronophagia and cellular infiltrations), which may extend into the dorsal root ganglia of the same area of the spinal cord. Cellular infiltrations are usually mononuclear in character and are often perivascular and perineural. They are minimal if the patient dies after a short disease but are more extensive when the disease is prolonged.

Rabies virus produces a specific cytoplasmic inclusion, the Negri body, in infected nerve cells. The demonstration of such inclusions is pathognomonic of rabies. The inclusions are eosinophilic, sharply demarcated, and more or less spherical, measuring 2–10 nm in diameter. Several may be found in the cytoplasm of large neurons. They occur throughout the brain and spinal cord but are most frequently found in Ammon's horn of the hippocampus. Negri bodies have been found to contain rabies virus antigens.

Paralysis and death due to allergic encephalomyelitis may follow a course of killed or attenuated rabies vaccine made from infected brain and spinal cord or even from duck embryo tissue. Therefore, histopathologic examination of the brain and spinal cord in fatal paralytic cases must reveal specific inclusion (Negri) bodies before rabies can be established as the cause of death. Serologic tests are useless here, since antibodies would have been formed either in the course of the disease or by the vaccination procedure.

The virus multiplies outside the CNS. When found in the salivary glands, it is accompanied by cellular interstitial infiltrations and by necrosis of the acinar cells of mucus-secreting tissue. The adrenal medulla, the acinar epithelium of the pancreas, and the renal tubules may also show acute degeneration.

The latent virus infection can be reactivated by the administration of corticotropin and by stress in experimental animals.

Clinical Findings

The usual incubation period in dogs ranges from 3–8 weeks, but it may be as short as 10 days. Clinically, the disease in dogs is divided into 3 phases: prodromal, excitative, and paralytic. The prodromal phase is characterized by fever, sluggish corneal reflexes, and a sudden change in the temperament of the animal; docile animals may become snappy and

irritable, whereas aggressive animals may become more affectionate. The excitable phase lasts 3–7 days, during which the dog shows symptoms of irritability, restlessness, nervousness, and exaggerated response to sudden light and sound stimuli. At this stage the animal is most dangerous because of its tendency to bite. The animal has difficulty in swallowing, suffers from convulsive seizures, and enters finally into a paralytic stage characterized by paralysis of the whole body followed by coma and death. Sometimes the animal goes into the paralytic stage without passing through the excitative stage.

The incubation period in man varies from 2–16 weeks but may be even longer. In the USA from 1955–1962, about 40% of the 18 fatal cases recorded developed symptoms between 14–21 days after exposure, while the median incubation period was 35 days. It is usually shorter in children than in adults. The clinical spectrum can be divided into 4 phases: a short prodromal phase, a sensory phase, a period of excitement, and a paralytic or depressive phase. The prodrome, which lasts 2–4 days, begins with malaise, and any of the following may also be present: anorexia, headache, nausea and vomiting, sore throat, and fever. Usually there is an abnormal sensation around the site of infection. The patient may show increasing nervousness and apprehension. General sympathetic overactivity is observed, including lacrimation, pupillary dilatation, and increased salivation and perspiration. The act of swallowing precipitates a spasm of the throat muscles. Because of the patient's fear of water, the disease has been known as hydrophobia since ancient days. A patient may allow saliva to drool from his mouth simply to avoid swallowing and the associated painful spasms. This phase is followed by convulsive seizures and death, usually 3–5 days following onset. If the patient survives this acute excitement phase, he becomes listless, stuporous, and finally comatose. Progressive paralytic symptoms may intervene before death but are not common. A form of Landry's ascending paralysis was the predominant clinical feature in cases of rabies transmitted by vampire bats in Trinidad and Latin America.

Vaccination against rabies with material made from infected brain tissue may result in a paralysis which is difficult to distinguish from paralysis due to the infecting virus.

Since the disease may be transmitted through a minor wound from an apparently healthy dog, a history of exposure is not always obtainable.

Hysteria may simulate certain features of rabies, particularly in persons who have been near a rabid animal or have been bitten by a nonrabid one.

Laboratory Diagnosis

A. Histopathology of Animals: The diagnosis of rabies is based on the finding of cytoplasmic inclusions (Negri bodies) in the nerve cells of a naturally infected patient or animal or in the brains of animals inoculated in the laboratory. Impression preparations of brain tissue (Ammon's horn) are often used in the microscopic examination for Negri bodies. If Negri bodies cannot be found in the brain of a dog suspected of having rabies, a suspension of the brain or submaxillary salivary gland should be passed to other animals (mice, rabbits, hamsters). Tissues infected with rabies virus can be identified by means of the fluorescent antibody technic, which is the method of choice as regards speed and accuracy of identification. The method is outlined in Chapter 28.

Specific antirabies hamster serum labeled with fluorescent dyes has been shown to be superior to horse serum for detecting rabies virus antigen in infected tissues. An indirect fluorescent antibody technic has also been used successfully for the demonstration of antirabies antibodies in human sera.

Even after an apparently healthy dog bites a person, it should be isolated and watched for the next 7 days. If the dog does not show signs of rabies within this time, the person has presumably not been exposed to the virus. If signs of rabies do develop, the dog should be held in isolation for a few more days to permit the Negri bodies, which increase in number as the disease progresses, to accumulate in the brain. If the animal is dead, the brain should be examined for Negri bodies which are located in the cytoplasm. The matrix of Negri bodies is acidophilic, and basophilic granules are distributed in the matrix. The Negri bodies should be distinguished from nonrabies inclusions occasionally encountered in dogs infected with distemper virus (measles type inclusion). The nonrabies inclusions lack internal structure.

B. Recovery of Virus: The virus should be sought in the patient's saliva, which should be taken from under the tongue in order to obtain material originating in the submaxillary salivary gland. After the bacteria have been inactivated with penicillin and streptomycin, the saliva is inoculated into mice (intracerebrally) or hamsters (intramuscularly). Brain tissue should be collected from fatal cases and inoculated in a similar fashion. Next to the nervous tissue, the submaxillary glands are the best source of virus. Inoculated mice usually develop flaccid paralysis of the legs and then die. Their brains should be examined for Negri bodies. If Negri bodies cannot be found, the virus should be identified by its neutralization by specific antiserum or the tissue examined for rabies antigen by the fluorescent rabies antibody test.

C. Serology: Because patients with rabies do not recover, serologic tests are of little value. However, antibodies may develop in an unvaccinated person during the course of the disease. Neutralizing and complement fixing antibodies may develop after vaccination. The indirect fluorescent antibody test may be used for the detection of antirabies antibodies in unvaccinated and vaccinated individuals.

Immunity & Vaccines

Only one antigenic type of virus is known. All infections are held to be fatal. Preexposure or postexposure prophylaxis must provide, therefore, effective levels of antibodies to prevent the multiplication and spread of rabies virus. Two types of vaccine are presently used in the USA: duck embryo vaccine (DEV) and nerve tissue vaccine (NTV). DEV is prepared in embryonated duck eggs infected with the Pasteur rabbit brain fixed virus, and is then inactivated with propiolactone. NTV is a rabbit brain tissue preparation infected with a fixed virus and inactivated by phenol and incubation at 37° C (Semple type) or ultraviolet irradiation.

Canines are presently immunized with an attenuated rabies virus which has been adapted to chick embryos (Flury strain). Its failure to multiply in man and the low viral titers obtained (small antigenic mass) make this vaccine unsuitable for postexposure prophylaxis in man, although the high-egg-passage (HEP) variant has been used for preexposure prophylaxis.

An experimental attenuated live virus vaccine has been developed by propagating the virus in human diploid cells. The tissue culture adapted virus is not pathogenic when tested in monkeys, and is highly antigenic. Inactivated vaccine prepared from tissue culture adapted virus has proved to be highly antigenic in animals and, at the same time, free of material responsible for sensitizing the subjects to allergic encephalitis. However, this tissue culture vaccine has not yet undergone field trials in man.

Vaccines prepared from nerve tissue (Semple vaccine) are dangerous because the foreign brain material may sensitize the person being vaccinated and produce an allergic encephalitis and paralysis. This accident occurs in about one out of every 4000–8000 persons vaccinated. In certain instances, the chances of allergic encephalitis or paralysis from the vaccine may be greater than the chances of contracting rabies. Death has occurred in a ratio of 1:35,000 persons treated.

Allergic encephalitis is the result of an in vivo antigen-antibody (delayed hypersensitivity) reaction. The foreign brain material in the vaccine stimulates antibodies against nerve tissue which react with brain antigens of the vaccinated individual. Such reactions occurring in the nervous system give rise to inflammation and degeneration. Allergic encephalitis is more likely to occur in persons previously vaccinated against rabies.

Duck embryo vaccine is the most frequently used commercial vaccine in the USA for immunization and treatment. The serologic responses are not significantly different from those due to conventional vaccines of brain tissue origin. Although this vaccine markedly reduces the chances of encephalitis, acute anaphylactic reactions and posttreatment paralysis have been reported.

Treatment (See Tables 33–1 and 33–2.)

Every case should be individually evaluated and treatment begun as soon as possible after exposure. Assessment of the extent and location of the wound is often helpful in deciding appropriate management. Severe wounds are designated as multiple or deep, or located on the head, neck, or upper extremities. Mild degrees of exposure are designated as scratches or

TABLE 33–1. Check list of treatments for animal bites.*

1. Flush wound immediately.
2. Thorough wound cleansing under medical supervision.
3. Antirabies serum and/or vaccine as indicated.
4. Tetanus prophylaxis and antibacterial treatment when required.
5. No sutures or wound closure advised.

*From *Immunization Against Disease,* 1966–67. National Communicable Disease Center.

lacerations in areas other than those mentioned above, or possible contamination of open wounds and abrasions with saliva. Bites from rodents and adequately vaccinated animals seldom require specific antirabies prophylaxis.

Since rabies virus is assumed to multiply in the muscle, or connective tissue, and to become fixed to nerve tissue soon after exposure, and since the interval between exposure and onset of symptoms is frequently less than 21 days, the importance of early, adequate local wound therapy supplemented by antiserum and vaccine is emphasized. Immediate scrubbing and flushing of the wound with soap and water or quaternary ammonium compounds is one of the most effective measures for preventing rabies. If hyperimmune antirabies serum is indicated (Table 33–2), some should be infiltrated around and into the wound. Tetanus prophylaxis should be administered as indicated.

Postexposure vaccination in combination with hyperimmune serum is recommended for all bites by rabid animals, in those exposures designated as severe, and in the victims of unprovoked attacks by wild carnivores and bats (Table 33–2). Because antibody responses are more rapid and achieve higher levels when the vaccine is given daily, a course of 14–21 single daily injections is recommended, followed by 2 booster doses, 10 and 20 days after the primary course. This schedule also counteracts the suppressed immune response frequently associated with passive-active immunization procedures. Homologous rabies immune globulin appears to be as effective as equine antibody in animal protection tests and produces less interference with the subsequent stimulation of antibody by the vaccine. In addition, since 16% of all patients receiving heterologous antirabies serum are reported to develop serum sickness (46% over the age of 15), the advantages of a human source of rabies immune globulin are apparent. However, the only commercial source of rabies immune globulin presently available in the USA is of equine origin.

The usefulness of hyperimmune rabies antiserum, in addition to its local virus-neutralizing capability, is its ability to markedly prolong the incubation period. This provides a longer period of time for development of vaccine-stimulated antibody, which can then appear before the passively administered antibody disappears.

Epidemiology

Rabies occurs all over the world but especially in India, Africa, and parts of Europe. Since 1963, only 1–2 cases of rabies have been reported annually in the USA. However, several thousand cases of rabies have been reported in domestic and wild animals. The incidence of animal rabies dropped from 1946 to

TABLE 33–2. Guide for postexposure antirabies prophylaxis.*

The following recommendations are intended only as a guide. They may be modified according to knowledge of the species of biting animal and circumstances surrounding the biting incident.

Biting Animal		Treatment		
		Exposure		
Species	Status at Time of Attack	No Lesion	Mild	Severe
Dog or cat	Healthy	None	None†	S†
	Signs suggestive of rabies	None	V‡	S+V‡
	Escaped or unknown	None	V	S+V
	Rabid	None	S+V	S+V
Skunk, fox, raccoon, coyote, bat	Regard as rabid in unprovoked attack	None	S+V	S+V
Other	Consider individually			

V = Rabies vaccine S = Antirabies serum
*From *Immunization Against Disease,* 1966–67. National Communicable Disease Center.
† = Begin vaccine at first sign of rabies in biting dog or cat during holding period (preferably 7–10 days).
‡ = Discontinue vaccine if biting dog or cat is healthy 5 days after exposure, or if acceptable laboratory negativity has been demonstrated in animal killed at time of attack. If observed animal dies after 5 days and brain is positive, resume treatment.

1960, but since then it has been on the rise. Rabies in domesticated animals has declined since 1953. Since 1960, more cases of rabies have occurred in wildlife than in domestic animals (dogs, cats, and livestock), with the latter group accounting for only 25% in 1968. Cases in foxes and skunks constitute 82% of the wildlife rabies. Nearly 300 cases of rabies in bats were also reported in 1968. Rabies in domestic animals included cattle (40%), dogs (33%), cats (17%), and horses (7%). The fox has become the predominant host in the southern and eastern United States, while the skunk is most commonly involved in Texas, Ohio, California, and the Midwest. Rabid raccoons are frequently reported from Georgia and Florida. Epizootics of rabies can occur in any climate at all seasons of the year.

Most human cases are caused by the bite of an infected animal. Man is an accidental host, and is not a reservoir of infection. Infection from man to man is quite rare, one reason being that patients are usually kept under heavy sedation.

The spread of rabies is limited by the ability of the virus to reach and to propagate in the salivary glands of the infected animal. Only about 50% of rabid dogs have the virus in their saliva.

In Russia and the eastern European countries, wolves carry the infection to man. In India and South Africa, jackals and mongooses play a similar role. In South America, in the vicinity of Trinidad, rabies is transmitted by the vampire bat. This animal usually feeds on cattle and may cause large epizootics among them. However, it may also bite man. The infection is also present in fruit-eating bats, which serve as a reservoir of virus for the vampires.

Rabies has recently been discovered in colonial and noncolonial frugivorous and insectivorous bats in the USA. Bats are able to transmit the disease both to quadrupeds and to human beings. Virus occurs in colonial Mexican free-tailed bats, and antibodies are found in a large percentage of normal healthy bats. Rabies-infected insectivorous bats are known to inhabit caves also inhabited by vampire bats. Transmission from one bat species to the other may account for the infection of Mexican free-tailed bats, since the latter may winter in Mexico—within the range of the vampire bat.

The virus carrier rate may be high in bats. Although 1% or more of apparently healthy bats may carry virus, as many as 9% of those with abnormal signs have proved to be positive. Virus may be found both in the brain and in the salivary glands, especially if the bats appear abnormal. However, in normal bats virus may be present only in the salivary glands.

The importance of the bat in the epidemiology of rabies lies not so much in the occasional animal that responds to infection with overt symptoms and is incited to abnormal behavior and contact with man, but rather in the great number of healthy carriers in bat populations which maintain ever-shifting foci of rabies infection, providing a constant source of infection for wildlife predators, domestic animals, and man,

and offering a means of persistence of the virus in nature. In addition, aerosol transmission of rabies by bats has recently been proved, adding to the problem of rabies control especially among those who explore caves inhabited by bats.

Control

Rabies is best controlled by destroying stray dogs in cities and by compulsory vaccination of all others. During outbreaks and for at least 6 months after each case, all dogs should be muzzled. Imported dogs should be quarantined for 6 months.

Dogs that have bitten human beings should be isolated for at least 5 days, preferably 7–10 days. If rabies is suspected after that period has passed, the animal should be killed for diagnosis.

Within the past few years, bat rabies has been found to be widespread in the USA. Antirabies treatment appears indicated for all persons or animals bitten by bats. The need for treatment on the basis of the brain smear of the bat cannot be relied upon, as almost 50% of infected bats have no detectable inclusion (Negri) bodies by this procedure, and many harbor the virus only in their salivary glands or brown fat.

Preexposure prophylaxis is recommended for persons subjected to a high risk, eg, veterinarians, animal caretakers, mailmen, field personnel, and certain laboratory workers. DEV is most frequently used. The schedule for immunization is either 2 doses 1 month apart followed by a third dose in 6 months, or 3 weekly injections with a fourth dose 3 months later. Booster immunizations should be obtained every 2–3 years and effectiveness confirmed by a serum neutralization test.

In areas where vampire bats or foxes transmit rabies, prophylactic vaccination of cattle should be carried out.

ASEPTIC MENINGITIS

This disease is characterized by acute onset, fever, headache, and stiff neck. There is pleocytosis of the spinal fluid consisting largely of mononuclear cells. The fluid is bacteria-free, has a normal glucose content, and normal or slightly elevated protein.

Etiology

Aseptic meningitis may be caused by a variety of agents: (1) primarily neurotropic viruses (poliomyelitis, lymphocytic choriomeningitis, and arthropod-borne encephalitis viruses); (2) viruses not primarily neurotropic (enteroviruses, mumps, herpes simplex, herpes zoster, infectious mononucleosis, infectious hepatitis, varicella, and measles); (3) spirochetes (*Treponema pallidum* and leptospirae); (4) bacteria, as in silent brain abscess and inadequately treated bacterial meningitis; and (5) mycoplasmas or chlamydiae.

Diagnosis

The diagnosis of aseptic meningitis is made by exclusion of bacterial causes of the symptom complex. Specific etiologic causes of aseptic meningitis can usually be determined only by isolation of the agent or the demonstration of a rise in specific antibodies. However, epidemiologic features have diagnostic value. (See discussions of specific agents.)

Laboratory Findings

The peripheral white count is usually normal, but in lymphocytic choriomeningitis eosinophilia may appear a few days after onset. There is pleocytosis of the CSF; polymorphonuclear cells often predominate during the first 24 hours, but a shift to lymphocytes usually occurs thereafter. In mumps and poliomyelitis, the usual range is 50–300 cells, but more may be found. In herpes simplex and leptospiral meningitis, up to 300 cells is usual. In lymphocytic choriomeningitis there may be 500–3000 cells or more. Protein levels of the spinal fluid are often elevated.

LYMPHOCYTIC CHORIOMENINGITIS

Lymphocytic choriomeningitis is an acute disease characterized usually by the aseptic meningitis syndrome or by a mild systemic influenza-like illness but occasionally by a severe encephalomyelitis or a fatal systemic disease. The incubation period is usually 18–21 days but may be as short as 1–3 days. The mild systemic form, which is rarely recognized clinically, is characterized by fever, malaise, generalized muscle aches and pains, low backache, weakness, and, in some patients, respiratory symptoms, including sore throat and cough. The temperature returns to normal after 3–14 days, and the patient is well by that time.

The LCM virus recently has been shown to be identical morphologically, and to cross-react serologically, with arboviruses of the Tacaribe complex, which includes the Junin and Machupo viruses of South American hemorrhagic fevers. A new taxonomic group of these RNA-containing, enveloped viruses has been proposed: the **Tacaribe-LCM group.**

Diagnosis

Specific diagnosis can be made by the isolation of virus from spinal fluid or blood during the acute phase and by serologic tests demonstrating a rise in antibody titer between acute and convalescent serum specimens. Complement fixing antibodies rise to diagnostic levels by the third or fourth week, fall gradually over the ensuing weeks, and reach normal levels after several months. Neutralizing antibodies appear later and are not present at diagnostic levels until 7–8 weeks after onset; they persist for as long as 4–5 years.

Laboratory Findings

In the prodromal period (or mild systemic form), leukopenia with relative lymphocytosis is frequently present. In patients with the meningitic form, occasional leukocytosis up to 20,000 with an increase mainly in polymorphonuclear leukocytes is seen. CSF pleocytosis is higher than in most other forms of aseptic meningitis, ranging between 100 and several thousand cells; about half of patients have counts greater than 600. The cells are predominantly lymphocytes. The average protein content is about 100 mg/100 ml. Abnormal CSF findings persist for several weeks.

Epidemiology & Control

The disease is endemic in mice and other animals (dogs, monkeys, guinea pigs) and is occasionally transmitted to man. There is no evidence of person-to-person spread. Infected gray house mice, probably the most common source of human infection, excrete the virus in urine and feces. The virus may be harbored by mice throughout their lives, and females transmit it to their offspring, which in turn become healthy carriers. The mode of transmission in man is not known, but contaminated dust and food are probably vehicles. *Trichinella spiralis* can be infected experimentally, and it has been suggested that this parasite may serve as a means of conveying the virus from one animal to another and perhaps through an intermediate host such as the pig to man.

Mice should be eliminated from the home.

ENCEPHALITIS LETHARGICA
(Von Economo's Disease)

Several thousand cases of this acute type of encephalitis occurred during the winter seasons between 1915 and 1926. Epidemics did not occur after that time, and the disease has not been seen in recent years. The etiology is presumed to have been viral. Pathology was similar to that produced by the neurotropic viruses. Onset was gradual, with malaise, headache, fever, and aching of joints and muscles; this was followed by signs suggesting mesencephalic involvement. Somnolence and stupor were common. The case fatality rate was about 40%. Neurologic sequelae (eg, paralysis agitans) are common in survivors.

EPIDEMIC NEUROMYASTHENIA
(Benign Myalgic Encephalomyelitis)

A number of outbreaks of epidemic neuromyasthenia has been reported in Europe and the USA. No etiologic agent has been isolated, although viruses are believed to play a role. The main features of the disease are fatigue, headache, intense muscle pain, slight and transient paresis, mental disturbances, and objective evidence of diffuse involvement of the CNS. The illness is sometimes confused with poliomyelitis. Young and middle-aged adults are principally afflicted. Sporadic cases have also been reported.

MENGO FEVER
(Columbia-SK Infection, Encephalomyocarditic Virus Infection)

This virus has been recovered in eastern USA and in Uganda. It appears to infect man only rarely, producing a mild febrile illness (3-day fever with spinal fluid lymphocytosis). Only one case has been proved by virus isolation. The patient had fever, headache, nuchal rigidity, photophobia, vomiting, and short periods of delirium. The virus was isolated from the blood on the first and second days of illness, and antibodies appeared during convalescence. A few instances have been recorded in which sera from individuals suffering from CNS diseases neutralized the virus.

The virus is pathogenic for many animals, including mice, guinea pigs, monkeys, and chick embryos. It has been isolated in nature from the cotton rat, mongoose, rhesus monkey, baboon, chimpanzee, and Taeniorhyncus mosquitoes. Neutralizing antibodies are present in wild rats collected in certain areas of the USA and Uganda, but they are rarely found in man. The virus can cause lesions in the CNS and in striated and cardiac muscle. An outbreak of fatal myocarditis in pigs caused by this virus has been observed.

The agent belongs to the picornavirus group. It has a diameter of about 25 nm and contains 30% RNA. It is a satisfactory antigen in the complement fixation test and also agglutinates sheep erythrocytes. Antibodies can be measured by neutralization, complement fixation, and hemagglutination inhibition methods.

CHRONIC VIRAL DISEASES OF THE CNS & OTHER PROGRESSIVE DEGENERATIVE DISORDERS
(Kuru, Amyotrophic Lateral Sclerosis, Slow Virus Diseases)

Studies of certain animal viruses have established that viruses are capable of producing chronic infections of the CNS which may be manifest as progressive degenerative disorders. These diseases include scrapie in sheep in England and Scotland and visna of sheep in Iceland. The progressive neurologic diseases produced by these 2 different viruses may have incubation periods of up to 5 years before the clinical manifestations of the infections become evident.

The agent of **scrapie** has been found to be unusually resistant to inactivation by heat, formalin, nucleases, and ultraviolet irradiation—properties that have led some investigators to consider it a member of an entirely new class of agents different from true viruses. Scrapie, which behaves as a recessive genetic trait in sheep, shows marked differences in genetic susceptibility of different breeds. Susceptibility to experimentally transmitted scrapie has been found to range from zero to over 80% in sheep, whereas goats are almost 100% susceptible.

Visna virus is an RNA lipid-containing virus morphologically similar to the viruses which cause leukosis in chickens (see Chapter 40). The virus infects all of the organs of the body of the infected sheep; however, pathologic changes are confined primarily to the brain, lungs, and reticuloendothelial system. There is a long incubation period, and virus can be recovered from the animal at least 4 years after inoculation. Infected animals develop antibodies to the virus; these can be detected in the CSF as well as the serum of sick animals.

Spongiform encephalopathies of man also appear to be of viral etiology. Spongiform degeneration of neurons is observed in Alpers disease (progressive diffuse cerebral degeneration of infants), Creutzfeldt-Jakob disease (subacute presenile dementia), and kuru, an unusual degenerative disease of the CNS found among certain tribes of New Guinea. Brain material from patients afflicted with kuru and Creutzfeldt-Jakob disease has been shown to produce similar diseases when injected into chimpanzees. Furthermore, the passage of diseased chimpanzee brain into healthy animals successfully transfers the diseases to other chimpanzees. The incubation period of the diseases in chimpanzees is measured in months or years.

Kuru occurs only in the Fore tribe and the neighboring tribes of the eastern highlands of New Guinea. The disease consists of relentless progressive ataxia, tremors, dysarthria, and emotional lability without significant dementia. It occurs more frequently in women than in men, which coincides with the customs around cannibalism. The remains of the dead were eaten primarily by women and children. Since cannibalism has been outlawed, the incidence of the disease has decreased, and it is now felt that this was the primary mode of transmission of the agent.

Chronic virus infections may be associated with a number of less exotic progressive degenerative diseases of the CNS of man. Russian virologists have reported isolation of a virus responsible for **"amyotrophic lateral sclerosis"** which has been passed to monkeys. The experimental disease had an incubation period of 5 years, and the histopathologic changes produced were similar to those of the natural disease of human beings. **Subacute sclerosing encephalitis,** a fatal disease characterized by inflammatory cell infiltration, gliosis, and demyelination of the CNS, had been shown by electron microscopy to be associated with helical structures morphologically resembling and antigenically similar to the internal components of measles virus. Recently, measles virus has been isolated from infected brain tissue by co-cultivation of the living tissue with normal human cells which are highly susceptible to the virus. Similar helical structures suggestive of an incomplete paramyxovirus have been observed in muscle biopsies in chronic **polymyositis.** The lesions of **progressive multifocal leukoencephalopathy** (a CNS complication found in some patients suffering from chronic leukemia, Hodgkin's disease, lymphosarcoma, and carcinomatosis) have been found to contain papovavirus particles.

Many workers consider **multiple sclerosis** to be the result of a hypersensitivity phenomenon associated with a disturbance in the immune mechanism. However, recent studies with scrapie and other CNS diseases of sheep suggest a viral etiology. Four of 7 British investigators developed a syndrome resembling multiple sclerosis while studying a neurologic disease of sheep called **swayback**. The demonstration of a transmissible agent in kuru and in some cases of amyotrophic lateral sclerosis, the presence of virus-like particles in lesions of some "degenerative" CNS diseases, and the epidemiologic features of multiple sclerosis and certain forms of parkinsonism (especially the parkinsonian dementia encountered among the Chamorro population of Guam) suggest that chronic virus infections may play a major role in these disorders.

Slow viruses often produce their disease by forming virus-antibody complexes which continue to circulate for long periods of time. The manifestation of the disease may be the result of the virus-antibody complex being deposited in the affected organ (see Chapter 27).

• • •

General References

Gajdusek, D.C., & others: Transmission of experimental kuru to the spider monkey (*Ateles geoffreyi*). Science 162:693–694, 1968.

Johnson, H.N.: Rabiesvirus. Pages 321–353 in: *Diagnostic Procedures for Viral and Rickettsial Infections*, 4th ed. American Public Health Association, 1969.

Porter, D.D., Larsen, A.E., & H.G. Porter: The pathogenesis of Aleutian disease of mink. I. In vivo viral replication and the host antibody response to viral antigen. J Exper Med 130:575–593, 1969.

Winkler, W.G., Schmidt, R.C., & R.K. Sikes: Evaluation of human rabies immune globulin and homologous and heterologous antibody. J Immunol 102:1314–1321, 1969.

34...

Myxovirus Group
(Influenza)

The name **myxovirus** indicates virus with an affinity for mucins, and was originally proposed for the first members of the group, the influenza viruses. They contain RNA in the form of helical nucleoprotein which is surrounded by an ether-sensitive envelope. The viruses are pleomorphic in shape and vary from 80 to more than 250 nm in diameter. Other viruses, including mumps, measles, respiratory syncytial, and parainfluenza viruses, have been found to possess certain characteristics in common with the influenza viruses and have been placed in the myxovirus group. The myxoviruses have been divided into 2 subgroups on the basis of the size of their inner ribonucleoprotein (RNP) helix: 9 nm for the myxoviruses and 18 nm for the paramyxoviruses (see Chapter 35).

Recently, several viruses with some of the characteristics of the myxovirus group have been reported. Among these are several human respiratory viruses now classified as coronaviruses (see Chapter 39) that have been isolated in human embryonic tracheal organ cultures. The pneumonia virus of mice has been examined, and the virus particle possesses an internal RNP helix of 11–15 nm, a diameter between that of the myxoviruses and paramyxoviruses. As more new virus isolates are examined, it may be necessary to expand or otherwise alter the present 2 subgroups of the myxoviruses.

INFLUENZA

Influenza is an acute respiratory tract infection which usually occurs in epidemics. Three immunologic types of influenza virus are known: A, B, and C. Antigenic changes appear to be continually taking place within the A group of influenza viruses and perhaps to a lesser degree in the B group, while influenza C appears to be antigenically stable. In addition to human types, influenza A strains are known for pigs, horses, ducks, and chickens (fowl plague).

Properties of the Virus
A. Size of Virus and Its Components: Typical of myxoviruses, influenza virus consists of spherical to pleomorphic particles having an external diameter of about 110 nm and an inner electron-dense core of 70 nm. The surface of the spherical virus (or filamentous form; see below) is covered with projections about 10 nm long. The internal component is made up of a helical ribonucleoprotein (RNP) structure about 9 nm in diameter and 800 nm in length. Virus can be broken down by ether treatment into (1) hemagglutinating units consisting of spherical particles about 35 nm in diameter (containing protein but no nucleic acid), and (2) a soluble complement fixing ribonucleoprotein antigen consisting of rod-like structures of variable length (mean about 60 nm) and about 9 nm in diameter. The soluble antigen seems to be an RNA-containing helix in the form of a double chain having 2-fold symmetry parallel to the particle axis. The helix appears to consist of hollow rings, each containing 5 or 6 spherical protein subunits 3 nm in diameter. A complete turn of each helix is made up of 5 or 6 subunits, with 50 or 60 subunits (5 complete turns of the helix) making up an average soluble antigen particle.

Purified hemagglutinin contains rosettes made from units identical in size and shape with those forming the outer surface projections of the complete virus particle. Associated with the hemagglutinin in the envelope is the enzyme, neuraminidase (sialidase), which can cleave N-acetylneuraminic acid esters.

Nucleic acid of the influenza virus is not a single molecule, and 5 distinct and separable components have been resolved. The summed molecular weight of these RNA pieces total close to 2 million daltons per virion. Because of a divided genome, these groups of viruses exhibit several biologic phenomena like high recombination frequency, multiplicity reactivation, and ability to synthesize hemagglutinin and neuraminidase after chemical inactivation of viral infectivity.

When high concentrations of the virus are used as inocula, defective virus particles are produced that are not infectious (Von Magnus phenomenon). This may also indicate an uncoordinated replication of discrete segments of viral RNA.

B. Reactions to Physical and Chemical Agents: Influenza virus is relatively stable and may be stored at 4° C for a week and at 0° C for longer periods. Infectivity is destroyed by heating at 56° C for a few minutes, by ultraviolet irradiation, and by treatment with ether, formaldehyde, phenol, and other protein denaturants. The hemagglutinin and the complement fixing antigens are more stable to physical and chemical agents than the mature, infective virus. However, the infectivity of virus can be stabilized by 1 M $MgSO_4$ to such a degree that heating at 50° C for 30 minutes has hardly any deleterious effect.

The virus is less stable at −20° C than at +4° C. The infectivity is best preserved at −70° C or by lyophilization of the crude virus suspensions.

C. Animal Susceptibility and Growth of Virus: Human strains of the virus can infect a number of different animals; ferrets are more susceptible than other species. Serial passage in mice increases its virulence for this animal, producing extensive pulmonary consolidation and death. The developing chick embryo readily supports the growth of virus, but for most strains even a high level of infection fails to produce grossly detectable lesions.

From the A/WS influenza virus, mutants were derived which grow readily in the mouse brain and induce in these animals fatal encephalitis.

The influenza viruses do not grow well in tissue cultures. In most instances, only an abortive growth cycle occurs, ie, viral subunits are synthesized but no new infectious progeny, or very little, is formed. It is possible to select mutants which will grow well and induce cytopathic effect and plagues (under agar overlay) in rhesus monkey kidney cells or calf kidney cells from virtually all influenza strains. Several passages are usually necessary before such viruses are isolated. Striking exceptions are the fowl plague virus and neurotropic mutant of WS virus (NWS) which grow well in tissue cultures of divergent origin. It has also been shown that this property can be transferred from these viruses to other influenza viruses by means of genetic recombination.

The multiplication of several influenza viruses has been studied in tissue culture systems supporting their growth. The infectious virion attaches to the surface of the host cell, and for a brief period its infectivity in the cell population decreases rapidly, thus indicating degradation of the virion. This period in which little infectious material can be found is the "virus eclipse" phase and is similar to the infection of bacteria by their viruses. Synthesis of viral RNA in the nucleus starts between 1 and 2 hours after infection and reaches maximum level at 3 hours; the early stage of the replication seems to be dependent on the cellular genome. A strong indication has been obtained from biophysical studies that the RNA pieces replicate independently. About 3 hours after infection, a specific nuclear staining is obtained with fluorescein labeled antiribonucleoprotein (S) antibody. The nuclear fluorescence increases with time, and the immunofluorescent antigen then enters the cytoplasm. This transition requires synthesis of a new protein. About 4 hours after infection, an increase in the hemagglutinin or viral (V) antigen can be observed; unlike the S antigen, however, it is found exclusively in the cytoplasm. After their production, the 2 viral components diffuse to the cell margin, where they are assembled together with neuraminidase to become new infective virus particles by budding from the cell membrane. The site of synthesis of neuraminidase in the infected cell has not been determined. It is believed that its function is necessary for the last stage of virus growth, ie, for the release of infectious particles from the cells.

The rate of virus increase varies with the amount of virus inoculated. With large doses of seed virus, maximum levels are reached within 12–15 hours after inoculation, whereas with smaller doses the peak of virus activity is not attained until 48 hours after inoculation. Comparison of the virus levels ultimately reached has shown that the total amount of viral material produced—as measured by hemagglutinins—is virtually the same regardless of the multiplicity of infection. However, the amount of infective virus produced with large doses of inoculum is less than that produced in eggs infected with small doses of virus. The dissociation between fully infective particle and hemagglutinin becomes more marked on serial passage of undiluted allantoic fluid by the allantoic route. Under such circumstances large amounts of hemagglutinating but noninfective virus ("incomplete" virus) are produced. Such incomplete virus interferes with and inhibits multiplication of infective virus. This phenomenon is called the Von Magnus effect, after the investigator who discovered it.

Preparations of incomplete virus exhibit a higher degree of pleomorphy and most of the particles lack the electron-dense center where the RNA soluble antigen is located. The incomplete virus does not undergo multiplicity reactivation, suggesting that the missing part of the RNA might be the same in different incomplete virus particles.

The multiplication of influenza virus is inhibited by amantadine (see Treatment), dactinomycin, *p*-fluorophenylalanine, and mitomycin C.

D. Biologic Properties: Influenza viruses were the first found with the capacity to agglutinate erythrocytes. The reaction takes place in 3 stages: (1) adsorption of virus by the erythrocytes, (2) agglutination of the erythrocyte-virus aggregates, and (3) spontaneous dissociation of virus from erythrocytes. Red cells which have once combined with and released virus can no longer combine with the same or closely related virus strains but can combine with different virus strains. Yet the virus is not changed; if it is added to fresh erythrocytes, the cycle of adsorption, agglutination, and spontaneous dissociation can be repeated many times. The reaction is enzyme-like in nature. A mucoprotein substrate or receptor for the virus is present in the stroma of the red cell, and this is destroyed by the virus enzyme (neuraminidase). The enzyme has been identified with the protein rods projecting from the surface of the virus.

A cycle similar to that described for hemagglutination by influenza virus also occurs between the virus and cells of the respiratory tract. Virus is adsorbed and subsequently released spontaneously from the cells of the lung. This is the first stage of infection of a susceptible cell by influenza virus.

The soluble particles are not infective, are not adsorbed on red cells, and do not cause hemagglutination. The ribonucleoprotein component can be demonstrated only by complement fixation tests, in which it acts as a strong antigen. Antibodies to the soluble antigen usually develop only after infection and not after vaccination with killed virus.

Vaccine preparations containing large amounts of free ribonucleoprotein antigen were shown to induce antibody to this substance. Thus, the complement fixation test with ribonucleoprotein antigen is not a completely reliable means for differentiating between infection and antibody response due to vaccine administration.

The infectious virus particles induce in animals the development of virus neutralizing and other antibody, and the inoculated animals become resistant to infection. The virus particles also fix complement in the presence of immune serum, but this complement fixing antigen is different from that associated with the soluble substance. It is strain-specific. A similar antigenicity is exhibited in the complement fixation test by the hemagglutinin isolated after the virus is disrupted by ether treatment. However, there is evidence that the liberated viral subunit is antigenically broader than the intact particle. Influenza virus administered in large amounts is toxic for laboratory animals. The effect is apparently associated directly with the virus particles and can be prevented by specific antibody.

In addition to the spherical particles, elongated forms possessing the same surface projections have been observed. The filamentous forms react with erythrocytes in precisely the same way as do the spherical virus particles; they can be adsorbed onto the red cell membrane and then spontaneously eluted from it. After heat inactivation, both forms of virus are adsorbed together on the red cell membrane and neither is spontaneously eluted. Addition of homologous antiserum, however, removes both filamentous and round forms from the membrane, while heterologous serum has no such effect. Finally, studies using the darkfield microscope have shown that only homologous immune serum can agglutinate the filaments. They may represent a stage in virus multiplication, and it has been suspected that at least some of the spheres arise by segmentation of the long forms. In its early passages in chick embryos, the virus is usually in filamentous form, but with serial passage it takes on the spherical appearance described above. Whether the virus is spherical or filamentous in the human host is not known. Genetic studies demonstrated that the morphology of the virion is under the control of the viral genome.

Neuraminidase is closely related to hemagglutinin by its location but is antigenically distinct from it. Antibody against the neuraminidase does not neutralize the virus, but it modifies the infection by its effect on the release of virus from the cells. The antibody against the neuraminidase was found in sera of infected mice and also in sera of humans who experienced natural infection. It has been shown in mice that the presence of antineuraminidase antibody results in marked protection.

In the laboratory, genetic recombination between the different influenza strains is frequently observed. It can be achieved more easily with closely related than with distant viruses, and more so when one of the parent viruses has been inactivated by heat or by ultraviolet irradiation. In some of the crossings a much higher frequency of recombinants (up to more than 50%) was obtained than might be expected from the size of the influenza virus RNA. It has been suggested that this phenomenon may be due to the existence of viral RNA in several physical units which replicate independently and are then assembled into infectious virions.

Pathogenesis & Pathology

The virus enters the respiratory tract in airborne droplets. Viremia has been reported rarely. Virus is present in the nasopharynx from 1—2 days before to 1—2 days after onset of symptoms. The virus enzyme, neuraminidase, lowers the viscosity of the mucous film in the respiratory tract, laying bare the cellular surface receptors and promoting the spread of virus-containing fluid to lower portions of the tract. Even when antibodies are present in the blood they may not protect against infection. Antibodies must be present in sufficient concentration at the site of action of the virus, ie, at the superficial cells of the respiratory tract. This can only be achieved if the antibody level in the blood is high or if specialized antibody is secreted locally.

Inflammation of the upper respiratory tract is the usual extent of pathology. Pneumonia, when it occurs, may be followed by death. In such cases, the lungs show interstitial inflammation, with necrosis of bronchiolar and alveolar epithelium. The virus causes necrosis of the ciliated and goblet cells of the tracheal and bronchial mucosa but does not affect the basal layer of epithelium. The pneumonia is often associated with secondary bacterial invaders: staphylococci, pneumococci, streptococci, and *Hemophilus influenzae*.

Clinical Findings

The incubation period is only 1 or 2 days. Chills, malaise, fever, muscular aches, prostration, and respiratory symptoms may occur but are not pathognomonic. The fever persists for about 3 days, complications are not common, and in general the disease is not serious. The severity of the pandemic of 1918—1919 has been attributed to the fact that pneumonia developed, often secondary and of bacterial etiology. Infection due to influenza C virus appears to be much milder than that due to influenza A or B viruses.

When influenza appears in epidemic form, the clinical findings are consistent enough so that the disease can be diagnosed in most cases on this basis alone; sporadic cases are almost impossible to diagnose solely on clinical grounds. Mild as well as asymptomatic infections occur.

The pandemic of 1957—1958 was clinically a mild disease. However, during the early winter of 1957—1958, in 100 cities of the USA, deaths were 40,000 above expectancy. Of the associated pneumonias, the largest number were pneumococcal. However, the vast majority of pneumonia associated deaths were in the small (10%) staphylococcal group. Two to 3 months after the first wave of infections, a second wave of 20,000 influenza and pneumonia deaths occurred. In most of the fatal cases, typical influenza symptoms preceded the pneumonia; from a number of the cases studied, influenza virus was obtained from the lung tissue at autopsy. In young children, influenza A_2 (Asian type) has been associated with croup.

The lethal impact of an influenza epidemic is reflected in the excess deaths due to cardiovascular and renal diseases as well as those due to pneumonia and influenza. Pregnant women and older persons suffering from chronic diseases have a higher risk of death.

Laboratory Diagnosis

Influenza can be readily diagnosed by laboratory procedures. For antibody determinations, the first serum should be taken less than 5 days after onset and the second about 10–14 days later.

For rapid detection of influenza virus in clinical specimens, the detection of complement fixing antigens within infected tissues may be sought within 24 hours after inoculation. Another rapid method is the detection of positive smears from nasal swabs and washings by specific staining with fluorescein-labeled antibody.

A. Recovery of Virus: Throat washings or garglings are obtained within 3 days after onset and stored frozen. Penicillin and streptomycin are added to limit bacterial contamination, and embryonated eggs are inoculated by the amniotic route. Amniotic and allantoic fluids are harvested 2–4 days later and tested for hemagglutinins by the addition of 1% suspensions of chicken and guinea pig erythrocytes. If results are negative, passage is made to fresh embryos. If hemagglutinins are not detected after 2 such passages, the result is negative.

Primate cell cultures (human or monkey) have been reported to be even more susceptible than embryonated eggs, but only to certain human strains of influenza virus.

If a strain of virus is isolated—as demonstrated by the presence of hemagglutinins—it is titrated in the presence of type-specific influenza sera to determine its type. The new virus belongs to the same type as the serum which inhibits its hemagglutinating power.

The phenomenon of hemadsorption is utilized for the early detection of virus growth in cultures. Erythrocytes from guinea pigs or human O cells are added to the cultures 24–48 hours after the clinical specimens have been inoculated, and the reaction is viewed under the low power lens. When positive, characteristic patterns are formed, with the red blood cells firmly attached to the cell culture sheets as rosettes or chains of erythrocytes. Cultures which are negative at 24 hours can be reincubated for several more days with the red blood cell suspensions and examined periodically. The cytopathogenic effects of the influenza viruses are often minimal and difficult to detect in tissue cultures, and the production of hemagglutinin may be too low to permit its detection in the culture fluid. Hemadsorption provides a more sensitive testing procedure.

B. Serology: Paired sera can be used to detect rises in hemagglutination inhibiting, complement fixing, or virus neutralizing antibodies. Of these, the hemagglutination inhibiting antibody is most frequently employed. Normal sera often contain nonspecific mucoprotein inhibitors which must first be destroyed by treatment with RDE (receptor-destroying enzyme of *Vibrio cholerae* cultures), trypsin, carbon dioxide, or periodate. Because normal persons usually have influenza antibodies, a 4-fold or greater increase in titer is necessary to indicate influenza infection. Peak levels of antibodies are present 2 weeks after onset, persist for about 4 weeks, and then gradually fall during the course of a year to preinfection levels. When using the strain-specific complement fixation test (with V antigen), the peak antibody levels are found in the fourth week.

Within one type of influenza virus, strains may differ markedly in antigenicity. It is essential to use recently isolated strains, preferably strains isolated at about the time the patient whose sera are under test became ill.

Complement fixing antigens are of 2 types. One is the soluble substance (S antigen), which is antigenically type-specific but fails to show antigenic differences between strains of one type. The other is associated with the virus particle itself (V antigen) and is highly specific for different strains within each type; the reaction with viral antigen is at least as specific as that demonstrable by the hemagglutination inhibition test, and at times is even more specific. Furthermore, after infection with the Asian strain, it also proved more sensitive and should be used in diagnostic laboratories. It is of special advantage for demonstrating antibody rise when the first serum specimen was not taken early after the onset of the disease.

Immunity

Three distinct and immunologically unrelated types of influenza virus are known; they are referred to as influenza A, B, and C. In addition, the swine influenza viruses are antigenically related to the influenza A virus. Influenza C virus exists as a single and stable antigenic type, in contrast to the variations known among the influenza A and B viruses.

At least 18 different antigenic components have been determined in type A strains of influenza virus by quantitative adsorption methods. More undoubtedly exist, for only 29 strains have been adequately studied in this fashion. Strains share their antigenic components, but in varying proportions. For example, the 1947 strains known as A′ or A_1 possess major antigens in common with 1946–1950 strains and minor antigens in common with 1934 and 1953 strains. A strain generally shares its major antigens with strains prevalent within a few years of its isolation; its minor antigens, with strains prevalent several more years before or after its isolation. The wide sharing of antigenic components in some of the new isolates indicates that the antigenic components of strains prevalent several years ago have not completely disappeared, even though the most common antigens are of the most recent A_2 (Asian) set.

Two possible mechanisms for the antigenic variation of influenza virus have been suggested:

(1) All the possible configurations may be present in a pool of antigens which exist throughout the globe; from these, highly infectious strains arise and initiate epidemics. As antibody levels to recent strains are usually high in the human population, these will inhibit strains with major antigens which were dominant in recently prevalent strains and will select strains of different antigenic composition.

Serial passage of virus in mice vaccinated with the homologous strain yields a virus with an apparent rearrangement of antigens, or the appearance of new antigens. The passage virus multiplies more readily in mice vaccinated with the parent virus, and it evokes an antibody which reacts well with the passage virus but only poorly with the parent strain. The change in antigenic character evolves slowly on passage; a change of great magnitude involving almost all the antigenic components of the virus does not occur quickly.

(2) Antigenically different strains may be selected by means of genetic recombination induced by environmental factors such as passage in a partially immune host. When critical concentrations of 2 strains of influenza virus are simultaneously injected into mice or eggs, a new strain sharing the properties of each parent strain may be recovered; this has been attributed to genetic recombination. However, another interpretation of these findings is that the 2 "parent" strains may mutually interfere and prevent the multiplication of the characteristic major particles from each strain, thus allowing the minority particles of each strain to be selected for replication. This might result in the recovery of strains with antigens capable of reacting with one or both of the "parent" strains but featuring still other heretofore unrecognized components.

Antibodies are important in immunity against influenza, but they must be present at the site of virus invasion. Before antibodies can be detected in the respiratory secretions they must exist in high concentration in the serum. The transient immunity which exists in influenza probably reflects the fact that the infectious process is limited to the mucous membranes of the respiratory tract. Mucoids which may block enzymatically inactive virus particles from attaching to susceptible cells are present in respiratory secretions, but their role in resistance to influenza virus is imperfectly understood.

Treatment

In the past there was no specific treatment for influenza. Amantadine hydrochloride (Symmetrel), a symmetrical amine, is the first antiviral drug for systemic administration to be licensed in the USA. Although in laboratory test systems the compound inhibits many myxoviruses, including several influenza A and C strains, one parainfluenza strain, and rubella virus, its use is indicated only for A_2. The drug acts by blocking the penetration of influenza A_2 into cells, thereby preventing viral replication and cell destruction. Since the drug has no effect on virus per se, early administration after contact with persons suffering from influenza A_2 seems essential. The drug is not intended for treatment of the established disease or for use against influenzal or respiratory diseases other than influenza A_2. Strains of influenza B, Newcastle disease, mumps, most strains of parainfluenza, and measles virus are all resistant to the drug. Members of other major groups of RNA and DNA viruses have all been found to be resistant.

When doses in excess of those indicated are given, CNS manifestations such as nervousness, insomnia, dizziness, drunken feeling, slurred speech, ataxia, inability to concentrate, and some psychic reactions (including depression and feelings of detachment) may occur. The use of the drug in persons with CNS disease, particularly geriatric patients with cerebral arteriosclerosis and patients with a history of epilepsy or other "seizures," should be strictly controlled for possible adverse effects.

Amantadine inhibits the mitogenic action of phytohemagglutinin on human peripheral leukocytes. The question has been raised whether the low incidence of antibody responders in amantadine-treated persons exposed to influenza virus might be due to the inhibition of cellular proliferation of immunocytes by the drug.

Epidemiology

Influenza occurs in successive waves of infection, with peak incidences during the winter. Influenza A infections may vary from a few isolated cases to extensive outbreaks which within a few weeks involve 10% or more of the population, with rates of 50—75% in children of school age. The period between epidemic waves of influenza A is 2—3 years. Influenza B does not spread through a community as quickly as influenza A. Its interepidemic period varies from 3—6 years. Extensive pandemics have occurred. During the pandemic of 1918—1919, over 20 million people died following influenza infection, a large number from pneumonia due to secondary bacterial invaders.

About 80 million cases occurred during the 1957—1958 pandemic of Asian influenza (a new type A strain designated A_2). The illnesses were generally mild, but the estimated number of pneumonia-influenza deaths in the USA was about 60,000 above normal during the pandemic.

Asian strain influenza virus was disseminated extensively around the world within 3 months after the disease spread from the mainland of China to Hong Kong (spring of 1957). The seeding of virus in Europe and in the USA during the summer months prepared for the epidemic disease which occurred in the fall season. The pandemic occurred over the globe in a period of 6 months. Increased human mobility was responsible for the rapid spread. Many outbreaks in the early stages of the pandemic could be directly traced to passengers and crews of air and surface vessels which had recently arrived from epidemic regions.

The next cycle of epidemic influenza, in 1962, was caused by influenza B. At that time over 12,000 excess deaths occurred, all among the elderly (age 65 and over). In 1963, an epidemic of A_2 influenza occurred with 34,000 excess deaths. The deaths were mainly among the elderly. In the epidemics of the last 10 years, children under 1 year of age have almost never been involved.

In the summer of 1968, an outbreak of influenza was reported from Hong Kong which then spread rapidly around the world. In the USA there were an estimated 30 million cases with nearly 20,000 deaths. This epidemic was due to a new antigenic variant. Although the isolates were still classified as influenza A_2, they exhibited a greater dissimilarity from earlier A_2 strains than had been previously observed. The A_2 Hong Kong viruses exhibited a low reciprocal cross with influenza A equine type 2 strains, which was never observed with earlier isolates.

The main reason for the periodic occurrence of epidemic influenza is the accumulation of a sufficient number of susceptibles in a population which harbors the virus in a few subclinical or minor infections throughout the year. Epidemics may be started when the virus mutates to a new antigenic type which has survival advantages and to which antibodies in the population are low. Antibodies against the pandemic Asian strain were very rare prior to 1957 except in persons who were alive during 1889.

Studies in the serologic epidemiology of influenza have been revealing. Antibodies against swine influenza (believed by some to be related to the pandemic influenza strain of 1918) are not found in persons born after 1923. Persons born during 1923–1933 had their first influenza experience with a type A virus closely related to the 1933 WS strain, the first influenza virus to be isolated. Those born between 1934 and 1943 do not possess swine or WS antibodies, but have antibodies against another type A virus, PR-8.

Another antigenic change occurred among the A viruses in 1946. Strains occurring between 1946 and 1957 have been called A_1 strains because, although related to the older viruses, they had a major difference in antigenic constitution. The influenza antibodies in persons born between 1946 and 1957 are chiefly against the A_1 strains.

Most of the world's population probably has been immunized with the A_1 strains, because almost all sera contain detectable titers of A_1 antibody. However, during the 10-year period of A_1 prevalence there were many modifications of antigenic structure even within the A_1 group of viruses. With the widespread appearance of the type A_2 Asian strain in 1957, the A_1 set of viruses has been largely replaced, just as the PR-8 set of viruses disappeared when the A_1 set began its period of prevalence in 1947.

Type A_2 virus seems to be related to previous influenza viruses, in that sera in 1957 from people who were 70 years of age or older often contained antibody against A_2 isolates. Furthermore, anti-A_2 antibody increases were found in sera from this age group after injections of type A vaccine which did not contain the A_2 virus (anamnestic response). This indicates that viruses prevalent during the 1889 pandemic contained antigens shared with the 1957 Asian strains.

Influenza B type appears to be changing antigenically since almost all strains of type B influenza virus isolated in 1965–1966 were closely related to B/Singapore/3/64, which differs significantly from the formerly prevalent variant represented by B/Johannesburg/33/58 or B/Maryland/1/59.

In early years of life the range of the influenza antibody spectrum is narrow, but it becomes progressively broader in later years. The antibodies (and immunity) acquired from the initial infections of childhood are of limited range and reflect the dominant antigens of the prevailing strains. Later exposures to viruses of related but differing antigenic composition result in an antibody broadening toward a larger number of the common antigens of influenza viruses. Exposures later in life to antigenically related strains result in a progressive reinforcement of the primary antibody. The highest antibody levels in a particular age group therefore reflect the dominant antigens of the virus responsible for the childhood infections of the group. Thus, a serologic recapitulation of past infection with influenza viruses of different antigenic makeup can be obtained by studying the age distribution of influenza antibodies in normal populations.

Recent studies have been made on sera of isolated Pacific islanders whose only exposure to influenza occurred during the time of the 1918 pandemic. Neutralizing antibody titers were greatest to the human A strains (PR-8 and BH) which were isolated in 1934 and 1935; they were significantly lower to swine influenza virus (isolated in 1931), and absent to human type A viruses isolated in 1940–1946, to the later human types A_1 and A_2, and to the later equine A types 1 and 2. There is evidence that antibody to swine influenza virus in cosmopolitan populations may be the result of cumulative infections with a variety of human type A strains. Thus, antibodies to the swine strain in almost all persons born before 1923 might be the result of additional infections and broadening of the antibody response. The study in the Pacific islanders rests solely upon the single infection by the 1918 pandemic virus and indicates that the viruses circulating 17 years later were still antigenically related to the virus that caused the catastrophe of 1918.

Control

The subcutaneous inoculation of influenza virus, inactivated by formalin or ultraviolet irradiation, induces in man a relatively transient increase in resistance to infection with the same or with closely related strains. The experimental use of vaccines emulsified in mineral oil and injected intramuscularly has given higher and more lasting antibody responses.

In 1947, the encouraging results which had been achieved with influenza vaccination up to that time received a setback: Vaccines prepared with strains recovered earlier proved ineffective because of the appearance in that year of new so-called type A_1 strains. Since then, the vaccines available have been more effective for the epidemic strain of previous years than for those of future outbreaks. In addition to the changing antigenicity of influenza strains, there are other difficulties with vaccination. The currently available vaccines are made from infected chick embryos. They contain a high concentration of virus material which possesses toxic properties even though it is no longer infectious. It may cause distress in a fair number of persons, especially in children. Because it also contains chick materials, it may at times lead to sensitization or even to severe allergic reactions in persons already hypersensitive.

The recommended adult dose of polyvalent vaccine for 1969–1970 contains 400 chick cell agglutinating (CCA) units of Hong Kong strain 1968 antigen and 300 CCA units of type B 1966 antigen. Persons who have not previously been immunized should also receive a second dose of 1 ml about 2 months after the first injection. Persons previously immunized with polyvalent vaccine should be reinoculated with a booster dose of 1 ml subcutaneously when threatened by an influenza epidemic.

Children 6–12 years of age should receive 0.5 ml subcutaneously. Those not previously immunized should receive a second dose of 0.5 ml about 2 months after the first injection.

Preschool children over 3 months old should receive 2 initial doses of 0.1–0.2 ml subcutaneously at intervals of 1–2 weeks. A booster injection of the same strength should be given 2–3 months later. Since febrile reactions to vaccine in this age group may reach an incidence of 20%, it is suggested that aspirin be given unless contraindicated.

Vaccination should be performed as soon as practicable after September 1 and before the beginning of the usual influenza season in late December. Since a 2-week delay in the development of antibodies may be expected, it is important that immunization be carried out before epidemics occur in the area.

It is possible that the number of antigens might be finite even though they vary in proportions from one influenza strain to the next. If several strains of differing but broad antigenic composition are included in the vaccine, effective control against influenza might still become possible. Such a vaccine should yield an antigenic mass in which all known influenza antigens are adequately represented. On the other hand, the possibility of antigenic drift among these agents might be almost limitless, and the outlook for effective control dubious.

An attenuated live virus vaccine has been developed and used widely in the USSR. Attenuated strains have been prepared by serial transfer of influenza strains through embryonated eggs. They are antigenically identical with the virulent ones, but when administered intranasally in high concentrations they do not produce local or general symptoms in adults and produce only mild symptoms in children. However, they multiply in the upper respiratory tract and produce immunity.

It is strongly recommended that for immunization one should use commercially available vaccine made from **purified** virus which contains much less nonviral protein, or vaccine made from **subviral antigens**. For the latter, the intact virion is disrupted by ether treatment and the nucleic acid is selectively removed by precipitation, leaving the virus proteins. Such purified noninfectious viral antigens do not produce fever or other symptoms even in sensitive preschool children. Infants may be given 40 times the recommended permissible dose of the present vaccine with no ill effects but with a greater antibody response. Another possible advantage of this type of vaccine is that the ether disruption may expose antigenic components hidden in the intact virion, and consequently the antibody response may be broader than after administration of vaccines prepared from the intact virion.

Although older age groups have the lowest incidence of influenza, the case fatality rate is highest among them. This is particularly true in those who suffer from chronic debilitating disease, including cardiovascular, pulmonary, renal, or metabolic disorders. Such persons at high risk should receive commercial influenza vaccine on a regular basis (provided they are not hypersensitive to eggs or egg products).

• • •

General References

Kingsbury, D.W.: Replication and functions of myxovirus ribonucleic acids. Progr Med Virol 12:49–77. 1970.

Peck, F.B.: Purified influenza virus vaccine: A study of viral reactivity and antigenicity. JAMA 206:2277–2282, 1968.

Pereira, H.G.: Influenza: Antigenic spectrum. Progr Med Virol 11:46-79, 1969.

Robinson, R.Q., & W.R. Dowdle: Influenza viruses. Pages 414–433 in: *Diagnostic Procedures for Viral and Rickettsial Infections,* 4th ed. American Public Health Association, 1969.

Schulman, J.L.: Effects of immunity on transmission of influenza: Experimental studies. Progr Med Virol 12:128–160, 1970.

35...
Paramyxovirus Group
& Rubella Virus

The paramyxoviruses include the viruses of mumps, measles, parainfluenza, respiratory syncytial (RS) disease, and Newcastle disease. The group includes RNA viruses with an 18 nm inner helix. They possess an ether-sensitive envelope having a diameter ranging from 100–300 nm in size. Related members exist in other species; human measles virus is related to canine distemper and bovine rinderpest viruses. Simian, bovine, and bat parainfluenza viruses are known.

Rubella virus has been recently found not to belong to the paramyxovirus group; however, since the virus is presently unclassified, it will be considered in this chapter because of similarities of its epidemiologic and clinical features to those of certain paramyxoviruses. However, its physical and chemical characteristics place it in a newly defined group, the **togaviruses**.

MUMPS
(Epidemic Parotitis)

Mumps is an acute contagious disease characterized by a nonsuppurative enlargement of one or both of the parotid glands, although other organs may also be involved.

Properties of the Virus
A. Size: The RNA virus particles vary considerably in size, the mean diameter being about 175–200 nm. The helix diameter is 18 nm.
B. Reactions to Physical and Chemical Agents: The hemagglutinin, the hemolysin, and the infectivity of the virus are destroyed by heating at 56° C for 20 minutes. The allergic antigen and the complement fixing antigen are more heat stable, withstanding 65° C and 80° C respectively for 30 minutes.

The attenuated vaccine virus is stable for 1 year in the lyophilized state; when reconstituted, it is stable for 8 hours at 40° C.
C. Animal Susceptibility and Growth of Virus: In monkeys, mumps can produce a disease which is very much like that in human beings. Parotitis is produced by introducing the virus into Stensen's duct or directly into the gland by injection. The swollen gland is a good source of virus or of skin-testing antigen. By the use of fluorescent antibody, the virus has been located in the cytoplasm of acinar cells.

The virus also grows readily in embryonated eggs, especially in the amniotic sac. Passage of mumps virus generation after generation in such embryos so modifies the virus that its pathogenicity for man and monkeys is greatly decreased. This method of attenuation was used to prepare the live virus vaccine. The virus has also been grown in newborn hamsters and tissue culture, in which it may produce large multinucleated giant cells (syncytia).

D. Biologic Properties: Several types of activity are associated with mumps virus:

1. Ability to induce the disease in susceptible hosts. The intact virus particle is essential for this property to be manifest.

2. Hemagglutinin for chicken, human, and other erythrocytes is also associated with the virus particle. The hemagglutinin becomes adsorbed to red cells but elutes from them when the suspension is brought to 37° C. It appears to be related to the hemagglutinins of parainfluenza and Newcastle disease viruses. Sera containing mumps antibodies inhibit viral hemagglutination, and the hemagglutination inhibition test for the detection of antibodies is based on this reaction.

3. Hemolysin for chick erythrocytes. This is also a property of the virus particle but is distinct from the hemagglutinin.

4. Soluble (S) complement fixing antigen, which is smaller than the virus particle and found in tissue in which virus is actively multiplying (chorioallantoic membrane). The S antigen forms the core of the virion and can be released by treatment of the virus with ether.

5. Viral (V) complement fixing antigen, which is a property of the virus particle itself. The V antigen is found in allantoic fluid which receives mature virus liberated from infected cells.

6. A skin test antigen for determining hypersensitivity to mumps virus. A reaction of erythema and induration indicates immunity.

Pathogenesis & Pathology
Two theories exist regarding the pathogenesis of mumps. (1) The virus travels from the mouth by way of Stensen's duct to the parotid gland where it undergoes primary multiplication. This is followed by a generalized viremia and localization in testes, ovaries, pancreas, or brain. (2) Primary replication occurs in the superficial epithelium of the respiratory tract. This

is followed by a generalized viremia and simultaneous localization in the salivary glands and other organs.

Little tissue damage is associated with uncomplicated mumps. The ducts of the parotid glands show desquamation of the epithelium, and polymorphonuclear cells are present in the lumens. There is interstitial edema and lymphocytic infiltration. With severe orchitis, the testis is congested and punctate hemorrhage as well as degeneration of the epithelium of the seminiferous tubules is observed. Other than the increased number of lymphocytes in the CSF, the changes induced by the virus in the CNS are unknown.

Clinical Features

The incubation period ranges from 12–35 days but most commonly is 18–21 days. A prodromal period of malaise and anorexia is followed by rapid enlargement of one or both parotid glands as well as other salivary glands. Swelling may be confined to one parotid gland, or one gland may enlarge several days before the other. The gland enlargement is associated with pain, especially when tasting acid substances. The salivary adenitis is commonly accompanied by fever and lasts for approximately a week.

The testicles and ovaries may be affected, especially during puberty. Twenty percent of males over 13 years of age who are infected with mumps virus develop orchitis, which is often unilateral and does not usually lead to sterility. Because of the lack of elasticity of the tunica albuginea, which does not allow the inflamed testicle to swell, atrophy of the testicle follows pressure necrosis. Secondary sterility does not occur in women because the ovary, which has no such limiting membrane, can swell when inflamed.

Mumps accounts for 10–15% of aseptic meningitis observed in the USA and is more common among males than females. Meningoencephalitis usually occurs 5–7 days after the inflammation of the salivary glands; however, the CNS complication may occur simultaneously or in the absence of parotitis and is rarely fatal. The CSF usually contains leukocytes, ranging from 10 to over 2000/cu mm (average, 200–600/cm mm); the white cells present are chiefly lymphocytes. Pleocytosis may persist for weeks, even after the patient appears to have recovered.

Other rare complications of mumps include (1) a self-limiting polyarthritis which resolves without residual deformity; (2) pancreatitis associated with transient hyperglycemia, glycosuria, and steatorrhea; (3) nephritis; and (4) thyroiditis.

Laboratory Diagnosis

Laboratory studies are usually not required to establish the diagnosis of typical cases. However, mumps can sometimes be confused with suppurative enlargement of the parotids, enlargements resulting from foreign bodies in the salivary ducts, tumors, and other conditions involving the salivary glands. In cases without parotitis, particularly in aseptic meningitis, the laboratory can be particularly helpful, for it is impossible to diagnose mumps from clinical observations alone if the salivary glands are not involved.

A. Recovery of Virus: Isolation of virus from patients should be attempted only with saliva, CSF, or urine collected within 4 or 5 days after the onset of illness. The saliva should be taken near the orifices of Stensen's ducts. After treatment with antibiotics, the specimen is inoculated into the amniotic cavities of 8-day-old chick embryos. Five days later, the amniotic fluid is tested for virus by mixing a few drops with erythrocytes and looking for hemagglutination. The identity of the virus is established by suitable neutralization tests with known antisera.

Monkey kidney cells in culture are more sensitive than embryonated eggs to human strains of mumps virus. Virus present in inoculated tubes may be detected in 2–5 days by adsorption of chicken or guinea pig red cells by the infected cells. An 0.4% suspension of red blood cells is added to cell cultures, and hemadsorption is detected after incubation at room temperature for 3–5 minutes or at 4° C for 20–30 minutes.

B. Serology: Antibody rise may be detected by testing matched acute and convalescent sera, the first sample being taken as soon after the onset of illness as possible, the second about 2–3 weeks later. The complement fixation test is recommended for specificity and accuracy, although other antibody tests (especially hemagglutination inhibition) may be used. A 4-fold or greater rise in antibody titer is evidence of mumps infection.

A complement fixation test on a single serum sample obtained soon after onset of illness may serve for a presumptive diagnosis if both soluble (S) and viral (V) antibodies are measured. S antibodies develop early, within a few days after onset, and sometimes reach a high titer before V antibodies can be detected. In early convalescence, both S and V antibodies are present at a high level. Subsequently, S antibodies disappear more rapidly, leaving V antibodies as a long-term marker of previous infection. After several years, even V antibodies may be hardly detectable or present at low levels (1:4 serum dilution). The intradermal injection of ultraviolet- or heat-inactivated virus stimulates the reappearance of V antibodies in high titer. Neutralizing antibodies, which also appear during convalescence, can be determined in eggs, but more easily in tissue culture, using the degree of inhibition of viral cytopathogenicity as a measure of antibodies. Mumps virus and Newcastle disease virus have a common antigen which can be demonstrated by complement fixation or hemagglutination inhibition reactions.

C. Skin Test Antigen: The skin test is of no value in the diagnosis of mumps, for hypersensitivity is first noted during the convalescent period, about 3–4 weeks after onset. The skin test is useful to detect susceptible persons who have previously escaped infection. The reaction in the skin is read 2 days after the antigen is inoculated.

Immunity

Immunity is permanent after a single infection. Only one antigenic type exists. Passive immunity is transferred from mother to offspring; thus it is rare to see mumps in infants under 6 months of age.

The noninfective skin-testing antigen available commercially may induce antibody formation or increase titers which have fallen to low levels. The response is better in older age groups; it indicates that they had been exposed previously and that their response is a recall or anamnestic phenomenon.

Treatment

Gamma globulin, prepared from mumps convalescent serum, can decrease the incidence of orchitis when given immediately after parotitis is first noted. Gamma globulin from normal adults is of no value for this purpose, for the antibody levels found in normal adults are low.

Epidemiology

Mumps occurs throughout the world, endemically throughout the year. Epidemics are facilitated where crowding favors the dissemination of the virus. The disease reaches its highest incidence in children 5–15 years of age, but epidemics in army camps are not uncommon. The peak incidence occurs in winter and spring. Although morbidity rates are high, mortality is negligible, even when the nervous system is involved.

The only known reservoir of infection is man. It is believed to be transmitted by direct contact, airborne droplets, or fomites contaminated with saliva. The recent demonstration of mumps virus in urine raises the possibility of urine as a source of natural infection. The period of communicability is believed to be from about 4 days before to about a week after the onset of symptoms. More intimate contact is necessary for the transmission of mumps than for measles or varicella.

About 30–40% of infections with mumps virus are inapparent. Individuals with subclinical mumps acquire immunity. During the course of inapparent infection, they can serve as sources of infection for others.

Antibodies to mumps virus are transferred across the placenta and are gradually lost during the first 6 months of life. In urban areas, antibodies are then acquired gradually, so that the 15-year-old group has about the same prevalence of persons with antibodies as the adult group. Antibodies are acquired at the same rate by persons living under favorable or unfavorable socioeconomic conditions.

Control

Mumps is usually a mild childhood disease and immunization for prevention does not carry the same urgency as the more serious preventable diseases, ie, polio, diphtheria, and tetanus. However, a live attenuated virus vaccine is available, and its use is recommended for children over 1 year of age and for adolescents and adults who have not had mumps parotitis. A single dose of the vaccine given subcutaneously produces detectable antibodies in 95% of vaccinees. The long-term duration of immunity induced by the

vaccine is not known, but 3-year observations indicate continuing protection against natural infection.

MEASLES
(Rubeola)

Measles is an acute, highly infectious disease characterized by a maculopapular rash which often becomes confluent and blotchy.

Properties of the Virus

A. Size: An RNA virus about 140 nm in diameter as determined by ultrafiltration. The sensitive unit (determined by inactivation with high-energy electron bombardment) is 65 nm, or about 1/10 the volume determined by ultrafiltration. Negative staining in the electron microscope shows the virus to have the helical structure of a paramyxovirus with the helix being 18 nm in diameter. Particles vary in their diameter from about 100–150 nm.

B. Reactions to Physical and Chemical Agents: The virus is destroyed by heating at 56° C for 60 minutes, by 1:4000 formaldehyde after 4 days at 37° C, or after ultraviolet irradiation. Measles virus is destroyed by sonic oscillation at exposures which do not diminish the infectivity of poliovirus or the echoviruses. It remains infective when stored at subzero temperatures, and lyophilized. Measles virus, like other myxoviruses, can be stabilized by molar $MgSO_4$ so that it resists heating at 50° C for 1 hour.

C. Animal Susceptibility and Growth of Virus: The experimental disease has been produced in monkeys infected by various routes. They develop fever, catarrh, Koplik's spots, and a discrete papular rash. The virus has been grown in chick embryos, cultures of human, monkey, and dog kidney tissue, and in human continuous cell lines. In cultures, multinucleate syncytial giant cells form by fusion of mononucleated ones, and other cells become spindle-shaped in the course of their degeneration. Nuclear changes consist of margination of the chromatin and its replacement centrally with an acidophilic inclusion body. Measles virus is relatively unstable after it is released from cells. During the culture of the virus, the intracellular virus titer is 10 or more times the extracellular.

D. Antigenic Properties: Measles antigens can be detected in infected cells by the fluorescent antibody technic. Immunofluorescent antigens can be detected in tissue culture cells before antigens can be detected by complement fixation. The fluorescence is confined to the cytoplasm in the early stages, and only later appears in the nucleus. Measles, canine distemper, and bovine rinderpest share an antigen in common.

E. Biologic Properties: Several types of activity are associated with measles virus:

1. Production of disease in both man and monkeys. The intact virion is required for this activity.

2. Hemagglutinin activity for erythrocytes of various species of baboons or monkeys, but not for

cells of other species, including man. In contrast to most of the other myxoviruses, measles virus does not elute spontaneously from the red cells, and treatment of the monkey red blood cells with receptor destroying enzyme does not prevent hemagglutination. A small, noninfective hemagglutinin is commonly found in cultures of measles virus.

3. Hemadsorption of red blood cells to the surface of tissue culture cells infected with measles virus.

4. Hemolytic activity associated with both the virion and a soluble component. Also associated with this smaller component is a factor responsible for the fusion of cells, resulting in formation of giant cells.

5. Some information about the location in the virion of these activities–hemagglutination, hemolysis, and complement fixation–has been obtained by ether-Tween 80 disruption and electron microscopy (Fig 35–1). The intact virion possesses all 3 activities, which are presumably associated with the envelope, in addition to being infectious. After spontaneous disruption, only the viral infectivity is lost. Treatment of the virion with ether-Tween 80 results in the disruption of the virion into membrane fragments or rosettes which possess both hemagglutination and complement fixation activity, and the internal ribonucleoprotein helix, which has complement fixation activity. Disruption of the virion with ether-Tween 80 destroys the hemolysis activity.

Pathogenesis & Pathology

The virus enters by the respiratory pathway, becomes implanted, and multiplies there. By the time the prodromal catarrhal period and the rash appear, the virus is present in the blood, throughout the respiratory tract in nasopharyngeal and tracheobronchial secretions, and in the conjunctival secretions. It persists in the blood and nasopharyngeal secretions for 2 days after the appearance of the rash. Transplacental transmission of the virus appears to result in congenital measles.

Koplik's spots consist of vesicles in the mouth formed by focal exudations of serum and endothelial cells, which are followed by focal necrosis. In the skin the superficial capillaries of the corium are first involved, and it is here the rash makes its appearance. The appearance and spread of exudate in the epidermis is followed first by vacuolation and necrosis of epithelial cells and then by vesicle formation. Generalized lymphoid tissue hyperplasia occurs. Multinucleate giant cells are found in lymph nodes, tonsils, adenoids, spleen, and appendix. In the rare cases of encephalomyelitis, the histopathologic findings include diffuse petechial hemorrhage, lymphocytic infiltration, and, later, patchy demyelination in the brain and spinal cord. Virus has been recovered from spinal fluid in cases of measles encephalitis.

Defective measles virus genomes (nucleoprotein helical structures lacking the envelope of the mature virion) have been identified within the inclusion bodies found in brain nerve cells in **subacute sclerosing**

panencephalitis. The viral antigen can be detected by means of immunofluorescence.

Clinical Findings

The incubation period is about 10 days to onset of fever and 14 days to appearance of rash. When passive immunization has been attempted too late to prevent infection, the incubation period may be as long as 21 days. The prodromal period is characterized by fever, sneezing, coughing, running nose, redness of eyes, Koplik's spots (enanthems of the buccal mucosa), and lymphopenia. The fever and cough persist until the rash appears and then subside within 1–2 days. The rash spreads over the entire body within 2–4 days, becoming brownish in 5–10 days. Symptoms are most marked when the rash is at its peak but subside rapidly thereafter.

In measles the respiratory tract becomes more susceptible to invasion by bacteria, especially hemolytic streptococci; bronchitis, bronchial pneumonia, and otitis may follow. Bacterial complications are much more readily controlled since the advent of antibiotics.

Encephalomyelitis occurs in about 1:1000 cases. This appears to be due to direct invasion of the CNS by measles virus. Symptoms referable to the brain appear usually a few days after the appearance of the rash, often after it has faded. There is a second bout of fever, and the patient may be drowsy or have convulsions. There is pleocytosis of the CSF. Survivors may show permanent mental disorders (psychosis or personality change) or physical disabilities, particularly epilepsy. Encephalitis may be due to a variant of measles virus possessing neurotropic properties. The mortality rate in encephalitis associated with measles is about 10–30%, and many survivors (40%) show sequelae.

Measles virus appears to be responsible for a chronic degenerative brain disorder known as subacute sclerosing panencephalitis (Dawson's inclusion body encephalitis). The disease manifests itself in children and young adults by progressive mental deterioration, myoclonic jerks, and an abnormal EEG with periodic high voltage complexes. The disease develops a number of years following a regular illness of measles, and measles virus can be isolated from affected brain tissue by special co-cultivation technics.

Laboratory Diagnosis

Measles is usually easily diagnosed on clinical grounds. However, about 5% of cases may lack Koplik's spots. These cases are difficult to differentiate clinically from infection with rubella virus, certain enteroviruses, and adenoviruses.

A. Recovery of Virus: By means of tissue culture technics, measles virus can be isolated from the blood and nasopharynx of a patient in the early acute phase, within 24 hours after the appearance of the rash. Virus can also be isolated from 1 day before to 4 days after the onset of rash. Human amnion or kidney cultures are best suited for isolation of virus.

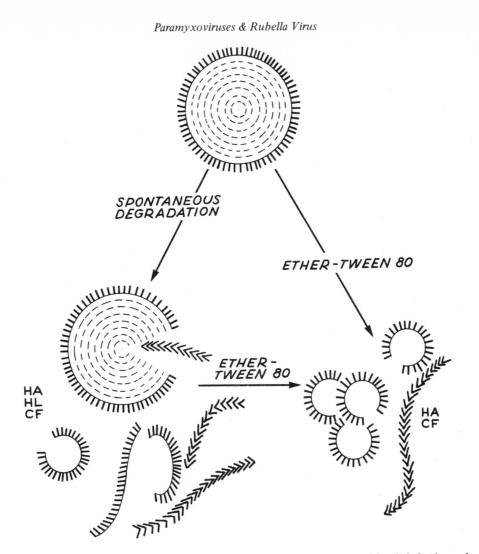

FIG 35–1. Disruption of measles virion into antigenic components. The intact virion is infective and contains hemagglutination, hemolysis, and complement fixation antigens. (After Waterson.)

B. Serology: Specific neutralizing, hemagglutination inhibiting, and complement fixing antibodies develop early in convalescent serum, with maximal titers sometimes achieved by the time of onset of rash. Neutralizing antibodies are measured in tissue culture; and hemagglutination inhibiting and complement fixing antibodies by using antigen grown in tissue cultures. Freeze-dried, noninfectious antigens are recommended for diagnostic purposes. Years after the clinical disease, both types of antibodies may be found, for there is only a gradual decline in antibody titer with age.

Immunity

There appears to be only one antigenic type of measles virus, as one attack generally confers lifelong immunity. Repeated attacks are rarely observed except in persons with immune disorders. Most so-called second attacks represent errors in diagnosis of the initial or the recurring illness.

Epidemiology

Measles is endemic throughout the world. In general, epidemics recur regularly; the inter-epidemic interval is about 2–3 years. The state of immunity of the population is the important factor in this regard. The disease flares up when there is an accumulation of susceptible children and continues in young children, for the most part, because older people are resistant from previous exposures. By the age of 20 years, over 80% have had an attack of the disease. The severity of the epidemic seems to be a function of the number of susceptibles; only about 1% of susceptible individuals fail to contract measles on their first close contact with a patient. Measles antibodies may occur naturally in monkeys, and virus has been isolated from these primates. Monkeys are highly susceptible and might become infected as a result of their human contacts.

The pattern of antibody development in a community coincides with the age-specific attack rate. Antibodies are acquired more rapidly in large families, but there is no relationship between antibodies and other socioeconomic factors (eg, class of housing).

When the disease is introduced into isolated communities where it has not been endemic, all age groups develop clinical measles. A classic example of this was the introduction of measles into the Faroe Islands in 1846; only old people over 60 years of age, who had been alive during the last epidemic, escaped the disease. In such places, where the disease strikes rarely, its consequences are often disastrous and the mortality rate may be as high as 25%.

The highest incidence of measles is in the late winter and spring. Infection is believed to be contracted by inhalation of droplets expelled in sneezing or coughing. Measles is spread chiefly by children during the catarrhal prodromal period; it is infectious from the onset of symptoms until a few days after the rash has appeared.

In view of the fact that measles and canine distemper share an antigen, measles patients develop antibodies which react with canine distemper virus during the course of their disease. Similarly, dogs, after infection with distemper virus, develop antibodies which fix complement with measles antigen. After inoculation with measles virus, dogs develop measles antibodies more readily than distemper antibodies; however, they become immune to virulent distemper virus challenge. Rinderpest virus has also been reported to be related to measles. All 3 agents appear in the urine, and for the animal diseases lesions are known to occur in the bladder and kidney.

Control

Live attenuated measles virus vaccine can effectively prevent measles and represents the most effective control measure. Prior to the introduction of the vaccine, over 0.5 million cases of measles occurred annually in the USA, eg, 763,094 in 1958. Following mass immunization, only 62,705 cases occurred in 1967. The incidence of measles has not decreased significantly further in 1968–1969, primarily because of the lack of immunization of children from certain segments of the population. In many areas of the USA, measles is now occurring in sporadic epidemics among nonimmunized children. In such epidemics, the attack rate for immunized and nonimmunized children is approximately 2% and 34%, respectively.

Less attenuated vaccine virus may produce fever and a modified skin rash in a fair proportion of vaccinees; this reaction can be prevented by the simultaneous administration of gamma globulin (0.01 ml/lb body weight) at a separate site from the vaccine. The further attenuated vaccine viruses do not produce symptoms and do not necessitate the use of gamma globulin. The different vaccine viruses appear to be equally effective in producing lasting immunity; however, the maximum duration of the immunity has not been determined.

Measles antibodies cross the placenta and protect the infant during the first 6 months of life. Vaccination with the live virus fails to take during this period and immunization is not recommended in early infancy. Vaccination is also not recommended in persons with febrile illnesses, allergies to eggs or other products used in the production of the vaccine, and in persons with congenital or acquired immune defects.

Killed measles vaccine should not be used, as certain vaccinees become sensitized and display local reactions when revaccinated with live attenuated virus or a severe illness upon contracting natural measles.

Measles may also be prevented or modified by administering antibody early in the incubation period. Commercial gamma globulin usually contains antibody titers of 200 to 1000 against 100 TCD_{50} of virus. With small doses, the disease can be made mild and immunity ensues. With a large dose of gamma globulin, the disease can be prevented; however, the person remains susceptible to infection at a later date. Antibodies given later than 6 days after exposure are not likely to influence the course of the disease.

PARAINFLUENZA VIRUS INFECTIONS

The parainfluenza viruses form a subgroup of the paramyxoviruses. They have a common size, are susceptible to ether, agglutinate mammalian or avian red blood cells, and (like the influenza viruses) contain a receptor-destroying enzyme. They grow well in primary monkey or human epithelial cell culture, but poorly or not at all in the embryonated egg. They produce a minimal cytopathic effect during primary tissue culture, but are easily recognized by the hemadsorption method. Like mumps virus, with which they share a common antigen, they differ from the influenza viruses in their slightly larger size (90–200 nm) and in their tendency to lyse as well as agglutinate erythrocytes. The parainfluenza viruses are relatively unstable, and activity falls off even at freezing temperatures. Laboratory diagnosis may be made by the hemagglutination inhibition, complement fixation, and neutralization tests.

Parainfluenza 1

Included here are **Sendai virus,** also known as the **hemagglutinating virus of Japan (HVJ)** or **influenza D,** and **hemadsorption virus type 2 (HA-2).** Sendai virus has been reported to be the etiologic agent of pneumonia in pigs and pneumonitis of newborn infants, but the endemicity of the virus in laboratory mice in which the isolations were made makes it difficult to evaluate the role of the virus as a cause of human illness. The most important member of this group appears to be the widespread HA-2 virus. Although it is not cytopathogenic for monkey kidney cultures, it is detected in such cultures by the hemadsorption test, ie, the clumping of guinea pig erythrocytes on the surfaces of the infected cells in the culture. It appears to be one of the main agents producing croup in children, but it can also cause coryza, pharyngitis, bronchitis, bronchiolitis, pneumonia, and undifferentiated upper respiratory illness. In adults it produces respiratory symptoms like those of the common cold, with reinfection occurring in persons with antibodies from earlier infections.

Immunization with inactivated parainfluenza type 1 vaccine stimulates antibody appearance in the blood but not in nasal secretions. Recipients of such a vaccine remain susceptible to reinfection. In contrast, infection stimulates antibody appearance in the nasal secretions and concomitant resistance to reinfection.

Parainfluenza 2

This group includes the **croup-associated (CA) virus,** also known as the acute laryngotracheobronchitis virus of children. The virus grows in human cells (HeLa, lung, amnion) and monkey kidney, in which syncytial masses are produced with loss of cell boundaries. The virus agglutinates chick and, to a lesser degree, human O erythrocytes. Adsorption and hemagglutination occur at 4° C, and elution of virus takes place rapidly at 37° C. However, the cells reagglutinate when returned to 4° C.

Antigenically, type 2 is unrelated to all the other myxoviruses except mumps. Mumps patients develop type 2 antibodies, as do also animals inoculated with mumps virus.

Parainfluenza virus 2 occurs spontaneously in monkey kidney cells grown in culture, as many as 30% of some culture lots being positive. Simian viruses 5 and 41 appear to be related antigenically to parainfluenza 2.

Parainfluenza 3

The viruses in this group are also known as **hemadsorption virus type 1 (HA-1).** As its name implies, it is detected in monkey kidney cultures by the hemadsorption technic. Serial passage in culture leads to cytopathic changes, but this effect is observed only several days after the hemadsorption reaction becomes positive. Multinucleated giant cell plaques are produced under agar on continuous line human cells.

The virus has been isolated from children with mild respiratory illnesses as well as from some children suffering from croup. Strains of type 3 virus have been isolated from nasal secretions of cattle ill with a respiratory syndrome known as "shipping fever." At least 70% of market cattle bled at slaughter have parainfluenza 3 antibodies. Infection is widespread in the USA; fall is the period of greatest acquisition of new infections.

After infection with parainfluenza 1 or 2, complement fixation titers rise not only to the infecting type but usually to type 3 as well. This reflects a sharing of antigens. Parainfluenza 3 infection is more prevalent and usually occurs earlier in life than does type 1 or 2 infection. Upon subsequent infection with type 1 or 2, a booster response is seen to type 3.

Parainfluenza 4

The M-25 strain is the parainfluenza 4 prototype. It has failed to produce any cytopathic effects, does not grow in embryonated eggs, and can be recognized only by the hemadsorption technic. As far as human disease is concerned, all that is known is that this virus is associated with malaise in young children.

Parainfluenza 1 and 3 differ from influenza in that they are ubiquitous endemic agents producing infections all through the year. Types 2 and 4 occur more sporadically. Types 1, 2, and 3 have a wide geographic distribution, whereas type 4 has only been recovered in the USA. They all infect early in life. About half of the first infections with parainfluenza 1 virus, 2/3 of those with parainfluenza 2, and ¾ of those with parainfluenza 3 produce febrile illnesses. The target organ of type 3 is the lower respiratory tract, with first infections frequently resulting in bronchial pneumonia, bronchiolitis, or bronchitis. While type 1 has been the chief cause of croup, the other types have also been involved to the extent that half of the cases of laryngotracheobronchitis can be shown to be caused by parainfluenza viruses. The incubation period for type 1 is 5–6 days; for type 3 it is 2–3 days.

Antibody surveys of normal populations in the USA indicate that type 3 infection generally occurs early in life, since most infants have type 3 neutralizing antibody by age 2. Acquisition of type 1 and type 2 neutralizing antibodies occurs at a slower rate, but most children possess such antibodies by the sixth to the tenth year.

Reinfection with these agents, particularly with type 3 virus, is a common occurrence. In children, preexisting low antibody levels reduce the likelihood of virus recovery but do not interfere with an antibody rise. Such children develop fever but only rarely develop lower respiratory tract illness. Preexisting high antibody levels limit but do not prevent reinfection. Children with high antibody levels, even when reinfected, have a low incidence of fever. Reinfection of adults results in minor illness indistinguishable from the common cold. These viruses have been isolated in 2–9% of college students and military personnel with upper respiratory illnesses. Parainfluenza viruses are responsible for about 18% of acute nonbacterial respiratory diseases in children requiring hospitalization.

RESPIRATORY SYNCYTIAL (RS) VIRUS

This agent appears to be an extremely labile paramyxovirus, about 90–140 nm in size, ether-sensitive, and producing a characteristic syncytial effect (pseudogiant cell) in serially propagated human cell cultures. It is the single most important agent causing infantile bronchiolitis and pneumonia.

A soluble complement fixing antigen can be separated from the virus particle by sedimenting the latter in the high-speed centrifuge. The virus is so labile that 90% of infectivity is lost by a single cycle of slow freezing and thawing. However, the virus is stable when it is rapidly frozen and stored at $-70°$ C.

RS virus has not been grown in eggs, nor has a hemagglutinin been demonstrated. It is not pathogenic for any of the laboratory rodents. It occurs spontaneously in chimpanzees and has been associated with coryza in these primates.

Of the paramyxoviruses which infect human beings, only measles, mumps, parainfluenza 2, and RS viruses produce syncytial changes in cell cultures. Antigenically, these viruses are distinct from each other, and all but RS possess a hemagglutinin.

A slight antigenic variation has been found in different isolates of RS virus, which resembles the variation found with influenza A and A$_2$ strains. Possibly the antigenic heterogeneity will be limited.

RS virus is recovered significantly more often from infants and children with respiratory illness than from controls free of such disease. The most striking association of RS infection with illness was observed in young infants (first 6 months of life) with bronchiolitis or pneumonia where the virus recovery rates were 39% and 23%, respectively, as against zero among hundreds of control infants without respiratory disease. Infection in older infants and children resulted in milder illness than that which occurred in the first half year of life. Upper respiratory tract disease associated with RS infection was not benign, however, since in 95% of instances a temperature elevation above $100°$ F was noted. The virus recovery rate indicates that RS virus is one of the major causes of bronchiolitis and is also an important cause of infantile and childhood pneumonia. About 25% of respiratory tract illnesses requiring hospitalization in Washington DC were associated with RS infection over a 4-year period of study.

The serologic response to infection of infants less than 7 months of age is relatively poor. Only 20% develop a complement fixing antibody rise and only 45% develop neutralizing antibody during convalescence. Infants over 6 months of age responded more often with an antibody rise.

RS virus spreads extensively in the childhood population every year during the winter months. The circumscribed yearly outbreaks of RS infection differ from the pattern of influenza A or B infections which characteristically recur at intervals of 2–3 years. The epidemiology of RS infection also differs from that of parainfluenza 1 and 3 viruses, which occur in the community during almost every month of the year.

RS virus infection in adult volunteers showed that reinfection occurs readily even though all the volunteers had moderate to high levels of neutralizing antibody prior to challenge. This antibody may have been responsible for the mild nature of the observed cold-like illnesses. However, serum neutralizing antibody does not seem to be very effective in providing resistance to severe lower respiratory tract disease of early life. Thus, bronchiolitis and pneumonia due to RS virus are common in infants in the first 3–4 months of life even though maternally transmitted antibody is present at significantly high levels. (Even in adults, antibody in nasal secretions is a better indicator of resistance to parainfluenza virus than serum antibody levels.)

The clinical disease in young infants may actually be the result of an antigen-antibody reaction that results when the infecting virus meets maternally transmitted antibody. For this reason, RS vaccines that produce antibodies in the serum but not in the nasal secretions may do more harm than good. Efforts to develop an attenuated vaccine that infects subclinically and produces nasal antibody are encouraging, but no commercial vaccine is as yet available.

NEWCASTLE DISEASE CONJUNCTIVITIS

Newcastle disease virus is a paramyxovirus that is primarily pathogenic for fowl. It produces pneumoencephalitis in young chickens and "influenza" in older birds. In man it may produce an inflammation of the conjunctivas. Recovery is complete in 10–14 days. The infection in man is an occupational disease, for it appears to be limited to laboratory workers and to poultry workers handling infected birds.

The virus grows readily in the embryonated egg, in chick embryo culture, or HeLa cells, and produces hemagglutination of the influenza virus type.

Human erythrocytes treated with the virus are agglutinated by specific serum against Newcastle virus and also by sera from certain patients with infectious mononucleosis and hepatitis. After contracting mumps, many persons develop antibodies which not only react with mumps virus but also cross-react with Newcastle disease virus.

Newcastle antibodies can be measured by the hemagglutination inhibition, complement fixation, and neutralization tests using chick embryos or tissue cultures. Normal human sera possess a heat-labile, nonspecific inhibitor which can be destroyed by heating at $56°$ C for 30 minutes.

GERMAN MEASLES
(Rubella)

Rubella is an acute febrile illness characterized by a rash and posterior and suboccipital lymphadenopathy which affects children and young adults. Infection in early pregnancy may result in serious abnormalities of the fetus.

Properties of the Virus

The virus is an RNA-containing, ether-sensitive virus which measures about 60 nm in diameter. Morphologically, the virus contains a 30 nm internal nucleoid with a double membrane; the virus forms by budding from the endoplasmic reticulum into intracytoplasmic vesicles and at the marginal cell membrane. There is a hemagglutinin which agglutinates red blood cells of day-old chicks, adult geese, or pigeons; there is no spontaneous elution, and hemagglutination is not affected by treating the erythrocytes with receptor destroying enzyme. The virus is relatively labile but can be kept viable by storing at $-70°$ C for several years. On the basis of physical and chemical characteristics, rubella virus belongs to the newly defined **togavirus group**.

Rubella virus can be propagated in tissue culture and commonly does not produce a characteristic cytopathic effect. However, in cultures of certain cells the virus produces sufficient cytopathology to be detected by experienced observers: These cells include human amnion cells, human thyroid cells, serial passaged lines of rabbit cornea (SIRC) and rabbit kidney (RK-13) cells and a line of monkey kidney (VERO) cells. In other cell culture systems, rubella virus replicates without causing a cytopathic effect; however, a rubella virus interference is induced which protects the cells against the cytopathic effect of other viruses. Thus, a standard method of isolating rubella virus consists of inoculating green monkey kidney cells with the specimen and, after 7–10 days of incubation, challenging the cultures with a picornavirus such as echovirus 11. If echovirus cytopathic effect develops, the specimen is considered negative for rubella virus; however, the absence of echovirus cytopathic effect implies the presence of rubella virus in the original specimen.

1. POSTNATAL RUBELLA

Pathogenesis

The route of infection is most likely through the mucosa of the upper respiratory tract. The virus probably replicates primarily in the cervical lymph nodes. After a period of 7 days, viremia develops which lasts until the appearance of antibody on about day 12–14. The development of antibody coincides with the appearance of the rash, suggesting an immunologic basis for the rash. During the viremic period, virus can be isolated from the urine and feces; however, after the rash appears, the virus remains detectable only in the nasopharynx.

Clinical Features

Rubella is usually heralded by the acute onset of malaise, low-grade fever, and a morbilliform rash appearing on the same day. Less often, systemic symptoms may precede the rash by 1 or 2 days, or the rash and lymphadenopathy may occur without systemic symptoms. The rash, which starts on the face and extends over the trunk and extremities, rarely lasts more than 3 days. Posterior auricular and suboccipital lymphadenopathy are consistent physical findings. Transient arthralgia and arthritis are commonly seen in adult females, whereas rare complications include thrombocytopenia and encephalitis.

Immunity

Rubella antibodies appear in the serum of patients as the rash fades, and the titer of antibody rises rapidly over the next 1–3 weeks. A sizable portion of the initial antibody consists of IgM which can be detected for 2–3 weeks following the illness. Although serologic diagnosis can best be accomplished by analysis of acute and convalescent sera, a single sample obtained 2 weeks after the rash may provide presumptive evidence of rubella by demonstrating rubella virus antibodies in the IgM fraction.

One attack of the disease confers lifelong immunity, as only one antigenic type of the virus exists. A history of rubella is not a reliable index of immunity. This can best be determined by assaying the serum for antibody. The presence of antibody at a 1:8 dilution implies immunity. Immune mothers transfer antibodies to their offspring, who are then protected for 4–6 months.

Treatment

There is no specific treatment unless the patient is pregnant. Rubella-like illness in the first trimester of pregnancy should be substantiated by isolation of the virus from the throat or by demonstrating a 4-fold rise in antibody titer to the virus by means of the hemagglutination inhibition, complement fixation, or neutralization test. Laboratory proved rubella in the first 10 weeks of pregnancy is associated with fetal infection in virtually 100% of cases. Therapeutic abortion is strongly recommended in laboratory proved cases to avoid the birth of malformed infants.

Gamma globulin has been used by some for pregnant women exposed to rubella during the first trimester. However, gamma globulin has been shown to have no inhibiting effect on viremia, and it is the virus in the blood that exposes the fetus. There is no convincing evidence that gamma globulin offers any benefit to the patient or the fetus.

2. CONGENITAL RUBELLA SYNDROME

Pathogenesis

Rubella infection during pregnancy may result in infection of the placenta and fetus. A limited number of cells of the fetus become infected. Although the virus does not destroy the cells, the growth rate and ultimate doubling potential of the cells are altered, which results in fewer than normal numbers of cells at birth. The earlier in pregnancy that infection occurs, the greater the chance of extensive involvement with the birth of an infant afflicted by severe anomalies. Infection in the first month of pregnancy results in abnormalities in about 80% of cases, while detectable defects are found in about 15% of infants acquiring the disease during the third month of gestation. The intrauterine infection is associated with a chronic persistence of the virus thought to be due to a defect in cellular immunity and lasting 12–18 months after birth.

Clinical Findings

Infants born with congenital rubella syndrome may have one or more abnormalities which include defects of the heart and great vessels (patent ductus arteriosus, pulmonary branch stenosis, pulmonary valvular stenosis, ventricular septal defect, and atrial septal defect), eye defects (cataracts, glaucoma, and chorioretinitis), and neurosensory deafness. Infants may also display intrauterine growth retardation, failure to thrive, hepatosplenomegaly, thrombocytopenia with purpura, anemia, osteitis, and an encephalitic syndrome leading to mild to severe cerebral palsy. The infants often have increased susceptibility to infection, and evaluation of their immunoglobulins may reveal abnormalities, most commonly elevated IgM with low levels of IgG and IgA.

There is a 20% mortality rate among congenitally virus-infected infants symptomatic at birth. Some virus-infected infants appearing normal at birth may manifest abnormalities at a later date. Those not requiring institutionalization generally function satisfactorily in adult life.

Immunity

While maternal antibody in the form of IgG is transferred to the infant with congenital rubella, the infant also produces antibodies to the virus and, as found with other intrauterine infections (syphilis, toxoplasmosis, and cytomegalovirus), the antibody is IgM. As is not the case with nonaffected infants who lose maternal antibody, antibody to the virus can be detected in the serum of congenital rubella infants after 4–6 months of age. Several investigators have recently suggested that persons with congenital rubella may lose their antibody in later life and become susceptible to postnatal rubella. This observation requires further study.

Epidemiology

The virus has been recovered from the nasopharynx, throat, blood, and urine, and it is believed that the infection is spread by respiratory pathways (droplets). Epidemics are not so frequent as those of measles, and the disease is accordingly more common in young adults. Rubella occurs chiefly in the spring.

As a result of the severe epidemic of rubella in the USA in the spring of 1964, the largest epidemic in at least 20 years, thousands of babies were born after September, 1964, with the congenital rubella syndrome. Advances in laboratory technics made possible extensive studies of these infants, and several important findings were documented. Most important, perhaps, is that infants continue to be infectious, with virus being found particularly in the throat and CSF, for up to 18 months after birth. The persistence of virus in the CSF may in part explain the progressive mental retardation and CNS disease observed in many of the infants. Virus has been recovered from almost all of the body tissues tested postmortem, and from antemortem specimens of throat swabs, urine, CSF, feces, peripheral blood, bone marrow, conjunctival sac fluid, middle ear fluid, and lens material.

Congenitally infected infants are capable of transmitting rubella to susceptible contacts such as nurses and physicians caring for the infants. This represents a serious hazard to women in the first trimester of pregnancy, who should avoid contact with these babies. Infants who appear normal but who shed virus have been born to mothers who had clinical rubella in the first trimester of pregnancy, or who were in contact with rubella during this period and who may have had subclinical infections. It is therefore advisable for all susceptible women in the first trimester of pregnancy to avoid unnecessary contact with all newborns until this problem has been further investigated.

Rubella without rash (rubella sine eruptione) may occur. This is of importance because it is now known that inapparent rubella infection (with viremia) acquired during pregnancy has the same deleterious effect on the fetus as rubella with the typical rash.

Control

It is anticipated that rubella can be controlled by mass vaccination of susceptible children. A live attenuated virus vaccine was licensed in the USA for use in 1969. A single subcutaneous injection of the vaccine is recommended for all children from age 1 to puberty. In postpubertal females, the vaccine produces self-limited arthralgia and arthritis in about 1/3 of the vaccinees; no information is available regarding the teratogenic potential of the virus if given during the first trimester of pregnancy. The vaccine should not be given to a postpubertal female unless she has been proved not to be pregnant, has been demonstrated serologically to be susceptible, understands that it is imperative not to become pregnant for at least 3 months after vaccination, and is adequately warned of the complications of arthralgia. Persons with abnormal immune functions or who are sensitive to chicken or duck proteins or to neomycin should not receive the vaccine.

•   •   •

General References

Chanock, R.M.: Parainfluenza viruses. Pages 434–456 in: *Diagnostic Procedures for Viral and Rickettsial Infections,* 4th ed. American Public Health Association, 1969.

Harris, R.W., Isacson, P., & D.T. Karzon: Vaccine-induced hypersensitivity: Reactions to live measles and mumps vaccines in prior recipients of inactivated measles vaccine. J Pediat 74:552–563, 1969.

Henle, W.: Mumps virus. Pages 457–482 in: *Diagnostic Procedures for Viral and Rickettsial Infections,* 4th ed. American Public Health Association, 1969.

Huygelen, C., Peetermans, J., & A. Prinzie: An attenuated rubella virus vaccine (Cendehill 51 strain) grown in primary rabbit kidney cells. Progr Med Virol 11:107–125, 1969.

Katz, S.L., & J.F. Enders: Measles virus. Pages 504–528 in: *Diagnostic Procedures for Viral and Rickettsial Infections,* 4th ed. American Public Health Association, 1969.

Parkman, P.D., & H.M. Meyer, Jr: Prospects for a rubella virus vaccine. Progr Med Virol 11:80–106, 1969.

Payne, F.E., Baublis, J.V., & H.H. Itabashi: Isolation of measles virus from cell cultures of brain from a patient with subacute sclerosing panencephalitis. New England J Med 281:585–589, 1969.

Rawls, W.E.: Congenital rubella: The significance of virus persistence. Progr Med Virol 10:238–285, 1968.

36...

Poxvirus Group

SMALLPOX & RELATED VIRAL INFECTIONS OF MAN

VARIOLA MAJOR
(Classical Smallpox, Asiatic Smallpox),
VARIOLA MINOR (Alastrim),
VACCINIA

Smallpox (variola major) is an acute infectious disease characterized by severe systemic involvement and a single crop of skin lesions which proceeds through macular, papular, vesicular, and pustular stages over a period of 5–10 days. A mild form (variola minor) also occurs. Vaccinia is a related poxvirus, attenuated for man, and has long been in use as (the first) live virus vaccine. Yaba virus, a simian poxvirus, induces benign histiocytomas in monkeys and can produce similar lesions in man.

Serologic and immunologic studies have shown that the viruses of variola major and variola minor are indistinguishable from each other and that they are differentiated only in minor ways from the viruses of vaccinia and cowpox, but they may be distinguished by ability to grow at different temperatures in eggs. The origin of the vaccinia virus is unknown. It is believed by some to have stemmed from cowpox, a natural disease of cows studied by Jenner in the 18th century. Others feel that vaccinia virus originated from variola virus.

Other poxviruses include 2 related agents: A virus that causes fibromas in rabbits and another, myxoma virus, that causes local gelatinous swelling in certain species of rabbit and a fatal disease in others.

Properties of the Virus
A. Size and Nucleic Acid: The DNA genome has a very large molecular weight, $160–240 \times 10^6$ daltons. Sufficient DNA is present to code for several hundred proteins.

Variola virus resembles other members of the pox group; its dimensions are about 200×300 nm. The virus particles are brick-shaped when visualized in dried films in the electron microscope, but are ellipsoid when seen in ultrathin sections of infected cells. A poxvirus consists of an outer membrane or coat surrounding the lateral bodies, and a dense nucleoprotein core which contains the viral DNA associated with an inner membrane.

Vaccinia virus has been purified. Its chemical composition resembles that of a bacterium. It contains protein, DNA, phospholipid, neutral fat, carbohydrate, copper, flavin, and biotin. Whether the latter constituents are really part of the virus or whether they represent adsorbed constituents of the host cell in which virus has grown has not yet been established.

B. Reactions to Physical and Chemical Agents: Both variola and vaccinia withstand drying for months, even when held at room temperature. They withstand lower temperatures for years. In the moist state the virus is destroyed at 60° C for 10 minutes, but in the dry state it can resist 100° C for 5–10 minutes. Acids (pH 3.0) destroy the virus within an hour. One percent phenol has little effect at 4° C but inactivates the virus at 37° C in 24 hours. Alcohol in 50% concentration or potassium permanganate in 0.01% concentration destroys the virus within 1 hour at room temperature.

C. Animal Susceptibility and Growth of Virus: The host range of variola virus is restricted to man and monkeys. Unlike vaccinia virus, it cannot be propagated in rabbits or mice. However, it grows readily on the chorioallantoic membrane of the 10- to 12-day-old chick embryo. It produces characteristic small, white lesions which are different from the large vaccinia lesions, having central depressions due to necrosis. The morphologic character of the lesion produced on the chick membrane can be used for rapid identification of variola virus in clinical specimens. Vaccinia virus grows readily in cultures of chick embryo or primate cells, producing necrosis of the cells. Monkey kidney cell cultures are much more sensitive than rabbit skin in vivo.

D. Antigenic Properties: Antigenic relationships among poxviruses are determined with the use of extracts of infected cells. Up to 20 antigens capable of forming precipitin lines with antiviral antiserum can be detected in the vaccinia-variola group of viruses and in the myxoma-fibroma group. Viruses of the vaccinia-variola group are very similar antigenically and differ by not more than one antigen by this technic. Viruses of the myxoma-fibroma group are not neutralized by antiserum to viruses of the vaccinia-variola group, and no major antigens in the respective cell extracts cross-react. However, the inner core of all poxviruses contains a common antigen, NP antigen, which can be released from the core by alkaline digestion.

In addition to structural antigens, poxviruses produce soluble antigens and hemagglutinins. Vaccinia virus contains a heat-labile (L) antigen which is destroyed at 60° C and a heat-stable (S) antigen which withstands treatment at 100° C. Both antigens may be present in soluble form in infected tissue. They appear to be different antigenic components of a complex LS antigen, an elongated protein with a molecular weight of about 240,000. In addition the virus contains deoxynucleoprotein (NP), which is also antigenic. Adsorption of immune sera with LS or NP antigens fails to remove neutralizing antibody. Upon the LS antigens depend the serologic tests for smallpox diagnosis. LS antigens from variola and from vaccinia virus have been shown to be antigenically similar, using either convalescent sera from smallpox patients or rabbit antivaccinia serum.

A third antigen has been isolated with a molecular weight of 100,000–200,000 which, unlike the other antigens studied, is capable of combining with virus-neutralizing antibody and when injected into animals confers some resistance to infection.

The hemagglutinin of vaccinia, variola, or of infectious ectromelia (mousepox) is not an integral part of the virion and can be obtained free from the much larger virus particles. The hemagglutination reaction with chicken red cells can be inhibited by vaccinia immune serum, convalescent smallpox serum, or infectious ectromelia immune serum. The hemagglutinin is a lipoprotein complex, associated with a particle 65 nm in diameter. It is heat-stable; it is distinct from the LS antigens, but does not exhibit receptor destroying (neuraminidase) activity.

Poxvirus Multiplication

Intracellular growth of various poxviruses has been intensively studied with immunofluorescence and with cytochemical, biochemical, and electron microscopic methods.

A. Virus Penetration and Uncoating: The intracellular uncoating of the virion is basically a 2-stage process. Virus particles establish contact with the cell surface and are then engulfed in phagocytic vacuoles of the cell. Inside the cell, a phagolysozome vacuole develops which initiates first stage uncoating, probably by means of hydrolytic enzymes in the vacuoles. Under control of the cell, this step results in degradation of the outer membrane and lateral bodies, releasing the nucleoprotein core into the cytoplasm. The second uncoating step involves degradation of the nucleoprotein core, liberating DNA and rendering it sensitive to deoxyribonuclease.

For second stage uncoating to occur there is a requirement for both RNA and protein synthesis which implies information transfer from DNA to RNA. When protein synthesis is inhibited either at the transcription stage (dactinomycin) or at the translational stage (fluorophenylalanine or puromycin), the breakdown of the virus occurs normally but it is not followed by liberation of naked DNA.

Until recently it was thought that both uncoating steps were required for viral DNA to transcribe RNA.

However, recent experiments have shown that some RNA can be transcribed from the poxvirus DNA even though it resides within the viral core and is resistant to deoxyribonuclease. This peculiarity of the poxviruses is apparently due to the fact that the virion carries within its core an RNA polymerase which mediates synthesis of poxvirus messenger RNA and can function while DNA is still enclosed in the core. This mRNA is transcribed within the virus core and is then released into the cytoplasm where it codes for the synthesis of a protein capable of directing the release of virus DNA from the core, thereby allowing expression of the entire virus genome. This concept is contrary to the hypothesis previously held, which proposed that a "viral inducer" protein released from the virion during the first stage of uncoating depressed the host genome, allowing the cell to synthesize an uncoating protein which facilitated release of viral DNA from the core. Additional evidence that the uncoating of the cores involves a viral function is the finding that uncoating of viral DNA was inhibited by interferon.

With the removal of the outer coat in the phagolysozome during the first stage of uncoating (1), the nucleoprotein core is released into the cell cytoplasm leading to the following sequence of events of the second stage of uncoating (Fig 36–1). The virion-associated RNA polymerase transcribes an mRNA while still within the core. The mRNA leaves the core to associate with ribosomes in the cell cytoplasm (2) and is translated into a protein (P1). P1 functions as an uncoating enzyme directly (3) by degrading the core and releasing the naked viral DNA (4). An alternative scheme rests on the possibility that a section of the cell genome contains genetic information necessary to code for a protein capable of completing the second stage of uncoating. P1 may act as an inducer protein by derepressing this section of the cell genome (5). This results in the synthesis of an mRNA coded by the cell DNA which directs the synthesis (6) of a protein (P2) capable of degrading the virus core (7) and releasing the naked viral DNA into the cell cytoplasm.

Poxviruses inactivated by heat can be reactivated either by viable poxviruses or by poxviruses inactivated by nitrogen mustards (which inactivate the DNA moiety). The reactivation is due to the stimulation of the uncoating protein. The heat-inactivated virus is no longer able to do this because of the heat lability of the DNA-dependent RNA polymerase. The significance of poxvirus reactivation lies in the fact that it embraces the whole of the poxvirus group and that any poxvirus can reactivate any other poxvirus, suggesting that all members of the poxvirus group carry the RNA polymerase in their cores.

B. Intracellular Sequence of Multiplication: The intracellular events in vaccinia virus replication have been characterized by cytochemical and immunofluorescence technics. The following sequence occurs: (1) Early increase in cytoplasmic RNA. (2) At 4 hours after infection, appearance of centers of viral DNA synthesis in cytoplasm and the formation of the LS antigen. (3) At 5–6 hours, the appearance of the NP

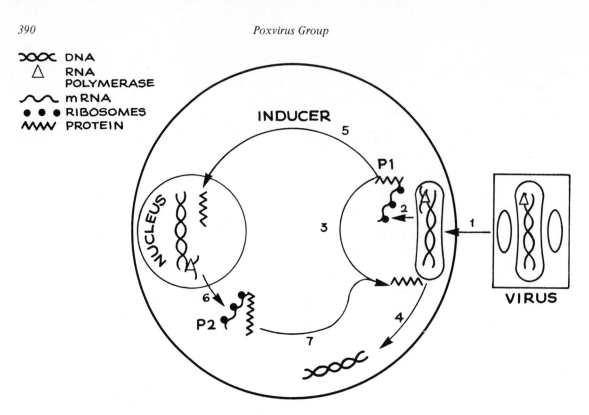

DNA
RNA POLYMERASE
mRNA
RIBOSOMES
PROTEIN

FIG 36–1. Sequence of events in the penetration and uncoating of poxviruses. (See text for description.)

antigen at the sites of DNA synthesis (classical pox inclusion body). (4) Both antigens are found only in the cytoplasm and precede the formation of infective virus, which first appears at 8 hours. (5) At 10 hours the hemagglutinin antigen develops. The analysis of the growth cycle shows that the sites of LS and NP antigen synthesis are separate in the cytoplasm until 8 hours after infection, when they are intimately mixed, at a time coinciding with the fragmentation of the inclusion body and with the first appearance of infective particles.

The structural proteins of vaccinia virus can be divided into 2 classes based on their time of synthesis within the infected cell. The "early" proteins are synthesized 1–3 hours after infection and prior to the onset of viral DNA replication. They are associated with the core of the virion and do not elicit production of virus neutralizing antibody. An additional "early" protein has been detected on the surface of vaccinia-infected cells by the direct fluorescent antibody test. Characterization as to a structural or nonstructural function of this antigen has not been obtained. The "late" proteins are synthesized after viral DNA replication and also have been divided into 2 classes. The first correspond to the above mentioned L and S antigenic complex and are located on the outer surface of the virion. The second class of "late" antigens also includes 2 proteins termed the G antigens. One of these antigens is associated with the viral core, whereas the other is in a subsurface location. Both proteins are basic in nature and do not elicit an antibody response.

Cells infected with vaccinia virus and treated with bromodeoxyuridine (BUDR) produce viral antigen in the cytoplasm and yield particles that have incorporated BUDR in their nucleic acid in place of thymidine. Such particles are malformed and noninfectious. This is similar to the effect of IUDR on herpesvirus-infected cells.

C. Maturation of Virus Particles: Electron microscopic studies of ultrathin sections of infected tissue have shown that poxviruses form developmental bodies preliminary to the production of the mature infectious virus. Developmental bodies, or immature forms, are round to oval, slightly larger than mature virus particles, less dense to electrons, and have a varied morphology. It has been suggested as a working hypothesis that the process of maturation of a virus particle takes place as follows: (1) In the earliest form the developmental bodies appear as hollow spheres embedded either in a very dense cytoplasmic mass constituting an inclusion or in a less dense matrix near the nucleus in cells without typical inclusion bodies. (2) The spheres become filled with a homogeneous material of low electron density. (3) A small, dense granule appears in each developmental body and grows at the expense of the low-density material. (4) Following growth of the granule, particles are found with the dimensions of mature viruses and having complex internal structures resembling bars or dumbbells. (5) Mature virions are ovoid and dense to electrons. Isolated, mature vaccinia virus particles, after pepsin treatment, contain a dense "nucleoid" and 2 thin outer membranes. The nucleoid is susceptible to deoxyribonuclease treatment. The mature virus is made up of a DNA-containing central body encased by double membranes, surrounded by protein, and all enclosed within 2 outer membranes.

Within an hour of adding virus to susceptible cells in culture, virus particles with their outer membranes intact are found within the cells. The immature forms appear 4–5 hours after infection, followed within 2 hours by the mature infective virus. The infection spreads gradually in the cell for the next 16 hours. Thus, thin sections observed in the electron microscope 24 hours after infection show that the virus is being manufactured throughout the cytoplasm.

D. Virus-Induced Enzymes: Infection of a cell by vaccinia virus leads to the synthesis of several enzymes that are under the control of the virus genome. The enzymes that have been described thus far are DNA polymerase, DNase, and thymidine kinase. Of these, thymidine kinase has been studied in some detail and mutants have been isolated that do not induce the formation of this enzyme even though virus multiplication proceeds at normal rates. Thymidine kinase activity first increases about 2 hours after infection and rises to 10 times the normal level by 10 hours after infection. The enzyme increase is completely inhibited under conditions inhibiting the synthesis of protein. Cellular DNA synthesis stops at the time viral DNA synthesis begins. The time course for synthesis of thymidine kinase and DNA polymerase indicates that the genetic code for thymidine kinase can be expressed before the breakdown of viral cores, whereas DNA polymerase can be synthesized only after the uncoating of the viral DNA. The DNA polymerases from vaccinia-infected cells and uninfected cells differ significantly with regard to ion exchange chromatographic properties, primer response, pH optimum, heat inactivation, and inhibition by vaccinia antiserum.

Pathogenesis & Pathology of Smallpox

The portal of entry of variola virus is through the mucous membranes of the upper respiratory tract. During the incubation period, the virus may propagate in lymphoid and other tissues. Inasmuch as there are no open lesions on the mucosal surface during incubation, the patient is not infectious during this period. After the entry of the virus, the following are believed to take place: (1) primary multiplication in the lymphoid tissue draining the site of entry; (2) transient viremia and infection of reticuloendothelial cells throughout the body; (3) a secondary phase of multiplication in these cells, leading to (4) a secondary, more intense viremia; (5) the clinical disease.

The skin lesion follows the localization of virus in the epidermis from the blood stream. The virus can be isolated from the blood in the early phases of the disease but not after the second day of fever (except in fatal cases). The clinical improvement which follows with the development of the skin eruption is held to be the result of the rapid appearance of antibodies. The pustulation of the skin lesions may give rise to a secondary fever; this is believed to be the result of the absorption of the products of cell necrosis rather than of a secondary bacterial infection.

Neither in mild nor in severe cases are bacteria found in the blood during the early viremic (pre-eruptive febrile) phase. In severe cases, bacteria may be found in the blood about the 8th to 12th days of disease during the pustular phase. Skin pustules may become contaminated, usually with staphylococci, sometimes leading to a number of bacterial complications (osteomyelitis, septic joints).

At the time of the skin eruption, there is a large amount of virus in the lower layer of the epidermis. However, because of the impermeable nature of this tissue, virus is not shed until the later rupture of vesicles and pustules. In the mouth and pharynx, this protective layer is absent; lesions therefore break down early, rapidly rendering the oropharyngeal fluid and saliva infective.

Early in the course of the illness (pre-eruptive phase), the disease is hardly infective. On the first or second day of disease, saliva is negative for virus, but by the sixth to ninth days it is usually positive. At this time lesions in the mouth tend to ulcerate and discharge virus into the oral cavity. Thus early in the disease infectious virus has its source in the lesions in the mouth and upper respiratory tract. Later, pustules break down; and virus in the environment of the smallpox patient is then derived from this source.

Histopathologic examination of the skin shows that proliferation of the prickle-cell layer occurs early and that these proliferated cells contain large numbers of cytoplasmic inclusions. There is infiltration of mononuclear cells, particularly around the vessels in the corium. Epithelial cells of the malpighian layer become swollen through distention of cytoplasm and undergo "ballooning degeneration." The vacuoles in the cytoplasm enlarge and distend the cell membrane. This finally breaks down, and the coalescence with neighboring, similarly affected cells results in the formation of vesicles. As the disease progresses, the vesicles enlarge and then become filled with white cells and tissue debris. In variola minor, the basilar layer is little involved, whereas in variola major and vaccinia all the layers are involved and there is actual necrosis of the corium. Thus scarring is seen after variola major and vaccinia but not after variola minor.

The cytoplasmic inclusions (Guarnieri bodies) are sometimes round or oval, homogeneous, and acidophilic, but often the inclusion body has a granular appearance with an irregular outline.

Clinical Findings

A. Variola Major (Smallpox): The incubation period is about 12 days. The onset may be gradual or sudden. One to 5 days of fever and malaise precede the appearance of the exanthems, which are papular for 1–4 days, vesicular for 1–4 days, and pustular for 2–6 days, forming crusts which fall off 2–4 weeks after the first sign of the lesion and leave pink scars which fade slowly. In each skin area affected, the lesions are generally found in the same stage of development. The temperature falls within 24 hours after the rash appears.

The nature and extent of the rash are functions of the severity of the disease. Vaccinated contacts may develop a febrile illness called **variola sine eruptione**. They have all the symptoms of the pre-eruptive stage of smallpox, but the disease progresses no further. In severe cases, the rash is hemorrhagic. The case mortality rate varies from 5% (discrete rash) to over 40% (confluent rash).

B. Variola Minor (Alastrim): The symptoms during the prodromal period are similar to those of variola major but not so severe. The distribution and course of the eruption are also similar, but the lesions are less profuse. The disease is like that of mild variola major in vaccinated persons. Mortality is under 1%.

Modified or mild smallpox may occur when the infecting virus is of low virulence, as in variola minor, or when the patient has some immunity, as in variola major in vaccinated individuals. In modified smallpox of either type, lesions are smaller and more superficial and develop more rapidly than in severe smallpox. The real difference between them lies in the disease transmitted to contacts: Variola minor invariably gives rise to a mild disease in the contacts, whereas modified variola major often gives rise to severe smallpox.

Laboratory Diagnosis

The tests which should be used at various stages of smallpox are shown in Table 36–1. They are especially important in previously vaccinated persons, in whom the clinical course may be atypical. They depend upon direct microscopic examination of material from skin lesions, recovery of virus from the patient, identification of viral antigen from the lesion, and demonstration of antibody in the blood. The direct examination of clinical material in the electron microscope can also be used for rapid identification of virus particles, and can readily differentiate smallpox from chickenpox.

The virus can sometimes be found in the blood in moderately severe cases during the first day or so of illness. However, in the severe, fulminating, hemorrhagic case, the virus is regularly present in the blood until the time of death. Complement fixing antigen may even be found in the serum in such cases. The virus is found regularly in the skin of all cases, and typical histopathologic findings are present in the skin of fatal cases.

A. Smears: In a high percentage of cases, carefully prepared and properly stained smears from lesions of the papular and vesicular stages give a positive result within 30 minutes after the sample is submitted. Smears on grease-free slides are made with material from papules or from the bases of vesicles by first removing the superficial epidermis and then scraping the lesion gently with the point of a knife or a needle. The smears are washed with distilled water and ether, fixed with alcohol, and stained as follows: A mixture of equal parts of 1% gentian violet and 2% sodium bicarbonate is filtered onto the slide and allowed to react for 5 minutes with steaming. If elementary bodies are seen in large numbers, a presumptive diagnosis of smallpox can be made. Negative microscopic findings in confirmed smallpox cases are frequently due to the unsuitable nature of the material submitted for examination. After the vesicular stage of the disease, this method gives unsatisfactory results.

B. Virus Culture: The detection of virus on the chorioallantoic membrane of the 12- to 14-day-old chick embryo is the most reliable laboratory test. It is the easiest way of distinguishing cases of smallpox from generalized vaccinia which may occur in vaccinated persons during an epidemic period, for the lesions produced by these viruses on the membrane differ markedly. The use of the chick embryo is more

TABLE 36–1. Laboratory tests in diagnosis of smallpox. (After Downie.)

Stage of Illness	Material to Be Examined	Microscopic Examination of Smears From Skin Lesions	Culture on Chick Embryo Chorioallantois or in Tissue Culture	Detection of Antigen by Agar Gell Diffusion or Complement Fixation	Detection of Antibody
Pre-eruptive illness	Blood		May be positive	May be positive	Usually negative
Macular and papular	Smears (on slides) from skin lesions	Usually positive	Usually positive	May be positive	
	Blood				Usually negative
Vesicular	Vesicle fluid and smears (on slides) from base of vesicles	Usually positive	Usually positive	Usually positive	
	Blood				Usually negative
Pustular	Pustule fluid	May be positive	Usually positive	Usually positive	
	Blood				May be positive
Crusting	Crusts	Usually negative	Usually positive	Usually positive	
	Blood				Usually positive
Later	Blood				Usually positive
Time required for completion of test		1 hour	1–3 days	3–24 hours	3–24 hours

reliable than the corneal inoculation of the rabbit (Paul's test), which may be followed by a specific keratitis. Penicillin may be added to the inoculum (from papules, vesicles, or crusts) in a concentration of 500 units/ml to suppress bacterial contaminants. The lesion becomes apparent in 2–3 days. Its specificity should be confirmed by histologic examination of the membranes and by hemagglutination inhibition and neutralization with antivaccinia serum on passage of the virus into other eggs.

Susceptible cultures may be prepared from human embryonic tissue, monkey kidney, or continuous cell lines. Three days are usually required for cytopathic changes to become evident, but virus may be detected 1–2 days earlier by hemadsorption with added chick cells, by development of typical cytoplasmic inclusions in stained coverslip preparations from the culture, or by immunofluorescence.

C. Antigen Detection: Antigen can be detected readily by the complement fixation test if sufficient material is collected from the skin lesion. It can also be detected by immunodiffusion.

D. Antibody Determination: Serum antibody can be detected in patients after the first week. Neutralizing, complement fixing, and hemagglutination inhibiting antibodies may be detected; only the last 2 tests are used regularly since they can be carried out in vitro. Antibody tests are of little value in recently vaccinated persons, even though antibody levels are slightly higher in smallpox patients than in vaccinated individuals. However, as the complement fixing antibody is transient and is rarely found more than 12 months after vaccination, the detection of this antibody is of diagnostic value in patients with variola sine eruptione who have been vaccinated over a year previously. Not all chickens provide suitable erythrocytes for the hemagglutination test. Screening of chickens is done by using cardiolipin antigen diluted 1:10,000; cells agglutinated by this antigen will be agglutinated by the variola-vaccinia group of viruses.

Differential Diagnosis

There are no laboratory methods for distinguishing variola major from variola minor. This must be done on epidemiologic grounds alone. Unusual cases of smallpox may be confused with varicella, pustular acne, meningococcemia, blood dyscrasias, drug rashes, and other illnesses associated with a skin eruption, but none of these illnesses yield materials which give positive laboratory tests for variola virus or its antibody (Table 36–1).

Vaccinia virus, cowpox virus, and herpesvirus can be distinguished from smallpox virus by the morphologic pattern of the pocks produced on the chorioallantois. Vaccinia virus pocks are large, with necrotic centers, while cowpox virus pocks are hemorrhagic. Herpesvirus pocks are smaller than those of variola virus. In addition, herpesvirus can be distinguished from the poxviruses by the intranuclear inclusions found in herpetic infection and by virus-specific serologic reactions.

Variola and alastrim can also be differentiated from other poxviruses (vaccinia, cowpox, rabbitpox, monkeypox) by the inability of variola major and minor to form plaques on monolayers of chick embryo fibroblasts. Another distinguishing property is that vaccinia, unlike variola, can be passed serially in rabbits by skin to skin passage.

Immunity

Children are born with maternal antibodies, but these are lost within a few months after birth. At that time artificial immunity should be produced by vaccination (see Control, below). Immunity is demonstrable 8 or 9 days following vaccination, reaches its maximum within 2 or 3 weeks, and is maintained at an appreciable level for a few years. Vaccination in infancy may be responsible for attenuation of the disease in later life. In endemic areas, vaccination should be repeated at least at yearly intervals. It should also be repeated yearly in persons apt to be exposed; these include quarantine officers, customs officers, health officers, and people working in infectious disease hospitals. In the USA, vaccination should be repeated about every 7 years to maintain immunity.

In those who recover from smallpox, active immunity persists for years.

The efficiency of passively conferred antibody in protecting unvaccinated persons from smallpox has been well established. Animal model studies have also demonstrated effective passive immunization with antisera against poxviruses. However, antibodies alone do not appear to be sufficient for recovery from primary poxvirus infection. In the human host, neutralizing antibodies develop within a few days after onset of smallpox but do not prevent progression of lesions, and patients often die in the pustular stage with high antibody levels. There is strong evidence that delayed hypersensitivity or some other aspect of cell-mediated immunity may be as important as circulating antibody. Patients with hypogammaglobulinemia generally react normally to vaccinations and develop immunity, despite the apparent absence of antibody. Immunity is accompanied by well-developed delayed cutaneous hypersensitivity to vaccinia. It also appears that patients who have defects in both cellular immune response and antibody response develop a progressive, usually fatal, disease upon vaccination.

Delayed Hypersensitivity

The major problem confronting attempts to determine the relative importance of cellular versus humoral immunity to poxviruses is the difficulty in separating the effects of a cellular response from the effects of an antibody response in in vivo studies. A number of in vitro tests have been recently developed which appear to be reliable indicators of delayed hypersensitivity reactions. One test, the macrophage migration inhibition test, has been used to measure delayed hypersensitivity to virus infections in vitro. If macrophages and lymphocytes pelleted in capillary tubes are placed in culture chambers, the macrophages migrate out of the tubes over the glass surface. If antigen is placed in the culture chamber, macrophages fail to migrate from the tubes. Inhibition of migration of the macrophages is apparently due to a factor produced by the sensitized lymphocytes upon contact with the antigen. Recent studies with fibroma virus, a poxvirus that produces benign tumors in rabbits, indicate that there is a good correlation between the onset of delayed hypersensitivity to fibroma infection and inhibition of migration (Fig 36–2). Tumor regression does not occur until several days after a positive skin test and a positive migration inhibition test are observed. Increase in tumor size after onset of delayed hypersensitivity is not due to spread of the infection but to a local immune reaction due to infiltration of inflammatory cells into the lesion. This is indicated by the observation that animals bearing tumors become resistant to reinfection on the fifth day after the primary infections, which correlates with development of delayed hypersensitivity.

In addition to a delayed hypersensitivity reaction which could suppress virus synthesis and spread at the site of infection (pathogenesis of the vaccinia skin lesion), production of interferon, which would block virus synthesis, is a possible defense mechanism. This is supported by the observations that irradiated animals,

without detectable antibody or delayed hypersensitivity, recovered from vaccinia infection as rapidly as untreated control animals.

Although the precise mechanism involved in immunity to poxviruses is not known, it is probable that active immunity is promoted through a combination of the different types of immunologic responses.

Treatment

Vaccinia immune globulin (VIG) is available for immediate shipment anywhere in the USA. The American Red Cross has established a program for the preparation and distribution of VIG in cooperation with the Armed Forces—newly vaccinated servicemen provide blood for the hyperimmune gamma globulin. Indications for use of VIG are accidental inoculation of vaccine in the eye, eczema vaccinatum, and preventing or diminishing the severity of the disease in contacts of smallpox cases. VIG should be given as soon as possible after exposure. After clinical smallpox is evident, VIG is of no value, since by that time in the course of the disease the patient has already made his own neutralizing antibodies and at levels higher than could be obtained by VIG administration.

Antibiotics have no effect in the early stages of smallpox but may be of value in preventing secondary bacterial infection in the pustular stage.

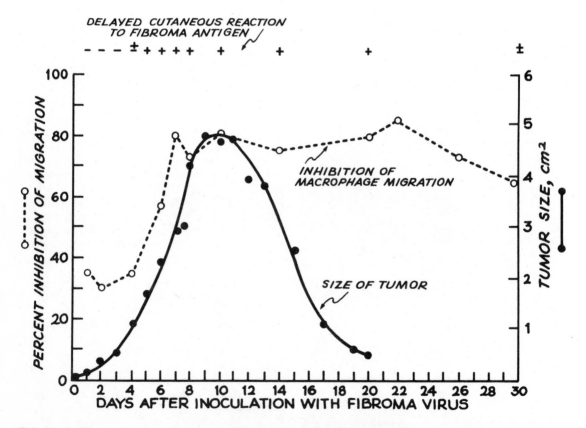

FIG 36–2. Temporal relationship between fibroma virus-induced tumor growth and regression and development of cell-mediated immune response as measured in vivo by skin testing and in vitro by macrophage migration inhibition. (From Tompkins and Rawls.)

Epidemiology

Smallpox is highly contagious. Transmission can often be traced to direct contact between cases. Indirect contact may also occur, as in the infection of laundry workers through infected bedclothes. The virus can survive for months; outbreaks in England have been initiated by cotton imported from Egypt.

Patients are not infectious during the incubation period. They first become infectious in the pre-eruptive stage, when virus appears in the throat. Lesions of the throat occur earlier than lesions of the skin. With the rupture of the vesicle or pustule, the skin lesions become infective and remain so throughout the disease. Early erosion of the lesions on the mucous membranes leads to heavy contamination of the oral, nasal, and bronchial secretions.

In the absence of vaccination, all human beings are susceptible to smallpox. The disease occurs at all seasons of the year but is less prevalent in summer.

When it occurs, the mild type of smallpox seems more difficult to control than the severe type. It has been suggested that virulent strains are quickly and effectively exterminated by proper control measures, whereas mild strains do not cause alarm, and quarantine and vaccination precautions are therefore not so rigorously enforced.

In the USA it is now a rare event for even one case of smallpox to be reported per year. In recent European outbreaks, the disease remained unrecognized until the third or fourth cycle of transmission, when over 20 cases had occurred, more than 10 weeks after the first imported case (usually a national returning home from an area of endemicity). When the disease is reintroduced into the USA, the course of events will probably be the same.

Control (Vaccination)

The introduction of living vaccinia virus into the skin dates from Jenner's work, published in 1798. Variolation, the introduction into the skin of variola virus obtained from mild cases of smallpox, had been used before this time for centuries by the Chinese. Vaccinia virus for vaccination is prepared from vesicular lesions ("lymph") produced in the skin of calves or sheep. (Recent experiments suggest that equally good virus for vaccination may be prepared in tissue cultures of bovine embryos. Tissue culture virus, like virus grown in chick embryos, can be harvested under bacteriologically sterile conditions.) The final product contains 40% glycerol and 0.4% phenol in order to destroy bacteria and keep the vaccine from freezing at its storage temperature of $-10°$ C. Commercial calf lymph vaccine of good potency should contain about 4×10^{10} virus particles per ml, which can be measured directly by electron microscopic counting methods. This should be the equivalent of about 10^8 infectious units per ml. WHO standards require that smallpox vaccines have a potency of not less than 10^8 pock forming units per ml.

Vaccine as issued to physicians can be stored for several weeks in the ordinary refrigerator without significant loss in potency. Once removed to room temperature, it should be used within a few days. Deterioration of vaccine is a problem in tropical countries, where it is often necessary to send vaccinators on long journeys from the base laboratory. For tropical countries, dried vaccinia virus is recommended. Stable lyophilized vaccinia virus has been prepared from the chorioallantoic membranes of hens' eggs. It should be reconstituted with 5% peptone, which has a protective effect on the virus and little capacity to sensitize the persons to be vaccinated. The availability of a jet injection instrument permits the rapid, effective administration of vaccine to large populations in a short period of time.

A. Time of Vaccination: Primary vaccination has usually been carried out in infants between 4 and 6 months of age. It has been pointed out recently, however, that eczema vaccinatum, unduly severe takes, progressive vaccinia, and other complications are all more commonly seen under the age of 1 year. It is therefore recommended that vaccinating between 1 and 2 years of age would be preferable to vaccinating in the first year of life. Primary vaccination gives the child a basic immunity and protects him against the risk of developing postvaccinal encephalitis when revaccination becomes necessary at a later time, for postvaccinal encephalitis has its lowest incidence after primary vaccination of young children. Infants suffering from skin diseases, or their healthy siblings, should not be vaccinated, because the vaccinia virus may localize in the lesions of the vaccinated child or of the contact (eczema vaccinatum).

Revaccination is done at regular intervals (before entering school and again at the age of 16 or so) or in the face of possible exposure to smallpox. In countries like India where smallpox is endemic, revaccination is recommended at yearly intervals or even oftener. It is possible that revaccination should be considered at regular 3-year intervals since resistance to infection falls off sharply 3 years after vaccination. All resistance to infection is felt to be gone 20 years following vaccination.

Smallpox may occur in spite of successful vaccination. Early allergic responses may be mistaken for immune reactions. In one study of 2000 Indians with smallpox, over 1800 had one or more vaccination scars. To afford real protection, vaccination must be successfully performed before exposure. When vaccination immediately follows exposure, it is much less protective.

B. Technic: The method of choice is that of multiple pressure. The skin on the arm over the lower part of the posterior border of the deltoid muscle is used. It is prepared by swabbing with acetone or ether or by washing with soap and water. After the area is dry, a drop of the vaccine is placed on the skin, and the side of the needle is then pressed firmly 10–20 times through the drop of vaccine into the superficial layers of the skin. The point of the needle should not draw blood. No dressing should be applied.

C. Reactions and Interpretations:

1. **Primary take**—In the fully susceptible person, no reaction is seen until the third or fourth day, at

which time a papule appears that is surrounded by a narrow areola of hyperemia. The papule increases in size until vesiculation appears (on the fifth or sixth day). The vesicle reaches its maximum size by the ninth day, and then becomes pustular, usually with some tenderness of the axillary nodes. Desiccation follows and is complete in about 2 weeks, leaving a depressed pink scar which ultimately turns white. The reading of the result is usually made on the seventh day. Virus which has been inactivated by storage at room temperature will not produce a primary take.

2. **Accelerated (vaccinoid) reaction**—This indicates partial immunity. A small vesicle appears on about the fifth day and becomes pustular within a few days; the entire reaction is complete by 10 days.

3. **Immediate (immune) reaction**—If the person is immune to smallpox, a small papule appears on the second day and disappears within 3 days. Virus which has become inactivated by storage at excessive temperatures will also produce this allergic reaction. Therefore, the fact that a vaccine lot produces an immune reaction is no proof that it contains live virus capable of producing primary takes in susceptible persons.

The term "immune reaction" may be misleading, for immunity does not always exist in persons giving this reaction. The WHO Expert Committee on Smallpox recommended that successful vaccination or revaccination reactions should be termed major reactions and all others should be termed equivocal.

A **successful revaccination** is one which on examination 1 week (6–8 days) later shows a vesicular or pustular lesion or an area of definite palpable induration or congestion surrounding a central lesion, which may be a scab or ulcer. These reactions should be termed "major reactions"; all others should be termed "equivocal reactions." A major reaction indicates virus multiplication with consequent development of immunity. An equivocal reaction may be the consequence of immunity adequate to prevent virus multiplication or may be an allergic skin response elicited by inactive vaccine or poor technic. Since these cannot be differentiated, vaccine potency should be checked and revaccination repeated. A second reading should be made after 6–8 days, and, if the result is still equivocal, revaccination should again be repeated. This should be done at a different site, preferably the highly susceptible forearm, using many pressures or even insertions into the skin. A new lot of vaccine should be employed.

Simultaneous administration of yellow fever and smallpox vaccines is feasible under special conditions (see pp 303 and 308).

D. **Complications of Vaccination:**

1. **Bacterial infection of the vaccination site**—This has been attributed to faulty technic at the time of vaccination or to subsequent infection of the vaccinal lesion. Tetanus is reported to occur only when the vaccinated area has been covered by a dressing.

2. **Generalized vaccinia**—This is manifested by the occurrence of crops of vaccinal lesions over the surface of the body. Following vaccination, virus may circulate in the blood; children suffering from eczematous conditions of the skin are therefore apt to develop vaccinal lesions on the eczematous areas (eczema vaccinatum). Unless the risk of smallpox is great, children with a current or past history of eczema should not be vaccinated, since the mortality in generalized vaccinia is 30–40%. Neither should children who have siblings with eczema be vaccinated, because of the danger of transmitting the virus and producing generalized vaccinia (often fatal) in the siblings. Generalized vaccinia can occur in the absence of eczema, but this is rare. The use of vaccinia immune globulin has reduced the fatality rate of eczema vaccinatum from 40% to 7%.

Recent trials with an attenuated vaccine in patients suffering from eczema or other skin disorders resulted in antibody production comparable to that of normal individuals receiving the standard vaccine. Local and systemic reactions were significantly less marked than in normal individuals receiving the standard vaccine. Secondary vaccinations of the eczematous patients with the standard vaccine resulted in marked modification in the reaction with no systemic or febrile complications.

Since the majority of postvaccinal complications are associated with primary vaccination, a strong case can be argued for use of such an attenuated vaccine for primary vaccination which would confer partial immunity and reduce the risk of complications and the severity of vaccination reactions with the standard strain.

3. **Postvaccinal encephalitis**—The mortality rate of this serious complication may be as high as 40%. However, the incidence among vaccinated persons is usually not over 1 per 100,000, but is higher in adults who receive vaccine for the first time. The onset is sudden about 12 days after vaccination. There is a pleocytosis of the CSF, the lymphocyte count being 100–200/cu mm. Focal lesions are widely distributed throughout the gray and white matter of the brain and cord. Perivascular infiltrations of mononuclear cells and areas of demyelination are the chief histologic lesions. The etiology is not clear. Several possibilities exist: (1) Vaccinia virus may invade the CNS. (2) Vaccination may activate a latent virus of the nervous system. (3) The reaction may be due to an antigen-antibody reaction which is allergic in character. Similar demyelinating disease may follow infection with variola, measles, and varicella, and vaccination against rabies. In small babies (and sometimes in adults), there may be an encephalopathy without demyelination.

Recent trials with an inactivated smallpox vaccine seem to offer hope of almost completely eliminating neural postvaccinal complications. The inactivated vaccine was given to over 16,500 adults who had never been vaccinated. This was followed by live virus vaccination. Only one case of mild postvaccinal encephalopathy was noted, while several cases of severe encephalopathy would have been expected in such an adult population receiving the live vaccine alone.

4. **Vaccinia necrosum or progressive vaccinia**—This results from inability to make antibody or to

develop cellular resistance, eg, in persons with lymphoma undergoing immunosuppressive chemotherapy. These children are sick 4–5 months and usually die. Treatment with vaccinia immune globulin may be of value.

As indicated above, smallpox vaccination is associated with a definite measurable risk. In a 1963 USA study involving 6 million primary vaccinees (chiefly young children) and 8 million revaccinees and their contacts, there occurred 12 cases of vaccinia encephalitis, 9 cases of vaccinia necrosum, and 108 cases of eczema vaccinatum, with 7 deaths among them. Virtually all of the vaccine-associated illnesses occurred among the primary vaccinees. Over half of the complications could have been prevented if the contraindications to vaccination had been observed.

Some have recommended delaying primary vaccination until adulthood and giving it only to persons at risk. The argument is that vaccination does not accomplish its intended purpose. While young children are protected against smallpox, they are not the most likely population to be exposed. On the other hand, young adults, a more crucial population in smallpox importation, have a relatively high rate of susceptibility. Vaccination of persons at risk would involve about 1–2 million primary vaccinees per year (military service, travelers, health workers), and the annual complications would probably be greater than those now being reported since the incidence of complications is higher in primary adult vaccinees. It would appear that the optimal time for primary vaccination is in the second year of life.

In England, compulsory vaccination is held to be unnecessary chiefly because smallpox is no longer endemic there; sanitary regulations at the ports have helped prevent introduction of smallpox into England. Material from suspicious cases aboard ship is sent ahead by air to London so that the diagnosis can be made before the ship arrives in Britain. However, importation of virus by air travelers (or in such material as cotton) makes it almost impossible to keep the virus out by even the most rigorous measures. When the disease occurs, control depends upon the prompt detection and isolation of cases and the tracing, vaccination, and observation of all contacts. Mass vaccination is not recommended by the British authorities.

Current research on more highly attenuated strains for vaccine suggests that in the near future the dangerous complications of vaccination will be eliminated. Mass protection will be accomplished by providing a minimum primary antigenic experience with a modified less virulent strain at an early age.

E. Drug Prophylaxis: Methisazone (N-methylisatin-β-thiosemicarbazone, Marboran) has been shown to provide transitory protection in an individual who has been exposed to smallpox. In this situation the drug is of value, but it is by no means a substitute for vaccination. It is of no value in the treatment of the disease once the patient has become febrile. A note of caution appears in the observation that drug-resistant strains have been produced in the laboratory.

Rifampin, an antibiotic which functions by preferentially inhibiting RNA polymerase of bacteria over that of animal cells, has recently been applied to poxvirus infections. The reason for this is that poxviruses contain their own RNA polymerase which is needed to transcribe the viral DNA into viral messenger RNA, and rifampin preferentially inactivates the viral RNA polymerase also. Field trials against smallpox are under way.

COWPOX

This disease of cattle is milder than the pox diseases of other animals, the lesions being confined to the teats and udders. Infection of man occurs by direct contact during milking, and the lesion in milkers is usually confined to the hands. In unvaccinated persons the disease is more severe than in the vaccinated. The local lesion is associated with fever and lymphadenitis, and generalized eruption is rare.

Immunologically and in host range, cowpox virus is similar to vaccinia virus. It is also closely related immunologically to variola virus, which is the foundation of Jenner's observation that those who have had cowpox are immune to smallpox. However, British workers believe that cowpox virus is distinct from that of vaccinia. Cowpox virus can be readily distinguished from vaccinia virus by the deep red hemorrhagic lesions which cowpox virus produces on the chorioallantoic membrane of the chick embryo. The strains of vaccinia virus used for vaccination of man are of uncertain origin. If originally derived from cowpox strains, their artificial passage in laboratory animals has resulted in new properties.

YABA MONKEY VIRUS

This simian poxvirus causes benign histiocytomas 5–20 days after subcutaneous or intramuscular administration to monkeys. These tumors regress after about 5 weeks; this is ascribed to the cytopathic effect of the virus itself. Intravenous administration of the virus causes the appearance of multiple histiocytomas in the lungs, heart, and skeletal muscles. The virus is easily isolated from tumor tissue, and characteristic inclusions are found in the tumor cells.

Monkeys of various species and human beings are susceptible to the oncogenic effect of the virus. Newborn mice, hamsters, guinea pigs, rabbits, cats, dogs, and developing chick embryos have proved insusceptible, though the virus has been administered in various ways. When tumors have been developed experimentally, they have always been of the same type. Under natural conditions the virus is possibly transmitted by blood-sucking vectors (as is myxoma, a poxvirus of rabbits).

In morphology, the Yaba virus particles are similar to vaccinia and molluscum contagiosum virions. No immunologic relationship has been found between Yaba virus and other representatives of the poxvirus group, including monkeypox and infectious simian dermatitis viruses. The virus multiplies in cultures of monkey kidney cells (Cercopithecus) with cytopathic and proliferative effects, and characteristic eosinophilic inclusions in the cytoplasm of the cell have been found. The virus usually occurs intracellularly in cultures and appears to be transmitted directly from cell to cell. Multiplication in cultures has been accomplished only in cells of monkey origin.

Recent studies have characterized the Yaba virus DNA. The DNA has a guanine plus cytosine content of 32.5%, which is significantly different from the 36% G + C of vaccinia, rabbitpox, cowpox, and ectromelia viruses.

MOLLUSCUM CONTAGIOSUM

The lesions of this disease are small, pink, wartlike tumors on the face, arms, back, and buttocks. The disease occurs throughout the world, in both sporadic and epidemic forms, and is more frequent in children than in adults. It is spread by direct and indirect contact (eg, by barbers, common use of towels).

Histologically, inclusions form in basal layers of the epithelium, gradually enlarge, crowd the nucleus to one side, and eventually fill the cell.

The virus has not been transmitted to animals but has been studied, particularly by electron microscopy, in the human lesion. The purified virus is more or less oval or brick-shaped, having a major axis of 330 nm and a minor axis of 230 nm.

In ultrathin sections of infected cells, the inclusion bodies are divided into compartments by extremely thin walls with nests of mature virus particles filling the cavities between the septa. The matrix of the cytoplasm surrounding the cavities appears to be honeycombed and to be undergoing segmentation into spherical objects which are larger than the virus itself. The virus appears to form within this larger sphere.

The virus is cytopathic for human and monkey cell cultures but has not yet been serially transferred in culture. Virus particles in extracts from lesions of molluscum contagiosum interfere with the growth of heterologous viruses in cultures of mouse embryo cells. This interference action can now be used to study biologic properties of the virus. Thus it was found that the pattern of adsorption of molluscum virus with respect to time, temperature, and inoculum volume is similar to that already described for adsorption of vaccinia virus infective units to cells in culture.

● ● ●

General References

Downie, A.W., & C.H. Kempe: Poxviruses. Pages 281–320 in: *Diagnostic Procedures for Viral and Rickettsial Infections,* 4th ed. American Public Health Association, 1969.

Dumbell, K.R.: Laboratory aids to the control of smallpox in countries where the disease is not endemic. Progr Med Virol 10:388–397, 1968.

Joklik, W.K.: The poxviruses. Ann Rev Microbiol 22:359–390, 1968.

Lane, J.M., & others: Complications of smallpox vaccination, 1968. New England J Med 281:1201–1208, 1969.

37 . . .

Adenovirus Group

The adenovirus group consists of over 30 antigenic types, some of which cause acute respiratory diseases or the febrile catarrhs. Some adenoviruses also cause certain external diseases of the eye (conjunctival sac). Certain adenoviruses serve as models of cancer viruses because they produce tumors in hamsters.

Properties of the Virus

A. Nucleic Acid: DNA. The DNA content is specific for each adenovirus type, and ranges from 11.6–13.5%. Base ratio determinations revealed 3 distinct groups of adenoviruses: those with a low guanine + cytosine (G + C) content (48–49%); those with an intermediate G + C content (50–53%); and those with a high G + C content (56–60%). The strongly oncogenic adenovirus types 12, 18, and 31 are the only members of the group with low G + C, while certain adenoviruses in the intermediate group (types 3, 7, 21) are mildly oncogenic.

B. Size: The infective virus particles, 60–85 nm in diameter, are icosahedrons with shells (capsids) composed of 252 subunits (capsomeres). No outer envelope is known. Three major soluble antigens are separable from the infectious particle by differential centrifugation. These antigens, a group-specific antigen common to all adenovirus types, a type-specific antigen unique for each type, and a toxin-like material which also possesses group specificity, are felt to represent virus-structural protein subunits produced in large excess of the amount utilized for synthesis of infectious virus.

C. Reactions to Physical and Chemical Agents: These viruses are ether-resistant but are heat-labile, being destroyed at 56° C for 30 minutes. They are considerably more stable to pH alterations and to temperatures between 4° and 50° C than are the myxoviruses (influenza, mumps, Newcastle disease). They are relatively stable when exposed to temperatures ranging from 4–36° C, and type 4 shows less than a 2 log unit reduction when heated at 50° C for 20 minutes. They are resistant to the common antibiotics. The viruses are stable in the pH range from 6.0–9.0, less so in the pH range of 3.0–6.0, and are destroyed at pH 2.0 or below and at pH 10.0 or above. The viruses are usually stored frozen. One type has been lyophilized without loss of activity.

D. Animal Susceptibility and Transformation of Cells: The virus does not commonly produce disease in laboratory animals but has been shown to produce fatal infections in newborn hamsters (type 5), bronchopneumonic lesions in young, colostrum-deprived pigs, and tumors in newborn hamsters (types 3, 7, 12, 14, 16, 18, 21, 31). Although virus cannot be recovered from adenovirus-induced hamster tumors, a new antigen induced by the virus can be detected by complement fixation or immunofluorescence. This antigen, called tumor or T antigen because of its association with tumor or transformed cells, can also be detected in the cytolytic cycle of the virus. Hamster cells can be transformed in vitro by the oncogenic human adenoviruses. These cells contain the adenovirus tumor antigen, do not contain infectious virus, and will product tumors when inoculated into adult hamsters. Adenovirus messenger RNA (mRNA) can be detected in the cytoplasm and nucleus of either transformed or tumor cells. This mRNA has a guanine plus cytosine (G + C) content of 47–48%, even in tumor cells induced by adenovirus 7 or 16, both of which have a G + C content of 50–52% in their DNA. This suggests that viral DNA regions containing 47–48% G + C are those integrated in the tumor cells or that such regions are preferentially transcribed. However, the mRNA from tumor cells induced by the highly oncogenic adenoviruses (types 12 and 18) will not hybridize with DNA from the weakly oncogenic adenoviruses (types 7 and 16) and vice versa. Apparently, different viral-coded information is involved in carcinogenesis by the 2 different groups of adenoviruses.

Although no tumors have been produced in animals following inoculation of the nononcogenic human adenoviruses (eg, types 1, 2, 5), rat embryo cells have been successfully transformed in tissue culture by these agents. The transformed cells contain adenovirus tumor antigen and mRNA specific for the nononcogenic adenoviruses. Again, the mRNA contains only 49–51% G + C, although the DNA of this group averages 56–60% G + C. However, the cells have failed to produce tumors upon transplantation into adult animals to date.

E. Replication of Virus: Adenoviruses are cytopathic for human cell cultures, particularly primary kidney and continuous epithelial cells. Growth of virus in tissue culture is associated with a stimulation of acid production (increased glycolysis) in the early stages of infection. The viruses are epitheliotropic, growing and causing changes in human epithelial cells more rapidly than in fibroblasts. The cytopathic effect usually consists of marked rounding and aggregation of affected cells into grape-like clusters. It is noteworthy that adenoviruses 3, 4, 7, 14, and 21 are the greatest disease producers, and these in tissue cultures have shorter growth cycles than types 1, 2, 5, and 6. Monolayer cultures infected with adenoviruses take up neutral red just like healthy living cells. The infected cells do not lyse, even though they round up and leave the glass surface on which they have been grown. The chromatographic behavior of the soluble antigens (see below) on the anionic exchange resin DEAE-cellulose allows a similar subdivision into the 2 subgroups indicated by their biologic properties (enumerated above).

In HeLa cells infected with adenoviruses, rounded intranuclear inclusions, which progress from eosinophilic and Feulgen-negative to basophilic and Feulgen-positive, are prominent features. With types 3, 4, and 7 the amount of deoxyribonucleic acid increases in the nuclei of infected cells. Electron microscopic observations of thin sections of HeLa cells infected with these 3 types show that the virus particles develop in the nucleus and frequently exhibit crystalline arrangement in a cubic body-centered lattice. The crystals are strongly Feulgen-positive, indicating that the virus particles themselves contain deoxyribonucleic acid. A large proportion of cells infected with type 5 virus also contain crystals, but these crystals are not composed of viral particles. The crystals often exceed 30 μm in length and are readily visible in the light microscope. They are composed of protein and are devoid of nucleic acid. The crystalline protein has not been identified.

The tumor antigen (referred to in the preceding section) is induced early during the replicative cycle of the virus, prior to the synthesis of viral DNA and viral capsid proteins. There is recent evidence that adenovirus specific proteins are synthesized in the cytoplasm of infected cells and then moved rapidly into the nucleus where viral maturation occurs. In the adenovirus growth cycle in human epithelial cells, new virus particles can be detected about 16–20 hours after inoculation, and continue to be formed at a uniform rate for the next 24 hours. About 7000 virus particles are produced per infected cell, and most of them remain intracellular unless means are taken to release them. Particles having a density of 1.34 are highly infectious (1 particle in 5 is infectious), whereas those having densities of less than 1.30 are practically non-infectious (only 1 particle in 1000 is infectious) and are devoid of the DNA core. Crude infected cell lysates show huge quantities of capsomeres, sometimes partially assembled into viral components. In addition, strands whose width is equal to the diameter of the capsomeres can be seen associated with the developing virion.

In cells derived from heterologous species, the human adenoviruses undergo an abortive replicative cycle. Adenovirus tumor antigen, mRNA, and DNA are all synthesized, but no capsid proteins or infectious progeny are produced. This has resulted in problems in vaccine production (see Prevention & Control, p 403).

F. Antigenic Properties: At least 31 antigenic types have been isolated from human hosts, and in addition a number of different types have been isolated from other animals. At the present time, a number of distinct serotypes are known for simian, bovine, canine, murine, and avian species. They are specific by cross-neutralization tests. However, complement fixation tests reveal cross-reactions among the types. Virus preparations treated with heat or formalin to kill their infectivity still contain complement fixing antigen.

Adenoviruses contain 4 complement fixing antigens—A, B, C, and P—whose characteristics are described in Table 37–1. The hexon antigens form the majority of the capsomeres of the adenocapsid (240) and are 8 nm in diameter. The penton antigens are found at the 12 vertices of the capsid and are also 8 nm in diameter. Associated with the penton antigen is a toxin-like activity which causes tissue culture cells to detach from the surface on which they are growing. Attached to each penton is a fiber antigen. For adenovirus type 5, the fiber antigen consists of a rod (2 X 20 nm) attached to the penton with a 4 nm knob at the end. However, the dimensions of the fiber antigen vary with the adenovirus type. The P antigen of adenoviruses is an internal antigen, which is released upon virus disruption and is very unstable. The hemagglutinating activity of adenovirus is associated with the penton and fiber antigens.

In addition, polyacrylamide gel electrophoresis of purified adenovirus and adenovirus subunits after disruption by detergent (sodium dodecyl sulfate) and urea has revealed 9 virus-specific polypeptides. The hexon capsomere is composed of 3 molecules of a single type (component II) which comprises about 50% of the total virion. Groups of these hexon capsomeres ("groups of nine") are associated with 2 additional minor polypeptides (components VIII and IX). The penton base is composed of a single type of peptide (component III), as is the fiber antigen (component IV) also. The internal core released by treatment of the virion with 5 M urea contains the viral DNA in association with 3 arginine rich peptides (components V, VI, VII) which comprise some 20% of the total virion protein. In addition, there is a very small polypeptide (component X) whose location in the virion and role remain unknown.

A hemagglutinin has been used to separate the human viruses into 3 subgroups. Group A (types 3, 7, 11, 14, 16, 20, 21, 25, 28) agglutinates rhesus but not rat erythrocytes; group B (8, 9, 10, 13, 15, 17, 19, 22, 23, 24, 26, 27, 29, 30) agglutinates rat cells but not (or hardly) rhesus cells; group C (1, 2, 4, 5, 6) fails to agglutinate rhesus cells and only partially agglutinates rat cells. Types 12, 18, and 31 do not usually agglutinate, but some strains partially agglutinate rat cells. The hemagglutination-inhibition test is being used for type-specific identification.

Some cross-reactions have been noted, particularly between types 3 and 7; 7, 11, and 14; 10 and 19; 15 and 28; 14 and 16; and 12, 18, and 31.

TABLE 37–1. Comparative data on adenovirus type 2 morphological, antigenic, and polypeptide subunits.

Appearance	Name	Number Per Virion	Molecular Weight	Antigen	Specificity	Protein Components
Virion	DNA		23,000,000			
Virion	Protein		150,000,000			
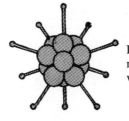 O	Hexon	240	210,000 400,000 320,000 360,000	A	Group	II
Hexons	Hexons	20	3,600,000			II, VIII, IX
Penton	Penton	12	280,000 1,100,000			III, IV
O	Penton Base	12	210,000	B	Subgroup	III
Fiber	Fiber	12	70,000	C	Type	IV
Core	DNA	1	23,000,000	P		V, VI, VII
	Protein		29,000,000			
	Protein		13,000			VIII, IX
	Protein		7,500			X

Dodecon: Hemagglutinin made up of 12 pentons with their fibers.

G. Adenovirus-SV40 "Hybrid": An adenovirus grown in monkey kidney cell cultures was found to be contaminated with papovavirus SV40. After removal of all infectious SV40 by passage in the presence of specific SV40 antiserum, the virus still contained the tumorigenic properties of the papovavirus SV40, and has been called an adenovirus-SV40 "hybrid." Although the virus population can be completely neutralized by type-specific adenovirus antiserum, it still contains SV40 genetic material. (See Chapter 40, Oncogenic Viruses, for further discussion.)

H. Adenosatellite Virus: During the course of biophysical studies on adenoviruses, a 20 nm particle was found in several adenovirus preparations. These particles contain DNA and appear to possess a protein coat which exhibits icosahedral symmetry. The particles have been named adenosatellite virus or adeno-associated virus. Adenosatellite virus appears to be a defective virus since it thus far has been unable to replicate in the absence of adenoviruses. However, the adenosatellite virus does not seem to be antigenically related to the adenovirus group. Four antigenic types of satellite virus are recognized. Types 1–3 naturally infect man; type 4 infects monkeys. They are not known to be pathogenic.

Pathogenesis & Pathology

At least 5 adenovirus types have been demonstrated in the tissues of adenoids and tonsils removed at surgery, by growing epithelium from such tissue for prolonged periods in culture. The viruses could not be isolated from nasopharyngeal swabs or from suspensions of adenoids and tonsils of the same persons by the conventional method of inoculating such material into highly susceptible cell cultures. One possible explanation of the greater sensitivity of the first procedure is that patients who yielded these viruses have usually possessed serum antibodies against the virus type later recovered from them. Such antibodies have also been demonstrated in suspensions of adenoidal and tonsillar tissue. It is likely that these antibodies were gradually washed from the culture tube and thus from the outgrowing cells during several weeks of biweekly changes of tissue culture fluid. The question has been raised whether these agents play a role not only in acute diseases but also in chronic diseases (hypertrophy of tissues) of the nasopharynx that result in the necessity of surgical removal of adenoids and tonsils.

Viruses of this group were found in the adenoids or tonsils (or both) of 57% of children whose tissues were cultured. However, the groups were selected because of the pathology of these tissues, and no conclusions can yet be drawn about the prevalence of the viruses in tissues of children lacking the clinical indications for tonsillectomy or adenoidectomy. Conversely, the association or coexistence of the virus with adenoid-tonsillar pathology cannot be considered of etiologic significance.

In human volunteers, conjunctivitis caused by adenovirus infection occurs primarily in the eye that has been inoculated (by swabbing the palpebral conjunctiva with 100 TCD_{50}).

Clinical Findings

The acute illness, sometimes called febrile catarrh, is characterized by a basic syndrome of fever, pharyngitis, and cough, often with conjunctivitis, rhinitis, otitis, laryngitis, tracheobronchitis, or pneumonitis, accompanied by constitutional symptoms. Adenovirus diseases include syndromes designated as undifferentiated acute respiratory disease, pharyngoconjunctival fever, nonstreptococcal exudative pharyngitis, and primary atypical pneumonia unassociated with the development of cold or streptococcus MG agglutinins.

Pharyngoconjunctival fever may be caused by any of several adenovirus types. It is characterized by fever, conjunctivitis, pharyngitis, malaise, and cervical lymphadenopathy. The conjunctival features of the disease are readily reproduced when any adenovirus types are swabbed onto the eyes of volunteers. However, under natural conditions only types 3 and 7 regularly cause outbreaks in which conjunctivitis is a predominating symptom. Other types which have produced sporadic cases of conjunctivitis are types 1, 2, 5, and 6. Even when large numbers of the latter infections are occurring, conjunctivitis is an infrequent finding.

Type 8 is the cause of epidemic keratoconjunctivitis (shipyard eye). The disease is characterized by an acute conjunctivitis, with enlarged, tender preauricular nodes, followed by keratitis which leaves round, subepithelial opacities in the cornea for up to 2 years. Type 8 infections have been characterized by their lack of associated systemic symptoms; only in infants have systemic signs been observed. Intussusception of infancy has been reported to be caused by adenoviruses 1, 2, 3, and 5, which readily spread by the enteric route.

Laboratory Diagnosis

A. Recovery of Virus: The viruses are isolated by inoculation of tissue cultures of human cells, in which a characteristic series of cytopathic changes is produced. The viruses have been recovered from throat swabs, conjunctival swabs, rectal swabs, and stools of patients with acute pharyngitis and conjunctivitis. Virus isolations from the eye are obtained almost exclusively from the one with conjunctivitis.

B. Serology: In almost all cases, the neutralizing antibody responses of infected persons show a 4-fold or greater rise against the type recovered from the

patient, and in general no response, or much lesser response, to other types. Neutralizing antibodies are measured in human cell cultures using the cytopathic endpoint in tube cultures, or by the color test in panel cups or tubes under oil. The latter test depends upon the phenomenon that growth of adenovirus in HeLa cell cultures is accompanied by an excess production of acid over that of the uninfected control cultures, and that this viral lowering of pH can be prevented by immune serum. The pH is measured by incorporating phenol red into the medium and observing the color changes after 3 days of incubation. Serum and cell control cultures reach a pH of 7.4; virus activity is indicated by a pH of 7.0; and neutralization is presumed to have occurred where the pH is 0.2 units above that of the virus control.

Infection of human beings with a single adenovirus type stimulates a rise in complement fixing antibodies to adenovirus antigens of all types. The complement fixation test is of less value in identifying infections due to a particular type of virus. However, there is good evidence that responses to the common antigen are not produced by other agents; the complement fixation test, using the common antigen, is thus of considerable value as an easily applied method for detecting infection by a member of the group. Complement fixing antibody levels often go from negative to titers of 128.

Immunity

Studies in human volunteers contributed the following information: Type-specific neutralizing antibodies protect against the disease, but the protection is not absolute. It was possible to superimpose the infectious process in 27% of persons with evidence of previous infection with the same type as that given. Infections with the viruses were frequently induced without the production of overt illness.

The cumulative occurrence of neutralizing antibodies against one or more types in different age groups shows that antibodies may be present in over 50% of the infants 6–11 months of age. In one study a substantial increase in antibodies occurred in persons 2 years of age, but very little additional increase occurred in the children 3–5 years old. Marked increases were observed in the 6–15 and 16–34 age groups, in which the majority of persons had antibodies to 3 or more types. Normal healthy adults were found to have antibodies to at least 4–5 types of 6 tested.

The antibodies to types 1 and 2 were found to be especially prevalent in younger age groups, positive reactions occurring in 56 and 72%, respectively, of persons 6–15 years of age. Antibodies against types 3 and 4 were significantly less prevalent in persons in young adulthood than those for types 1 and 2.

Infants are usually born without complement fixing antibodies but develop these by 6 months of age. Older individuals with neutralizing antibodies to 4 or more strains frequently give completely negative complement fixation reactions. The complement fixing antibodies usually disappear long before the neutralizing antibodies. It is likely that the latter persist for life. Recent studies have shown that complement fixing antibodies may persist for varying periods of time, ranging up to at least 7 years. The variation in persistence may result from a number of factors, such as repeated exposure to the same or other adenoviruses, or perhaps the presence of the virus in a latent form. In studies of military populations it was shown that the incidence of infection (especially due to types 3 and 4) among recruits was not influenced by the presence or absence of group complement fixing antibodies on entrance into the new environment.

Epidemiology

Man is commonly infected with these agents, the virus being readily spread from person to person. Many of the types have been recovered by culture of adenoids and tonsils. In civilian populations only 2–4% of acute respiratory diseases are caused by adenoviruses, but in military groups the incidence of respiratory disease caused by these viruses is high.

Type 3 has been recovered commonly from patients with acute pharyngitis and conjunctivitis, a 5-day illness that occurs endemically in the general population, as well as in sharp outbreaks. The virus is found in almost all stools (as well as throat cultures) in the acute phase of the illness, the concentration of virus being as high as 10 million infectious doses per gram of stool. Some patients continue to excrete virus in the feces for at least 2 months. The virus has also been isolated from sewage during epidemic prevalence.

Type 1, 2, and 5 infections occur chiefly during the first years of life, and are associated with illnesses characterized by fever and pharyngitis. These are the types most frequently obtained from the adenoids and tonsils.

Respiratory disease due to types 3, 4, 7, 14, and 21 occurs commonly and widely among military recruits within the USA and elsewhere. Adenovirus disease causes great disability when large numbers of men are being inducted into the Armed Forces, and consequently its greatest impact is during periods of mobilization. During a 1-year study at an induction post, 10% of the 58,000 men given basic training were hospitalized for a respiratory illness caused by an adenovirus. During the winter, incidence of respiratory disease in recruits was about 20 per 1000 per week, and adenovirus accounted for 72% of all the respiratory disease. During the summer, incidence fell to 2 per 1000, and only 12% of these illnesses were caused by adenovirus. In contrast, adenovirus disease is not a serious problem in seasoned troops, the rates in recruits being 33 times higher. In another study, in which 80% of recruits became infected, 25% had a severe disease requiring hospitalization, while the disease in another 25% was sufficiently mild to permit treatment at the dispensary. The remaining 50% suffered either a very mild or an inapparent infection. Type 4 infections in troops were much less frequent during the summer than in the winter. Thus, only 10%

of the men showed a significant rise in antibody titer during their first 2 months in the company during the summer, in contrast to the 80% finding in the winter.

In children, type 7 has been associated with acute respiratory illnesses (high fever and involvement of nose, throat, conjunctivas, cervical lymph nodes, and lungs) and also with gastroenteritis, and type 21 has been associated with bronchitis and bronchial pneumonia. A large number of adenovirus types has been isolated in a small percentage of infants with diarrhea in different parts of the world, but their etiologic relationship to the disease has not been established.

A possible relationship of adenovirus to rubelliform exanthem exists. Among military recruits, types 4 and 7 were isolated from the sera of 9% and the urine of 35% of patients, as well as from throat and rectal swabs.

The conjunctivitis caused by certain adenoviruses, and the evident association of types 3 and 7 cases with swimming pools, suggest a relation with swimming pool conjunctivitis. However, the systemic clinical findings, the duration and character of the ocular findings, and the absence of inclusions in conjunctival smears distinguish these illnesses from swimming pool and inclusion conjunctivitis.

Epidemic keratoconjunctivitis caused by adenovirus type 8 is often spread by ophthalmologists in the course of examining and treating an infected eye. Minor injuries to the eye may predispose to infection. Epidemic keratoconjunctivitis was unknown in the USA until 1941, when it spread from Australia via the Hawaiian Islands to California and the Pacific Coast. There it spread rapidly through the shipyards and other industries, thence to the East Coast, and finally to the Midwest. In the USA the incidence of neutralizing antibody to type 8 adenovirus in the general population has been about 1%, whereas in Japan it has been over 30%. In Japan an effective vaccine has been developed. In the USA the incidence of the disease is regarded as too low to warrant vaccination.

At least 13 antigenic types were isolated in a study of conjunctival specimens in Saudi Arabia, with most of the strains being isolated during the summer from children under 2 years. Three of the types (16, 17, and strain 931) proved to be pathogenic for man, producing acute follicular conjunctivitis.

Canine hepatitis virus has recently been established as an adenovirus. It is therefore understandable why human beings infected with adenoviruses develop complement fixing antibodies against canine hepatitis virus.

Prevention & Control

A commercial trivalent vaccine produces neutralizing antibodies and immunity in human subjects. The vaccine was prepared by growing type 3, 4, and 7 viruses in monkey kidney cultures and then inactivating the viruses with formalin. Because adenovirus epidemics have been almost limited to the military, the vaccine was widely and effectively used in such populations. However, it has never been recommended for general use in civilian populations.

Since certain vaccine strains have been found to be contaminated genetically with the papovavirus SV40 tumor determinants, and since most strains of "clean" adenoviruses do not grow well in monkey kidney cells, vaccine made from contaminated strains was withdrawn from use in the USA in 1964. New experimental vaccines are under study. The first is made from adenovirus capsid protein, and thus circumvents the problem of contaminated genetic material. The second is made of noncontaminated live virus, and is given orally in a coated capsule to liberate the virus into the intestine. By this route the live vaccine has produced a subclinical infection which has conferred a high degree of immunity against wild strains and has the desirable property of not spreading from the vaccinated person to his contacts.

• • •

General References

Fujinaga, K., & M. Green: Mechanism of viral carcinogenesis by DNA mammalian viruses. 5. Properties of purified viral-specific RNA from human adenovirus-induced tumor cells. J Molec Biol 31:63–73, 1968.

Huebner, R.J.: Pages 149–163 in: *Malignant Transformation by Viruses.* Kirsten, W.H. (editor). Springer-Verlag (New York), 1966.

Maizel, J.V., Jr., White, D.O., & M.D. Scharff: The polypeptides of adenovirus. Soluble proteins, cores, top components and the structure of the virion. Virology 36:126–136, 1968.

Norrby, E.: The structural and functional diversity of adenovirus capsid components. J Gen Virol 5:221–236, 1969.

Rapp, F., & J.L. Melnick: Papovavirus SV40, adenovirus and their hybrids: Transformation, complementation, and transcapsidation. Prog Med Virol 8:349–399, 1966.

Rose, H.M.: Adenoviruses. Pages 205–226 in: *Diagnostic Procedures for Viral and Rickettsial Infections,* 4th ed. American Public Health Association, 1969.

Schmidt, N.J., Lennette, E.H., & C.J. King: Neutralizing, hemagglutination-inhibiting and group complement-fixing antibody responses in human adenovirus infections. J Immunol 97:64–74, 1966.

38 . . .

Herpesvirus Group

At least 20 viruses have been placed in the herpesvirus group. They all contain a core of DNA surrounded by a protein coat that exhibits icosahedral symmetry, which in turn is enclosed in an envelope. The envelope contains essential lipids, as the viral infectivity is sensitive to ether. The enveloped form is 180 nm in diameter; the "naked" virion is 110 nm in diameter and contains 162 capsomeres.

The molecular weight of the DNA of herpesviruses varies from $3-9 \times 10^7$ daltons. The guanine plus cytosine content also varies, the range being 33–73% for different members.

Herpes simplex virus types 1 and 2, varicellazoster virus, EB virus, and cytomegalovirus infect man. Herpes simplex virus is readily found in the fluid phase, but the other members of the group are more firmly associated with the cell. Although varicella and zoster strains have been grown in a number of tissue cultures, they have not yet been obtained free in the fluid phase (except when grown in cells from human thyroid). The EB (Epstein-Barr) herpesvirus appears to replicate only in human lymphoid cell cultures.

Herpesviruses that infect animals are B virus of Old World monkeys, marmoset virus of New World monkeys, pseudorabies virus of pigs, virus III of rabbits, infectious bovine rhinotracheitis virus, equine rhinopneumonitis (equine abortion) virus, canine herpesvirus, infectious laryngotracheitis virus of fowls, and cytomegalovirus of monkeys, guinea pigs, mice, and other animal species. Herpesviruses are also known for cold-blooded animals (frogs, snakes).

HERPES SIMPLEX
(Herpes Febrilis, Herpes Labialis, Herpetic Gingivostomatitis, Eczema Herpeticum, Herpes Genitalis)

Infection with herpes simplex virus (*Herpesvirus hominis*) may take several forms and is often inapparent. The clinical response is usually a mild vesicular eruption of the skin or mucous membranes. This eruption is both grossly and microscopically similar to herpes zoster; however, the viruses are unrelated antigenically and biologically (different host range). Herpes simplex may also cause severe illnesses, such as stomatitis, Kaposi's varicelliform eruption, sometimes fatal meningoencephalitis, and generalized, usually fatal, neonatal disease.

Properties of the Virus

A. Nucleic Acid: DNA. Molecular weight of DNA, $5-7 \times 10^7$ daltons. Density, 1.727 in CsCl. Guanine + cytosine content, 68%.

B. Size: When stained by phosphotungstate, the virus can be shown to consist of a DNA-containing core imbedded in a protein capsid surrounded by an outer membrane. The polyhedral core has a diameter of 78 nm; the capsid, 110 nm; and the envelope, 180 nm. The icosahedral capsid is made up of 162 units (capsomeres) arranged in an orderly manner (5:3:2 axial symmetry). Each capsomere is an elongated, chiefly hexagonal prism about 9×12 nm with a hole of 4 nm running down the middle. The envelope frequently shows periodic projections from its surface, and is in part derived from the nuclear membrane of the infected cell. It seems essential for infectivity. The envelope is rapidly removed by ether treatment.

The events that occur during the process of virus envelopment at the nuclear membrane and of subsequent virus release into extracellular fluid are described in Chapter 27.

C. Reactions to Physical and Chemical Agents: Suspensions of infected tissue may be stored in the frozen state. Long considered as exceedingly thermolabile, herpesvirus has recently been shown to become stabilized by 1 M Na_2SO_4 so that it withstands heating at 50° C, but the virus is not protected by 1 M $MgSO_4$ or 2 M NaCl. In contrast, herpesvirus is extremely thermosensitive at isotonic concentrations of any salt, but again becomes stable as the virus is diluted with distilled water. Thus, once removed from the isotonicity of the tissue culture medium in which it is grown, and suspended in distilled water, herpesvirus turns out to be a relatively stable virus. In the dry state herpes simplex virus may withstand temperatures as high as 90° C. It is destroyed by ether, 1% phenol, and 0.5% formaldehyde.

D. Animal Susceptibility and Growth of Virus: The virus has a wide host range and can infect rabbits, guinea pigs, mice, hamsters, rats, and the chorioallantois of the embryonated egg.

In rabbits, herpesvirus produces a typical vesicular eruption in the skin of the inoculated area. Generalized disease and meningoencephalitis develop in some cases, depending upon the type of animal and virus strain used. Corneal inoculation results in dendritic keratitis and in most instances keratoconjunctivitis. With some strains, the corneal involvement is regularly followed by encephalitis. Whether or not encephalitis has been manifest, the virus may be found several months after inoculation in the brains of survivors. During the period of viral latency, anaphylactic shock will precipitate an acute relapse of encephalomyelitis. In rabbits, corneal inoculation of virus produces herpetic keratitis followed by healing. Sensitization of the animals to horse serum and induction of an Arthus reaction in the healed cornea results in repeated recovery of infective herpesvirus.

In mice, stress imposed by avoidance-learning or by restraint induces an increased susceptibility to infection with the virus.

The chorioallantoic membrane is particularly susceptible to infection; lesions become obvious in 1–2 days and reach their maximum in 3–4 days. They are small, raised white plaques, and their number is directly proportionate to the concentration of virus particles. The virus also grows readily in tissue culture, producing typical inclusions; inclusion body formation is followed by necrosis of cells (cytopathic effect). The virus growth is suppressed by omitting the amino acid arginine from the tissue culture media. Human kidney or amnion or rabbit kidney cultures are the cells of choice.

Herpesviruses cause a rapid increase in the DNA-synthesizing enzyme thymidine kinase in infected cells. Enzymes produced by 2 different herpesviruses—one of man and one of pigs—are serologically different from each other and different from thymidine kinases in uninfected cells. The most likely explanation is that the genome of each virus codes for its own thymidine kinase. The enzyme adenosine triphosphatase may be carried by the virus from the plasma membrane of the cell. In Chinese hamster cells, which contain only 22 chromosomes, the virus causes aberrations which are usually restricted to breaks in region 7 of chromosome No. 1 and in region 3 of the X chromosome. The Y chromosome is unaffected.

E. Antigenic Properties: Associated with the growth of the virus is the production of a smaller, soluble complement fixing antigen. This antigen is also capable of eliciting the dermal hypersensitivity response in persons with herpes antibodies.

The human viruses in the herpes group are antigenically distinct except for types 1 (oral) and 2 (genital), which show cross-reactivity. They are readily distinguished, however, by the use of sera with high homotypic titers and by their preferential growth in different cell species.

Pathogenesis & Pathology

The lesion in the skin is similar to that of varicella and zoster: proliferation, ballooning degeneration, and intranuclear acidophilic inclusions. In fatal cases of herpes encephalitis, there is meningitis, perivascular infiltration, and nerve cell destruction, especially in the cortex. Intranuclear inclusions are found in glial cells and, less frequently, in nerve cells. Neonatal generalized herpes infection is characterized by multiple areas of focal necrosis with a mononuclear reaction and formation of intranuclear inclusion bodies in all organs (particularly the liver), and often extensive destruction of the adrenals. Permanent damage has been reported in survivors.

The fully formed inclusion is typical of the Cowdry type A inclusion body. During the early stages of its formation, it is rich in deoxyribonucleoprotein (Feulgen-positive, stains blue with hematoxylin and eosin) and virtually fills the nucleus, compressing the chromatin to the nuclear margin. When it has completely developed, the inclusion loses its deoxyribonucleoprotein (Feulgen-negative, stains pink with hematoxylin and eosin) and is separated by a halo from the chromatin at the nuclear margin. Viral antigen is present in the nucleus only in the early stages of infection; the fully developed intranuclear inclusion is devoid of virus.

Clinical Findings

Herpesvirus may cause various clinical entities, and these have been classified as primary and recurrent attacks. Primary infections, occurring in persons without antibodies, are sometimes characterized by systemic involvement which may be serious and even fatal. Antibody production invariably accompanies the infection. The primary infection in most individuals is not recognized. Recurrent infections, which occur in persons having circulating antibodies, are characterized by local lesions and by a lack of systemic involvement. Such recurrent attacks often follow nonspecific stimuli, such as fever accompanying certain infections, artificially produced fever, menstruation, or emotional disturbances.

Neonatal herpes infection is usually transmitted during birth from herpetic lesions in the birth canal. The agent is usually herpesvirus type 2. Premature infants are more often affected than full-term babies. Vigorous gamma globulin therapy of babies born of mothers with antepartum herpes infections has been suggested but has not definitely been proved effective. Most affected newborns have died, and permanent brain damage has been shown in at least one survivor. Transplacental infection has also been postulated.

The clinical entities attributable to herpesvirus include:

A. Herpes Simplex (Herpes Febrilis, Herpes Labialis): This is the most common disease produced by herpes type 1. Crops of localized vesicles occur again and again in the same area, usually at mucocutaneous junctions of the mouth and lips. Recurrent keratitis may also occur due to herpesvirus.

B. Eczema Herpeticum (Kaposi's Varicelliform Eruption): This is a severe herpetic infection in skin areas affected by chronic eczema.

C. Acute Herpetic Gingivostomatitis (Aphthous Stomatitis, Vincent's Stomatitis): This is the most common clinical entity caused by primary infection with herpesvirus. It occurs most frequently in infants and small children (6 months to 3 years of age). It is a severe febrile disease. In addition to the vesicular eruption of the mouth, there is regional lymphadenitis. The gums are also involved. The incubation period is short, about 3—5 days. The disease must be differentiated from bacterial tonsillitis and from herpangina caused by certain of the coxsackieviruses.

D. Meningoencephalitis: The virus may produce a benign aseptic meningitis or a severe form of encephalitis. Pleocytosis (chiefly of lymphocytes) is present in the CSF. Fluorescent antibody may reveal herpesvirus antigen in formalin-fixed paraffin-embedded blocks of frontal cerebral cortex, even when typical herpes inclusions may be absent. In such cases the most extensive neuropathologic lesions may not be fluorescent, which suggests that the virus has already been removed from the scene of damage.

E. Keratoconjunctivitis: This may occur as a primary or as a recurrent herpetic infection. Herpetic keratitis or keratoconjunctivitis is suggested by typical dendritic corneal ulcers or when vesicles appear on the eyelids and palpebral conjunctivas. In either primary or recurrent keratitis there may be progressive involvement of the deeper layers of the cornea (corneal stroma) with permanent opacification. The disease is often self-limiting, and it is possible that interferon induced by the virus restricts spread of the disease.

F. Genital Herpes: Herpesvirus type 2 is the cause of this common infection in men and women. Recurrent lesions often occur. Patients with cervical cancer have a high incidence of type 2 antibodies (80%), but it is not known whether this is a co-variable or an etiologic association.

Laboratory Diagnosis

A. Recovery of Virus: The virus may be isolated from tissues exhibiting herpetic lesions (skin, conjunctivas, or brain). It may also be found in the throat, saliva, and stools. In the primary infection, it may be present for as long as 2—3 weeks in the throat and for an equal period of time in the stools. Because it may be isolated at times from the throats of apparently healthy carriers, the isolation of herpesvirus is not in itself sufficient evidence to indicate that this virus is the etiologic agent of the disease under investigation.

Inoculation of tissue cultures, of the chorioallantois of the chick embryo (12 days old), or of the cornea of the rabbit is used for virus isolation. The appearance of typical intranuclear inclusion bodies in cell cultures or of typical pocks (or plaques) on the membrane or of corneal opacity suggests the presence of herpesvirus. Identification of the agent as herpesvirus is established by demonstrating intranuclear inclusions in histologic specimens and by neutralization of the virus by specific herpes antiserum. With tissue cultures, a provisional diagnosis can be made 24 hours after receipt of the specimen.

B. Serology: Antibodies may be measured quantitatively by neutralization tests on the chorioallantois of the chick embryo (pock-counting method), in mice, or in cultures.

A soluble complement fixing antigen of considerably smaller size than the virus can be prepared from infected chorioallantoic membranes. The soluble antigen of herpesvirus may be used to detect a dermal hypersensitivity in previously infected persons. There is a good correlation between dermal hypersensitivity and the presence of serum antibodies.

As early as the fourth or fifth day after a primary infection, neutralizing and complement fixing antibodies appear. They reach their peak in about 2—3 weeks. They may be retained for life, perhaps as the result of repeated stimulation by recurrent infections with the virus. An increase in antibody titer is essential for establishing a diagnosis. The presence of antibody in a single sample of serum is of little value, for the majority of adults have antibodies in their blood at all times.

About 30% of patients with herpes simplex infections show heterologous increases in preexisting complement fixing and neutralizing antibody titers to varicella-zoster virus. The heterologous reactions occur most often in patients who experienced a recent varicella-zoster infection. Infection with varicella-zoster virus is followed less frequently by an increase in herpes simplex antibody. This heterologous antibody response can be detected usually by complement fixation but not by neutralization.

Immunity

Children are usually born with passively transferred maternal antibodies. This antibody is lost during the first 6 months of life, and the period of greatest susceptibility to primary herpes infection occurs between 6 months and 2 years. Only one main antigenic type of virus is known, although antigenically overlapping subgroups exist.

After recovery from a primary infection (inapparent, mild, or severe), the virus is often carried in a latent state, even in the presence of antibodies. Antibodies appear after the primary infection but may fall in titer after a few months. A series of recurrent attacks may be required to maintain antibodies at high levels.

The early stage of the primary immune response is characterized by the appearance of neutralizing antibody detectable only in the presence of fresh complement. This antibody is of short duration and is replaced by neutralizing antibody that can function independently of complement.

Herpesvirus strains isolated from the genitalia have been found to differ in antigenic and certain growth properties from strains isolated from the lip. Antibodies to type 2 (genital herpesvirus) are not acquired in the general population until the age of adolescence and increased heterosexual activity.

Treatment

There is no specific treatment. Secondary bacterial infections of lesions in the mouth occur and may be controlled by antibiotic or chemotherapeutic agents.

Idoxuridine (5-iodo-2-deoxyuridine, IUDR) and cytosine arabinoside have been reported to be effective against herpes simplex keratitis if given early in the course of the disease. They are instilled locally, 1−2 drops in each eye every 1−2 hours day and night. These agents inhibit replication of virus in vitro and in vivo, but drug-resistant variants may appear. Treatment of acute herpetic epithelial keratitis with IUDR results in prompt suppression of clinical manifestations in a majority of cases. About three-fourths of patients treated with IUDR are asymptomatic within 1 week after onset, whereas only half of patients treated with curettage and cauterization of the cornea are asymptomatic in the same period. However, the virus is not eradicated by treatment, and the rate of relapse appears to be similar in IUDR treated and untreated individuals. IUDR apparently acts by suppressing, but not eradicating, virus production. This also limits interferon production; after therapy is discontinued, virus synthesis thus can recur. Some strains of virus are not affected by the drug. IUDR has little or no effect on stromal disease. Recently, massive doses of IUDR (400 mg/kg) have been used in cases of herpesvirus encephalitis. This treatment has led to complete recovery.

Epidemiology & Control

Herpes simplex virus is probably more constantly present in man than any other virus. Primary infection occurs early in life when maternal antibodies decline, often taking the form of a vesicular stomatitis. Even though antibodies develop, the virus is not eliminated from the body; a carrier state is established which lasts throughout life and is punctuated by transient attacks of herpes. If primary infection is avoided in childhood, it may not occur in later life; this is because adults may be less susceptible to primary herpetic infection (perhaps as a result of their thicker, more resistant epithelium), and also because the likelihood of picking up infection in the home may not be so great for adults as for children (less exposure to salivary contamination).

The highest incidence of type 1 virus carriage in the oropharynx of healthy persons occurs among children 6 months to 3 years of age. The virus is found less often in children 4–14 years of age, and rarely in persons 15 years of age and older or in infants under 6 months of age. A corollary of this is the observation that 70−90% of adults have type 1 antibodies.

Type 1 virus is transmitted more readily in families of the lower socioeconomic groups; the most obvious explanation is their more crowded living conditions and their lower hygienic standards. The virus is believed to be spread by direct contact (saliva or stools) or indirectly from utensils contaminated with the saliva of a virus carrier. The source of infection for children is usually a parent who has had a recurrence of the herpetic lesion a few days before the onset.

Type 2 virus is spread venereally. Infection begins after puberty and may involve 20−25% of the adult population.

No specific control measures are recommended. However, patients with eczema should be protected from sources of infection.

VARICELLA-ZOSTER VIRUS

VARICELLA
(Chickenpox)
ZOSTER
(Herpes Zoster, Shingles, Zona)

Varicella (chickenpox) is a mild, highly-infectious disease, chiefly of children, which is characterized by a vesicular eruption of the skin and mucous membranes. The etiologic agent is a virus which is morphologically and antigenically similar to the virus of zoster.

Zoster (shingles) is a sporadic, incapacitating disease of adults (rare in children) which is characterized by an inflammatory reaction of the posterior nerve roots and ganglia, accompanied by crops of vesicles (like those of varicella) over the skin supplied by the affected sensory nerves.

Properties of the Viruses

A. Varicella Virus: Morphologically identical with herpes simplex virus. A DNA icosahedral virus composed of 162 capsomeres surrounded by an envelope. Vesicular fluid of early lesions is capable of inducing typical varicella infection in children inoculated intradermally. The virus propagates in cultures of human embryonic tissue and, in so doing, produces typical intranuclear inclusion bodies. Supernatant fluids from such infected cultures have contained a complement fixing antigen but have been free of infective virus. Fluids harvested from infected thyroid cells have yielded infectious virus. The virus has not been propagated in laboratory animals.

B. Herpes Zoster Virus: Particles of the same size and shape as those of varicella can be obtained from vesicular fluid of zoster patients and even from the CSF in cases of zoster manifesting a lymphocytic pleocytosis. Like varicella virus, zoster virus fails to induce disease in laboratory animals; in cultures of human embryonic tissue, however, it does produce inclusion bodies and cytopathic changes which can be carried in serial passage. Intranuclear inclusions also develop in human skin grafted onto the chorioallantoic membrane of the chick embryo. The virus has a colchicine-like effect on human cells. Arrest in metaphase, overcontracted chromosomes, chromosome breaks, and formation of micronuclei are often seen.

Inoculation of vesicle fluid of zoster into children produces vesicles at the site of inoculation in about 10 days. This may be followed by generalized skin lesions precisely like those of varicella. Generalized varicella may occur in such inoculated children without local vesicle formation. Contacts of such children develop typical varicella after a 2-week incubation period. Children who have recovered from zoster virus-induced infection are resistant to varicella, and those who have had varicella are no longer susceptible to zoster virus.

Pathogenesis & Pathology

A. Varicella: The route of infection is not known. Most likely it is through the mucosa of the upper respiratory tract. The virus probably circulates in the blood and localizes in the skin lesions. Swelling of epithelial cells, ballooning degeneration, and the accumulation of tissue fluids result in vesicle formation. In nuclei of infected cells, particularly in the early stages, eosinophilic inclusion bodies are found.

B. Zoster: In addition to skin lesions, histopathologically identical to those of varicella, there is an inflammatory reaction of the dorsal nerve roots and ganglia. Often only a single ganglion may be involved. As a rule the distribution of lesions in the skin corresponds closely to the areas of innervation from an individual root ganglion. There is cellular infiltration, necrosis of nerve cells, and inflammation of the ganglion sheath. Destruction of the sensory nerve fibers from the corium has been demonstrated, with degeneration of the corresponding fibers of the spinal cord.

One explanation of the relationship of zoster to varicella is that there are 2 different viruses with overlapping antigenicity. Another hypothesis which has been advanced is that in some cases varicella virus may be neurotropic and enter and remain within nerve cells for long periods; years later, various insults (exposure to cold, pressure on a nerve) may cause a flare-up in the virus along posterior root fibers, whereupon zoster vesicles appear.

Clinical Findings

A. Varicella: The incubation period is usually 12–16 days. Malaise and fever are generally the earliest symptoms; these are soon followed by the rash, first on the trunk and then on the face, the limbs, and at times even in the buccal and pharyngeal mucosa. Successive fresh vesicles appear in crops during the next 3–4 days, so that all stages of papules, vesicles, and crusts may be seen at one time. The eruption is found together with the fever and is proportionate to its severity. Complications are rare, although encephalitis does at times occur about 5–10 days after the rash. Mortality is much less than 1% in uncomplicated cases. In neonatal varicella (contracted from the mother just before or just after birth) the mortality may be as high as 20%. In varicella encephalitis, mortality is about 10% and another 10% are left with permanent injury to the CNS. Chromosome breaks have been observed in leukocytes from children with chickenpox.

Children with leukemia should avoid exposure to varicella, as chickenpox in such children is severe and often fatal. This may be due to the leukemia itself or to the drugs used in its treatment (adrenal steroids, mercaptopurine), which may inhibit the immune response.

B. Zoster: The incubation period is 7–14 days. Malaise and fever are soon followed by severe pain in the area of skin or mucosa supplied by one or more groups of sensory nerves. The inflammatory reaction which typically is found in the dorsal nerve roots and ganglia occasionally spreads to the anterior horn cells, resulting in a paralysis which is usually temporary. Within a few days after onset, a crop of vesicles appears over the skin supplied by the affected nerves. Usually the eruption is unilateral; the trunk, head, and neck are most commonly involved. Lymphocytic pleocytosis in the CSF may be present.

Laboratory Diagnosis

Antibodies develop during the course of the infection. They have been detected by the agglutination with convalescent serum of elementary bodies found in vesicle fluid. Complement fixing antigen has also been demonstrated in vesicle fluids. The demonstration of cytopathogenicity of varicella and of zoster viruses in tissue culture and the detection of a soluble complement fixing antigen in the culture fluids now form the basis of more readily performed serologic tests. A precipitation test in agar gel has also been described which indicates the identity of varicella and zoster antigens, and the test has been used to follow the development of precipitating antibodies in patients. Antibodies in human serum can also be demonstrated using the immunofluorescence technic. The sera are reacted with infected tissue cultures and then the antigen-antibody complex is exposed to antihuman globulin labeled with fluorescein isothiocyanate.

Laboratory tests are also of value in differential diagnosis. Failure to obtain positive complement fixation with vesicle fluid or crust suspension when mixed with vaccinal antiserum and failure to grow and produce lesions on the chorioallantoic membrane of the chick embryo suggests varicella rather than smallpox. Herpes simplex can be readily differentiated from zoster by recovering from herpes simplex lesions a virus which infects chick embryos, rabbits, and mice.

Immunity

Laboratory studies also indicate a relationship between varicella and zoster viruses. Inoculation of zoster virus into children induces varicella. Zoster virus particles can be agglutinated by serum from patients convalescent from zoster or from varicella. The viruses produce similar cytopathic changes accompanied by the appearance of intranuclear inclusion bodies in cultures of human embryonic tissue.

Previous infection with varicella or zoster leaves the patient with an enduring immunity to the homologous virus. However, zoster may occur in persons who have contracted varicella at an earlier date.

Individuals with a recent history of varicella or zoster infection respond to infection with herpes simplex virus with a concomitant complement fixing antibody rise to herpes simplex and varicella-zoster viruses.

Treatment

Gamma globulin prepared from pooled plasma of patients convalescing from herpes zoster can be used to prevent varicella in children. Standard immune serum globulin is without value because of the lower titer of varicella antibodies.

Idoxuridine and cytosine arabinoside inhibit replication of the viruses in vitro, but they have not proved of value clinically.

Epidemiology

Zoster occurs sporadically, chiefly in adults, and without seasonal prevalence. In contrast, varicella is one of the common epidemic diseases of childhood (peak incidence is in children 2–6 years of age), although adult cases do occur. It is more common in winter and spring than in summer.

Varicella readily spreads, presumably by droplets as well as by direct or indirect contact with the skin surface. Contact infection is rare in zoster, perhaps because the virus is absent in the upper respiratory tract.

Adults exposed to varicella develop zoster more often than children do. Zoster, whether in children or adults, can be the source of varicella in children and can initiate large epidemics.

Control

None is available. The use of ultraviolet light in schools is said to reduce the explosive nature of varicella epidemics, but it does not prevent completely the transmission of the disease.

.   .   .

CYTOMEGALOVIRUS
(Cytomegalic Inclusion Disease, Salivary Gland Virus Disease)

Cytomegalic inclusion disease is a generalized infection of infants caused by intrauterine or early postnatal infection with the cytomegaloviruses, also known as salivary gland viruses. (Indigenous cytomegaloviruses occur among several animal species.) The disease is characterized by large basophilic (or sometimes eosinophilic) intranuclear inclusions and small cytoplasmic inclusions which occur in the salivary glands as well as in the lungs, liver, pancreas, kidneys, endocrine glands, and, occasionally, in the brain. Most fatalities occur in children under 2 years of age. Inapparent infection is common during childhood and adolescence.

Properties of the Virus

A. General Properties: Morphologically, cytomegalovirus is indistinguishable from herpes simplex or varicella-zoster virus. The virus contains DNA, as shown by the following: (1) In the electron micro-scope, the core of the virus particle stains with uranyl acetate. (2) The inclusions of infected cells in culture stain yellow-green when treated with acridine orange dye. (3) The DNA antagonist 5-fluorodeoxyuridine inhibits viral replication. The molecular weight of the DNA has been reported as $3–4 \times 10^7$ daltons, with a density of 1.716 gm/ml in CsCl and a guanine + cytosine content of 58%.

The virus has been studied in infected human fibroblasts by means of the electron microscope. Virus particles are synthesized in the nucleus. The outer of the 2 coats of the virus is derived from the inner nuclear membrane in a manner similar to that in which other viruses acquire a coat at the plasma membrane. The growth cycle of the virus is slower than that of herpes simplex virus. As with herpes simplex virus, the growth of cytomegalovirus is inhibited in the absence of arginine.

B. Reaction to Physical and Chemical Agents: Cytomegalovirus loses its infectivity when heated at 56° C for 30 minutes, when exposed to 20% ether for 2 hours, or when kept at pH below 5.0. It is relatively stable when stored at −90° C in the presence of 35% sorbitol.

In the presence of isotonic saline solutions containing bicarbonate, the virus is (paradoxically) inactivated at a faster rate at 4° C than at 37° C. The virus is more stable when suspended in distilled water.

C. Animal Susceptibility: All attempts to infect animals with human cytomegalovirus have failed. A number of animal cytomegaloviruses exist, all of them species-specific. Experimental passage of cytomegalovirus disease within the same species has been accomplished with mice and guinea pigs, both in vivo and in tissue cultures of the homologous species. Histopathologic studies indicate that a similar infection occurs in rats, hamsters, moles, rabbits, and monkeys. The virus isolated from monkeys has been shown to propagate in cultures of monkey as well as human cells.

Pathogenesis & Pathology

In infants, cytomegalic inclusion disease is congenitally acquired, probably as a result of primary infection of the mother during pregnancy. The virus can be isolated from the urine of the mother at the time of birth of the infected baby, and typical cytomegalic cells, 25–40 μm in size, can be found in the placental chorionic villi of the infected neonate.

Foci of cytomegalic cells are found in fatal cases in the epithelial tissues of the liver, lungs, kidneys, gastrointestinal tract, parotid gland, pancreas, thymus, thyroid, adrenals, and other regions. The cells can be found also in the urine sediment, gastric washings, or adenoid tissue of healthy children. The route of infection in older infants, children, and adults is not known.

The incidence of typical inclusions within salivary glands of 10–33% of routine autopsies in children, and the isolation of the virus from urine and from tissue cultures of adenoids of healthy children, strongly suggest subclinical infections at a relatively young age. The virus may persist in the salivary glands and other organs for long periods in a latent state or as a chronic infection.

Inclusions are rarely found in adult salivary glands. This is in agreement with the failure to recover virus from the mouths of adults. The disseminated occurrence of inclusions in older children and adults has usually been observed in association with other severe diseases.

Clinical Findings

Congenital infection may result in death of the fetus in utero or may produce the clinical syndrome of cytomegalic inclusion disease with signs of prematurity, jaundice with hepatosplenomegaly, thrombocytopenic purpura, pneumonitis, and often evidence of CNS damage which may be associated with microcephaly, periventricular calcification, chorioretinitis, optic atrophy, and mental or motor retardation. Congenital cytomegalic inclusion disease was once believed to result invariably in death, but the availability of technics to establish the diagnosis during life has made it increasingly apparent that infants with the disease may survive initial infection and live for many years. Cases with milder symptoms have also been reported. Microcephaly, motor disability, and mental retardation are common sequelae in surviving infants. Recent studies suggest that a significant proportion of unexplained microcephaly and mental retardation may be caused by congenital cytomegalovirus infection.

Acquired infection with cytomegalovirus is extremely common and usually inapparent. In children, acquired infection may result in subacute or chronic hepatitis, interstitial pneumonitis, or acquired hemolytic anemia.

Recently cytomegalovirus has been associated with an infectious mononucleosis-like disease without heterophil antibodies. "Cytomegalovirus mononucleosis" occurs in children and adults, either spontaneously or after transfusions of large quantities of fresh blood during major surgical interventions ("postperfusion syndrome"). The incubation period appears to be about 30–40 days. Appearance or rise of cytomegalovirus antibody and cytomegaloviruria are common features of the disease. Cytomegalovirus has been isolated from the peripheral blood leukocytes of such patients. Hence, it is presumed that the postperfusion syndrome is caused by cytomegalovirus harbored in the leukocytes of the blood donors.

Patients with malignancies or immunologic defects or those undergoing immunosuppressive therapy for organ transplantation may develop cytomegalovirus pneumonitis or hepatitis and occasionally generalized disease; the relative importance of primary infection versus reactivation of a latent infection in such cases remains to be clarified.

Laboratory Diagnosis

A. Recovery of Virus: The virus can be recovered from mouth swabs, urine, liver, adenoids, kidneys, and peripheral blood leukocytes by inoculation of human fibroblastic cell cultures. Attempts to grow it on human epithelial cultures have failed. The incubation period in cultures is usually 1–2 weeks or longer. The early cytologic changes consist of small foci of swollen, rounded, translucent cells which, upon staining, show large eosinophilic or amphophilic intranuclear inclusion bodies, margination of chromatin, halo formation, and sharply defined nuclear membranes. The cytoplasm may contain several small basophilic bodies. Cell degeneration progresses slowly, and the virus concentration is much higher within the cell than in the fluid. Prolonged serial propagation is needed before the virus reaches titers sufficient for performance of the usual serologic procedures.

B. Serology: Antibodies in human sera, as well as in sera of monkeys and baboons immunized with human cytomegalovirus, may be measured quantitatively by neutralization tests in tissue culture. Hyperimmune antiserum from these primates neutralizes cytomegalovirus only in the presence of fresh complement. (Herpes simplex antiserum made in these animals does not require complement.) A soluble complement fixing antigen of considerably smaller size than the virus can be prepared from infected human embryonic fibroblast cultures. In contrast to the infectious virus, the complement fixing antigen is less stable at 37° than at 4° C. Antibodies in human sera can also be demonstrated using the immunofluorescence technic.

The virus of each species was thought to be made up of a single but distinctive antigenic type. The cytomegalovirus of the monkey shares complement fixing antigens with some but not all human strains. An antigenic heterogeneity has been suggested for the human viruses on the basis of neutralization tests with sera from congenitally infected infants. More recent findings indicate that the human viruses form an antigenic spectrum rather than falling into distinct serotype groups.

Immunity

Complement fixing and neutralizing antibodies have been found in a high proportion of human sera. In young children possessing complement fixing antibodies, virus may be detected in the mouth and in the urine for many months, long after antibodies make their appearance. Evidence of reinfection is suggested by an antibody rise, superimposed on the preexisting antibody level, which may occur at the time of virus isolation.

Virus may occur in the urine of children even though serum neutralizing antibody has been present for as long as 2 years. This suggests that the virus may propagate in the urinary tract rather than being passively excreted from the blood stream. Virus is not present in young children who have not yet acquired complement fixing antibody.

Intrauterine infection may occur and produces a serious disease in the newborn. Infants infected during fetal life may be born with antibody which continues to rise after birth in the presence of persistent virus excretion. (This is similar to the situation in congenital rubella infection.)

Treatment

There is no specific treatment. The merit of steroid therapy has been questioned. Administration of immune gamma globulin has been suggested for generalized infections accompanying debilitating diseases.

Epidemiology & Control

Except for the congenital infection, the mechanism of virus transmission in older children and adults remains unknown. Widespread infection with cytomegaloviruses occurs, as indicated by the increase in the rate of antibody appearance with age. This reaches 80% in individuals over 35 years of age. The rate of virus excretion among institutionalized children has been found to be 10 times that in children of comparable age in the population at large, suggesting virus transmission by close contact.

Specific control measures are not available. Isolation of newborns with generalized cytomegalic inclusion disease from other neonates is advisable.

EB HERPESVIRUS
(Infectious Mononucleosis, Burkitt Lymphoma, Nasopharyngeal Carcinoma)

The presence of EB (Epstein-Barr) virus, a new and antigenically distinct member of the herpes-group, was initially detected by means of electron microscopy in a small proportion of cells in continuous lymphoblastoid cell lines derived from Burkitt's lymphoma (a tumor indigenous for children in Central Africa). The virus—called also HL (herpes-like) or HT (herpestype)—has also been detected in lymphoblastoid cell lines derived from nasopharyngeal carcinomas or peripheral blood leukocytes of patients with infectious mononucleosis or other illnesses as well as from normal individuals. EB virus is suspected of being the etiologic agent of infectious mononucleosis and has been associated to a high degree with Burkitt's lymphoma and nasopharyngeal carcinoma.

Properties of the Virus

A. **Morphology and Size:** Under the electron microscope the virus is indistinguishable in size and structure from the other human herpesviruses. Most of the particles seen in infected cells are without the central core, and few possess an envelope. Only about 10% of the extracellular virus is enveloped.

In sucrose gradients, EB viral DNA has recently been found to have a density of 1.720, the same as that of the DNA of herpes simplex virus.

B. **Virus Growth:** Attempts to infect or transform human or animal cells of fibroblastic or epithelial origin with EB virus has thus far been unsuccessful, possibly because most of the virus particles are defective. Nor has it been possible to induce infection or tumor formation in animals inoculated with the concentrated virus particles or virus-containing lympho-

blastoid cells. The virus appears to have a distinct predilection for lymphoblastoid cells, in which it is found in a carrier state. In such cells, EB virus is detected either by means of electron microscopy or by immunofluorescence, using acetone-fixed cells and EB antibody-positive human sera. Both virus particles and immunofluorescence antigen reside in the same cell.

The content of EB virus in various lymphoblastoid cell lines differs markedly. In some it is present only in rare cells; in others, as many as 10% of the cells may contain the virus. The virus content also varies within the same line. As a rule, the percentage of cells harboring the EB virus drops with increasing number of cell passages; however, the opposite has also been reported. Cultivation of cells in media deprived of arginine—or cell maintenance at subnormal temperature—increases the virus content in some lines. The virus genome seems to be present not only in the cells containing the EB virus, or EB viral antigens, but also in the majority of the cells within the cultures, possibly in all of them; this has been revealed by tests with cloned cell lines which produce progeny cultures that possess all the properties of the parent cultures.

It is not yet clear whether EB virus is a passenger virus or whether it is the agent responsible for the lymphoblastoid transformation of peripheral blood leukocytes in culture. Only leukocytes that contain the EB viral genome have been assumed to have the capacity to replicate in vitro. Co-cultivation of lethally irradiated EB virus-positive cells of male origin with peripheral blood leukocytes of female origin (that by themselves could not initiate permanent cultures) yielded permanent female lymphoblastoid cultures that contain the virus. Similar transformation has also been obtained when human fetal leukocytes were inoculated with cell-free EB virus preparations. However, it remains to be seen whether EB virus is essential for establishment of continuous lymphoblastoid cell lines, for lines have been described which lack EB virus particles and immunofluorescent antigen.

C. **Antigenic Properties:** EB virus is distinct from all the other human herpesviruses. It has been reported, however, to share a common precipitating antigen with the frog herpesvirus which induce Lucké adenocarcinoma in frog kidneys. No evidence is available on the possible antigenic differences between the HT viruses carried by different lymphoblastoid cell lines.

Immunity

The most widely used serologic procedure for EB virus infection is the indirect immunofluorescence test with acetone-fixed smears of cultured Burkitt's lymphoma cells. The cells containing the EB virus are those which exhibit the fluorescence after treatment with fluorescent antibody. By this technic, antibody to EB virus has been demonstrated in many human sera from different parts of the world. In another type of serologic test, semipurified virus particles extracted from the cells have been used as complement fixing antigen. Good agreement exists between the immunofluorescence test and complement fixation test with the viral antigen, although the immunofluorescence test is more sensitive for detecting low levels of antibody. Detectable levels of both types of antibody seem to persist for many years.

Other antigens can be demonstrated in the lymphoblastoid cells, some of which are most probably virus-induced but nonstructural antigens. Among these are the soluble antigens demonstrable by complement fixation and precipitation tests in cell extracts of different lymphoblastoid cell lines, and the antigens demonstrable by immunofluorescence on the surface of viable cells obtained by biopsy of Burkitt's tumors and on the surface of cells propagated in cultures of the tumor. The nature of these antigens and their relationship to EB virus are not clear.

Epidemiology

Seroepidemiologic studies using the immunofluorescence technic and complement fixation reaction indicate that infection with EB virus is common in different parts of the world and that it occurs early in life. In some areas, including urban USA, about 50% of children 1 year old, 80–90% of children over age 4, and 90% of adults have antibody to EB virus. The mechanisms of virus transmission remain unknown; it is possible that some of the infections occur during intrauterine life.

Antibody to EB virus is also present in nonhuman primates, and it is probable that some of these animals were infected in nature. EB virus has also been detected in lymphoblastoid lines derived from peripheral leukocytes of normal chimpanzees.

EB Virus & Human Disease

The great majority of the EB virus infections are clinically inapparent. Antibodies to the virus develop in the course of infectious mononucleosis. This suggests that the EB virus is the etiologic agent of this disease; however, it is also possible that in the course of the disease the antigenic stimulus may result from the excessive growth of lymphoid cells which already harbor the virus or which are susceptible to the virus present in a few cells in occult form.

EB virus is suspected to be the cause of 2 human malignant diseases: Burkitt's lymphoma and postnasal (nasopharyngeal) carcinoma. The following observations favor the etiologic association:

(1) The virus is frequently detected in cell lines derived from Burkitt's lymphomas.

(2) The incidence of antibody is more frequent and the antibody titers are higher among patients with Burkitt's lymphoma and postnasal carcinoma than in healthy matched controls or individuals suffering from other types of malignancies.

(3) The virus has been reported to induce the lymphoblastoid transformation of leukocytes.

(4) Herpesviruses morphologically similar to EB virus have been linked with malignant diseases of lower animals: (a) frog, Lucké adenocarcinoma of kidney; (b) chick, Marek's lymphoma; (c) rabbit, Hinze's lymphoma; (d) monkey, Melendez' lymphoma of owl monkeys and marmosets caused by a latent herpesvirus of the squirrel monkey.

INFECTIOUS MONONUCLEOSIS
(Glandular Fever)

Infectious mononucleosis is a disease of children and young adults characterized by fever and enlarged lymph nodes and spleen. Epidemics are common in institutions where young people live.

The total white blood count may range from 10,000–80,000, while polymorphonuclear leukocytes may drop to low levels, about 2000/cu mm. Monocytes and large lymphocytes are increased and show morphologic abnormalities.

During the course of infection, 50–80% of patients develop heterophil antibodies. These antibodies are of diagnostic importance and are measured by their ability to agglutinate sheep erythrocytes. The test can be made more specific by adsorbing nonspecific substances with guinea pig kidney and with boiled beef erythrocytes. The heterophil antibody in normal human serum is adsorbed by the guinea pig kidney, whereas the antibody of infectious mononucleosis is adsorbed only by the boiled beef erythrocytes.

Bone marrow cells or peripheral blood leukocytes from patients with infectious mononucleosis, grown in culture, develop into permanent lymphoblastoid cell cultures. Circulating atypical mononuclear cells in such patients are capable of active DNA synthesis and mitotic activity.

It has not been clearly demonstrated, even with human volunteers, that this disease can be transmitted artificially. It is generally considered to be caused by a virus, but its infectious nature is not well documented.

Patients with infectious mononucleosis develop antibodies against the EB herpesvirus as measured by immunofluorescence with virus-bearing cells derived from patients with Burkitt's lymphoma. Similar cell lines have been obtained from the peripheral blood and bone marrow of patients with infectious mononucleosis or leukemia, as well as from some normal individuals. Antibodies appear early in the acute disease, rise to peak levels within a few weeks, and remain high during convalescence. Unlike the short-lived heterophil antibodies, those against EB virus persist for years.

However, the evidence that EB virus causes mononucleosis is not yet conclusive. Although mononucleosis patients develop antibodies to EB virus, the disease is characterized by the production of a variety of antibodies—against red cells of sheep and cows, against syphilitic antigen, and sometimes against the patient's own red cells and platelets. EB virus is also associated with other lymphoid diseases, eg, Burkitt's lymphoma, and with nasopharyngeal tumors which are heavily infiltrated with lymphocytes. Thus, the virus may simply have an unusual affinity for lymphocytes, explaining its presence in lymphoproliferative disorders.

Mononucleosis may be a self-limited form of leukemia in which a new kind of cell growth develops, stops, and then reverses itself. The numerous antibodies formed in the course of mononucleosis help distinguish the disease from leukemia. If this antibody production accounts for the self-limited nature of mononucleosis, the speculation may be made that leukemia could be controlled by inducing an immune response against the disease.

B VIRUS
(Herpesvirus of Old World Monkeys)

B virus infection of man is an acute ascending myelitis. Cases have followed the bites of apparently normal monkeys, which were healthy carriers of the virus, or contact with materials (tissue culture fluids) derived from monkeys. Human cases are rare but are increasing as the number of persons handling monkeys and preparing vaccines from kidney cultures increases. The virus has been recovered from rhesus and cercopithecus monkeys.

The size of the virus is about 110 nm. It may be preserved in 50% glycerol at 4° C or may be stored at −20° C or below, or in the lyophilized state.

Because B virus infection occurs naturally in monkeys, the virus has been named *Herpesvirus simiae*. It is related to herpes simplex and pseudorabies viruses. The virus is transmissible to monkeys, rabbits, and guinea pigs. Mice are susceptible, but only in the first few weeks of life. The virus grows in the chick embryo, producing pocks on the chorioallantoic membrane. Experimentally infected animals exhibit intranuclear inclusions and multinucleated giant cells. The same cytologic lesion is produced in cultures of rabbit, monkey, or human cells.

The virus enters through the skin and localizes at the site of the monkey bite, producing vesicles and then necrosis of the area. From the site of the skin lesion, the virus enters the CNS by way of the peripheral nerves. The picture is predominantly that of a meningoencephalomyelitis; there is also focal necrosis of the lymph glands, spleen, and adrenals.

About 3 days after exposure the patient develops vesiculopustular lesions at the site followed by regional lymphangitis and adenitis. About 7 days later motor and sensory abnormalities occur; this is followed by acute ascending paralysis, involvement of the respiratory center, and death.

Virus can be recovered from the brain, spinal cord, and spleen of fatal cases. Suspensions of these tissues are inoculated into rabbit kidney tissue cultures or interdermally into rabbits; a necrotic lesion of the skin occurs, and the rabbit develops myelitis. The agent is established as B virus by the histopathologic findings (intranuclear inclusion bodies) and by serologic identification. Herpes antiserum neutralizes B virus hardly at all, whereas B virus antiserum neutralizes both herpes simplex and B viruses equally well.

Because of the fatal outcome of B virus infections in man, serologic tests for neutralizing and complement fixing antibodies are of little value for diagnostic purposes.

There is no specific treatment once the clinical disease is manifest. However, because of the antigenic crossing between herpes simplex and B virus, antibodies against B virus may occur in certain individuals. For this reason, gamma globulin (if known to contain B virus antibodies) is recommended in large doses as a preventive measure immediately after the patient is bitten by the monkey. Infiltration of the wound with B virus antiserum has been suggested.

B virus infection occurs in monkeys as a latent infection much as herpes simplex occurs in man. The virus has been recovered from monkey saliva, brain, spinal cord, and from many lots of monkey kidney culture (the starting material for preparing poliomyelitis and other vaccines for human use). Antibodies may be present in healthy monkeys. The virus has been transmitted to man only through the bite of the monkey, or through contact with monkey tissue cultures.

MARMOSET HERPESVIRUS
(Herpesvirus of New World Monkeys)

A herpes virus has been recovered from South American marmoset monkeys (*Tamarinus nigricollis*) which has all the properties of a herpesvirus. It is highly virulent for marmoset monkeys and for mice; it produces pocks on the chick chorioallantoic membrane. Antigenically, this virus of New World monkeys is different from classical herpes simplex virus and from B virus of Old World monkeys, with no detectable cross-reactivity. The virus appears to have its natural habitat in squirrel monkeys, in which it sets up latent infections.

By using primary kidney cell cultures of rabbit and of green and rhesus monkeys, it is possible to distinguish among the primate herpesviruses of the simplex type on the basis of differing cell susceptibility. Rhesus cultures are susceptible only to the herpesvirus of Old World monkeys (B virus); green monkey cultures, to the herpesvirus of both Old and New World monkeys; and rabbit cultures, to the herpesviruses of both kinds of monkeys and of man.

•   •   •

General References

Bell, T.M.: Viruses associated with Burkitt's tumor. Prog Med Virol 9:1–34, 1967.

Benyesh-Melnick, M.: Cytomegalovirus. Pages 701–732 in: *Diagnostic Procedures for Viral and Rickettsial Infections,* 4th ed. American Public Health Association, 1969.

Darlington, R.W., & L.H. Moss: The envelope of herpesviruses. Prog Med Virol 11:16–45, 1969.

Niederman, J.C., & others: Infectious mononucleosis: Clinical manifestations in relation to EB virus antibodies. JAMA 203:205–209, 1968.

Plummer, G.: Comparative virology of the herpes group. Prog Med Virol 9:302–340, 1967.

Roizman, B.: The herpesviruses: A biochemical definition of the group. Curr Top Microbiol Immunol 49:1–79, 1969.

Tokumaru, T.: Herpesviruses. Pages 641–700 in: *Diagnostic Procedures for Viral and Rickettsial Infections,* 4th ed. American Public Health Association, 1969.

Weller, T.H.: Varicella-zoster virus. Pages 733–754 in: *Diagnostic Procedures for Viral and Rickettsial Infections,* 4th ed. American Public Health Association, 1969.

39...

Diplornavirus (Reovirus), Coronavirus, & Other Viral Infections of Man

DIPLORNAVIRUS GROUP

The diploravirus group is made up of the double-stranded RNA viruses which have a core about 40 nm in size. Their nucleic acid has a molecular weight of about 10×10^6 daltons. Some members of the reovirus subgroup possess both an outer and an inner capsid, whereas other diplornaviruses possess only the inner capsid. Diplornaviruses are known for invertebrates and plants.

REOVIRUSES

The reoviruses are a group of respiratory (R) and enteric (E) orphan (O) viruses previously classified as echovirus type 10.

Properties of the Viruses

The reoviruses are about 70 nm in diameter and are ether-resistant. They are morphologically identical to the wound tumor virus which produces tumors in plant stems and leaves that have been subject to trauma. Reoviruses exhibit icosahedral symmetry of the T=9 pattern. Their structural protein appears to be arranged in the form of a double capsid: an inner capsid component 45 nm in diameter and an outer layer of 92 hollow columnar capsomeres (4 capsomeres on each edge of the triangular faces of the associated icosahedron). The nucleic acid of this group of viruses is RNA; however, it is unique in that it appears to fit a model of a double-helical polynucleotide with complementary strands running in opposite directions, similar to the polynucleotides of double-stranded DNA.

Some arboviruses—eg, bluetongue virus, African horsesickness virus, and a number of others—have been shown to contain double-stranded RNA and to have some structural and developmental characteristics resembling reovirus and wound tumor virus. By analogy to the picornavirus group, a new group, **diplorna** (double-stranded RNA) viruses, has been suggested to contain the reoviruses of mammals, wound tumor and rice dwarf viruses of plants, and these arboviruses. This recently discovered subgroup to which bluetongue virus belongs has a diameter of about 40 nm, the size

of the inner capsid of reovirus. Bluetongue virus possesses 32 capsomeres but no reovirus-like outer capsid.

The double-strandedness of the reovirus RNA results in characterization of the nucleic acid by its melting in a narrow temperature range, only slight reactivity with formaldehyde, resistance to hydrolysis by pancreatic ribonuclease, and a general appearance and stiffness on electron microscopic examination similar to double-stranded DNA. The reovirus genome is composed of structural units of double-stranded RNA linked end to end. The RNA occurs in 3 major size classes with molecular weights of 0.8×10^6, 1.4×10^6, and 2.4×10^6 daltons. The molecular weight of the whole genome is at least 10×10^6 daltons. Corresponding to each class of double-stranded RNA, 3 classes of virus-specific single-stranded messenger RNA of equivalent length are synthesized in infected cells. An adenine-rich single-stranded RNA has also been isolated from reoviruses, but its function and location in the intact virion are currently unclear.

Dactinomycin, an antibiotic which inhibits cellular RNA but not viral RNA synthesis, has been used to study the formation of the unique RNA of reovirus. Infected cells treated with dactinomycin produce 2 types of RNA. One type of RNA is resistant to ribonuclease and in this respect has the characteristics of the viral (double-stranded) nucleic acid. The other type of RNA, which constitutes about 60% of the total RNA produced, is sensitive to ribonuclease, and probably represents the RNA which directs the formation of virus protein coat constituents and enzymes necessary for viral replication.

The double-stranded RNA of reovirus which is resistant to ribonuclease is a very efficient inducer of interferon. (See Chapter 27.)

By the use of the negative staining technic and electron microscopy, it has been found that about 25–50% of the virus population is made up of empty protein coats. Separation of these particles from the complete forms by density gradient sedimentation makes it possible to determine that infectivity is associated with the complete rather than the coreless particles.

A unique property of reoviruses has recently been described. These viruses, in the presence of high concentrations of magnesium ions (0.5 M $MgCl_2$), are activated and their infectivity titer increased by heating at temperatures of $37°$–$55°$ C. This treatment has no effect on the titer of the viral hemagglutinin. On the other hand, exposing the virus to subzero temperatures, especially between $-20°$ C and $-40°$ C, in the presence of 0.5 M $MgCl_2$, almost completely destroys the infectivity titer of the virus and also inactivates its hemagglutinin. Thermal activation of the virus yields a particle to infectivity ratio close to unity, whereas before heating this ratio is 15:1.

Increase in infectivity can also be obtained by treating the virus with the proteolytic enzymes chymotrypsin and pancreatin. This treatment results in partial and eventually complete removal of the outer layer of capsomeres. If care is taken, infectivity need not be lost during this procedure.

Growth of Virus

Reovirus has a prolonged growth cycle and a tendency to accumulate within the cell. Reovirus protein replication has been shown to occur within the cytoplasm, and with the aid of fluorescent antibody staining and electron microscopy this has been selectively localized with intracytoplasmic structures (spindles and centrioles) which are involved in cell mitosis. Although these structures seem to have the capacity to concentrate the viral antigen selectively, abolition of spindle tubules by colchicine does not affect total virus production but only alters the site of progeny virus formation.

Reoviruses produce a distinctive cytopathic effect in monkey kidney cultures, in which cells separate from the sheet. At this stage, the nuclei are intact but the cytoplasm contains inclusion bodies in which the virus particles are found. The viruses also grow in kidney cultures of guinea pigs, cats, dogs, pigs, and less rapidly in kidney cultures of calves and rabbits. The viruses grow in newborn mice, some producing signs of overt disease, with lesions of the nerve cells, myocardium, and liver. Inoculated monkeys develop lesions in the ependymal lining of the ventricles and choroid plexus. A strain isolated from a chimpanzee with rhinitis produced the common cold syndrome when passed by nasal instillation into other chimpanzees. The virus also multiplies in chick embryos.

Inoculation of pregnant mice with reovirus may lead to a prolonged virus infection of the developing fetus and embryopathy. Some offspring develop severe illness (interstitial pneumonia, renal tubular necrosis) soon after birth. Some of the congenitally infected mice develop later illnesses (growth retardation and eye signs). Finally, some offspring develop no apparent illness but have a prolonged tolerant infection with immune paralysis.

Wound tumor virus not only multiplies in plant cells but also replicates in the nervous system and other organs of its insect vector, the leafhopper.

Antigenic Properties

Three distinct but related types of reovirus are demonstrable by neutralization and hemagglutination inhibition tests. All 3 types share a common complement fixing antigen. Reoviruses contain a hemagglutinin for human O erythrocytes. Type 3 reovirus, in addition, agglutinates bovine erythrocytes. The human red cell receptors for the reovirus hemagglutinin are not affected by the receptor-destroying enzyme of *Vibrio cholerae* but are destroyed by 1:1000 potassium periodate. However, receptor-destroying enzyme renders bovine red cells inagglutinable by reovirus type 3.

Epidemiology

The reoviruses have been found in human beings, chimpanzees, Asian and African monkeys, wild mice, laboratory mice, and domestic cattle. Antibodies are also present in guinea pigs, rabbits, dogs, and cats, a finding which suggests that these species may also be naturally infected. However, studies of the quokka, an Australian marsupial, have provided evidence that susceptible animals can become infected on contact with man.

All 3 types have been recovered from healthy children. In addition, type 1 virus has been recovered from young children during an outbreak of minor febrile illness occurring in winter, and also from monkeys. Type 2 virus has been recovered from children with diarrhea or steatorrheic enteritis; from chimpanzees with epidemic rhinitis; and from the lung of a monkey dying of pneumonia. Type 3 has been recovered from children with a febrile upper respiratory disease or with diarrhea, and from naturally infected cattle. Reovirus has also been recovered from an adult with a common cold. A number of strains have been recovered with some regularity from patients in Africa with Burkitt's lymphoma.

Human volunteer studies have failed to demonstrate a clear cause and effect relationship between virus and disease in man. When 27 young adult volunteers were inoculated intranasally with the 3 strains of reovirus, only a few individuals developed mild, afebrile illness which could not be definitely attributed to the inoculated virus. These studies did demonstrate, however, that reovirus is recovered far more readily from feces than from the nose or throat. No virus was found in the urine. In addition, it was shown serologically that almost all of the volunteers infected with reovirus type 1 developed heterotypic hemagglutination-inhibition antibodies to types 2 and 3, while those infected with reovirus type 3 developed only homotypic antibody. Much work remains to be done before there is a clear picture of the relationship between reoviruses and clinical disease in man.

COLORADO TICK FEVER VIRUS

Details about this virus and the disease that it causes may be found in Chapter 30. Recent work has shown that Colorado tick fever virus has the same size and morphology as reovirus. However, its nucleic acid has not yet been characterized. Unlike reovirus, Colorado tick fever virus is sensitive to ether, low pH, and heat. The differences in properties may be explained by a lipid-containing envelope essential for infectivity of Colorado tick fever virus. Reovirus does not possess such as envelope.

CORONAVIRUS GROUP

This is a newly recognized group of viruses that include the human "IBV-like" viruses, avian infectious bronchitis virus (IBV), mouse hepatitis virus (MHV), and rat pneumotropic virus. The human strains have been associated with acute upper respiratory illnesses in adults.

Properties of the Viruses

Negatively stained electron micrographs reveal round to elliptical particles with distinct wide-spaced, club-shaped surface projections 20 nm long. The diameter is variable, but usually between 80 and 160 nm, although the longest diameter may approach 250 nm (including the projections). They contain essential lipid (they are sensitive to ether and chloroform) and are acid-labile. The nucleic acid content appears to be RNA. Their density is between 1.18 and 1.19 gm/ml.

Growth of Virus

The human coronaviruses are extremely fastidious in their growth requirements, making routine isolation difficult. Some strains grow in human embryonic tracheal and nasal organ cultures, whereas others require human embryonic intestine or kidney cell cultures. These isolation systems are less sensitive than serologic methods. Occasional strains have been adapted to suckling mouse brain. Progeny virus forms by budding into cytoplasmic vesicles or from membranes of the endoplasmic reticulum.

Antigenic Properties

The human prototype strain is 229E. Other human isolates grown in tissue culture show a strong antigenic relationship to this strain, but only a limited relationship to the organ culture grown strains or MHV. Conversely, several of the strains grown in organ cultures are more broadly reactive, demonstrating a strong antigenic relationship to certain MHV strains. A rat coronavirus is widely prevalent in colony-reared and wild rats. It can be isolated from the lungs of adult animals, and it induces a fatal pneumonitis in newborn rats. It is also related to MHV. Avian IBV appears to have no antigenic relationships to the human or murine agents.

The agar gel diffusion technic has revealed at least 3 separate antigens for IBV and 2 antigens for strain 229E. A complement fixing antigen is present, but a hemagglutinin has been detected only with the avian IBV.

Clinical & Laboratory Findings

The human coronaviruses produce an acute upper respiratory tract illness in adults characterized by coryza, nasal congestion, sneezing, and sore throat. Most of the patients are afebrile. The majority of patients are in the 20–40 year age group. The diagnosis is suggested by isolating the virus, and confirmed by demonstrating a significant rise in complement fixing or neutralizing antibody titer to the agent in acute and convalescent serologic specimens.

Immunity & Epidemiology

The complement fixation test is a more sensitive index of human coronavirus infections than is virus isolation with the tissue culture or organ systems presently in use. Confirmation of infection by significant increases in antibody titer is more frequently successful using the complement fixation test than the neutralization test. These coronaviruses do not appear to be an important cause of acute respiratory illness in the pediatric age groups.

However, serologic evidence supports the hypothesis that these agents are a major cause of respiratory illness in adults during some winter months when the prevalence of colds is high but the isolation of rhinoviruses or other respiratory viruses is low.

. . .

WARTS
(Verrucae, Human Papovavirus)

Human wart virus belongs biologically to the papovavirus group, which includes papilloma viruses of rabbits, cattle, and man, polyoma and K viruses of mice, and vacuolating virus of monkeys. These viruses produce tumors in their natural host or in another species. (See Chapter 40 for discussion of oncogenic viruses.) They are ether-resistant DNA viruses, 40–55 nm in diameter, and contain 72 or 42 capsomeres in their outer shell. They are relatively resistant to heat, except in the presence of high concentrations of divalent cations.

Wart virus has been reported to produce proliferative changes in tissue cultures of human embryonic skin and muscle. These changes include the focal transformation of the well organized monolayer of fibroblasts into disorganized accumulations of epithelioid cells. Similar tissue culture changes are produced by the Shope rabbit papilloma virus, another member of the papovavirus group.

Warts can be spread by autoinoculation, through scratching; or by direct or indirect contact. A filtrable agent recovered from warts has reproduced warts in volunteers. Crystalline virus-like particles with a diameter of 45–55 nm can be obtained from those warts which have intranuclear inclusions in their rete cells. Thin sections of such papillomas have revealed the crystalline masses within the nucleus. Warts without intranuclear inclusions have not revealed the elementary bodies. By electron microscopic counting procedures, warts have been found to contain their highest concentration of virus particles when they are about 6 months old. There is no conclusive evidence that the virus can be transmitted to animals or that it can be grown in tissue culture.

The nuclei of normal skin cells are uniform in size, and the DNA content shows little variation from one cell to the next (being twice that contained in haploid human sperm). In contrast, wart-infected skin exhibits large and variable nuclear sizes, and also much higher and more variable DNA values which cannot be explained by increased polyploidy or by increased cell division.

Eosinophilic intranuclear inclusions occur with greater frequency in plantar warts (43%) than in common verruca vulgaris (4%).

Patients carrying warts possess specific 19 S (IgM) antibodies directed against the human papovavirus. This suggests that the antigenic stimulus which is persistent in the wart remains low, or that there is some immunopathologic involvement of the lymphoid system.

Papovaviruses have also been associated with progressive multifocal leukoencephalopathy. Large numbers of virus particles can be seen under the electron microscope in infected brain cells. This may be a late complication of chronic lymphocytic leukemia, Hodgkin's disease, and lymphosarcoma.

The papovaviruses have been used as models of oncogenic viruses. This aspect is discussed in Chapter 40.

EXANTHEM SUBITUM
(Roseola Infantum)

Exanthem subitum is a mild, nonfatal disease occurring almost exclusively in infants between 6 months and 3 years of age. At times it is confused with rubella. The causative agent is found in the serum and throat washings during the febrile period. In infants, the artificially induced disease is typical. The febrile disease but without rash can be transmitted to monkeys with serum which has been passed through bacteria-tight filters.

The incubation period is about 10–14 days. The onset is abrupt; the temperature may rise to 105 or 106° F (40.4–41° C), sometimes with convulsions. Fever may last 5 days. There is usually lymphadenopathy. The rubelliform rash characteristically follows the disappearance of fever by a few hours and affects most of the body, but not the face. There is leukopenia with a relative lymphocytosis. Roseola sine eruptione is the same disease without the rash.

All patients recover promptly without any specific therapy.

The disease increases in the spring and fall and may occur in mild epidemics. As a rule, only single cases occur in families; while this suggests to some that the disease is not contagious, it suggests to others that there may be many inapparent infections in families, especially in older siblings.

EPIDEMIC VIRAL GASTROENTERITIS

Epidemic viral gastroenteritis is a clinical syndrome characterized by (1) the absence of bacterial pathogens; (2) a clinical course of gastroenteritis with rapid onset and recovery, and relatively mild systemic signs; and (3) an epidemiologic pattern of a highly communicable disease which spreads rapidly with no particular predilection for age, season, or geography.

The syndrome appears to be distinct from that of epidemic diarrhea of the newborn, which is clinically more severe, is of longer duration, and in part is bacterial in etiology. In instances of infantile diarrhea where bacterial pathogens have not been recovered, certain enteroviruses and adenoviruses have been associated with nursery outbreaks and community cases. However, the viral etiology of infantile diarrhea has not yet been established, particularly because, in areas of high prevalence, enteroviruses and adenoviruses are found in the feces of the majority of normal children as well as those with infantile diarrhea.

Epidemic viral gastroenteritis is also distinct from the sporadic cases of diarrhea which have been sometimes associated with numerous other viral agents such as enteroviruses, reoviruses, infectious hepatitis viruses, and herpesviruses.

Two viruses that cause gastroenteritis have been recovered from human cases, and the disease has been reproduced by feeding bacteria-free fecal suspensions to human volunteers. The viruses appear distinct in that they produce different clinical pictures and lack cross-immunity. One virus, after an incubation period of 2 days, produces an afebrile illness of which diarrhea is the principal clinical manifestation. Recovery occurs after 4 days. The second virus, after a 1-day incubation period, causes a febrile illness of 1 day's duration characterized by persistent abdominal cramps and only mild diarrhea. Reinoculation experiments in volunteers indicate that, after an attack of afebrile nonbacterial gastroenteritis, specific immunity develops and lasts for at least 1 year. Since cases recur at yearly intervals in families and communities, it is necessary to postulate that there may be more than one antigenic type. Difficulty in growing these agents in animals and tissue culture has hindered efforts to clearly define their properties.

Clinically, malaise, anorexia, vomiting, dizziness, chills, fever, muscular aches, gastric pain, and diarrhea have been noted. The diarrhea is usually watery, but this is variable. The onset is rapid, and recovery occurs within 2–3 days. Fatalities are rare. There is no specific laboratory test, and the diagnosis depends upon negative bacteriologic findings and the clinical and epidemiologic characteristics of the disease. Treatment is symptomatic. Because of the infectious nature of stools, care should be taken in their disposal.

Although the syndrome is usually described in epidemic forms, frequent sporadic cases occur. Epidemics affect all age groups, occur during all seasons, and have been reported in widespread geographic areas. Outbreaks are common in public institutions and small communities.

CAT SCRATCH FEVER
(Benign Lymphoreticulosis)

Cat scratch fever is characterized by malaise, fever, and regional lymphadenitis. A cat scratch, cat bite, or merely contact with cats generally occurs a few days before onset. The primary reaction may be a cutaneous or vesicular lesion at the site of the scratch, followed by inflammation, and frequently suppuration, of the regional lymph nodes. Lymphadenitis may persist for 1–3 weeks or longer. An ocular manifestation takes the form of the oculoglandular symptom complex, similar to that which may occur in leptothricosis, tularemia, and tuberculosis.

The agent may have been transmitted to monkeys, which develop nodules at the sites of the intradermal inoculations and generalized lymphadenopathy.

Heat-inactivated suspensions of infected lymph nodes or heat-inactivated pus from a bubo serve as skin-test antigens. They yield a tuberculin-type of erythematous reaction about 24 hours after inoculation into convalescents.

The agent may belong to the psittacosis-lymphogranuloma venereum group of agents. Stained sections of infected lymph nodes in some cases were reported to contain elementary bodies similar in appearance to those of psittacosis. Furthermore, convalescent sera from patients with cat scratch fever sometimes fix complement in the presence of the psittacosis-LGV group antigen.

The disease is frequently not diagnosed, being confused with other infections of the lymph nodes. It occurs throughout the world. Although all age groups are susceptible, cases usually occur in children and young adults. In addition to transmission by contact with cats, cases have followed pricks from plant thorns, wood splinters, laceration while cutting meat, and insect bites. Cats are believed to be merely mechanical transmitters of the infection. They do not become ill.

The tetracycline antibiotics have been reported to shorten the course of the disease and prevent suppuration. However, even without treatment, recovery is complete within a few months.

• • •

General References

Bellamy, A.R., & others: Studies on reovirus RNA. I. Characterization of reovirus genome RNA. J Molec Biol 29:1–18, 1967.

Kapikian, A.Z.: Coronaviruses. Pages 931–946 in: *Diagnostic Procedures for Viral and Rickettsial Infections,* 4th ed. American Public Health Association, 1969.

Mayor, H.D., & others: Reoviruses. II. Structure and composition of the virion. J Bact 89:1548–1556, 1965.

Shatkin, A.J.: Replication of reovirus. Advances Virus Res 14:63–87, 1969.

Spendlove, R.S.: Unique reovirus characteristics. Progr Med Virol 12:161–191, 1970.

Verwoerd, D.W.: Diplornaviruses: A newly recognized group of double-stranded RNA viruses. Progr Med Virol 12:192–210, 1970.

40...

Oncogenic Viruses*

Although a viral origin for cancer has not been demonstrated in man, it would be illogical to suppose that the human species is unique in the animal world in escaping virus-induced malignant tumors. There are several reasons for believing that proof of the viral etiology of at least some types of human cancer will be forthcoming: (1) the well established viral etiology of benign warts and of molluscum contagiosum of man; (2) the many clinical, pathologic, and epidemiologic similarities between other human tumors and those of lower animals which have been shown to be caused by viruses; (3) the unquestionable role of numerous ordinary animal viruses, including human adenoviruses, in producing experimental cancer in animals; and (4) the biophysical, biochemical, and antigenic similarities between animal tumor viruses and viruses of man. Thus it is hoped that continuing research into the mechanism of viral oncogenesis with known tumorigenic animal viruses will provide models for the investigation of the possible viral etiology of cancer in man.

Although the first known malignancy of viral origin, avian leukemia, was discovered early in this century, the field of viral oncology has only recently received wide attention. Intensified research has led to the discovery of the viral etiology of many common tumors in lower animals. The recent contributions have been made largely because of technologic advances in tissue culture methods, the use of newborn animals for assay, and the application of modern biophysical, biochemical, and immunologic methods.

The tumor-inducing viruses can be classified into 2 main groups with differing physical, chemical, and biologic properties: Those which contain RNA as their genetic material, and those which contain DNA (Table 40–1).

This review is concerned with in vivo and in vitro carcinogenesis by representative members of the 2 groups of viruses, for they serve as models in the quest for knowledge of viral carcinogenesis in man.

General Properties of Tumor Viruses

Ample evidence obtained by research on transformation of single cells in vitro indicates that cancer originates as a single cell phenomenon. Once altered, the cell possesses new abnormal properties which are genetically transmitted to daughter cells. These genetic changes may be expressed as measurable morphologic,

metabolic, and antigenic alterations. In the animal the outcome of these phenomena may be one of 2 kinds: Either the altered cells invade surrounding tissue and metastasize to distant organs and tissues, resulting in host death; or the host may retain its homeostasis through humoral or cellular immune control mechanisms. Thus, a **tumor** may be defined as a permanently or temporarily uncontrolled growth of cells. It may be generalized or metastatic, culminating in the death of the animal (malignant tumor), or may remain localized and eventually regress (benign tumor).

How tumor viruses render cells malignant and how they differ in this respect from ordinary cytocidal viruses are questions which have not yet been fully answered, but the application of quantitative methods to the study of virus-cell interactions in tissue culture has brought some understanding of the mode of action of tumor viruses.

Virus infection of a cell has been described as the penetration of one genetic system into the sphere of action of another. Infection of a cell by a cytocidal virus results exclusively in cell death, but infection by a tumor virus leads to a synchronous virus-cell coexistence resulting in profound change in the properties of the infected cells (Figs 40–1 and 40–2). This phenomenon, called **cell transformation**, has been best studied in vitro.

Transformation may be recognized by an increase in the rate of cellular metabolism and multiplication and by a change in the appearance of the cells or of their arrangement in culture, usually as a result of lack of contact inhibition. When a virus induces transformation, small foci of cells resembling microtumors often appear in the culture. Statistical considerations show that a focus is produced by a single virus particle; the number of foci is thus a measure of the transforming titer of the virus. The most reliable test of true oncogenic transformation of an in vitro system is the ability of transformed cells to produce a tumor when injected into the proper animal host. This is not always possible, however, and one must then use the heritable changes in cellular appearance, pattern and rate of growth, metabolism, antigenic composition, or karyotype as criteria of transformation. It is important to realize that such changes in themselves do not always indicate oncogenic properties. Furthermore, such changes are not necessarily induced by a virus, since

*By Matilda Benyesh-Melnick, MD, Professor of Virology and Epidemiology, Baylor College of Medicine, Houston, Texas.

TABLE 40–1. Properties of RNA- and DNA-containing tumor viruses.

Virus	Host of Origin	Natural Tumors (Host of Origin)	Experimental Host Range: In Vivo Tumor	Experimental Host Range: In Vitro Cell Transformation	Size (nm)	Structure	Site of Virus Maturation	Persistence of Infected Virus in Tumor	Virus Induced Tumor Antigens: Transplantation (Surface)	Virus Induced Tumor Antigens: Nuclear (T)
RNA VIRUSES										
Avian leukosis complex:										
Lymphomatosis	Chicken	Yes	Chicken, turkey							
Myeloblastosis	Chicken	Yes	Chicken	Chicken						
Erythroblastosis	Chicken	Yes	Chicken	Chicken						
Rous sarcoma	Chicken	Yes	Chicken, duck, rat, guinea pig, turkey, mouse, hamster, monkey	Chicken, duck, rat, hamster, bovine, monkey, man	70-100	Pleomorphic, variable size and shape	Budding at cell membrane	Yes	Yes	No
Murine leukosis complex:										
Leukemia (many strains)	Mouse	Yes	Mouse, rat, hamster	Mouse, rat, hamster						
Sarcoma	Mouse	No								
Murine mammary tumor (Bittner)	Mouse	Yes	Mouse							
Feline leukosis complex:										
Leukemia	Cat	Yes	Cat							
Sarcoma	Cat	Yes	Cat, dog, rabbit, monkey	Cat, dog, monkey, man						
DNA VIRUSES										
Papovaviruses:										
Papilloma										
Human	Man	Yes	Man		40-55	Icosahedral symmetry	Nucleus	No	Yes	Yes
Rabbit	Rabbit	Yes	Rabbit							
Bovine	Cow	Yes	Cow	Bovine						
Canine	Dog	Yes	Dog							
Polyoma	Mouse	No	Mouse, hamster, rat, guinea pig, rabbit, ferret	Mouse, hamster, rat	70-80	Icosahedral symmetry	Nucleus	No	Yes	Yes
SV40	Monkey	No	Hamster	Hamster, mouse, monkey, man						
Adenoviruses:										
Human types 3, 7, 11, 12, 14, 16, 18, 21, 31	Man	No	Hamster, rat, mouse	Hamster, rat, man						
Simian (some)	Monkey	No								
Bovine type 3	Cow	No								
Avian (CELO)	Chicken	No								
Herpesvirus:										
Lucké carcinoma	Frog	Yes	Frog		100	Icosahedral symmetry	Nucleus	No		
Marek's disease	Chicken	Yes	Chicken							
Poxviruses:										
Fibroma-myxoma	Rabbit Squirrel Deer	Yes	Rabbit, squirrel, deer		230 X 300	Complex symmetry	Cytoplasm	Yes		
Yaba	Monkey	Yes	Monkey							
Molluscum contagiosum	Man	Yes	Man							

spontaneous changes of the kind mentioned above sometimes occur upon prolonged cultivation of cells in culture.

The mechanisms of carcinogenesis are probably not the same for all tumor-inducing viruses since both RNA and DNA viruses, which differ profoundly in their mode of replication, can induce tumors or cell transformation.

RNA-CONTAINING TUMOR VIRUSES

The viruses listed as RNA-containing tumor viruses in Table 40–1 are similar in structure, chemical composition, reaction to chemical and physical agents, and mode of growth. Another common property of these agents is that they are known to cause natural tumors in the host of origin. They can be divided into 4 groups on the basis of host range and type of malignancy.

(1) The avian leukosis complex of viruses: A group of antigenically related avian agents which are found to cause mainly leukemias (lymphomatosis viruses [ALV], myeloblastosis viruses [AMV], erythroblastosis viruses [AEV]) or mainly sarcomas (Rous sarcoma viruses [RSV]). However, a more comprehensive classification of these agents, based on antigenic studies (see below), is now evolving.

(2) The murine leukosis complex of viruses: Many different strains, some antigenically related and some not, have been associated with a variety of leukemias in mice. They remain "classified" by the name of the investigator first reporting the strain such as Gross, Friend, Graffi, Rauscher, and Moloney. The complex also includes the antigenically related murine sarcoma viruses (MSV) capable of inducing rhabdomyosarcomas.

(3) Murine mammary tumor virus: (Also known as milk factor or Bittner virus.) A virus transmitted through the milk and responsible for mammary carcinomas in certain strains of mice.

(4) The feline leukosis complex of viruses: A newly evolving group of feline leukemia viruses (FeLV), which can cause leukemias in the cat, and feline sarcoma (FeSa) viruses, which cause sarcomas in the cat as well as in other species such as dogs, rabbits, and monkeys.

Properties of the Viruses*

A. Morphology and Size: Electron microscopic studies of infected cells reveal virus particles only in the cell cytoplasm, with budding forms at the cellular membrane and mature particles in intracellular spaces (Figs 40–1 and 40–3). The particles range in size from 70–100 nm. The mature particle consists of an RNA-containing, electron dense nucleoid which can be either central (in C type particles) or eccentric (in B

*For general properties of viruses, see Chapter 27.

type particles): The nucleoid is separated from a single or double outer membrane (envelope) by an electron lucid area (halo). The nucleoid of immature (A type) particles is electron transparent because of the absence of nucleic acid. Biologic activity has been associated only with mature particles–C type in the case of the viruses of murine leukemia and of avian leukosis, and B type in the case of mammary tumor virus.

Particles extracted from affected organs from the plasma of viremic animals or from cells infected in vitro and stained with phosphotungstic acid (negative staining) reveal a superficial similarity with myxoviruses. Most of the particles lack the internal helical structure typical for myxoviruses, and only occasional particles reveal spikes on the outer membrane (envelope). Fixation in osmic acid or formalin before negative staining reveals particles with dense nucleoids.

B. Nucleic Acid: The nucleic acid isolated from these viruses is single-stranded RNA with an unusually high molecular weight of about 1×10^7 daltons. However, recent evidence suggests that these large RNA molecules may actually be composed of smaller subunits of $2–3 \times 10^6$ daltons held together by heat-labile hydrogen bonds.

C. Reactions to Chemical and Physical Agents: Being enclosed in a lipid-containing envelope, the RNA tumor viruses are sensitive to ether. They are readily inactivated by heating (56° C for 30 minutes), by mild acid treatment (pH 4.5), and by formalin at 1:4000. Like other viruses, they can be inactivated by light in the presence of basic dyes that combine with nucleic acid. The RNA tumor viruses can be preserved at −70° C or lower temperatures.

D. Antigenic Properties: Immunity to the RNA tumor viruses is associated with serum antibodies, but as a whole they are relatively weak antigens. Neutralizing and complement fixing antibodies are found in tumor-bearing animals or in animals immunized with live or killed virus.

1. The avian leukosis viruses have been recently classified into 4 antigenic subgroups (A–D), each including different leukemia-inducing viruses and different Rous sarcoma viruses (Table 40–2). This classification, based on antigenic cross-reactions in neutralization and immunofluorescence tests with antisera prepared in chickens, is in agreement with a classification based on virus host range and virus interference in cells of genetically defined avian species. In susceptible cells, viruses within the one antigenic subgroup interfere with each other but do not interfere with viruses of the other antigenic subgroup. All avian leukosis viruses share a group-specific antigen which can be detected with sera of rodents bearing Rous sarcoma tumors in a COFAL (complement fixing avian leukosis) test, in an immunofluorescence test, or in an immunodiffusion test. (Such animals do not develop antibodies against the virus coat protein, for the tumors are free of infectious virus.) Similar to the situation for the myxoviruses (see Chapters 34 and 35), the group-specific antigen of the avian leukosis viruses is soluble and represents an internal component of the

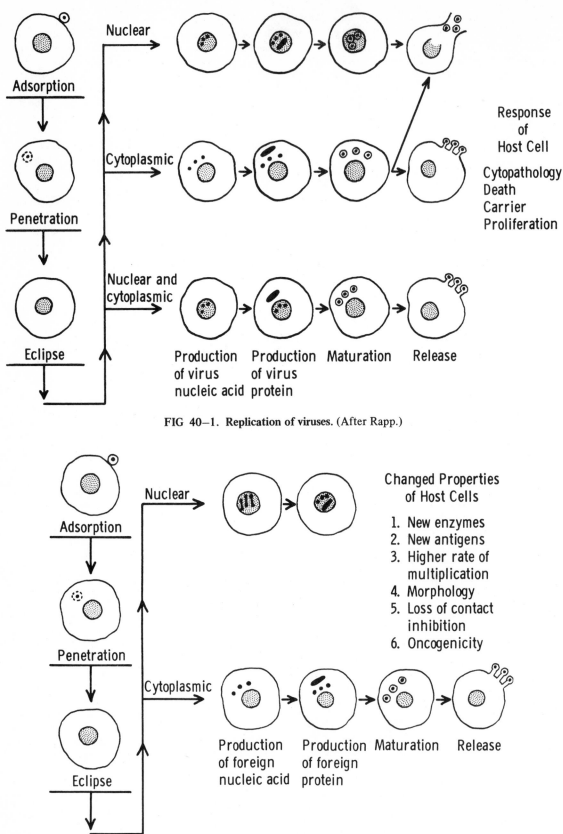

FIG 40–1. **Replication of viruses.** (After Rapp.)

FIG 40–2. **Transformation of cells by viruses.** (After Rapp.)

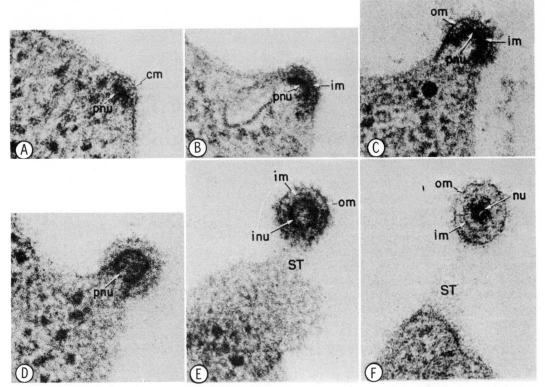

FIG 40–3. Virus budding at cell membrane of different leukemic myeloblasts either from circulating blood or tissue culture after various periods in vitro. (X 215,000.) Micrographs show different stages in increased size of dense prenucleoid (**pnu**), first beneath cell membrane (**cm**) in (A) and subsequent involvement of cell membrane in (B) and (C). Structures suggestive of outer (**om**) and inner particle membranes (**im**) are in buds in (B) and (C). A later stage of the bud is shown in (D). (E) shows typical "immature" avian tumor virus particle before nucleoid (**inu**) condensation. (F) shows dense nucleoid (**nu**) characteristic of "free" particles. The surface of buds and particles peripheral to outer membrane is irregular and indistinct. **ST** = stalk. (Courtesy of De Thé, G., Becker, C., & J.W. Beard: J Nat Cancer Inst 32:201, 1964.)

TABLE 40–2. Classification of avian leukosis viruses.

Antigenic Subgroup	Viruses*		Ability of Viruses to Grow in Genetically Defined Chick Embryo Cells				
	Leukemia Strains	Rous Sarcoma (RSV) Strains	C/O	C/A	C/B	C/AB	C/BC
A	RAV-1 RAV-3 RAV-4 RAV-5 RIF-1 AMV-1 FAV-1	Bryan Standard (BS-RSV) Schmidt-Ruppin-A (SR-RSV-A) Fuginami (FSV) Mill-Hill (MH-RSV) Prague-A (PR-RSV-A) Carr-Zilber-A (CZ-RSV-A)	Yes	No	Yes	No	Yes
B	RAV-2 RIF-2 AMV-2	Harris (HA-RSV) Schmidt-Ruppin-B (SR-RSV-B) Prague-B (PR-RSV-B)	Yes	Yes	No	No	No
C	RAV-7 RAV-49	Carr-Zilber-C (CZ-RSV-C) Prague-C (PR-RSV-C) B-77	Yes	Yes	Yes	Yes	No
D	RAV-50 CZAV	Carr-Zilber-D (CZ-RSV-D) Schmidt-Ruppin-D (SR-RSV-D)	Yes	Yes	Yes	Yes	Yes

*Abbreviations: RAV (Rous associated virus) = leukosis viruses used as "helper" viruses for the defective Bryan "high titer" (BH-RSV) strain of RSV; RIF (resistance inducing factor) = field strains of avian leukosis viruses that interfere with the focus-forming capacity of RSV; AMV = avian myeloblastosis virus; FAV = leukosis virus associated with the Fuginami sarcoma virus. CZAV = leukosis virus associated with the Carr-Zilber sarcoma virus; B-77 = a recent sarcoma virus isolate.

virion. Rabbits immunized with disrupted virions (but not those immunized with whole virus) develop precipitating antibodies to the group-specific antigen. Recent immunodiffusion studies indicate the existence of several distinct but cross-reacting, group-specific antigens.

2. The murine leukosis viruses have not been sufficiently characterized. However, recent studies indicate that they can be divided into 2 antigenic groups: one carrying the protein coat antigens of the Friend-Moloney-Rauscher (FMR) viruses and the other the antigens of the Gross (G) virus. Like the avian leukosis viruses, all the murine leukosis viruses share a group-specific soluble antigen that represents an internal component of the virion and can be detected with sera of rats bearing MSV-induced sarcomas (and free of neutralizing antibody) in complement fixation or immunodiffusion tests. As with the avian leukosis system, rabbits immunized with disrupted virions develop antibodies to the group-specific antigen.

3. For the mammary tumor virus one antigenic type, distinct from the murine leukemia viruses, has been reported.

4. The antigenic properties of the feline leukosis viruses are not well defined as yet. However, preliminary evidence suggests that they may share a group-specific antigen with the murine leukosis viruses.

Tumor Induction With RNA-Containing Tumor Viruses
A. Avian Leukosis Complex:
1. **Leukosis (leukemia-inducing) viruses**—Leukemic diseases are common in chickens, and the leukemia-inducing viruses are widely spread in normal as well as in diseased chicken populations. The main types of viral leukemias encountered are lymphoid, myeloid, and erythroid. They derive their names from the characteristic primitive cells (lymphoblast, myeloblast, erythroblast) found in large quantities in the blood of the diseased animal, and from this terminology the names of the viruses have evolved: avian lymphomatosis virus (ALV), myeloblastosis virus (AMV), and erythroblastosis virus (AEV).

Infectious virus and physical particles of the virus may be found in high concentration in tumor cells, peripheral blood, and other organs of the affected animals, a phenomenon not encountered with the DNA tumor viruses. Myeloblasts or erythroblasts taken from diseased birds and grown in tissue culture continue to release virus, which in turn can induce the malignancy on inoculation into chickens.

Malignancy can be induced in newborn or adult animals by inoculation with cell-free virus derived from diseased animals, or from leukemic cells grown in culture. Serial transplantation can also be made with leukemic cells; the resulting malignancy is eventually composed of cells of the recipient host, which suggests that it is virus-induced.

As mentioned above, the leukosis viruses are widely distributed in nature. Indeed, almost all flocks of chickens have been found to be infected with the various leukosis viruses, especially visceral lymphomatosis virus. The virus is transmitted horizontally through the saliva and feces, producing an infection in the adult animal characterized by transitory viremia and enduring antibodies. Relatively few adult birds develop clinical disease. Vertical transmission has been demonstrated from the viremic hen but not from the viremic rooster. It results in congenitally infected viremic chickens, tolerant to the virus, free of antibodies and permanent shedders of the virus. The incidence of leukemia in congenitally infected animals is much higher than in animals infected by contact.

2. **Rous sarcoma viruses**—Rous sarcoma virus has undergone countless passages experimentally since it was first isolated in 1911, and it probably now differs from the naturally occurring virus. Several strains of Rous virus exist which differ in their oncogenicity, antigenic structure, and host range. The most common laboratory strains are listed in Table 40–2.

Rous virus causes sarcoma in birds of all ages and in chick embryos; unlike lymphomatosis virus, however, it is not naturally transmitted. Rous virus also induces tumors in ducks, turkeys, pigeons, and other birds; certain virus variants (Schmidt-Ruppin and other strains) also induce tumors when inoculated into newborn rats, Syrian and Chinese hamsters, rabbits, mice, guinea pigs, and even monkeys. The presence of infectious virus and of physical particles of the virus is a common finding in avian but not in mammalian tumors.

B. Murine Leukosis Complex:
1. **Leukemia viruses**—To date numerous leukemogenic murine viruses have been isolated. The types of leukemia vary. For example, in mice of certain lines the Graffi virus causes mainly myeloid forms of leukemia, whereas in others lymphatic leukemia occurs in a high percentage of cases. In certain experiments Gross virus causes almost all known types of leukemic disease: lymphatic, stem cell, myeloid, and monocytic leukemia, erythroblastosis, chloroleukemia, lymphosarcoma, and reticulum cell sarcoma. Most leukemia viruses have proved pathogenic in rats, and the Moloney virus in hamsters as well.

Newborn animals are most susceptible to the effect of leukemogenic viruses, but the disease can also be produced in young and adult animals. Genetic factors play an important role in the susceptibility of mice to the virus, the nature of the disease caused, and the transmission of the virus. Thymectomy reduces the attack rate of lymphatic leukemia but not that of the myeloid forms. Thymectomy has no effect on the multiplication of the viruses in other organs.

In infected animals large amounts of infectious virus and of virus particles occur in the blood and in tumor tissue. It is known that some mouse leukemia viruses can be transmitted through milk, pass across the placenta, and be transmitted through the ovum.

2. **Murine sarcoma virus (MSV)**—Three strains (Harvey, Moloney, and Kirsten) have been isolated to date. The agents are antigenically related to some of the murine leukemia viruses and cause rhabdomyosarcomas in newborn mice, rats, and hamsters.

C. Murine Mammary Tumor Virus (Bittner Virus): The Bittner virus is found naturally in certain "high-cancer" lines of mice. It multiplies in the mammary gland and is present in large quantities in milk. Large amounts of infectious virus and of virus particles are found in tumor tissue. The virus has also been demonstrated in the organs of male and female mice of high-cancer lines, but this is apparently due to the content of virus in the blood of such animals.

The virus induces adenocarcinomas of the mammary gland only, and only in mice of susceptible lines. The latent period is 6–12 months. Newborn and suckling mice are susceptible to the virus if it is administered by the oral, subcutaneous, or intraperitoneal routes. Adult animals are considerably more resistant, but this resistance can be overcome by administering massive doses of virus. Animals that do not develop tumors remain infected subclinically and transmit the virus to their progeny. The main pathway of spread of the virus is through the milk, but it can also be transmitted by other routes in both males and females. The virus is not present in the excreta of mice of high-cancer lines. The natural frequency of mammary gland tumors in mice of some high-cancer lines may exceed 90%. The mammary tumor virus is also found in wild mice.

Electron microscopic investigations have revealed particles similar to the Bittner virus in lines of mice with a low incidence of cancer and supposedly free of the virus but in which mammary gland tumors can be induced by various carcinogens, perhaps working in concert with the virus.

D. Feline Leukosis Complex: Several isolates of feline leukemia virus (FeLV) and feline sarcoma (FeSa) virus have been derived to date from cats with leukemia and fibrosarcoma, respectively. When inoculated into newborn kittens, FeLV induces transmissible leukemia and FeSa virus induces transmissible fibrosarcoma. The virus is found in the tumor cells, bone marrow cells, and blood of the infected animals. The FeSa virus causes sarcomas also in dogs, rabbits, and monkeys.

Vegetative Growth & Cell Transformation With RNA Tumor Viruses

A characteristic property of the RNA tumor viruses is that they are not cytocidal during their period of vegetative growth. The infected cell produces new virus, continues to multiply, and may or may not undergo malignant transformation depending upon the virus or the cell used. Infectious virus and virus particles are readily detected in most of the tumor cells or cells transformed in vitro (Fig 40–2).

As shown by electron microscopic and tissue culture studies, the viruses multiply in the cell cytoplasm and mature at the cellular membrane; they are continuously released from the cell by budding from the cellular membrane.

Recent studies with cells transformed by and chronically infected with the murine sarcoma virus (MSV) indicate that the site of viral RNA synthesis is the cell nucleus rather than the cell cytoplasm; RNA complementary to the viral RNA was detected by hybridization procedures only in the nuclear but not in the cytoplasmic fractions of these cells.

Studies with some of the avian leukosis and murine leukosis viruses indicate that active host-cell DNA synthesis is required for the initial incorporation of the viral RNA genome in cells chronically infected with or transformed by these viruses.

A. Avian Leukosis Complex:

1. Leukosis (leukemia-inducing) viruses—Most of the leukosis viruses multiply in cultures of chick embryo fibroblasts without causing any cytopathic change or cell transformation. Virus replication in such cells can be detected by means of an immunofluorescence focus assay with type-specific chicken antisera or by failure of the cells to transform when exposed to Rous sarcoma virus, a phenomenon termed **interference**. The interfering property of the leukosis viruses is utilized to measure their activity in tissue culture in an RIF (resistance-inducing factor) test. Cells chronically infected with leukosis viruses can be propagated in serial passage, yielding large quantities of virus capable of inducing neoplasia in vivo or of inducing interference with Rous sarcoma virus in vitro.

Morphologic transformation of susceptible mesenchymal target cells into myeloblast-like cells has been achieved only with the avian myeloblastosis virus (AMV). The transformed cells multiply exponentially and produce new virus which in turn is capable of producing neoplasia in vivo or transformation in vitro. This in vitro transforming ability of AMV is used as a means of quantitatively assaying the virus.

Another distinctive feature of AMV is that it incorporates the enzyme adenosine triphosphatase (ATPase) during multiplication in cells which naturally synthesize the enzyme. For example, AMV particles released in the blood by the circulating myeloblasts contain high concentrations of the enzyme, but the same virus lacks the enzyme when the virus is isolated from kidney tumors whose cells cannot manufacture the enzyme. This ability of AMV to incorporate ATPase has led to a convenient assay for the virus, for there is a direct correlation between ATPase activity and infectivity of the virus.

2. Rous sarcoma virus (RSV)—Unlike the leukosis viruses, with which they share many physical and antigenic properties, the Rous sarcoma viruses are unique among tumor viruses in the speed and high frequency with which they induce malignant transformation of the infected cell. Infection of chick embryo cells with RSV results in foci of transformed cells, the morphology of which varies for the virus strain used. Virus activity is measured as the number of focus-forming units (FFU) per unit volume. In vitro, transformed chick or duck cells usually continue to release virus; both transformed cells and virus released from them can induce tumors in vivo.

The Schmidt-Ruppin (SR-RSV) and the Prague (PR-RSV) strains, which have been shown to induce tumors in mammals (including macaque and marmoset monkeys), can induce transformation in chick embryo cells as well as in mouse, rat, or hamster embryo fibroblast cells. The transformed chick embryo cells continue to produce infectious virus. Infectious virus cannot be demonstrated in cell-free extracts from transformed cells of mouse, rat, or hamster by conventional methods. However, infectious virus in such transformed cells can be elicited either by planting viable cells on chick embryo cell monolayers or by implanting viable cells into chickens (usually in the presence of a cell-fusing agent, such as inactivated Sendai virus). Transformation of human embryo, bovine embryo, and monkey cells has been reported with some of the RSV viruses.

Recent studies indicate some unique features of RSV-cell interaction: (1) Cell transformation is a function of the RSV genome, whereas (2) host range and sensitivity to specific interference by other leukosis viruses are governed by the protein coat in which the RSV genome is encapsidated. This was first revealed from work with the defective Bryan "high titer" (BH-RSV) strain. It was found that the BH-RSV was contaminated with a nontransforming leukosis virus—hence the term Rous-associated virus or RAV. Detailed studies of the symbiosis between RAV and RSV revealed that the BH-RSV actually contains 10 times more RAV than RSV. When selective pressures were applied to obtain infection with the RSV component alone, it turned out that pure RSV can induce cell transformation but cannot reproduce new, infectious virus (Fig 40–4); hence the term "defective."

Cells transformed in vitro or in vivo (tumors) by RSV alone fail to produce infectious virus or protein coat antigen, and such cells are called nonproducers (NP cells). However, NP cells, capable of multiplying for many generations, contain the group-specific avian leukosis antigen and the RSV genome. When superinfected with an RAV "helper" virus, which as indi-

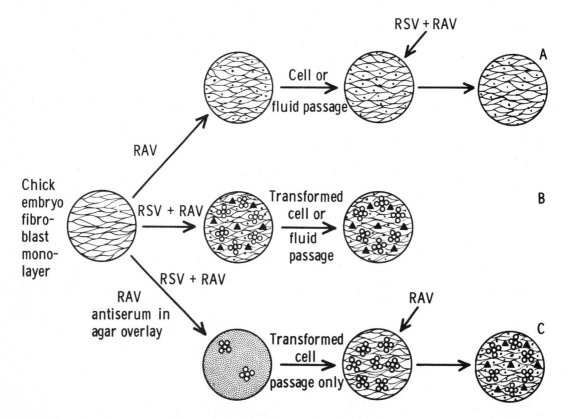

FIG 40–4. A: Interference. Chick embryo fibroblasts infected with RAV never transform, continue to produce infectious virus (black dots), and are resistant to superinfection with the (RSV + RAV) "high titer" Bryan strain of RSV. **B: Transformation.** Chick embryo fibroblasts infected with the (RSV + RAV) "high titer" Bryan strain of RSV undergo transformation (foci of rounded cells). The transformed cells release both RSV (black triangles) and RAV (black dots). Transformation of new cultures can be achieved by either passage of intact transformed cells or virus-containing tissue culture fluid. **C: Selection of NP cells.** Limiting dilution of the (RSV + RAV) "high titer" Bryan strain plated on chick embryo fibroblasts under an agar overlay containing RAV antiserum forms foci of transformed NP (free of infectious virus) cells. Transformation of new cultures can be achieved only by passage of intact NP cells. NP cells superinfected with a "helper" RAV release both infectious RSV and infectious RAV.

cated above does not possess transforming capacity, NP cells yield infectious RSV capable of transforming new cells in vitro or inducing sarcomas in vivo. Detailed analysis of this phenomenon revealed the following:

(1) Although RSV produces its own genetic material in solitary infection, it is dependent upon the "helper" virus for synthesis of its protein coat.

(2) As a result of this dependency, RSV bears the protein coat, and therefore the antigenic identity, of its helper virus. NP cells can be superinfected with various RAV viruses, and the resulting infectious RSV always has the antigenicity of the helper virus used. Several antigenically distinct helpers have been used: RAV-1, RAV-2, RAV-3, RAV-50, AMV-1, AMV-2, and the resulting mixed populations RSV (RAV-1), RSV (RAV-2), RSV (RAV-3), RSV (RAV-50), RSV (AMV-1), RSV (AMV-2) possess the genetic material of RSV but the antigenic make-up of the appropriate RAV.

(3) The ability of RSV to infect chicken cells of a given genetic constitution depends upon the coat of the helper and not on the RSV genome.

(4) The ability of the leukosis viruses to interfere with RSV depends upon the antigenic make-up of the RAV helper virus used to superinfect NP cells. For example, RAV-1 will interfere with RSV (RAV-1) and with RSV (RAV-3), both of which bear a protein coat antigenically related to RAV-1, but not with RSV (RAV-2), which has an RAV-2 coat unrelated to RAV-1.

More recent findings show that the BH-RSV is defective only in a quantitative sense. In addition to the avian leukosis group-specific antigen found in all NP cells, more than 90% of the different NP cell lines studied have been shown to carry virus particles as detected by electron microscopy. These particles were shown to contain the same large molecular weight RNA characteristic of the RAV or RSV (RAV) viruses. The particles, termed RSV (0), were found to be infectious but only for certain types of avian cells that had not been used in the past. Thus, the BH-RSV virus does not appear to be defective in the classical sense of lacking the function of coat formation, but the nature of the coat is such that the host range is limited. However, more recent evidence indicates the existence of 2 genetically different RSV (0) particles in NP cells: one, RSV β (0), able to replicate in certain avian cells; and a second, RSV α (0), unable to replicate in any known cell. It remains to be seen whether the latter represents the RSV genome in the protein coat of another yet uncharacterized helper RAV virus or whether it represents a true nondefective RSV population in BH-RSV strain.

The experimental exchange of protein coats of various RSV genomes has led to further evidence that the host range of RSV is completely dependent upon its protein coat. The enclosure of the genome of the Schmidt-Ruppin (SR-RSV) strain of RSV in the viral protein coat of RAV-1 (SR-RSV [RAV-1]) renders it incapable of inducing tumors in mammals. Conversely,

enclosure of the genome of the BH-RSV in the protein coat of a newly isolated leukosis virus RAV-50 (BH-RSV [RAV-50]) allows it to acquire the property of tumor induction in mammals. However, such alteration in the viral envelope does not cause a heritable stable change of the virus genome. Infection of chick embryo cells with SR-RSV (RAV-1) in the presence of RAV-1 antiserum leads to the occurrence of transformed cells that yield infectious SR-RSV capable of inducing tumors in mammals or transforming mammalian cells in vitro. Unlike SR-RSV, the BH-RSV genome present in the mammalian cells cannot be rescued by the mere co-cultivation of mammalian cells and chick embryo cells but can be elicited upon superinfection of the co-cultivated cell mixture with RAV virus, yielding infectious BH-RSV (RAV) virus.

B. Murine Leukosis Viruses:

1. **Leukemia viruses**—Laboratory strains of the FMR group can be propagated in vitro in mouse embryo fibroblasts of unrestricted genotype. On the other hand, the Gross virus and naturally occurring (field) leukemia viruses have been found to replicate only in cells of certain strains of mice. With some exceptions (see below), virus replication in infected tissue cultures is vegetative with no detectable change in cell morphology. The infected cells contain the group-specific antigen and continue to release infectious virus particles. However, the particles obtained from infected tissue cultures are about 10,000 times less infectious than the particles circulating in the blood of leukemic animals. The infected cells are resistant to transformation by the murine sarcoma virus (MSV), a situation similar to the resistance to RSV conferred upon chick embryo fibroblasts by the avian leukosis viruses. In vitro transformation of mouse, rat, and hamster embryo cells has been recently reported for some of the leukemia viruses (Friend, Gross, and Rauscher). The transformed cells contain the group-specific antigen, continue to release infectious virus, and are tumorigenic.

2. **Murine sarcoma virus (MSV)**—A great similarity exists between MSV and the defective Bryan "high titer" strain of Rous sarcoma virus (BH-RSV). Infection of mouse, rat, or hamster embryo cells with MSV results in foci of transformed cells, and virus activity can be measured in focus-forming units (FFU) per unit volume. Like the BH-RSV, the MSV preparations were found to contain a large quantity of nontransforming murine leukemia virus. However, unlike BH-RSV, MSV appears to require the helper leukemia virus not only for induction of protein coat synthesis but also for its focus-forming capacity. MSV preparations can induce fibrosarcomas in hamsters. The resulting tumor cells are free of the accompanying leukemia virus but contain the defective MSV genome, a state similar to the BH-RSV nonproducer (NP) transformed cells. Co-cultivation of the hamster tumor cells with mouse embryo cells in the presence of a nontransforming leukemia virus results in the production of infectious MSV capable of transforming cells in vitro or inducing tumors in vivo. Any one of the murine leukemia

TABLE 40–3. Terminology in tissue transplantation experiments.

Genetic Relatedness of Host and Donor Animal	Synonym Used to Identify the Animal	Synonym Used to Identify the Graft
The same animal	Autologous = autogenous	Autograft
Genetically compatible animals of the same inbred strain	Isologous = isogeneic = syngeneic	Isograft = syngeneic graft
Animals of the same species but genetically incompatible	Homologous = allogeneic	Homograft = allogeneic graft
Animals of different species	Heterologous = xenogeneic	Heterograft = xenograft

viruses can be used in these rescue experiments, and the resulting infectious MSV bears the protein coat of the helper virus used. The terminology MSV (MLV), MSV (RLV), MSV (FLV), and MSV (GLV) has been suggested for the MSV pseudotypes obtained when Moloney, Rauscher, Friend, or Gross leukemia viruses, respectively, are used as the helper virus.

In recent experiments the feline leukemia virus (FeLV) has been used as a helper for the defective MSV, with a resulting MSV (FeLV) pseudotype capable of transforming feline cells but not mouse cells. Substitution of the FeLV protein coat with that of the Moloney murine leukemia virus (MLV) results in an MSV (MLV) pseudotype infectious for mouse cells. These genetic interactions between RNA tumor viruses of unrelated species deserve further study and confirmation, for it may indeed open avenues to elucidate possible defective viral genomes in human tumor cells.

C. Murine Mammary Tumor Virus: Attempts at in vitro propagation of these agents by conventional tissue culture methods have not been successful. It has been possible, however, to demonstrate virus growth in organ cultures of the mammary glands of the mouse embryo.

D. Feline Leukosis Viruses: Information on the propagation of these viruses in tissue culture is very recent. Preliminary evidence indicates that the leukemia virus (FeLV) undergoes vegetative replication in feline, canine, and human cells. The infected cells remain morphologically unaltered and continue to release infectious virus, leukemogenic for the newborn kitten. The sarcoma (FeSa) virus has been found to transform in vitro cell cultures of feline, canine, monkey, and human origin.

Virus-Induced Tumor Antigens

One of the principal characteristics of carcinogenesis by the RNA tumor viruses is the continuous release of infectious virus from most of the in vivo or in vitro transformed cells. This property has made the assessment of new virus-induced but nonvirion antigens in these cells more difficult than in the case of cells transformed by DNA-containing viruses for the latter cells are usually free of infectious virions (see below).

However, work with virus-induced leukemias in highly inbred strains of mice indicates that the leukemic cells possess new antigens specific for the virus strain inducing the leukemia. These experiments are based on the principles of graft rejection among unrelated mice (Table 40–3). Thus, mice of one genetically defined strain accept autologous and syngeneic grafts. However, they reject allogeneic grafts and develop immunity against transplantation antigens in the allogeneic graft. Animals that have rejected allogeneic grafts still accept subsequent syngeneic grafts which lack the foreign transplantation antigens.

Transplantation immunity has been demonstrated in several of the virus-induced murine leukemias. Tumors induced in various strains of mice by one of the leukemia viruses share a common antigen, presumably under the genetic direction of the virus. Highly inbred mice inoculated with allogeneic Moloney virus-induced leukemic cells (homografts) develop immunity to the normal transplantation antigens and consequently reject these cells. At the same time, however, immunity also develops to the tumor-specific antigen as shown by the resistance of these mice to a subsequent challenge with sygeneic Moloney virus-induced leukemic cells (isograft).

Nonimmunized mice accept such isografts. The same type of immunity can be induced by subthreshold doses of viable syngeneic cells (isografts) or by large doses of irradiated syngeneic cells which do not grow in the recipient host. This finding strengthens the assumption that the tumor cells not only contain infectious virus but also acquire new virus-induced antigens.

Transplantation antigens in virus-induced leukemia cells can also be measured by in vitro tests which employ autologous or syngeneic cells and sera of tumor-bearing animals or sera of animals immunized by one of the methods mentioned above.

By means of this system the presence of reacting antigens has been demonstrated in murine leukemia cells induced by several of the murine leukemia viruses. The tests most commonly utilized are the indirect immunofluorescence test and the cytotoxic test. In the immunofluorescence test the surface of the reacting cells stains in the presence of the specific antiserum. In the cytotoxic test antibody directed against cellular antigens reacts with the cell possessing these antigens in the presence of complement. The antibody-cell reaction results in cell death which can be measured in vivo by the failure of the antibody-treated cells to grow when inoculated into a syngeneic host. The reaction can also be measured in vitro. Thus one can count the dead cells when stained with dyes like trypan blue, or one can measure the release of ^{51}Cr from damaged cells that have been prelabeled with ^{51}Cr. As with the in vivo transplantation immunity, the in vitro reactions are specific for all the leukemias induced by the same virus. Cross-reacting antigens exist in leukemia cells induced by the Friend, Moloney, or Rauscher (FMR group) viruses. However, the reactions are mono-specific for the Gross or Graffi virus-induced leuke-mias.

Transplantation antigens cross-reacting with those induced in leukemic cells by the FMR leukemia viruses have also been found in mouse sarcomas induced by the murine sarcoma virus (MSV). This cross-reaction is due to the fact that all preparations of infectious MSV contain murine leukemia virus with the antigenicity of the FMR group. Preimmunization of mice with irradi-ated virus-induced syngeneic sarcoma cells results in transplantation resistance to challenge with unirra-diated sarcoma cells or syngeneic leukemia cells induced by the viruses of the FMR group. The reverse is also true.

The transplantation antigen in MSV-induced sarcoma cells can also be detected in vitro by a colony inhibition test. This test measures the ability of either serum (in the presence of complement) or lymph node cells from animals in which the tumors have regressed (immune animals) to inhibit in vitro the plating effi-ciency of MSV-induced sarcoma cells. Lymph node cells of mice with progressively growing MSV-induced sarcomas (nonimmune animals) can also inhibit in vitro the colony formation of their own tumor cells, indi-cating an effective cellular immunity in such animals. However, tumor-bearing animals have circulating anti-body that appears to coat and thus protect the tumor cells from destruction by immune lymph node cells in the colony inhibition test. It is thus possible that these same humoral antibodies play a similar tumor-protecting role in vivo in animals with progressive tumors.

Transplantation type antigen similar to that described for the murine leukemias has been recently demonstrated for some mouse sarcomas induced by the Schmidt-Ruppin strain of RSV (SR-RSV). Inbred mice immunized with allogeneic sarcoma cells induced by SR-RSV or with irradiated syngeneic cells induced by the same virus develop transplantation resistance to challenge with syngeneic cells. Immunization with the virus alone, free of cells, does not confer this type of resistance.

DNA-CONTAINING TUMOR VIRUSES

This portion of the chapter is limited to the papovaviruses and adenoviruses, since they appear to serve as the best understood models of virus-induced but virus-free solid tumors. As demonstrated in Tables 27–1 and 40–1, viruses in these 2 subgroups share many properties such as cubic symmetry, naked virions, lack of essential lipids, resistance to ether and mild acid (pH 3.0), and multiplication in the cell

nucleus. They differ, however, in size, in number of capsomeres, and in antigenic structure. (For general properties of viruses, see Chapter 27.)

Papovaviruses

The name papova is derived from the first 2 let-ters of the names of the oncogenic viruses included in this group: papilloma viruses of man, rabbit, cow, and dog; polyoma virus of mouse; and vacuolating (SV40) virus of monkeys. (Two other viruses, rabbit vacuo-lating virus and murine K virus, also belong to the papovavirus group, but there is no evidence that they are oncogenic.)

A. Morphology and Nucleic Acid: Papovavirus particles exhibit icosahedral symmetry, have a naked capsid composed of 42 (or 72) capsomeres, and diameters of 40–55 nm. They contain double-stranded DNA with a molecular weight of 3×10^6 daltons for polyoma and SV40 viruses and 6×10^6 daltons for the papilloma virus. Infectious DNA has been isolated from all 3 viruses.

DNA extracted from all 3 viruses has been shown to exist as circular molecules. Upon analytical ultra-centrifugation, the DNA sediments into 2 components with sedimentation constants of 20 S and 16 S (polyoma, SV40) or 28 S and 21 S (papilloma). The heavier component has a twisted circular form that may convert to the lighter (circular or linear) compo-nent when single-strand breaks are introduced. For polyoma virus, both of these DNA components are known to be infectious, transform cells in vitro, and produce tumors in vivo. In addition, polyoma virus DNA has a third linear component with a sedimenta-tion coefficient of 14 S that appears to represent frag-ments of host-cell DNA enclosed in some of the virions.

There is evidence for some similarity between the DNA of the oncogenic papovaviruses and mammalian cell DNA: (1) The guanine + cytosine (G + C) content of the DNA of these viruses varies between 41–49%, which is very similar to mammalian host-cell DNA (40–42% G + C). (2) Hybridization of viral DNA with cell DNA on nitrocellulose membranes reveals that there is complementarity, though in various degrees, of base sequences between viral DNA and host-cell DNA. (3) Analysis of nearest neighbor base sequences reveals that the doublet pattern of the viral DNA closely resembles that of the host-cell DNA with a rarity of the G + C doublet.

B. Reaction to Chemical and Physical Agents: Papovaviruses are resistant to heating (50° C for 1 hour), ether, and acid treatment (pH 3.0). SV40 and polyoma viruses can be inactivated at 50° C in the presence of high concentrations of $MgCl_2$; thermal inactivation in the presence of molar $MgCl_2$ has been used to eliminate SV40 virus from stocks of oral polio-vaccine, since the infectivity of poliovirus is stabilized under these conditions. Papovaviruses can be stored at −20° C for long periods with no loss of infectivity. Infectivity of the viruses is decreased by 1:4000 for-malin solution, but they are not inactivated as readily as poliovirus and adenovirus. Consequently, live SV40 has been recovered from several lots of killed poliovirus and killed adenovirus vaccines.

C. Antigenic Properties: Each of the papovaviruses is antigenically distinct. The viruses induce the production of specific neutralizing and complement fixing antibodies. Only the polyoma virus has been shown to hemagglutinate red blood cells.

Adenoviruses

Adenoviruses comprise a large group of agents that occur widely in human beings, monkeys, cattle, dogs, mice, and chickens. Over 30 antigenic types exist for the human species alone; of these, types 3, 7, 11, 12, 14, 16, 18, 21, 31, and perhaps others cause tumors in newborn animals, particularly hamsters. All these viruses were isolated from human beings, and serologic surveys show that infection is common with types 3, 12, 14, 18, 21, and 31 and almost universal with type 7.

Recent studies have shown that several simian adenoviruses, bovine adenovirus type 3, and the avian adenovirus CELO (an acronym for chick embryo lethal orphan virus) are tumorigenic when inoculated into newborn hamsters.

The oncogenic adenoviruses are similar in structure to other adenoviruses and have naked capsids 70–80 nm in diameter, with 252 capsomeres arranged in icosahedral symmetry. Infectious nucleic acid has not been isolated as yet from any of the adenoviruses, but it has been shown that they contain double-stranded DNA in an amount corresponding to a molecular weight of 2.3×10^7 daltons.

The oncogenic human adenoviruses may be classified into 2 subgroups: highly oncogenic (types 12, 18, and 31) and weakly oncogenic (types 3, 7, 11, 14, 16, and 21). Those in the highly oncogenic subgroup are the only adenoviruses with a low G + C content in their DNA (48–49%; a value similar to that of the papovaviruses and cellular DNA). The weakly oncogenic types have an intermediate G + C content of 50–53%. A third subgroup of adenoviruses (types 1, 2, 5, and 6), that are nononcogenic but transform rat embryo cells in vitro, have a high G + C content (55–61%). A further relatedness between members within each of the 3 subgroups stems from DNA-DNA or DNA-messenger RNA (mRNA) homology studies. Maximal DNA-DNA or DNA-mRNA hybridization is attained only between viruses within a subgroup with negligible intersubgroup hybridization. (It should be noted that a highly oncogenic simian adenovirus [SA 7] has a high G + C content, similar in value to the nononcogenic human adenoviruses.)

Tumor Induction With Papovaviruses & Adenoviruses

A. Papilloma Viruses: Papilloma viruses are the only members of the papovavirus group known to cause natural tumors in their hosts of origin. They cause warts or papillomas in human beings, rabbits, cows, and dogs. The ecology of these viruses is not known, but they are found in large quantities in papillomas. Although the human wart virus was the first virus transmitted experimentally from host to host, only the rabbit papilloma virus has been studied extensively for its tumor-inducing properties. In the natural host, the wild cottontail rabbit, the virus causes large benign skin papillomas which, on rare occasions, become malignant carcinomas. When inoculated into the domestic rabbit the virus also produces benign skin papillomas which may either regress or develop into malignant carcinomas. Tumors can be induced in both rabbit species with the DNA isolated from the virus. Infectious virus can be readily recovered from the papillomas of cottontail rabbits but not from their carcinomas; virus cannot be isolated from either papillomas or carcinomas of domestic rabbits. However, infectious DNA has been isolated from such tumors. Transplantation of carcinoma cells results in carcinomas in the new host.

B. Polyoma Virus: Latent infection with polyoma virus is widespread among laboratory and wild mice. Young mice are infected naturally in the first few weeks by contamination with urine and saliva of adults. Intrauterine infection is not known to occur. Not a single natural tumor of mice, the host of origin, has been uncovered. However, the virus is highly tumorigenic when inoculated into newborn mice or hamsters, which develop tumors within a few weeks of inoculation of large doses of virus. Newborn rats, rabbits, guinea pigs, and ferrets are also susceptible. Infectious DNA isolated from the virus has been shown to be tumorigenic. The commonest tumors are spindle cell sarcomas, but epithelial tumors also occur in mice. The tumors appear in a number of sites, hence the name polyoma. The tumors are usually free of infectious virus or virus particles. As few as 10 tumor cells transplanted into a susceptible adult animal result in new tumors which can be further transplanted. Tumor cells can be serially grown in vitro and retain malignancy.

C. SV40 Virus: Simian vacuolating virus, or SV40, is commonly found in uninoculated cultures of rhesus and cynomolgus monkey kidney cells in which the virus apparently grows without causing a cytopathic effect. Introduction of fluids from such cultures into renal cell cultures derived from the green African or grivet monkey (*Cercopithecus aethiops sabaeus*) is followed by prominent cytoplasmic vacuolization; hence the name vacuolating virus. Isolation of the virus was quickly followed by demonstration of its oncogenic potential when introduced into newborn hamsters. It is not known, however, whether tumors develop in monkeys as a result of natural infection. Realization that millions of people have been exposed to this virus as a contaminant of viral vaccines, both live and inactivated, and that after ingestion of live poliovaccine many children continued to excrete SV40 for as long as 5 weeks, has spurred research on this agent. SV40 virus (as well as its infectious DNA) causes sarcomas at the site of inoculation in newborn hamsters. In addition, ependymomas have been produced. The tumors are usually free of infectious virus and virus particles. Tumor cells can be serially passed in adult hamsters and cause the same type of tumors as those induced by the virus itself. Both primary and transplanted tumors can be serially propagated in tissue culture and retain malignancy.

D. Adenoviruses: Adenoviruses types 12, 18, and 31 cause undifferentiated sarcomas at the site of inoculation, and less commonly at other sites, in newborn hamsters, rats, and mice. Adenovirus type 7 also causes tumors in newborn hamsters, but the latent period has generally been more than 160 days (compared to less than 90 days for tumors induced by types 12 and 18). Less than 25% of animals inoculated with type 7 develop tumors, and except for a few undifferentiated sarcomas the tumors are usually malignant lymphomas or lymphosarcomas. With adenoviruses 3, 11, 14, 16, and 21, the latent period before the appearance of sarcomas in newborn hamsters is even longer than that for type 7. Adenoviral tumors contain no infectious virus. Tumors can be maintained in serial passage by means of transplantation of tumor cells into adult animals of the appropriate species; tumor cells may also be grown serially in tissue culture and retain malignancy.

Cell Transformation With Papovaviruses & Adenoviruses

Unlike the RNA tumor viruses, which can grow vegetatively in susceptible cells without killing them, the DNA tumor viruses can either multiply and kill the cell in the process of making more virus, or they can transform the cell without subsequent virus production (Figs 40-1 and 40-2). One or the other may predominate, depending upon the cell and not the virus. The 2 activities do not normally take place in the same cell, for with the DNA viruses vegetative growth is cytocidal, leading to cell death which is incompatible with the process of cellular transformation and continued growth. Yet these 2 states are not always mutually exclusive since virus production with cell lysis may occur when polyoma-transformed cells are superinfected with polyoma virus.

Recent studies suggest that there is a common pathway following cell infection with DNA tumor viruses, presumably involving the synthesis of messenger RNA from viral DNA. There is probably a choice of pathways leading to either replication of the virion or to cellular transformation. For several reasons, it appears that fewer genes of the virus seem to be involved in transformation than in viral replication: (1) With polyoma virus it has been determined that only about 50% of the viral DNA responsible for cytocidal infection is involved in the transformation process. The cytocidal activity of the virus was found to be inactivated (ultraviolet light, x-ray, and other agents) at a rate twice that of its transforming ability. (2) Cells transformed by either papovaviruses or adenoviruses do not contain the viral capsid antigen or infectious viral nucleic acid. (3) Cells can be transformed by a defective mutant of SV40 virus which is unable to direct the synthesis of capsid protein. It is therefore

assumed that cell transformation by DNA viruses is either an expression of a function of defective viral genomes or that genetic repression occurs.

The papilloma viruses have not been successfully propagated in culture; the adenoviruses, which induce cytocidal infection in a variety of cells, can transform hamster, rat, and human cells in vitro but with limited success. The polyoma and SV40 viruses, however, have a marked cell-transforming potential, and they have been most extensively studied.

Infection of mouse embryo cells with polyoma virus is mainly cytocidal, but infection of hamster embryo cells with the same virus results mainly in cell transformation. Similarly, SV40 almost always undergoes cytocidal multiplication in green monkey kidney cells, but infection of hamster, mouse, or human fibroblast cells frequently results in cell transformation.

Hamster or mouse cells transformed in tissue culture by either polyoma or SV40 viruses can produce tumors when inoculated into the appropriate host, even when as few as 10-100 cells are used as inoculum.

The time required for transformation of cells by DNA tumor viruses may differ widely for different viruses and for different cells. In some systems, transformation occurs in a matter of days, and in other cases it may take place slowly and become apparent only several weeks after the culture has been inoculated with the virus. Polyoma virus usually causes transformation soon after it penetrates the cell, so that the susceptible cells exposed to polyoma virus promptly produce clones made up entirely of the newly transformed cells. In such an instance, the transformation takes place before a single new cell division occurs. With SV40 and with adenovirus, obvious transformation may not take place for weeks, because only a tiny fraction of the cell population seems responsive to the transforming ability of the virus added to the culture. Even with polyoma virus, however, a very large amount of virus is required to induce transformation. Since the dose response of cell transformation by polyoma virus is linear—a reflection of a one hit curve—a single effective particle is sufficient to cause transformation. It should be noted that with many viruses one infectious unit is equivalent to more than one virus particle (in some cases up to 10,000). With polyoma virus 40-100 virus particles are equivalent to one infectious (replicating) unit. For transformation of hamster fibroblasts, the most sensitive system known, one transforming unit is equivalent to 1 million particles. Presumably only one of these million particles is effective in the transformation process, just as one of the 40 particles is effective in initiating cytocidal infection. It has been recently found that karyotypically abnormal cell cultures from human patients with homozygous and heterozygous Fanconi's anemia (a rare autosomal recessive disease) or with Down's syndrome (trisomy 21) are 10-50 times more susceptible to transformation by SV40 virus as well as by SV40-adeno hybrids than diploid cell cultures derived from normal humans. It is of interest that both types of patients have an unusually high risk of developing malignancies.

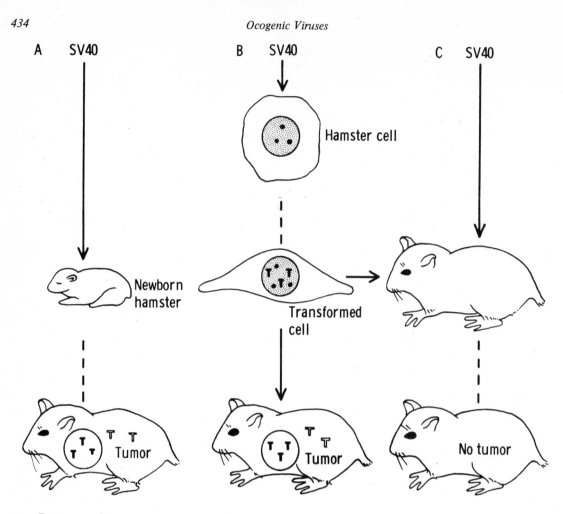

T   Tumor antigen

Т   Antibody specific to tumor antigen

FIG 40–5. Tumor (T) antigen. (A) Newborn hamsters inoculated with SV40 often develop tumors. **(B)** Similarly, hamster cells grown in culture and transformed by SV40—meaning that they were given permanent heritable changes—can induce tumors when transplanted to young adult hamsters. The tumor cells as well as the transformed cells contain the T antigen and the tumor-bearing animal develops antibodies to the T antigen. **(C)** Transplantation immunity. A hamster into which transformed cells are transplanted after the animal has been inoculated with SV40 virus resists the tumor-causing effect of transformed cells. The virus acts as a vaccine, inducing in certain of the animal's cells a new antigen ("transplantation antigen"); this in turn elicits an immune response, and the animal eliminates the cells bearing the new antigen. The animal also rejects cells that have been transformed in vitro which evidently carry the same "transplantation antigen." (From: *The Footprints of Tumor Viruses,* by Fred Rapp & Joseph L. Melnick. Copyright [©] 1966 by Scientific American, Inc. All rights reserved.)

Cells transformed in vitro by papovavirus or by adenovirus, or cells of tumors induced in vivo by these viruses, may release infectious virus for a short time, and then virus-free transformed cells and tumors emerge. Reproduction of infectious virus is not essential for maintenance of neoplastic characteristics. However, in some instances the situation resembles that of the Rous sarcoma virus genome in mammalian cells; thus, in hamster or mouse cells transformed by SV40, infectious virus may be produced when the virus-free cells are grown with virus-susceptible cells under conditions favoring fusion of the 2 types of cells.

As mentioned earlier, the virus-free transformed cells do not contain detectable infectious DNA or viral capsid protein. However, viral DNA has been detected in cells transformed by either papovaviruses or adenoviruses but in a state that is noninfectious. It has been estimated that the amount of polyoma or SV40 viral

DNA present in transformed cells varies between 7 and 60 molecules per cell, as compared to over 1 million DNA molecules per cell during cytocidal infection in permissive cells. In bacterial cells, permanent genotypic changes may be induced by viruses (see Transduction, Chapter 4, and Lysogenic Conversion, Chapter 9). In such cases the virus, in the form of provirus, is integrated with the cell genome by direct incorporation of viral nucleic acid or by the incorporation of virus-associated genetic material carried over from an earlier cell in which the virus had replicated. Experimental data have not as yet shown that a similar state exists in the virus-free transformed cells, for they have not manifested the classical properties of a bacterial lysogenic system: spontaneous and random release of virus from cells, induction of virus release by radiation or mutagenic chemicals, and resistance of provirus-containing cells to superinfection.

The possibility still exists that neoplastic cells contain the whole or a large part of the virus genome in a more highly integrated state than exists in the bacteria-virus system. It has been recently shown that tumor cells transformed by adenoviruses as well as by papovaviruses (polyoma and SV40) contain a small but highly specific fraction of viral messenger RNA (mRNA). This mRNA can be detected by its ability to hybridize with viral DNA. The mRNA is specific for the virus that had originally induced the transformation, since it is not found in normal cells nor in cells transformed by a different virus.

Additional evidence for the presence of an integrated viral genome or at least a portion of it in papovavirus- or adenovirus-transformed or tumor cells comes from the discovery in such cells of new **nonviral cellular antigens** specified by the virus inducing the transformation. This is most important since it permits recognition of the specificity of viral transformation.

Papovavirus- & Adenovirus-Induced Antigens in Transformed or Tumor Cells

Two principal types of new antigens have been recognized based on the methods used for their demonstration:

A. Transplantation Antigen: (See Fig 40–5.) A transplantation type of antigen can be detected by measuring the resistance of virus-immunized animals to challenge with neoplastic cells. Adult animals immunized with active virus are resistant to challenge of large doses ($10^5 - 10^6$) of virus-free transformed or tumor cells, whereas nonimmune animals develop tumors when inoculated with as few as 10–100 cells.

This type of immunity has been found to be unrelated to circulating viral antibodies but to be specifically associated with an antigen at the cell surface. It is presumed that this immunity occurs because the active virus induces this new antigen in some cells of the adult animal, and the new antigen in turn elicits a humoral and cellular immune response resulting in subsequent rejection of transformed cells carrying the same antigen.

In certain transformed cells which are not oncogenic in animals, virus-specific transplantation antigen can be demonstrated by its ability to block viral carcinogenesis. Thus, tumors fail to develop in hamsters inoculated at birth with oncogenic virus if the non-oncogenic transformed cells are injected during the latent period.

Another antigen has been reported for SV40-transformed hamster cells: a **cell surface (S) antigen** which can be detected in immunofluorescence and colony inhibition tests with sera of SV40-immunized hamsters that have resisted challenge with virus-free transformed cells. A cell surface (S) antigen can also be detected in polyoma virus-transformed cells reacted with sera of mice that had rejected allogeneic polyoma virus-induced (but virus-free) tumor cells. This S antigen may be related to the transplantation antigen, but the final proof of this assumption awaits further work.

Evidence is accumulating that a transplantation type immunity exists also in the rabbit papilloma system. Rabbits bearing transplanted virus-free carcinomas fail to produce papillomas when injected with virus. Virus-induced papillomas regress much more rapidly in animals preimmunized with virus-free papilloma tissue than in nonimmunized animals. In addition, rabbits whose primary virus-induced papillomas have regressed fail to develop tumors when inoculated with infectious nucleic acid, whereas rabbits bearing persistent primary virus-induced papillomas or carcinomas respond to such nucleic acid inocula with new tumors as readily as previously uninfected control rabbits.

The colony inhibition test has been used to detect transplantation antigens in virus-induced papilloma or carcinoma cells with results identical to those described for the MSV system.

B. Tumor or T Antigen: Tumor (T) antigen appears in the nucleus of tumor cells or cells transformed in vitro. It can be measured by means of immunofluorescence or complement fixation tests employing antibodies which develop in sera of animals bearing large primary or transplanted tumors. This antigen has been demonstrated for polyoma, SV40, and adenoviruses. (Adenovirus T antigen can be detected not only in the nucleus but also in the cytoplasm.)

The T antigens are unrelated to viral capsid (V) antigens but are specific for the inducing virus and are the same in cells of different species transformed by the same virus. Thus, both hamster and human cells, when transformed by SV40, contain the same antigens.

T antigens immunologically identical to those found in in vitro transformed cells or tumor cells are also synthesized by the papovaviruses (polyoma and SV40) and adenoviruses (including nontumorigenic strains) during cytocidal infection in susceptible cells. T antigen is formed in the nucleus early during the replicative cycle prior to the synthesis of viral DNA and viral capsid protein (see example with SV40 virus in Fig 40–6). The formation of the T antigen is not inhibited by drugs which prevent DNA synthesis (cytosine arabinoside) or drugs which induce the formation of faulty DNA (idoxuridine). However, its induction is inhibited by drugs which prevent synthesis of DNA-

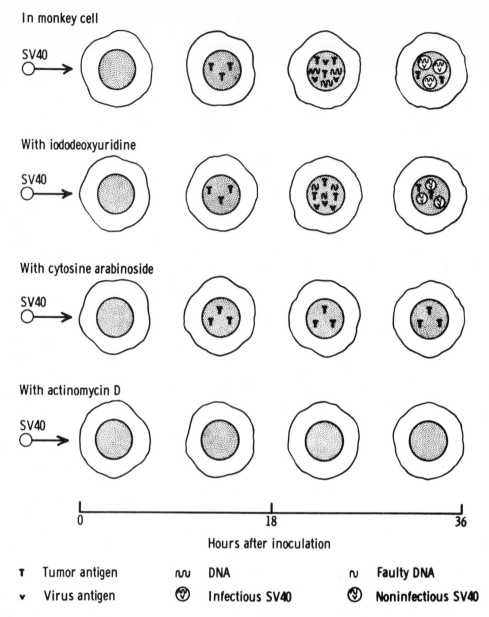

In monkey cell

SV40 →

With iododeoxyuridine

SV40 →

With cytosine arabinoside

SV40 →

With actinomycin D

SV40 →

| 0 | 18 | 36 |

Hours after inoculation

| т | Tumor antigen | ∿∿ | DNA | ∿ | Faulty DNA |
| ᴠ | Virus antigen | Ⓥ | Infectious SV40 | Ⓥ | Noninfectious SV40 |

FIG 40–6. **Evolution of SV40 virus under various conditions.** Injected into a monkey cell, SV40 virus replicates in about 30 hours, producing tumor antigen and viral DNA at earlier stages. The use of various inhibitors indicates the timing and sequence of events. For example, the synthesis of tumor antigen does not require viral DNA whose production is blocked by cytosine arabinoside. (From: *The Footprints of Tumor Viruses,* by Fred Rapp & Joseph L. Melnick. Copyright [©] 1966 by Scientific American, Inc. All rights reserved.)

dependent RNA (dactinomycin) or protein synthesis (cycloheximide) or by interferon treatment of the cells prior to infection.

T antigen is synthesized also during abortive virus infection in certain resistant cells such as hamster cells for polyoma virus, mouse cells for SV40 virus, and monkey kidney cells for the adenoviruses. Virus infection of these cells results in the production of T antigen but not of infectious virus or viral capsid antigen.

The biologic function of the virus-induced T antigens remains unknown. Although their appearance during cytocidal or abortive virus infection parallels the appearance of early enzymes (thymidine kinase, DNA polymerase, and others) required for DNA synthesis, there is no indication that T antigen is one of these enzymes.

Recently several mutants of defective SV40 virus have been isolated which induce the synthesis of T antigen in the cytoplasm rather than the nucleus of the cell. These mutants may prove to be useful in elucidating the biologic function of the T antigen.

Incorporation of SV40 Into Adenoviruses

In resistant cells derived from monkey kidney, virtually all adenoviruses are "defective"; they induce the production of T but not of V antigen. If SV40 virus is added to the system, infectious adenovirus is formed abundantly. SV40 virus probably induces enzymes essential for the replication of adenovirus in the resistant cells.

The emergence of a stable SV40-adenovirus "hybrid" in a population of adenovirus type 7 that had been grown in the presence of papovavirus SV40 has been recently established. This "hybrid" is capable of multiplying in monkey kidney cells and inducing the synthesis of the SV40 T antigen as well as the adenovirus T antigen; it does not induce the SV40 V antigen in any of the cell systems tested, but it readily induces the adeno-7 V antigen.

In newborn hamsters the "hybrid" produces tumors containing not only the adenovirus T antigen but also the SV40 T antigen. Furthermore, vaccination of adult hamsters with SV40-adenovirus "hybrid" (but not with adenovirus alone) confers protection against cells transformed by SV40 virus alone; this indicates that the SV40 determinant in the "hybrid" is not only responsible for the induction of the intranuclear T antigen but also for the induction of the transplantation antigen.

All these properties of the "hybrid" can be neutralized only with adenovirus type-specific serum but not with hamster serum prepared against the SV40 T antigen or monkey serum prepared against the SV40 viral capsid antigen. Thus the "hybrid" has the coat protein of only the adenovirus.

This "hybrid" population was found to be comprised of 2 types of particles, one being the adenovirus type 7 and the other containing SV40 genetic material encased in an adenovirus type 7 protein coat. The adenovirus particle can readily multiply in human kidney cells but not in monkey kidney cells. The second particle has been named PARA (particle aiding the replication of adenovirus). PARA has properties normally associated with SV40: It induces the synthesis of SV40 tumor and transplantation antigens (the adenovirion does not), and it aids the replication of adenovirus in monkey kidney cell cultures (Fig 40-7).

When the PARA-adenovirus type 7 population is inoculated at a limiting dilution into human kidney cell cultures, only the adenovirus particle replicates and forms plaques; PARA does not. Therefore, the progeny derived from such plaques are free of the SV40 genome and behave in every way as nonhybridized adenovirions. They no longer can induce the production of SV40 T antigens.

Recent investigation has shown that the PARA particle (similar to the "high titer" Bryan strain of Rous sarcoma virus) is defective. By itself PARA cannot replicate in monkey kidney cells; it requires a helper adenovirus which provides the protein coat. It has also been found that the adenovirus type 7 coat of the PARA particle in the PARA-adenovirus type 7 population can be exchanged for the specific protein coat of unrelated adenovirus types (such as types 1, 2, 3, 5, 6, 12, 16, etc), by a process termed transcapsidation (Fig 40-7).

Like the original PARA-adenovirus type 7 population, all PARA-adenovirus serotypes induce the SV40 T antigen and the SV40 transplantation antigen. The transfer of the SV40 determinant of the PARA particle into the protein coats of nononcogenic adenoviruses has resulted in the acquisition of oncogenic properties by these viruses. Thus PARA-adenovirus types 1, 2, 5, and 6 readily induce tumors in newborn hamsters, whereas the parental serotypes do not.

Transcapsidation of PARA bears a great similarity to the acquisition of coat proteins of different helper RAV viruses by the defective genome of the Bryan "high titer" RSV. The exact mechanism of the phenomena is not known, but it seems unlikely that the same pathways will be at work in both the DNA and RNA tumor virus systems even though RSV may require DNA synthesis for its replication.

VIRUSES & HUMAN CANCER

The recent progress in understanding viral carcinogenesis in animals has offered new avenues in the quest for the viral etiology of at least some human cancers. Based on the new knowledge of animal tumor-virus model systems, several approaches are being extensively explored.

Leukemia

Avian and murine leukemias induced by RNA viruses have served as one model for the study of leukemia in man. The advantages of working with this model are manifold: (1) Infectious virus of distinct structure can be readily identified in vivo throughout the life span of the diseased animal, either circulating in the blood or in the malignant cells themselves. (2) The malignant cells can be propagated in vitro, and the resulting cultures continue to produce infectious virus. (3) Virus can also be detected throughout the life span of cultures that have undergone malignant transformation in vitro. (4) Virus can also be detected by its ability to interfere with the multiplication of related viruses in susceptible cells.

Studies on human leukemia have revealed findings similar to those observed in virus-induced leukemias of animals. Electron microscopic examination revealed particles similar to the avian and murine leukemia RNA viruses in the cells or plasma of leukemia patients. Their significance is still undetermined, for it has not been demonstrated as yet that these particles possess biologic activity similar to the virus particles found in animal leukemias.

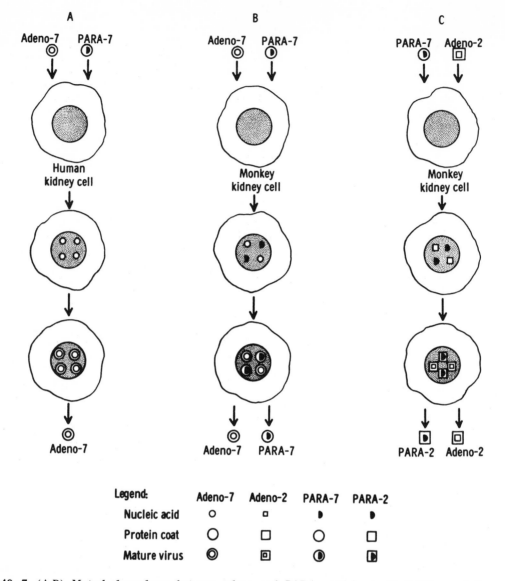

FIG 40–7. (A,B) **Mutual dependence between adeno and PARA particles in "hybrid" populations.** The synthesis of SV40 tumor antigen by a "hybrid" requires the multiplication of both adeno and PARA particles. In human kidney cells (left), only the adeno particle multiplies; in monkey kidney cells (center), both adeno and PARA particles multiply and the SV40 tumor antigen is formed. **(C) Transcapsidation.** PARA-7 particles (from an SV40-adenovirus type 7 "hybrid") grown in monkey kidney cells in the presence of adenovirus type 2 acquire the protein coat of the helper adenovirus. This results in an SV40 adenovirus type 2 "hybrid" population containing both pure adeno-2 and PARA-2 particles.

Another similarity between human leukemia and the virus-induced leukemias of animals has been demonstrated by tissue culture studies. Numerous cell lines have been derived from bone marrow aspirates or peripheral blood leukocytes of patients with lymphocytic or myelogenous leukemias. As with cells derived from animals suffering from RNA virus-induced leukemias, the human cell cultures can be propagated in vitro indefinitely. However, whether the human cultures are indeed comprised of potentially virus-induced malignant cells remains undetermined.

Many attempts have been made to demonstrate a cytopathic, interfering, or cell-transforming agent in human leukemia cells, but all have been unsuccessful. Thus, in contrast to the virus-induced animal leukemias, in which infectious virus can be demonstrated with relative ease, work on human leukemia has been suggestive of viral etiology but actual isolation of an active biologic agent etiologically related to the disease has not been possible. Some of the reasons for this failure may be as follows: (1) There is the obvious drawback of the lack of a susceptible host for in vivo experiments. The current trials with newborn laboratory primates may yield results in the years to come. (2) The concentration of infectious virus in the naturally occurring disease of man may be very low. (3) The tissue culture systems used to demonstrate the transforming capacity of materials derived from the patient or from cell lines grown in culture may not be sensitive enough. As shown with AMV, only specific target cells may undergo transformation. (4) If human leukemia is indeed caused by a virus, the responsible virus may be incomplete, as demonstrated for some of the avian and murine sarcoma virus strains. Thus, many avenues remain open for the elucidation of a viral agent in human leukemias, utilizing the model offered by the RNA tumor viruses of animals.

Recent electron microscopic studies reveal yet another type of virus-like particle, ie, particles indistinguishable from papovaviruses, in autopsy material from patients suffering from progressive multifocal leukoencephalopathy (a disease superimposed on chronic lymphatic leukemia or other diseases of the reticuloendothelial system). The interpretation of these observations also awaits further tests to determine whether specific biologic activity accompanies the morphologic findings of virus-like particles.

Solid Tumors

In view of the finding that, with few exceptions, solid tumors induced in experimental animals by papovaviruses and adenoviruses are free of infectious virus or of infectious nucleic acid, it is not surprising that innumerable attempts to isolate viruses from a variety of solid human tumors have met with complete failure.

Following the findings on the presence of virus-specific messenger RNA (mRNA) in DNA virus-induced (but virus-free) tumors, a search in human tumor tissues for mRNA hybridizable with the DNA of the known oncogenic virus is being attempted. Special attention is being given to the adenoviruses since they are oncogenic in experimental animals and are so widespread in man. However, the results to date have failed to give indication that any of the human tumors examined contain adenovirus-specific mRNA. Further study with these and other human viruses, especially the herpesviruses known to exist in a latent state in man, may yield more definitive information. Cell fusion is also being investigated in an attempt to demonstrate a defective virus in cancer cells by fusing them with normal susceptible cells in which the virus can replicate.

The new knowledge of virus-induced T antigens in tumors (or in transformed cells) and of T antibodies in the tumor-bearing animals has led to similar immunologic studies in cancer of man. Attempts made to test the sera of cancer patients for the presence of complement fixing or immunofluorescence antibodies to the T antigens of SV40 or adenovirus have thus far yielded negative results.

Recent studies have revealed that patients with melanomas, osteosarcomas or liposarcomas develop antibodies that react by immunofluorescence with a cytoplasmic antigen present in imprints of autochthonous and homologous tumors. The antibody has been found to react by immunofluorescence and complement fixation (employing human complement) with antigens derived from cells of such tumors propagated in tissue culture. Similar reactivity has been found in sera of the patients' family contacts with a much greater frequency than in sera of the population at large. The latter finding suggests that the antibody reactions attained may be directed to a viral antigen present in the tumor cells rather than a T-type antigen. Preliminary evidence suggests the presence of leukemia virus (C type) particles in liposarcoma cultures and a capacity of supernatant fluids from such cultures to transform normal human embryo fibroblasts. However, the significance of these findings awaits further study.

The knowledge that transplantation type antigens in virus-induced tumors can be detected by an in vitro colony inhibition test has been recently applied to the elucidation of similar antigens in some human tumors. Lymphocytes from children bearing neuroblastomas have been found to inhibit the plating efficiency of their tumor cells grown in culture. Lymphocytes of their mothers but not from unrelated controls had the same inhibitory effect. The reaction observed is reminiscent of that mentioned above for the virus-induced animal tumor systems. However, evidence is still lacking that the antigens being measured in the neuroblastoma cells are indeed virus-induced.

Herpesviruses & Human Malignancies

In recent years a great deal of attention has been focused on herpesviruses of man as potential oncogenic agents. The recently isolated and characterized herpes simplex virus type 2 has been found to be venereally transmitted in man (see Chapter 38 for details). Following seroepidemiologic studies revealed a high degree of association between infection with this virus and invasive carcinoma of the cervix in the USA. The prevalence of herpes type 2 antibody in women with the disease was found to be much higher than that of matched controls. Preliminary evidence suggests that women with cervical dysplasia and carcinoma in situ (considered by some to be premalignant lesions leading to invasive carcinoma) have also an increased prevalence of herpes type 2 antibody. Careful serologic follow-up of such patients as well as extensive seroepidemiologic surveys of different populations may shed further light as to whether the association found is co-variable or etiologic.

A high degree of association has been recently observed between the EB (Epstein-Barr) virus, a new member of the herpesvirus group (see Chapter 38 for details), and 2 human malignancies: Burkitt's lymphoma, a tumor with a predilection for the jaw and peculiar for children in Central Africa; and postnasal (nasopharyngeal) carcinoma, found in Chinese male populations in Southeast Asia with an incidence greater than in other populations. The virus was detected initially by electron microscopy and subsequently by immunofluorescence in cultured Burkitt's lymphoma cells (but not in the original tumor) that maintain their lymphoid character upon continuous in vitro propagation. The finding of a high incidence and high titers of EB antibody (detectable by immunofluorescence, complement fixation, and gel diffusion tests) in patients with Burkitt's lymphoma and postnasal carcinoma led to the assumption that the association may be etiologic. However, subsequent seroepidemiologic surveys showed that infection with EB virus in normal populations is widespread not only in Africa and Asia but all over the world. Furthermore, it was demonstrated that EB virus has an extreme predilection for cells of lymphoid origin. The virus has been detected with great regularity in cell lines derived not only from Burkitt's lymphoma and postnasal carcinoma but also those derived from peripheral blood leukocytes of patients with infectious mononucleosis and various other disease entities as well as from normal individuals. A much stronger case has been made for the etiologic association between EB virus infection and infectious mononucleosis, a benign immunoproliferative disorder (see Chapter 38), for such patients reveal a seroconversion to EB virus. Thus, the question as to whether EB virus is etiologically related to the above 2 malignancies or represents a passenger virus present in lymphoid cells trapped within the tumor, remains at present unanswered. Indeed, other viruses, such as herpes simplex virus and reovirus, have been frequently isolated from Burkitt's lymphomas. On the other hand, one cannot exclude the possibility that EB virus is indeed the prime agent responsible for the induction of malignant cells in vivo. Recent in vitro experiments reveal that the virus can convert virus-free normal peripheral blood leukocytes or fetal bone marrow cells into virus-positive cells capable of continuous growth. The lack of a susceptible animal host precludes at present the assertion that these cells are malignant.

Evidence is accumulating on the association between herpesviruses of lower animals and malignant disease. A latent herpesvirus has been found in neurolymphoma (Marek's disease) of chickens and in a frog (Lucké) adenocarcinoma of the kidney. In addition, a rabbit herpesvirus appears to be capable of inducing a lymphoma (Hinze) when inoculated into weanling cottontail (but not domestic) rabbits and a latent herpesvirus of the squirrel monkey has been found to induce lymphoma (Melendez) in owl monkeys and marmosets. Further work with these model systems may indeed open avenues for the understanding of the elusive relationship between herpesviruses and malignancy in man.

The technics for searching for viruses in human cancer have become more sophisticated than those currently used in the virus diagnostic laboratory. However, investigators must still contend with the problem of identifying "passenger" viruses present in the cancer but not in a causal relationship. Of even greater concern is the converse, the problem of identifying a virus no longer present in the cancer that it may have caused. Some of the modern approaches that have proved fruitful in the study of animals suffering from virus cancers have been outlined in this chapter.

●   ●   ●

General References

Black, P.H.: The oncogenic DNA viruses: A review of in vitro transformation studies. Ann Rev Microbiol 22:391–426, 1968.

Dulbecco, R.: Cell transformation by viruses. Science 166:962–968, 1969.

Habel, K.: Antigens of virus-induced tumors. Advances Immunol 10:229–250, 1969.

Haughton, G., & D.R. Nash: Transplantation antigens and viral carcinogenesis. Progr Med Virol 11:248–306, 1969.

Hellström, K.E., & I. Hellström: Cellular immunity against tumor antigens. Advances Cancer Res 12:167–223, 1969.

Huebner, R.J.: The murine leukemia-sarcoma virus complex. Proc Nat Acad Sc 58:835–842, 1967.

Ito, Y. (editor): Subviral Carcinogenesis. First International Symposium on Tumor Viruses. Sponsored by the Research Institute, Aichi Cancer Center, and the Japanese Cancer Association, 1967. NISSHA Printing Company (Mibu, Nakagyo-ku, Kyoto, Japan), 1967.

Rapp, F., & J.L. Melnick: Papovavirus SV40, adenovirus and their hybrids: transformation, complementation, and transcapsidation. Progr Med Virol 8:394–399, 1967.

Vigier, P.: RNA oncogenic viruses: Structure, replication and oncogenicity. Progr Med Virol 12:240–283, 1970.

Appendix:

*Medical Parasitology**

Although all of the medically significant micro-organisms considered in this *Review* are, of course, parasitic in their human hosts, the biomedical discipline of **parasitology** has traditionally been concerned only with the parasitic protozoa, helminths, and arthropods. This chapter offers no more than a brief survey of the protozoan and helminthic parasites of medical importance, with particular attention to those forms whose identification depends upon microscopic study. The chapter is designed as a first point of reference; the text is supplemented by tabular materials and by several pages of illustrations. The following texts are recommended for detailed reference.

Medical Parasitology

Belding, D.L.: *Textbook of Parasitology*, 3rd ed. Appleton-Century-Crofts, 1965.

Brown, H.W., & D.L. Belding: *Basic Clinical Parasitology*, 2nd ed. Appleton-Century-Crofts, 1964.

Chandler, A.C., & C.P. Read: *Introduction to Parasitology*, 10th ed. Wiley, 1961.

Dogiel, V.A.: *General Parasitology*. Oliver & Boyd, 1964.

Faust, E.C., Beaver, P.C., & R.C. Jung: *Animal Agents and Vectors of Human Disease,* 2nd ed. Lea & Febiger, 1962.

Faust, E.C., & P.F. Russell: *Clinical Parasitology*, 7th ed. Lea & Febiger, 1964.

Russell, P.F., & others: *Practical Malariology,* 2nd ed. Oxford, 1963.

Clinical Aspects

Adams, A.R.D., & B.G. Maegraith: *Clinical Tropical Diseases,* 3rd ed. Blackwell, 1964.

Audy, J.R., Dunn, F.L., & R.S. Goldsmith: Infectious diseases: Protozoal, Chap 24, pp 719–731, in: *Current Diagnosis & Treatment.* Brainerd, H., Krupp, M., Chatton, M.J., & S. Margen (editors). Lange, 1970.

Cahill, K.M.: *Tropical Diseases in Temperate Climates.* Lippincott, 1964.

Dunn, F.L., Audy, J.R., & R.S. Goldsmith: Infectious diseases: Metazoal, Chap 25, pp 732–751, in: *Current Diagnosis & Treatment.* Brainerd, H., Krupp, M., Chatton, M.J., & S. Margen (editors). Lange, 1970.

Hunter, G.W., III, Frye, W.W., & J.C. Swartzwelder: *A Manual of Tropical Medicine,* 4th ed. Saunders, 1966.

Maegraith, B.: *Exotic Diseases in Practice: The Clinical and Public Health Significance of the Changing Geographical Patterns of Diseases with Particular Reference to the Importation of Exotic Infections into Europe and North America.* Elsevier, 1965.

Manson-Bahr, P.: *Manson's Tropical Diseases,* 15th ed. Williams & Wilkins, 1960.

Medical Entomology

Gordon, R.M., & M.M.J. Lavoipierre: *Entomology for Students of Medicine.* Blackwell, 1962.

CLASSIFICATION

The parasites of man in the phylum Protozoa may be classified in 4 groups designated, by various authors, as subdivisions and classes (see Chapter 1), classes, or subphyla:

(1) Mastigophora or flagellates, with one or more whip-like flagella and, in some cases, an undulating membrane (eg, trypanosomes). These include intestinal and genitourinary flagellates (giardia, trichomonas, embadomonas, enteromonas, chilomastix) and blood and tissue flagellates (leishmania, trypanosoma).

(2) Sarcodina, typically ameboid, are represented in man by species of Entamoeba, Endolimax, Iodamoeba, and Dientamoeba.

(3) Sporozoa, which undergo a definite life cycle, often involving 2 different hosts (eg, arthropod and vertebrate). Hemogregarines, piroplasms (eg, tick-borne babesia, which causes serious infections of livestock and pets), and microsporidia (eg, nosema, which infect bees) are not dealt with here. The coccidia, a subclass of essentially intestinal sporozoa (family Eimeridae), and the hemosporidians, including the malaria parasites (plasmodium, family Plasmodidae) are represented in man. Sarcocystis, infecting animals and sometimes man, and toxoplasma, a common human parasite, are distinct simple forms of uncertain relationships; they are probably not sporozoa, but are conveniently placed in the artificial class Acnidosporidia.

*By J. Ralph Audy, MB, BS (Lond.), PhD–Director, G.W. Hooper Foundation, Chairman, Department of International Health, and Professor of Tropical Medicine and Human Ecology, University of California School of Medicine (San Francisco); and Frederick L. Dunn, MD, DTM&H–Professor of Epidemiology and Medical Anthropology, G.W. Hooper Foundation and Department of International Health, University of California School of Medicine (San Francisco). The illustrations on pp 460–470 are by P.H. Vercammen-Grandjean, DSc.

(4) **Ciliophora** or **Ciliata**, internally complex protozoa bearing cilia characteristically distributed in rows or patches, with 2 kinds of nuclei in each individual. *Balantidium coli*, a mammalian intestinal ciliate, is the only representative of this group in man.

The parasitic worms, or helminths, of man belong to 2 phyla:

(1) **Platyhelminthes** (flatworms), which lack a body cavity and are characteristically flat in dorsoventral section. All medically important species belong to the classes **Cestoda** (tapeworms) and **Trematoda** (flukes). The tapeworms or cestodes are hermaphroditic, band-like, segmented, and have no digestive tract. The flukes or trematodes are typically leaf-shaped and hermaphroditic, but the schistosomes (Schistosoma species) are more elongated and have separate sexes. The important cestodes of man belong to the following genera: Diphyllobothrium, Taenia, Echinococcus, Hymenolepis, and Dipylidium. Medically important trematode genera, in addition to Schistosoma, include Paragonimus, Clonorchis, Opisthorchis, Fasciolopsis, Heterophyes, Metagonimus, and Fasciola.

(2) **Nemathelminthes** (roundworms), represented in man by many parasitic species in the class Nematoda. All are wormlike, unsegmented, round in body section, with a body cavity, well-developed digestive system, and separate sexes. Many families of roundworms have parasitic species which infect man.

These are tabulated in Table 4 together with the other parasitic helminths. An essential procedure in diagnosis of many helminthic infections is microscopic recognition of ova or larvas in feces, urine, blood, or tissues. Diagnostically important stages are illustrated on pp 465, 467, and 468; certain important characteristics of the microfilariae, or larval filariid worms, are also presented in tabular fashion (see Table 5).

GIARDIA LAMBLIA

Giardia lamblia is a flagellated protozoon of the duodenum and jejunum of man, the cause of flagellate diarrhea or giardiasis.

Morphology & Identification

A. Typical Organisms: The trophozoite of *G lamblia* is a pear-shaped, bilaterally symmetric organism, 10–18 μm in length. There are 4 pairs of flagella, 2 nuclei with prominent central karyosomes, 2 axostyles, and a single or double parabasal body. A large concave sucking disk occupies much of the ventral surface. The swaying or dancing motion of giardia trophozoites in fresh preparations is unmistakable. In an unfavorable environment the parasite encysts. These cysts, 10–14 μm in length, are ellipsoid, thick-walled, and contain 2–4 nuclei and various structures of the trophozoite.

B. Culture: This organism has not been cultivated on artificial media.

Pathogensis & Clinical Findings

Giardia lamblia is usually weakly pathogenic or nonpathogenic for man. Cysts may be found in large numbers in the stools of entirely asymptomatic persons. In some persons, however, large numbers of parasites attached to the bowel wall may cause irritation and low-grade inflammation of the duodenal or jejunal mucosa, with consequent acute or chronic diarrhea. The stools may be watery, semisolid, or bulky and foul-smelling at various times during the course of the infection. Malaise, weakness, weight loss, abdominal cramps, distention, and flatulence may occur. Some of these symptoms may be due to interference with fat absorption as well as to mechanical irritation of the bowel. The bile ducts and gallbladder may also be invaded, causing a mild catarrhal cholangitis and cholecystitis. Children are more liable to clinical giardiasis than adults.

Diagnostic Laboratory Tests

Diagnosis depends upon finding the distinctive cysts in formed stools, or cysts and trophozoites in liquid stools. Concentration methods may be necessary to detect asymptomatic infections, but the parasite is usually abundant in the stool when gastrointestinal symptoms are present. Examination of the duodenal contents may be necessary to establish the diagnosis when the symptoms relate only to the biliary system.

Treatment

Administration of quinacrine hydrochloride (Atabrine) will cure about 90% of *G lamblia* infections. Metronidazole (Flagyl) is an alternative. The course of treatment may be repeated if necessary. Only symptomatic patients require treatment.

Epidemiology

G lamblia is cosmopolitan and common, especially in young children. Man is infected by ingestion of fecally contaminated water or food containing giardia cysts.

TRICHOMONAS

The trichomonads are flagellate protozoa with 3–5 anterior flagella, an axostyle, and an undulating membrane. Of the 3 species infecting man only *Trichomonas vaginalis* is pathogenic, causing trichomoniasis.

Morphology & Identification

A. Typical Organisms: *Trichomonas vaginalis* is pear-shaped, with a short undulating membrane extending to mid-body, and 4 anterior flagella. It normally measures 15–20 μm in length, but may reach 30 μm. The organism moves with a characteristic wobbling and rotating motion. The nonpathogenic trichomonads, *T hominis* and *T tenax*, cannot readily be distinguished from *T vaginalis* when alive. When fixed and stained, *T tenax* measures 6–10 μm in length; in other respects it is identical with *T vaginalis*. *T hominis* measures 8–12 μm, and bears 5 anterior flagella and a long undulating membrane extending the full length of its body. The parabasal body is small or absent. For all practical purposes, trichomonads found in the mouth are *T tenax;* in the intestine, *T hominis;* and in the genitourinary tract (both sexes), *T vaginalis.*

B. Culture: *T vaginalis* may be cultivated in a variety of solid and fluid cell-free media, in tissue cultures, and in the chick embryo. *T tenax* and *T hominis* will grow particularly well in sheep serum in saline; media used for culturing the intestinal amebas are also satisfactory. *T vaginalis* requires more specialized media for optimal growth. CPLM (cysteine-peptone-liver-maltose) medium is one of the most satisfactory. Simplified trypticase serum is usually used for semen cultures.

C. Growth Requirements: *T vaginalis* grows well under anaerobic conditions, somewhat less well aerobically. The pH optimum is 5.5–6.0; the temperature optimum is 35–37° C. The following substances appear to be essential for optimal growth: cysteine, a fermentable carbohydrate, 20% animal serum, 0.1% agar, and a heat-labile factor destroyed by autoclaving.

Pathogenesis, Pathology, & Clinical Findings

T hominis and *T tenax* are generally considered to be harmless commensals. *T vaginalis* is capable of causing low-grade inflammation, particularly when the infection is heavy. The organisms have a toxic action on tissue culture cells, and will produce extensive lesions in germ-free animals. The intensity of infection, the pH of vaginal and other secretions, the physiologic status of the vaginal and other genitourinary tract surfaces, and the accompanying bacterial flora are among the factors affecting pathogenicity. The organisms cannot survive at normal vaginal acidity of pH 3.8–4.4; nor can they survive at the nearly neutral vaginal pH found in young girls and elderly women.

In the female the infection is normally limited to the vulva, vagina, and cervix; it does not usually extend to the uterus. The mucosal surfaces may be tender, inflamed, eroded, and covered with a frothy yellow or cream-colored discharge. In the male the prostate, seminal vesicles, and urethra may be infected. Signs and symptoms in the female, in adition to profuse vaginal discharge, include local tenderness, vulval pruritus, and burning. About 10% of infected males have a thin, white urethral discharge.

Diagnostic Laboratory Tests

A. Specimens and Microscopic Examination: Vaginal or urethral secretions or discharge should be examined microscopically in a drop of saline or Trichomonas Diluent for characteristic motile trichomonads. Dried smears may be stained with hematoxylin or one of the Romanowsky stains for later study.

B. Culture: Culture of vaginal or urethral discharge, of prostatic secretion, or of a semen specimen may reveal organisms when direct examination is negative.

Immunity

Infection confers no apparent immunity. Little is known about the immune responses to trichomonads.

Treatment

Successful treatment of vaginal infections requires the destruction of the trichomonads, the restoration of normal vaginal epithelium and acidity, and measures to ensure that reinfection will not occur. The patient's sexual partner should be examined, and treated simultaneously if necessary. Postmenopausal patients may require treatment with estrogens to improve the condition of the vaginal epithelium. For vaginal infections treatment with metronidazole (Flagyl), Floraquin (a mixture containing diiodohydroxyquinoline, dextrose, lactose, and boric acid), or furazolidone-nifuroxime (Tricofuron) is usually effective. Prostatic infection can be cured with certainty only by systemic treatment with metronidazole.

Epidemiology & Control

T vaginalis is a common cosmopolitan parasite of both males and females. Infection rates vary greatly but may be quite high in some populations, particularly where the quality of female hygiene is poor. Coitus is the common mode of transmission, but contaminated towels, douche equipment, examination instruments, and other objects may be responsible for some new infections. Infants may be infected at birth. Most infections, in both sexes, are asymptomatic or cause inconsequential symptoms. Control of *T vaginalis* infections requires detection and treatment of the infected male sexual partner at the same time that the infected female is treated; mechanical protection (condom) should be used during intercourse until the infection is eradicated in both partners.

T hominis is also cosmopolitan and common, particularly in the tropics. Transmission is by the fecal-oral route.

T tenax, apparently transmitted directly from mouth to mouth, is found throughout the world. The incidence in some populations reaches 10–20%.

OTHER INTESTINAL FLAGELLATES

Embadomonas intestinalis, Chilomastix mesnili, and *Enteromonas hominis* are nonpathogenic intestinal parasites of man which must be distinguished in the laboratory from the pathogenic amebas and flagellates.

Embadomonas Intestinalis

This cosmopolitan but rare parasite lives as a commensal in the human intestine. The trophozoite is small, ovoid, and 4–9 μm long, with a single nucleus, a cytostome, and 2 flagella, one anterior and one lying in the cytostomal cleft. The oval or pear-shaped cyst, 4–7 μm long, has a single nucleus, sometimes dumbbell-shaped, and fibrils which represent the margins of the cytostome. The organism can be cultivated in media suitable for the trichomonads. Laboratory diagnosis depends upon detection of the cysts or trophozoites in stool specimens. Transmission presumably takes place by ingestion of the cysts.

Enteromonas Hominis

Human infections with this very small intestinal flagellate have been reported in many parts of the world. Although it is generally rare, high infection rates have been recorded in some populations. The oval trophozoite is 4–10 μm long, uninucleate, and bears 4 flagella (3 anterior, one posterior). There is no cytostome. The cyst is oval, 6–8 μm long, with 1–4 nuclei. When quadrinucleate, the nuclei are arranged in pairs at the poles. Cultivation is easy on ordinary flagellate media. Laboratory diagnosis and transmission are as for *Embadomonas intestinalis.*

Chilomastix Mesnili

This parasite, which can be confused with trichomonas in the laboratory, is more common than *Embadomonas intestinalis* and *Enteromonas hominis.* It is found throughout the world. Some workers consider it to be mildly pathogenic but there is little evidence to support this. The trophozoite is pear-shaped, 6–24 μm long, with 3 anterior flagella, a large cytostome bearing a fourth flagellum, and a large single nucleus. The spiral motion of the trophozoite is unlike that of trichomonas. The distinctive cyst is lemon-shaped, uninucleate, 7–9 μm long, with conspicuous fibrils representing the margins of the cytostome. Cultivation, laboratory diagnosis, and transmission are as for the 2 flagellates discussed above.

THE HEMOFLAGELLATES

The hemoflagellates of man include the genera Trypanosoma and Leishmania. There are 2 distinct groups of Trypanosoma: (1) African, causing sleeping sickness and transmitted by tsetse flies (Glossina): and (2) American, causing Chagas' disease and transmitted by cone-nosed bugs (Triatoma, etc). (Another species, *T rangeli* of South America, infects man without causing disease.) There are 3 species of Leishmania, causing cutaneous or mucocutaneous lesions or systemic disease (oriental sore, espundia, kala-azar). All are transmitted by sandflies (Phlebotomus). Most of the hemoflagellates have animal reservoirs and all have insect vectors.

Forms of Trypanosoma appearing in the blood are always fully developed trypanosomes with elongated bodies supporting a lateral undulating membrane and a flagellum which lies in the free edge of the membrane and emerges at the anterior end as a whip-like

process. The kinetoplast, present in all forms, is a darkly-staining body lying immediately adjacent to the tiny node (blepharoplast) from which the flagellum arises with or without its accompanying membrane. The forms in the mammalian tissues show one or more of the stages of the life cycle detectable in the insect vectors, ie, (1) a leishmanial rounded cell (see below and p 462); (2) flagellated leptomonad, lanceolate, without a membrane, with a kinetoplast at the anterior end; (3) a crithidium, more elongated, with a short undulating membrane and a kinetoplast placed more posteriorly but still anterior to the nucleus; and (4) a trypanosome with a posterior kinetoplast and a full membrane. In leishmania the life-cycle includes only the first 2 stages.

1. LEISHMANIA

The genus Leishmania, widely distributed in nature, comprises 3 morphologically indistinguishable species: *Leishmania donovani* (causing visceral leishmaniasis); *L tropica* (cutaneous leishmaniasis); and *L braziliensis* (mucocutaneous leishmaniasis). All are transmitted by sandflies (Phlebotomus) from animal and human reservoirs.

Morphology & Identification

A. Typical Organism: The Leishmania are indistinguishable from the 2 earliest stages of trypanosomes (see p 463). Only the first stage, the nonflagellated ovoid Leishman-Donovan (LD) bodies (see p 462) occur in the mammalian host; both stages occur in the gut of the sandfly, which transmits the infective flagellated leptomonads by bite. The leishmanial bodies are oval, 2–6 × 1–3 μm, with a laterally placed oval vesicular nucleus and a distinct dark-staining kinetoplast, usually rod-like. They are often packed into aggregates within cells, following multiplication.

B. Culture and Growth Characteristics: In NNN medium the flagellated leptomonad forms predominate. *L donovani* grows slowly, the leptomonads forming tangled clumps in the fluid. *L tropica* grows quickly, leptomonads forming small rosettes in the fluid and giving it a fine granular appearance with a distinct surface film. *L braziliensis* produces a distinct wax-like surface. In tissue cultures, leishmanial forms may be obtained in addition to leptomonads.

C. Variations: Strain differences in virulence, tissue tropism or predilection, biologic and pharmacodynamic characteristics, and adaptability to different vectors have been observed with all 3 species. There is consequent overlap in pathology and clinical pictures.

Pathogenesis, Pathology, & Clinical Findings

L donovani, the causative organism of kala-azar, spreads from the site of inoculation to multiply in reticulo-endothelial and parenchymal cells, especially in the spleen, liver, lymph nodes, and bone marrow.

This is accompanied by vascularity and marked hyperplasia, especially of the spleen. Progressive emaciation is usually accompanied by remarkably little prostration in spite of growing weakness. There is irregular fever, sometimes remittent.

L tropica causes dermal lesions at the site of inoculation by the sandfly: cutaneous leishmaniasis, oriental sore, Delhi boil, etc. Mucous membranes are rarely involved. The dermal layers are first affected, with cellular infiltration and proliferation of leishmania both intracellularly and extracellularly, until the organisms penetrate into the epidermis and cause ulceration. Satellite lesions may be found. These are tuberculoid, with few or no parasites, and are regarded as allergic leishmanids.

L braziliensis causes mucocutaneous or nasopharyngeal (naso-oral) leishmaniasis, which is known by many local names (including espundia). The pathologic findings are the same as those of *L tropica* infections, but the initial lesions are more superficial and tend to metastasize (or spread by direct extension) to mucous surfaces, where they may form polypoid growths and fungating destructive lesions. This is the characteristic clinical picture of espundia. At high altitudes the clinical features tend to resemble oriental sore, although mucous involvement is more frequent. In Mexico the ears are frequently involved, usually with an indolent infection without ulceration and few parasites.

Diagnostic Laboratory Tests

A. Specimens: Lymph node aspirates, scrapings, and biopsies are important in the cutaneous forms; lymph node aspirates, blood, and spleen or liver puncture are important in kala-azar. Purulent discharges are of no value for diagnosis.

B. Microscopic Examination: Giemsa-stained smears and sections may show LD bodies, especially in material from kala-azar and the edges of oriental sores.

C. Culture: NNN medium is the medium of choice. Blood culture is satisfactory only for *L donovani;* lymph node aspirates are suitable for all forms; and tissue aspirates, biopsy material, scrapings, or small biopsies from the edges of ulcers are useful for the cutaneous forms (and often for kala-azar also). A blood-agar culture medium is also popular. Only leptomonads can be cultivated in the absence of living cells.

D. Serology: The valuable formol-gel (aldehyde) test of Napier depends on an elevated serum globulin in kala-azar: 1 drop of commercial formalin in 1 ml of serum forms an opalescent gel.

Specific and nonspecific complement fixation tests are valuable for all forms of leishmaniasis.

Immunity

Recovery confers a solid and permanent immunity. Natural resistance varies greatly among individuals, between different ages and sexes, and among various species of mammals. Vaccination significantly reduces the incidence of oriental sore, especially the more florid "wet" type.

Treatment

Single lesions may be cleaned, curetted, treated with antibiotics if secondarily infected, and then covered and left to heal. Antimony sodium gluconate, pentavalent (Pentostam, Solustibostan), is the drug of choice for all forms.

Epidemiology, Prevention, & Control

Kala-azar is found focally in all tropical and subtropical countries except Australia. Its focal distribution is related to the prevalence of sandfly vectors, and in middle Asia and South America, domestic and wild canine reservoirs. Control is aimed at destroying breeding places and dogs and protecting people from bites. Oriental sore is essentially Asiatic, also occurring in the Mediterranean region and North Africa. The "wet" type is rural, and burrowing rodents are the main reservoir; the dry type is urban, and man is presumably the only reservoir. For *L braziliensis* there are a number of wild but apparently no domestic animal reservoirs. Sandfly vectors are involved in all forms.

2. TRYPANOSOMA

Hemoflagellates of the genus Trypanosoma occur in the blood of mammals as mature elongated trypanosomes with lateral undulating membranes. The earlier developmental stages of the life cycle sometimes take place in mammalian tissues but always occur in the alternative host, an insect vector. Trypanosomes cause trypanosomiasis (sleeping sickness, Chagas' disease, and asymptomatic trypanosomiasis) in man. The parent form in Africa is *T brucei* (causing nagana in livestock and game animals, with antelopes as a natural reservoir), and the 2 human forms are regarded by some as subspecies of *T brucei* because all 3 are indistinguishable morphologically.

Morphology & Identification

A. Typical Organisms: The African *T gambiense* and *T rhodesiense* are identical, both varying in the size and shape of the body and the length of the flagellum (12–42 μm, usually 15–30 μm). Slender forms 25–30 μm long usually predominate over stumpy forms with short flagella. The same forms are seen in blood as in lymph node aspirates. Somewhat stumpy forms with posterior (as opposed to central) nuclei occur rather more frequently in *T rhodesiense* than in *T gambiense*. The blood forms of the American *T cruzi* are present during the acute stage, and at intervals thereafter in smaller numbers. They are typical trypanosomes, varying about a mean of 20 μm, frequently curved in a C-shape when fixed and stained. The tissue forms most common in heart muscle, liver, and brain, however, develop from agglomerations of leishmanial forms which have multiplied to crithidia which in turn, after being transformed into trypanosomes, again enter the blood. *T rangeli* of South America infects man without causing disease and must therefore be carefully distinguished from the pathogenic species.

B. Culture: *T cruzi* and *T rangeli* are readily cultivated (3–6 weeks) in fluid or diphasic media. The various developing forms may also be recognized in clean triatomids (reduviids) which have fed on patients (xenodiagnosis), in which case the 2 species can be distinguished by the fact that *T cruzi* is confined to the hind-gut whereas *T rangeli* is usually present in the salivary glands also.

C. Growth Requirements: *T cruzi* requires at least hemin, ascorbic acid, and certain unidentified but dialyzable substances present in serum. The African forms require at least these for development, but neither these nor other known substances suffice to support development to the infective trypanosomal stage. The blood of some apparently uninfected persons inhibits growth of the African species.

D. Variation: The African blood forms are polymorphic, as noted above. The blood trypanosomes of *T cruzi* are monotypic, but the tissue forms practically repeat the developmental stages seen in the reduviid vector. Variations in virulence are well recognized: *T rhodesiense* is usually regarded as a virulent form of *T gambiense,* either fixed or periodically mutating. *T gambiense,* in contrast to *T rhodesiense,* is of low virulence to laboratory animals, but by passage can be made to rival the latter in virulence. Strains of *T cruzi* of low virulence to laboratory animals and apparently also to man are recorded mostly from the southern USA.

Pathogenesis, Pathology, & Clinical Findings

Infective trypanosomes of *T gambiense* and *T rhodesiense* are introduced through the bite of the tsetse fly and multiply at the site of inoculation to cause variable induration and swelling (the primary lesion), which may progress to form a trypanosomal chancre. Infective forms of *T cruzi* pass to humans by inoculation of infected bug feces into the conjunctiva or a break in the skin; at the site of inoculation they progress from the leishmanial to the leptomonad to the crithidial stage, multiply to cause variable induration and swelling, and may form a chagoma. Chagas' disease is common in infants, who show such dramatic acute responses that it is sometimes described as if it were a purely pediatric disorder. Particularly in children, unilateral swelling of the eyelids (Romaña's sign) is frequent and characteristic at onset. The primary lesion is accompanied by fever, acute regional lymphadenitis, and dissemination to blood and tissues. The parasites can usually be detected within 1–2 weeks as trypanosomes in the blood. Subsequent developments depend upon the organs and tissues most affected and on the nature of multiplication and release of toxins. The African forms multiply extracellularly as trypanosomes in the blood as well as in the tissues; but *T cruzi* multiplies mostly within reticuloendothelial cells, going through a cycle starting with large agglomerations of

leishmanial bodies. In all forms, multiplication in the tissues is punctuated by phases of parasitemia with later destruction of the blood forms, accompanied by characteristic bouts of intermittent fever gradually decreasing in intensity. Parasitemia is more commonly found in *T rhodesiense;* is intermittent and scant with *T cruzi.*

The release of toxins explains much of the systemic as well as local or tissue reactions (eg, blood vessels and lymph sinuses in African forms; around infected reticuloendothelial and other cells in the American form). The organs most seriously affected are the CNS and heart muscle. Interstitial myocarditis is marked in Chagas' disease and is the most common serious element in the clinical picture. It is least evident in the chronic gambian infection. The opposite is the case with CNS involvement, except that untreated rhodesian infection often leads to death before brain damage occurs. *T rhodesiense,* a virulent organism, appears in the CSF in about 1 month and *T gambiense* in several months, but both are present in small numbers. *T gambiense* infection is chronic and leads to progressive diffuse meningoencephalitis ("sleeping sickness"). The more rapidly fatal *T rhodesiense* produces the same condition of somnolence and coma during the final weeks of a terminal infection. Other organs affected are the liver and spleen, especially with chronic *T cruzi* infection, which produces a vigorous reticuloendothelial system response often simulating kala-azar (splenomegaly, hepatomegaly, bone marrow hyperplasia and engorgement).

Invasion of nerve plexuses in the alimentary tract walls leads to megaesophagus and megacolon. All 3 trypanosomes are transmissible through the placenta, and congenital infections are reported in hyperendemic areas.

Diagnostic Laboratory Tests

A. Specimens: Blood (thick and thin films, for culture, and for serology), preferably collected when the temperature rises; CSF, lymph node aspirate, and sometimes marrow primary lesion aspirates or splenic puncture are valuable for diagnostic tests. Uninfected triatomid bugs are required if xenodiagnosis of *T cruzi* is intended.

B. Microscopic Examination: Fresh blood (or aspirated tissue in saline) is kept warm and examined immediately for the actively motile trypanosomes. Thick films may be stained by Field's rapid method or with Giemsa's stain. Thin films stained with Giemsa's stain are necessary for confirmation. Centrifugation may be necessary. Tissue smears must be stained for identification of the pretrypanosomal stages. Centrifuged CSF should be similarly examined; there is seldom more than one trypanosome per ml. The most reliable tests are blood examinations for *T rhodesiense;* gland puncture for *T gambiense;* and CSF examination for *T rhodesiense* and advanced *T gambiense.*

C. Culture: Any or all of the specimens required for microscopic examination may be inoculated into media such as Tobie's, Wenyon's semisolid, NNN, or

Senekji's medium for attempted culture of *T cruzi* or *T rangeli*. The organisms are grown at 22–24° C and subcultured every 1–2 weeks, centrifuged material being examined microscopically for trypanosomes. However, trypanosomes are usually very scanty in the blood in Chagas' disease except perhaps in the acute phase. Culture of the African forms is unsatisfactory.

D. **Animal Inoculation:** *T cruzi* and *T rangeli* may be detected by inoculating blood intraperitoneally into a number of mice (when available, pups and kittens are animals of first choice). *T rhodesiense* is often detectable (and *T gambiense* with some effort) by this procedure in mice. Trypanosomes appear in the blood in a few days after successful inoculation.

E. **Serology:** A positive complement fixation (Machado's) test may give confirmatory support in *T cruzi* infection. African forms cause serologic reactions, but these are of limited diagnostic value.

F. **Xenodiagnosis:** This is the method of choice in suspected Chagas' disease if other examinations are negative. About 6 clean laboratory-reared triatomid bugs are fed on the patient, and their droppings examined in 7–10 days for the various developmental forms. Defecation follows shortly after a fresh meal, or it may be forced by gently probing the anus and then squeezing the bug's abdomen—taking care that the anus is in contact with a drop of saline or serum to prevent accidental self-infection by a sudden spray from the anus. Xenodiagnosis is impracticable for the African forms.

G. **Differential Diagnosis:** *T rhodesiense* and *T gambiense* are morphologically identical but may be distinguished by their behavior in man (since they cause different clinical pictures and are differentially distributed in tissues and blood) and in rats (*T rhodesiense* is usually more virulent in rats). The differentiation of *T cruzi* from *T rangeli* (*T ariarii*, *T guatemalense*) is practicable and important since *T rangeli* is innocuous. The points of differentiation are shown in Table 1.

Immunity

Man apparently shows some individual variation in natural resistance to all 3 pathogenic trypanosomes. Strain-specific complement-fixing and protecting antibodies can be detected in the plasma, and these presumably lead to the disappearance of blood forms. The tissue forms are apparently less accessible, and it is significant that each relapse of African trypanosomiasis is apparently due to a strain serologically distinct from the preceding one. Apart from such relapses, Africans free from symptoms may be found to have trypanosomes in the blood (cf premunity in malaria, pp 452–453).

Treatment

There is no effective drug treatment for American trypanosomiasis, although Bayer-7602 may temporarily relieve some patients with trypanosomes in the blood. African trypanosomiasis is treated principally with suramin sodium (Naphuride, Antrypol) or pentamidine isethionate (Lomidine), the former preferably

TABLE 1. Differentiation of *T cruzi* and *T rangeli*.

	T cruzi	*T rangeli*
Blood forms		
Size	20 μm	Over 30 μm
Shape	Often C-shaped in fixed preparations	Rarely C-shaped
Posterior kinetoplast	Terminal, relatively large	Distinctly subterminal, small
Developmental stages in tissues	Leishmanial to crithidial	Not found (only trypanosomes)
Triatomid bugs		
In salivary gland and/or proboscis	Always absent	Usually present
In hind-gut or feces	Present	Present

for gambiense and vice versa. Late disease with CNS involvement requires melarsoprol (Mel B), as well as suramin or tryparsamide in the presence of parasitemia and active infection of lymph nodes.

Epidemiology, Prevention, & Control

African trypanosomiasis is restricted to recognized tsetse fly belts. Broadly, *T gambiense*, transmitted mostly by the stream-side tsetse *Glossina palpalis*, extends from west to central Africa and produces a relatively chronic infection with progressive CNS involvement. *T rhodesiense*, transmitted mostly by the woodland-savannah *G morsitans*, is more restricted, being confined to the south and east of Lake Tanganyika, and therefore causes smaller numbers of cases; but it is more virulent. Game and domestic animals may serve as a reservoir of *T rhodesiense*, and domestic animals as a reservoir of *T gambiense*. Control depends upon searching for and then isolating and treating patients with the disease; controlling movement of people in and out of fly belts and the use of insecticides in vehicles; and by fly control, principally with insecticides and by altering habitats. Contact with reservoir animals is difficult to control.

Chemoprophylaxis, eg, with suramin sodium (Naphuride), is difficult because the drug must be given intramuscularly, but it may be considered in certain circumstances.

American trypanosomiasis (Chagas' disease) is important only in certain parts of Central and South America, although infection of animals with virulent or mild strains extends much more widely, eg, into the southern USA. Certain triatomid bugs become as domiciliated as bedbugs, and infection may be brought in by opossums or armadillos—which may themselves become domiciliated and then spread the infection to domestic animals. Since no effective treatment is known, it is particularly important to control the vectors with residual insecticides and habitat destruction and to avoid contact with animal reservoirs. Chagas' disease occurs only among people in poor economic circumstances.

•   •   •

ENTAMOEBA HISTOLYTICA*

Entamoeba histolytica is a parasite commonly found in the intestines of man, certain higher primates, and some domiciliated and commensal animals. It is probable that most cases are asymptomatic.

Morphology & Identification

A. Typical Organisms: Three stages are encountered in feces or tissues: the active ameba, the inactive cyst, and the intermediate precyst. The ameboid trophozoite is present in tissues during invasion and in fluid feces during amebic dysentery. Its size is 15–30 μm (range, 10–60 μm). About 2/3 of the cytoplasm is granular; it may contain red cells (pathognomonic) but no bacteria, and is distinct from the surrounding clear ectoplasm. Iron-hematoxylin staining shows the nuclear membrane to be lined by fine, regular granules of chromatin, forming a distinct regular profile around the periphery; the central karyosome is small and deeply staining. Movement in fresh warm material is relatively brisk and apparently purposeful. Pseudopodia are fingerlike and broad. Dying amebas are sluggish, with less clear differentiation of the ectoplasm but a more distinct nucleus. Precystic amebas do not move about, show no fingerlike pseudopodia and little ectoplasm, have no red cells or other debris, and are only slightly larger than the cysts. They may be present in fluid feces.

Cysts are present only in the lumen of the colon and in fluid and formed feces. Subspherical cysts of actively pathogenic amebas range from 10–20 μm, but smaller cysts (of debatable significance but generally accepted as cysts of a nonpathogenic form) range down to 3.5 μm. The small forms (average below 10 μm) are generally regarded as either a distinct species (*E hartmanni*) or as a distinct subspecies or variety (*E histolytica* var *hartmanni*). The cyst wall, 0.5 μm thick, is hyaline. The initial uninucleate cyst may contain a glycogen vacuole and distinctly staining chromatoid

---

*The type-species of Endamoeba Leidy, 1879, is *End blattae* from the cockroach, while that of Entamoeba Cas & Barb, 1895, is *Ent coli* from man. The current and published (1928) official ruling of the International Commission of Zoological Nomenclature is that the 2 genera are inseparable, therefore that Entamoeba is a synonym of Endamoeba, which has priority in time. Protozoologists who believe that *End blattae* is generically distinct from all the others have petitioned for a revision of the official decision. If a new opinion is published in favor of this view, the species histolytica and coli will officially be in Entamoeba.

---

bodies or bars. Division soon takes place within the cyst to produce the final quadrinucleate cyst, usually without chromatoid bodies or glycogen vacuoles; diagnosis rests on the characteristics of this cyst (see p 460). Stools will contain cysts with 1–4 nuclei. (See the Keys on pp 450–451.)

B. Culture: Trophozoites are readily studied in cultures, and both encystation and excystation can be controlled.

C. Growth Requirements: Growth is most vigorous in various rich complex media under partial anaerobiosis at 37° C and pH 7.0, and with a mixed flora or at least a single coexisting species, eg, of Streptobacillus. Growth in tissue culture is also best under partial anaerobiosis.

D. Variation: Variations in cyst size and the occurrence of small nonpathogenic forms are subject to debate because the small cysts may represent a race (minor), a mutant (minor) selected in the intestine from a polymorphic ameba, or a distinct species (*E hartmanni*). In addition, there is the controversial change in behavior between a possibly noninvasive commensal phase and invasive phases in the same individual.

Pathogenesis, Pathology, & Clinical Findings

Multiplication takes place among trophozoites and again (4-fold) within cysts. Trophozoites emerge from ingested cysts on entry into the colon. The greatest concentration of amebas is at the sites of greatest fecal stasis, ie, the cecum and lower ascending colon, sigmoid colon, and rectum. Mucosal invasion by amebas with the aid of proteolytic enzymes leads to discrete, tiny flask-shaped cavities containing cell debris, mucus, and the organisms. It is assumed that this process continues in asymptomatic cyst passers, but this is not known; some authorities believe that the trophozoites may exist in the intestinal lumen without being invasive (cf other intestinal amebas). Active invasion, however, leads to lateral invasion of the small cavities, with undermining of edges and production of ulcers, which may coalesce. This is accompanied by diarrhea or dysentery, trophozoites being carried out with mucus and a few red cells in the fluid feces. In the absence of gross inflammation, destruction and regeneration proceed simultaneously unless secondary infection supervenes. These processes may lead to appendicitis, perforation, hemorrhage, and occasionally stricture, amebic granuloma (ameboma, self-healing), or pseudopolyposis. The bowel wall is friable (surgery is contraindicated in the active stage).

Extraintestinal infection is assumed to be metastatic, since it rarely occurs by direct extension from the bowel. By far the most common form is amebic hepatitis or liver abscess (4% or more of clinical infections, with much variation in different populations), which is assumed to be due to microemboli, including trophozoites carried through the portal circulation. Abscess often develops without being clinically evident. It is assumed that hepatic microembolism (including trophozoites) is a common accompaniment of bowel lesions, but that the diffused focal lesions rarely progress; many authorities regard the slight hepatic enlargement and tenderness (and the chronically impaired liver function) encountered in acute, subacute, and chronic intestinal infection to be nonspecific. A true amebic abscess is progressive, nonsuppurative (but occasionally secondarily infected), and destructive without compression and formation of a wall. The contents are necrotic and typically sterile, active amebas being confined to the walls. More than half of patients with amebic liver abscess give no history of intestinal infection; and only 1/8 of them pass cysts in their stools. Amebic abscesses also occur rarely elsewhere (eg, lung, brain, spleen).

Diagnostic Laboratory Tests

A. Specimens: Fluid feces, fresh and warm for trophozoites, or preserved in polyvinyl alcohol or MIF (merthiolate-iodine-formaldehyde) fixatives for sending away; formed feces for cysts; fluid feces after saline purge—or high enema after saline purge—for cysts and trophozoites. Scrapings and biopsies may be obtained through a sigmoidoscope. Liver abscess aspirates should be collected in a series of approximately 20 ml samples for detection of trophozoites, and all discarded but the last. Blood is required for complement fixation tests and cell counts.

B. Microscopic Examination: If possible, always examine fresh warm feces for trophozoites. Otherwise, stain smears with iron-hematoxylin stain. The stools in amebic dysentry can usually be distinguished from those in bacillary dysentery by the fact that they contain much fecal debris; small amounts of blood, with red cells often degenerated and clumped; few polymorphonuclear cells, epithelial cells, or bacteria; scattered Charcot-Leyden crystals; and trophozoites. Although considerable experience is required to distinguish *E histolytica* from commensal amebas (see below and p 460), it is necessary to do so because misdiagnosis often leads to unnecessary treatment or overtreatment.

Further differentiation of *E histolytica* (H) and *E coli* (C), the most common other intestinal ameba, can be made on stained smear as follows (see also p 460):

1. Trophozoites—The cytoplasm in H is glassy, and contains almost no inclusions except perhaps red cells, and vacuoles, spherical when present; the cytoplasm in C is granular, with many bacterial and other inclusions and ellipsoidal vacuoles. The ectoplasm is usually clearly demarcated in H but not in C. The nuclei of H have very small central endosomes and regular fine chromatin granules lining the periphery (or sometimes in crescentic distribution); the nuclei of C have larger eccentric endosomes and the peripheral chromatin is more coarsely beaded and less evenly distributed, the nucleus at times apparently resting in a clear vacuole. Moribund trophozoites and precysts of H and C are generally indistinguishable.

2. Cysts—Glycogen vacuoles disappear during successive divisions. Nuclei resemble those of the trophozoites. Occasional cysts of H and C may have 8 and 16 nuclei, respectively. Cysts of H in many preparations contain many uninucleate early cysts; these are rarely seen with C. Chromatoid bodies in early cysts of H are blunt-ended bars; those of C are splinter-like, do not have blunt, rounded ends, and often occur in clusters. *E coli* is present in 15–20% of normal individuals.

C. Culture: Diagnostic cultures are made in a layer of fluid overlying a solid nutrient base, partial anaerobiosis being produced by appropriate incubation or by use of thioglycollate. Dobell's diphasic and Cleveland-Collier media are most often used for diagnosis, and media such as Balamuth's for investigation.

D. Serology: The complement fixation test is not always satisfactory because a good and highly specific antigen is not available. It is at present, therefore, a research technic still to be developed. This applies also to a hemagglutination technic, which shows promise for the future. Positive responses to both tests, however, may be of value in supporting a tentative diagnosis in doubtful cases of extraintestinal amebiasis.

Treatment

Diiodohydroxyquin with chloroquine (prophylactic), followed by glycobiarsol, is the treatment of choice for mild intestinal infections. Severe dysentery requires emetine (or dehydroemetine) with oxytetracycline, followed by the course for mild infections. Emetine (or dehydroemetine) and chloroquine are specific against extraintestinal amebas, preferably given in that order followed by diiodohydroxyquin.

Epidemiology, Prevention, & Control

Cysts are usually ingested through contaminated water or, less often, contaminated vegetables and food. Asymptomatic cyst passers are the main source of contamination, and flies may be intermediaries. A high-carbohydrate, low-protein diet favors the development of amebic dysentery both in experimental animals and in known human cases. Control measures consist of improving environmental and food sanitation. Treatment of carriers is controversial, although it is agreed that these people should be barred from food handling. Chemoprophylaxis with glycobiarsol (Milibis) and chloroquine (Aralen) is reported to suppress amebiasis (as well as malaria, in the case of chloroquine).

OTHER INTESTINAL AMEBAS

Entamoeba histolytica must be distinguished from 4 other amebas which are also intestinal parasites of man: (1) *E coli* (see also above), which is very common; (2) *Dientamoeba fragilis,* the only intestinal ameba other than *E histolytica* which has been suspected of causing diarrhea and dyspepsia, but in the manner of giardia and not by invasion; (3) *Iodamoeba bütschlii;* and (4) *Endolimax nana.* These amebas and their cysts are illustrated on p 460. To facilitate detection, cysts should be concentrated by the zinc sulfate flotation technic. Unstained, iron-hematoxylin-stained, and iodine-stained preparations should be systematically searched. Mixed infections may occur.

Key for Identification of Amebic Trophozoites

Examine fresh warm feces; or, if this is impracticable, feces which have been promptly preserved while still fresh and warm. Include exudate and flecks of mucus in the specimen.

(1) If all trophozoites have one nucleus, see paragraph (2), below.

If more than half of trophozoites have 2 nuclei, the organism is

Dientamoeba fragilis—a small (mostly 5−15 μm) rounded ameba with nuclei containing a large chromatin mass in a clear space; no peripheral chromatin and no cysts. *D fragilis* may be present in about 50% of populations (eg, institutions). Often overlooked.

(2) If nucleus has peripheral granules, see paragraph (3), below.

If the nucleus has no peripheral granules, and a subspherical endosome larger than the radius of the nucleus and surrounded by large light granules, the organism is

Iodamoeba bütschlii—an ameba with a characteristic cyst (see below). It is present in about 8% of the population.

(3) If the peripheral granules of the nucleus are regularly arranged and the endosome is small, see paragraph (4), below.

If the peripheral granules are scattered and scarce and the endosome is irregular and much larger than the radius of the nucleus, the organism is

Endolimax nana—a small organism present in 15−20% of the population.

(4) If the cytoplasm is not coarsely granular, nuclei are always invisible in saline preparations, trophozoites move steadily and in one direction by streaming into blunt pseudopods, and some contain erythrocytes undergoing digestion but not bacteria; or if in an iron-hematoxylin stained

preparation the nuclear membrane is delicate and lined with a single layer of fine chromatin granules, and the karyosome is minute and central, the organism is either

Entamoeba histolytica—The pathogenic trophozoites are present only in dysenteric or diarrheal fluid feces, and are usually large (20−60 μm). (Do not confuse with macrophages containing erythrocytes; these may also contain bacteria, and they do not progress in one direction with single blunt pseudopods.) Verify identification by examining a series of stool specimens and searching for identifiable cysts. Pathogenic trophozoites are most often found in flecks of mucoid exudate.

or *Entamoeba hartmanni* (*E histolytica* var *hartmanni,* or small race *E histolytica* of some authors)—nonpathogenic and present in fluid or formed feces, always small (8−15 μm). See Cysts, below.

If present in fluid, semiformed, or formed feces, cytoplasm is coarsely granular, nuclei are sometimes visible in saline preparation, trophozoites do not move progressively but protrude pseudopods in several directions simultaneously, cytoplasm contains bacteria but not erythrocytes; if in iron-hematoxylin preparations the nuclear membrane is distinct and lined with larger and more irregular chromatin granules; or if larger than 15 μm, the organism is

Entamoeba coli—a normal commensal which may be almost impossible to differentiate from *E histolytica* in a fluid stool, except in the cystic state (see below).

Key for Identification of Amebic Cysts

No cysts are known for *Dientamoeba fragilis.*

(1) If mature cysts have 4 nuclei, see paragraph (2), below.

If mature cysts have 1−2 large nuclei with a large eccentric karyosome with a granular cluster, and a large iodine-staining vacuole, the organism is

Iodamoeba bütschlii.

If mature cysts have 8 nuclei, the organism is

Entamoeba coli.

(2) If quadrinucleate cysts are oval or ellipsoid and the nuclei have distinct large chromatin masses, the organism is

Endolimax nana.

If the cysts are spherical and the nuclei have regular peripheral chromatin granules and a small karyosome, the organism is

Entamoeba histolytica or *E hartmanni* (mean diameters respectively above and below 10 μm).

THE PLASMODIA

The sporozoan protozoa of the genus Plasmodium are pigment-producing ameboid parasites in vertebrate animals (the intermediate hosts) with one habitat in the red cells and another in other tissues. The definitive hosts are various species of mosquitoes.

Morphology & Identification

A. Typical Organisms: There are at least 5 species of plasmodia which may infect man: *P vivax, P ovale, P malariae, P falciparum,* and *P knowlesi.* Natural transmission of *P knowlesi* to man has only recently been demonstrated in Malaya. In addition, at least 2 species of nonhuman primate plasmodia, *P cynomolgi* and *P brasilianum,* are transmissible to man experimentally and probably also in nature. The morphology and certain other characteristics of the 4 principal species which infect man are summarized in Table 3. (See also illustrations on p 463.) *P cynomolgi* is similar to *P vivax* in morphology and in erythrocytic cycle length. *P knowlesi,* morphologically distinct from the other species, is unique in having a 24-hour erythrocytic schizogonic cycle.

B. Culture: The human malaria parasites have been cultivated with limited success in fluid media containing serum, erythrocytes, inorganic salts, and various growth factors and amino acids. Such media will support the parasites through a few cycles of schizogony. Cultivation of certain other species has been more successful; the avian plasmodia, in particular, can be grown in tissue cultures and in chick or duck embryos. Studies in culture have provided much fundamental biologic information about these protozoa.

C. Growth Characteristics and Requirements: In host red cells the parasites convert hemoglobin to globulin and hematin, which becomes the characteristic malarial pigment. Globulin is split by proteolytic enzymes and digested. Oxygen, dextrose, lactose, and erythrocyte protein are also utilized. Growth requirements, in addition to carbohydrates, proteins, and fats, include methionine, riboflavin, ascorbic acid, pantothenic acid, and para-aminobenzoic acid.

D. Variation: Variations of strains exist within each of the 4 human species. Variations have been detected in morphology, pathogenicity, resistance to drug therapy, infectivity for mosquitoes, and other characteristics. Complete immunity is usually strain-specific.

Pathogenesis, Pathology, & Clinical Findings

Human infection results from the bite of an infected female Anopheles mosquito, in which the sexual or sporogonic cycle of development takes place. The first stage of development in man takes place in the liver (the pre-erythrocytic cycle). At the end of this cycle parasites escape from the liver and, as merozoites, invade erythrocytes. The parasites develop and multiply asexually in the red cells (the schizogonic erythrocytic cycle), finally escaping as the cells rupture. The new crop of parasites, again called merozoites, invades new red cells and the cycle is repeated. Several such cycles occur before symptoms appear. Thus the incubation period includes the pre-erythrocytic cycle and at least one or 2 erythrocytic cycles. For *P vivax* and *P falciparum* this period is usually 10–15 days, but it may be much longer (in some cases even months). The incubation period of *P malariae* averages about 28 days. *P falciparum* multiplication is confined to the red cells after the first liver cycle; without treatment, the infection will terminate spontaneously in less than 2–3 years (usually 6–8 months). The other 3 species continue to multiply in liver cells long after the initial blood stream invasion. These exoerythrocytic cycles coexist with erythrocytic cycles, and may persist after the parasites have apparently disappeared from the peripheral blood. *P vivax* and *P ovale* infections may persist without treatment for as long as 5 years. *P malariae* infections lasting 40 years have been reported.

TABLE 2. Time factors of the various plasmodia in relation to cycles.

	Length of Sexual Cycle (in mosquito)	Prepatent Period (in man) (Pre-erythrocytic Cycle)	Length of Asexual Cycle (in man)
P vivax (tertian)	7–16 days	8 days	48 hours
P malariae (quartan)	15–30 days	11 days	72 hours
P falciparum (malignant tertian)	15–30 days	5½ days	36–48 hours
P ovale (ovale)	9–20 days	9 days	48 hours

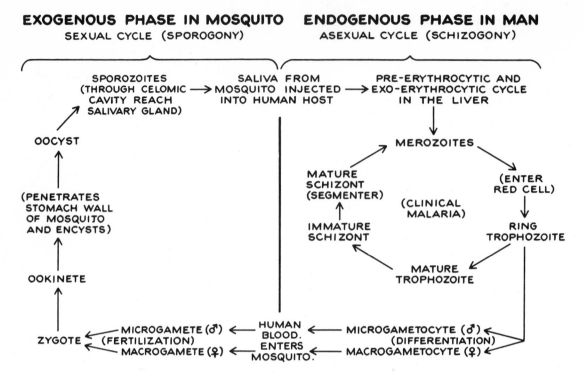

FIG 1. Life cycle of the malaria parasites.

During the erythrocytic cycles a few parasites become differentiated as male and female gametocytes. Thus the sporogonic or sexual cycle actually begins in the vertebrate host. For completion of this cycle, however, the gametocytes must be taken up and ingested by blood-sucking Anopheles mosquitoes.

P vivax, P malariae, and *P ovale* parasitemias are relatively low-grade, primarily because the parasites favor either young or old red cells but not both; *P falciparum* invades red cells of all ages, and the parasitemia may be very high. *P falciparum* also causes the parasitized red cells to agglutinate and adhere to capillary walls, with resulting obstruction, thrombosis, and local ischemia. *P falciparum* infections are therefore frequently more serious than the others, with a much higher rate of severe or fatal complications (cerebral malaria, malarial hyperpyrexia, gastrointestinal disorders, algid malaria).

The periodic paroxysms of malaria are closely related to events in the blood stream. The chill, lasting from 15 minutes to 1 hour, begins as a generation of parasites rupture their host red cells and escape into the blood. Nausea, vomiting, and headache are common at this time. The succeeding febrile stage, lasting several hours, is characterized by a spiking fever, sometimes reaching 104° F or more. During this stage the parasites presumably invade new red cells. The third or sweating stage concludes the episode. The fever subsides, and the patient falls asleep and later awakes feeling relatively well. In the early stages of infection the cycles are frequently asynchronous and the fever patterns irregular; later, the paroxysms may recur at regular 48- or 72-hour intervals. As the disease progresses, splenomegaly and, to a lesser extent, hepatomegaly appear. A normocytic anemia also develops, particularly in *P falciparum* infections.

Diagnostic Laboratory Tests

A. Specimens and Microscopic Examination: The thick blood film stained with one of the Romanowsky stains (usually Giemsa's stain) is the mainstay of malaria diagnosis. This preparation concentrates the parasites and permits detection even of light infections. Examination of thin blood films, also stained with Giemsa's stain, is necessary as a second step for parasite species differentiation.

B. Other Laboratory Findings: Normocytic anemia of variable severity, with poikilocytosis and anisocytosis, may be detected. During the paroxysms there may be transient leukocytosis; subsequently, leukopenia develops with a relative increase in large mononuclear cells. Hepatic function tests may give abnormal results during attacks, but liver function reverts to normal with treatment or spontaneous recovery. Children with *P malariae* infections sometimes suffer from a form of nephrosis, with protein and casts in the urine. In severe *P falciparum* infections renal damage may cause oliguria and the appearance of casts, protein, and red cells in the urine.

Immunity

The mechanisms of immunity in malaria deserve much more study. An acquired strain-specific complete immunity has been observed which appears to depend

TABLE 3. Some characteristic features of the malaria parasites of man (Romanowsky stained preparations).

	P vivax (Benign Tertian Malaria)	*P malariae* (Quartan Malaria)	*P falciparum* (Malignant Tertian Malaria)	*P ovale* (Ovale Malaria)
Parasitized red cells	Enlarged. Fine stippling (Schüffner's dots). Primarily invades reticulocytes; young red cells.	Not enlarged. No stippling (except with special stains). Primarily invades older red cells.	Not enlarged. Coarse stippling (Maurer's clefts). Invades all red cells regardless of age.	Enlarged. Fine stippling. Cells often oval or fimbriated.
Level of usual maximum parasitemia	8,000–20,000/cu mm of blood.	Less than 10,000/cu mm.	May reach 500,000/cu mm.	Less than 10,000/cu mm.
Ring stage trophozoites	Large rings (1/3–1/2 red cell diameter). Usually one chromatin granule; accolé forms rare.	Large rings (1/3–1/2 red cell diameter). Usually one chromatin granule.	Small rings (1/6 red cell diameter). Often 2 granules; often accolé forms; multiple infections common.	Large rings (1/3 red cell diameter). Usually one chromatin granule.
Older trophozoites	Very pleomorphic.	Occasional band forms.	Compact and rounded. Very rare in peripheral blood.	Compact and rounded.
Mature schizonts (segmenters)	More than 12 merozoites (12–24).	Less than 12 merozoites (6–12). Often rosette.	Usually more than 12 merozoites (8–32). Very rare in peripheral blood.	Less than 12 merozoites (6–12). Often rosette.
Gametocytes	Round or oval.	Round or oval.	Crescentic.	Round or oval.
Distribution	All forms in peripheral blood.	All forms in peripheral blood.	Only rings and crescents (gametocytes) in peripheral blood.	All forms in peripheral blood.

upon the presence of parasites in the blood stream of the host. This so-called **premunity** is soon lost after the parasites disappear from the blood. Exo-erythrocytic forms in the liver cannot alone support premunition; hence superinfection of the liver by homologous strains can continue to occur. Premunity is heavily dependent upon the reticuloendothelial system, which becomes extremely active in patent malaria infections (ie, infection with detectable blood form). In addition to acquired strain-specific immunity, natural genetically-determined partial immunity to malaria occurs in some populations, notably in Africa.

Treatment & Prevention

Chloroquine (Aralen) is the drug of choice for treatment of all forms of malaria during the acute attack. This drug will terminate *P falciparum* infections, in which there are no exo-erythrocytic forms. Primaquine, which disposes of the exo-erythrocytic tissue forms, must be used in conjunction with chloroquine to achieve complete cure of other forms of malaria. There is no satisfactory alternative to primaquine for eradication of tissue forms, but other compounds, eg, amodiaquine (Camoquin), quinine, and proguanil (Paludrine), are available for treatment of acute attacks. Resistant strains should be treated with quinine (intravenously in severe cases) with pyrimethamine and either sulfadiazine or dapsone.

Suppressive prophylaxis can be achieved with chloroquine diphosphate or amodiaquine plus primaquine.

Epidemiology & Control

Malaria today is generally limited to the tropics and subtropics; in years past transmission occurred in many temperate regions. Temperate zone malaria is usually unstable and relatively easy to control or eradicate; tropical malaria is often more stable. In the tropics malaria generally disappears at altitudes above 6000 feet. *P vivax* and *P falciparum*, the most common species, are found throughout the malaria belt. *P malariae* is also broadly distributed but considerably less common. *P ovale* is rare except in West Africa, where it seems to replace *P vivax*. All forms of malaria can be artificially transmitted by blood transfusion from an infected donor, but natural infection (other than transplacental transmission) takes place only through the bite of an infected female Anopheles mosquito.

Malaria control depends upon elimination of mosquito breeding places, personal protection against mosquitoes (screens, netting, repellents), suppressive drug therapy for exposed persons, and adequate treatment of cases and carriers. Eradication, a highly complex field, requires elimination of contact between Anopheles mosquitoes and man for a sufficient length of time to permit elimination, by treatment and spontaneous cure, of all cases in an area. At the end of this period a state of anophelinism-without-malaria will theoretically have been achieved.

THE ISOSPORA

Isospora belli and *Isospora hominis* are intestinal sporozoan protozoa of man, the causes of a disease known as coccidiosis or isosporosis. Numerous species of intestinal sporozoa or coccidia, some of them important pathogens, occur in other animals.

Morphology & Identification

A. Typical Organisms: Although all life cycle stages are known for many species of coccidia, only the elongated ovoid oocysts are known for *I belli* and *I hominis*. The life cycles of these parasites in man have never been adequately studied. The oocyst of *I hominis* measures about 16 X 10 μm; that of *I belli* is larger, 25–33 X 12–16 μm. The oocyst may contain a single sporoblast, 2 sporoblasts, or 2 sporocysts, each with 4 sporozoites. In fresh stool specimens *I belli* oocysts are often monosporoblastic; *I hominis* oocysts are more often disporoblastic or even disporocystic. In addition, the *I belli* oocyst wall is often asymmetric, whereas that of *I hominis* is smoothly ovoid or spherical.

B. Culture: These parasites have not been cultivated.

Pathogenesis & Clinical Findings

The isospora which infect humans are presumed to inhabit the small intestine, where schizogony probably takes place in the intestinal epithelial cells. The oocysts are shed into the intestinal lumen and pass out in the stools. Signs and symptoms of coccidiosis are apparently due to the invasion and multiplication of the parasites in the intestinal mucosa. Infections may be silent or symptomatic. About 1 week after ingestion of viable cysts, a low-grade fever, lassitude, and malaise may appear, followed soon by mild diarrhea and vague abdominal pain. The infection is self-limited and symptoms usually subside within 1–2 weeks. Symptomatic coccidiosis is more common in children than in adults. Chronic infections are rare, but have been recorded in poorly nourished populations living under insanitary conditions where continued reinfection is possible.

Diagnostic Laboratory Tests

Diagnosis rests entirely upon detection of the immature oocysts of *I belli* or the mature oocysts and sporocysts of *I hominis* in fresh stool specimens. Stool concentration technics are usually necessary.

Immunity

Apparently no immunity is conferred by infection. The many species of coccidia are notably host-specific.

Treatment

Treatment consists of bed rest and a bland diet for a few days. No specific treatment is necessary because the infection is self-limited.

Epidemiology

Human coccidiosis is usually sporadic, and most common in the tropics and subtropics. It is moderately endemic in parts of South Africa, several South American countries, and islands of the Southwest Pacific. More than 800 cases have so far been reported in the Western Hemisphere, including more than 40 from the USA (California and the southeastern states). The infection is easily overlooked on routine stool examination for parasites, and may be more common than the records indicate. New infections result from ingestion of viable cysts.

SARCOCYSTIS LINDEMANNI

Sarcocystis lindemanni of man and other species of Sarcocystis are protozoa of uncertain taxonomic position. These parasites, some species of which are pathogenic, are found in the muscles of many kinds of vertebrate animals.

Morphology & Identification

In the muscles the parasites develop in elongated cysts, known as sarcocysts or "Miescher's tubes," measuring from less than 1 mm to several cm in length. The sarcocyst is partitioned by septa into chambers containing many uninucleate crescentic spores or "Rainey's corpuscles." The mature spore, 10–15 μm in length, is pointed at one end and rounded at the other, with an oval vacuole near the pointed end. The spores, when set free by rupture of the cyst, are motile; they have occasionally been found in blood films from mammalian hosts. *S lindemanni* of man is morphologically indistinguishable from species found in other animals.

Pathogenesis & Clinical Findings

Heavy sarcocystis infections may be fatal in some species of animals (eg, mice, sheep, swine). Extracts of the parasite contain a toxin, sarcocystin, which is probably responsible for the pathogenic effects. This toxin is fatal when injected into rabbits. About 15 cases of human infection have been reported, mostly at autopsy following death due to other causes; however, inapparent infections are probably common. It is not clear that the parasite is pathogenic for man. Fleeting subcutaneous swellings, eosinophilia, and heart failure have, however, been attributed to *S lindemanni*. Sarcocysts have been found in man in the heart, larynx, tongue, and the skeletal muscles of the extremities.

Diagnostic Laboratory Tests

Since the infection ordinarily causes no symptoms or signs in man, it is usually detected only at autopsy. A reliable complement fixation test has been developed for detection of suspected infections.

Treatment

There is no known effective treatment.

Epidemiology

Sarcocystis shows little host specificity; cross-infections between various hosts can easily be produced. Since most Sarcocystis species are morphologically identical, it is likely that many of the described species (perhaps including *S lindemanni*) are not valid. Man is apparently an incidental and unsuitable host, probably being infected by ingestion of raw or poorly cooked infected lamb, beef, or other meats. Sarcocystis infections are particularly common in sheep, cattle, and horses.

TOXOPLASMA GONDII

Toxoplasma gondii is a protozoon of worldwide distribution which infects a wide range of animals and birds but may not cause disease in them. The organism causes either neonatal or postnatal toxoplasmosis in man.

Morphology & Identification

A. Typical Organisms: The organisms consist of boat-shaped, thin-walled cells, 4–7 X 2–4 μm when within tissue cells and somewhat larger (up to 10 X 4 μm) outside them. They stain lightly with Giemsa's stain; fixed cells sometimes appear crescentic. Packed intracellular aggregates may be seen (cf *Leishmania donovani*).

B. Culture: *T gondii* may be cultured only in the presence of living cells, in tissue culture or eggs. Typical intracellular and extracellular organisms may be seen.

C. Growth Requirements: Optimal growth is at about 37–39° C in living cells.

D. Variations: There is considerable strain variation in infectivity and virulence, possibly in part related to a degree of adaptation to a particular host. Variations in microscopic appearance are negligible.

Pathogenesis, Pathology, & Clinical Findings

The organism directly destroys cells, and has a predilection for parenchymal cells and those of the reticuloendothelial system. Man is relatively resistant, but a low-grade lymph node infection resembling infectious mononucleosis may occur. Neonatal infection leads to stillbirths, chorioretinitis, intracerebral calcifications, psychomotor disturbances, and hydrocephaly or microcephaly. In these cases the mother was infected during pregnancy.

Diagnostic Laboratory Tests

A. Specimens: Blood, bone marrow, CSF, and exudates for direct inspection; lymph node biopsy material; tonsillar and striated-muscle biopsies; and ventricular fluid (in neonatal infections) may be required.

B. Microscopic Examination: Smears and sections stained with Giemsa's stain may show the organism. Densely packed cysts ("pseudocysts") suggest chronic infection. Identification must be confirmed by isolation in animals.

C. Animal Inoculation: This is essential for definitive diagnosis. A variety of specimens are inoculated intraperitoneally into groups of mice which have been dye-tested to make certain that they are free from infection. If no deaths occur the mice are observed for about 6 weeks, and tail or heart blood is then tested for specific antibody. The diagnosis is confirmed by demonstration of cysts in the brains of the inoculated mice.

D. Serology: The Sabin-Feldman dye test is valuable for diagnosis and surveys. It depends upon the appearance in 2–3 weeks of antibodies which will render laboratory-cultured living *T gondii* unable to take up alkaline methylene blue. A complement fixation test may be positive (1:8 titer) as early as 1 month after infection, but it is valueless in many chronic infections. Frenkel's intracutaneous test is of limited clinical value but is useful for epidemiologic surveys.

Immunity

There are great variations in strains and hosts, and a degree of acquired immunity (or premunity in some cases) may develop. Antibodies in mothers, as detected in either blood or milk, tend to fall within a few months.

Treatment

No effective treatment has been established. Combined pyrimethamine (Daraprim) and trisulfapyrimidines, however, show great promise.

Epidemiology, Prevention, & Control

Transplacental infection of the fetus is the only mode of transmission which has been identified with certainty. Later infection is assumed to be via the upper respiratory tract or conjunctiva, but arthropods have been suspected also. No measures can be devised for prevention except occasionally to trace local concentrations of cases to some animal or avian source and then to eradicate the reservoir. Patients with acute congenital or severe acquired disease should be isolated.

TABLE 4. Diseases due to helminths.

(Some uncommon infections tabulated here are omitted from the text.)

C = cestode (tapeworm)	N = nematode (roundworm)		T = trematode (fluke)	
Disease and Parasite	**Location in Host**	**Mode of Transmission**	**Geographic Distribution**	**Treatment of Choice**
Angiostrongyliasis; eosinophilic meningo-encephalitis *Angiostrongylus cantonensis* (N)	Larvae in meninges	Eating raw shrimps, prawns; raw garden slugs.	Local in Pacific, especially SW	Thiabendazole (experimental)
Ascariasis *Ascaris lumbricoides* (N), common roundworm	Small intestine; larvae through lungs.	Eating viable eggs from feces-contaminated soil or food	Worldwide, very common	Piperazine, thiabendazole
Clonorchiasis *Clonorchis sinensis* (T), Chinese liver fluke	Liver	Uncooked fish	China, Korea, Indochina, Japan, Taiwan	Chloroquine
Cysticercosis (bladder worm) *Taenia solium* (larval) (C)	Subcutaneous; eye, meninges, brain, etc.	Regurgitation of gravid proglottid from lower GI tract	Worldwide	Surgical excision
Dipetalonemiasis *Dipetalonema perstans* (N) (*Acanthocheilonema perstans*) (nonpathogenic?)	Peritoneal and other cavities; micro-filariae in blood.	Bite of gnat Culicoides	Equatorial Africa; N coast of S America, Argentina, Panama, Trinidad.	Not treated
Dracontiasis *Dracunculus medinensis* (N), Guinea worm	Subcutaneous; usually leg, foot.	Drinking water with Cyclops	Africa, Arabia to Pakistan and India, New Guinea	Mechanical or surgical extraction; niridazole
Echinococcosis *Echinococcus granulosus*, *E multilocularis* (C)	Liver; lung, brain.	Contact with dogs	Worldwide but local; sheep-raising areas.	Surgical excision
Enterobiasis *Enterobius vermicularis* (N), pinworm, threadworm	Cecum, colon	Anal-oral; self-contamination and internal reinfection.	Worldwide	Piperazine or pyrvinium pamoate
Fascioliasis *Fasciola hepatica* (T), sheep liver fluke	Liver	Watercress, aquatic vegetation	Worldwide, especially sheep-raising areas	Emetine; dehydroemetine.
Fasciolopsiasis *Fasciolopsis buski* (T), giant intestinal fluke	Small intestine	Aquatic vegetation	E and SE Asia	Hexylresorcinol
Filariasis *Wuchereria bancrofti*, *Brugia malayi* (N)	Lymph nodes; microfilariae in blood.	Bite of mosquitoes; several species.	Tropical and sub-tropical, very local but widespread	Diethylcarbamazine
Filariasis, Occult *Dirofilaria* species	Lungs (larvae)	Contact with dogs?	India, SE Asia	Diethylcarbamazine
Gnathostomiasis *Gnathostoma spinigerum* (N)	Subcutaneous, migratory	Uncooked fish	E and SE Asia	Surgical excision; diethylcarbamazine.
Heterophyiasis *Heterophyes heterophyes* (T)	Small intestine	Uncooked fish (mullet)	China, Korea, Japan, Taiwan; Israel; Egypt.	Tetrachloroethylene
Hookworms *Ancylostoma duodenale*, *Necator americanus* (N)	Small intestine; larvae through lungs	Through skin, infected soil	Worldwide, warm countries	Bephenium; tetrachloroethylene; thiabendazole.
Larva migrans: Cutaneous, creeping eruption *Ancylostoma braziliense* and other domestic animal hookworms (N)	Subcutaneous, migrating	Contact with soil contaminated by dog or cat feces	Worldwide	Thiabendazole
Visceral *Toxocara* species, cat and dog roundworms (N)	Liver, lung, eye, brain, other viscera	Ingesting soil contaminated by dog or cat feces	Worldwide	Thiabendazole; corticosteroids.
Loiasis *Loa loa* (N)	Subcutaneous, migratory; eye.	Bite of deerflies, Chrysops	Equatorial Africa	Surgical removal; diethylcarbamazine.

TABLE 4 (cont'd). Diseases due to helminths.

Disease and Parasite	Location in Host	Mode of Transmission	Geographic Distribution	Treatment of Choice
Mansonelliasis *Mansonella ozzardi* (N) (nonpathogenic)	Body cavities; microfilariae in blood.	Bite of gnat Culicoides	Argentina, N coast of S America; Caribbean Islands; Panama, Yucatan.	Not treated
Metagonimiasis *Metagonimus yokogawai* (T)	Small intestine	Uncooked fish	As for Heterophyes plus USSR, Balkans, Spain	Tetrachloroethylene
Onchocerciasis *Onchocerca volvulus* (N)	Subcutaneous; larvae in skin, eyes.	Bite of black-fly Simulium	Equatorial Africa; C and S America.	Surgery; diethylcarbamazine.
Opisthorchiasis *Opisthorchis felineus,* *O viverrini* (T)	Liver	Uncooked fish	E Europe, USSR; Thailand.	Chloroquine
Paragonimiasis *Paragonimus westermani* (T)	Lung	Raw crabs	E and S Asia; N Central Africa; S America; animals in N America.	Bithionol; chloroquine.
Schistosomiasis: *Schistosoma haematobium* (T)	Venous capillaries, urinary bladder		Africa, widely; Madagascar; Arabia to Lebanon.	Niridazole; antimony Na dimercaptosuccinate, stibophen, lucanthone.
S japonicum (T)	Venous capillaries, intestine	Cercaria (larvae) penetrate skin in snail-infested water.	China, Philippines; Japan; potentially Formosa.	Antimony potassium tartrate.
S mansoni (T)	Venous capillaries, colon, rectum		Africa to Near East; parts of S America, Caribbean Tropics and Subtropics.	Stibophen, antimony Na dimercaptosuccinate, lucanthone
Sparganosis Diphyllobothrium (Spirometra) larva (sparganum) of pets	Intraorbital, etc	Native poultices such as infected raw frog flesh	Orient, occasionally other countries, including N and S America	Surgical removal
Strongyloidiasis *Strongyloides stercoralis* (N)	Duodenum, jejunum; larvae through skin, lungs.	Through skin and (rarely) by internal reinfection	Worldwide	Thiabendazole; pyrvinium pamoate.
Tapeworm disease (See also Cysticercosis, Echinococcosis, Sparganosis): *Dipylidium caninum* (C), dog tapeworm	Small intestine	Ingestion of crushed fleas, lice from pets	Worldwide	Quinacrine, niclosamide
Diphyllobothrium latum (C), fish tapeworm	Small intestine	Uncooked fish	Alaska, E Canada, Great Lakes area, N W Florida, parts of S America; N Europe, E Mediterranean, Asiatic USSR, Japan; Australia.	Quinacrine, niclosamide
Hymenolepis diminuta (C)	Small intestine	Indirectly from rats, mice via infected insects.	Worldwide	Quinacrine, niclosamide
H nana (C), dwarf tapeworm	Small intestine	Anal-oral transfer of eggs or accidental ingestion of infected insects	Worldwide	Niclosamide
Taenia saginata (C), beef tapeworm	Small intestine	Uncooked beef	Worldwide	Niclosamide, quinacrine
T solium (C), pork tapeworm (see also cysticercosis)	Small intestine	Uncooked pork	Worldwide	Quinacrine
Trichinosis *Trichinella spiralis* (N)	Larvae in striated muscle	Uncooked pork	Worldwide	Thiabendazole; corticosteroids.
Trichuriasis *Trichuris trichiura* (N), whipworm	Cecum; colon.	Ingestion of eggs from feces-contaminated soil	Worldwide	Hexylresorcinol; thiabendazole.

PNEUMOCYSTIS CARINII

Pneumocystis carinii appears to be a protozoon of uncertain relationships, probably widely distributed among animals in nature—including rats, mice, and dogs—but usually without causing disease in them. The organism may cause an interstitial pneumonitis in man, most often in infants.

Morphology & Identification

A. Typical Organisms: The most characteristic stage is the rosette of 8 pear-shaped sporozoites, each 1–2 μm, in a "cyst" 7–10 μm in diameter. Earlier stages consist of 1–4 nuclei in a mucoid sphere, respectively staining red and blue within a red-violet membrane when heavily stained with Giemsa's stain. Organisms are seen in large numbers packed in foamy material and among many plasma cells and eosinophils in the pulmonary alveoli and bronchioles of fatal cases. Some organisms may be within histiocytes. Pulmonary infections with pneumonitis have been reported in rats.

B. Culture: Not reported. Attempts should be made to culture in the lungs of cortisone-treated rats or mice.

Pathogenesis, Pathology, & Clinical Findings

Most infections in man are probably inapparent. Excessive multiplication leading to blocking of the alveolar respiratory surface appears to occur especially in premature or marasmic infants but also in those whose resistance has been lowered, ie, children and adults receiving corticosteroids, cytotoxic drugs, or antibiotics over extended periods, or those suffering from agammaglobulinemia. There is interstitial plasma cell pneumonitis (detectable in x-rays) with alveoli filled with organisms and foamy material.

Diagnostic Laboratory Tests

The organism is usually discovered after autopsy, but lung puncture biopsy has been reported to be successful. Staining is difficult. Heavy Giemsa staining should be used simultaneously with Böhmer's hematoxylin (30 minutes, without differentiation) and periodic acid-Schiff stain for mucopolysaccharides.

Treatment

Pentamidine isethionate and pyrimethamine are the drugs with most promise.

Epidemiology, Prevention, & Control

The mode of infection is unknown, but sporozoites, presumably inhaled, are derived from domestic rodents or pets (perhaps from carrier adults in nurseries).

BALANTIDIUM COLI

Balantidium coli, the cause of balantidiasis or balantidial dysentery, is the largest intestinal protozoon of man. Morphologically similar parasites are found in swine and lower primates.

Morphology & Identification

A. Typical Organisms: The trophozoite is a bulky, oval organism, 60 × 45 μm in average dimensions (occasionally almost twice as large). Its motion is characteristic, a combination of steady, boring progression and rotation around the long axis. The cell wall is lined with spiral rows of cilia which also extend into the deep and conspicuous anterior cytostome. The cytoplasm surrounds 2 contractile vacuoles, food particles and vacuoles, and 2 nuclei—a large, kidney-shaped macronucleus and a much smaller, spherical micronucleus. When the organism encysts it secretes a spherical or oval double-layered wall. The macronucleus, contractile vacuoles, and portions of the ciliated cell wall may be visible in the cyst, which ranges from 45–65 μm in diameter.

B. Culture: These organisms may be cultivated in a variety of simple media, including those used for cultivation of intestinal amebas.

Pathogenesis, Pathology, & Clinical Findings

When cysts are ingested by the new host, the cyst walls dissolve and the released trophozoites invade the mucosa and submucosa of the large bowel and terminal ileum. As they multiply, abscesses and irregular ulcerations with overhanging lips are formed. The number of lesions formed depends upon the intensity of infection and the degree of individual host susceptibility. Chronic recurrent diarrhea, alternating with constipation, is the commonest clinical manifestation, but attacks of severe dysentery with bloody mucoid stools, tenesmus, and colic may occur intermittently in light as well as heavy infections. Many light infections are asymptomatic.

Diagnostic Laboratory Tests

The diagnosis of balantidial infection, whether symptomatic or not, depends upon laboratory detection of trophozoites in liquid stools or, more rarely, of cysts in formed stools. There are no other constant and distinctive laboratory findings. Sigmoidoscopy may be useful for obtaining material directly from ulcerations for examination. Culturing is rarely necessary for diagnosis.

Immunity

Man appears to have a high natural resistance to balantidial infection. Factors underlying individual susceptibility are not known.

Treatment

A course of oxytetracycline may be followed by diiodohydroxyquin if necessary.

TABLE 5. Microfilariae.

Filariid	Disease	Distribution	Vectors	Microfilariae		
				Sheath	Tail Nuclei	Periodicity
Wuchereria bancrofti	Bancroftian and Malayan filariasis: lymphangitis, hydrocele, elephantiasis	Worldwide 41° N to 28° S	Culicidae	+	Not to tip	Nocturnal or nonperiodic
Brugia malayi		Oriental region to Japan	Culicidae	+	Two distinct	Nocturnal
Loa loa	Loiasis; Calabar swellings; conjunctival worms	Western and Central Africa	Chrysops, biting fly	+	Extend to tip	Diurnal
Onchocerca volvulus	Onchocerciasis: skin nodules, blindness, dermatitis	Africa, Central and South America	Simulium	-	Not to tip	Diurnal
Dipetalonema perstans	Dipetalonemiasis or acanthocheilonemiasis (minor disturbances)	Africa and South America	Culicoides midges	-	Extend to tip	Nocturnal or diurnal or nonperiodic
Dipetalonema streptocerca	Usually nonpathogenic	Western and Central Africa	Culicoides	-		In skin only
Mansonella ozzardi	Ozzard's mansonelliasis (benign), occasionally hydrocele	Central and South America	Culicoides	-	Not to tip	Nonperiodic

Epidemiology

B coli is found in man throughout the world, particularly in the tropics, but it is a rare infection. Only a few hundred cases have been recorded. Infection results from ingestion of viable cysts previously passed in the stools by humans and possibly by swine. Although it has been generally accepted that pigs are important sources of human infections, some epidemiologic evidence suggests that this may not be so.

HELMINTHS: OVA IN FECES & MICROFILARIAE IN BLOOD & TISSUES
(See also Table 4 and illustrations on pp 464, 465, and 470.)

Ova (pp 465 and 470) may be detected in feces (or urine, with *Schistosoma haematobium* and sometimes *S japonicum*), preferably after concentration by zinc sulfate centrifugal sedimentation, eg, formalin-triton-NE-ether technics (especially for operculated and schistosome eggs). Eggs of enterobius and taenia may be collected directly from the anal margins with cellulose tape on the end of a spatula.

Microfilariae (see Table 5 and p 464) are the larval stages of filariid worms in man.

PROTOZOA IN FECES (× 2000)

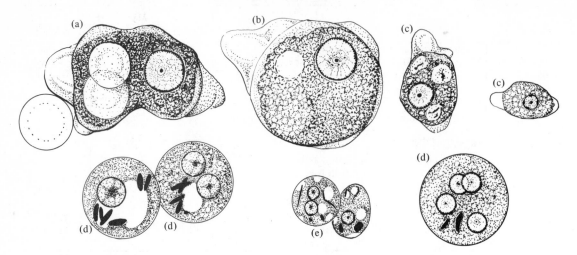

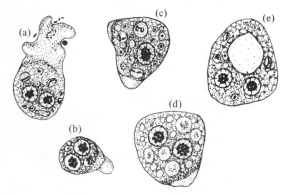

Entamoeba histolytica. (a-d) Trophozoite or vegetative form with ingested red cells; (b) with chromatid bodies; (c) small race (*E hartmanni*) trophozoite; (d) cysts with 1, 2, and 4 nuclei and chromatid bodies; (e) *E hartmanni* cysts.

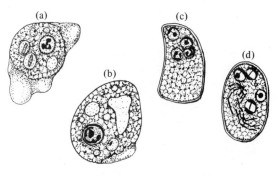

Endolimax nana. (a) Trophozoite; (b) precystic form; (c) and (d) cysts.

Dientamoeba fragilis. Trophozoites: (a) active, (b) small, (c) mononuclear, (d) and (e) resting. No cysts are found.

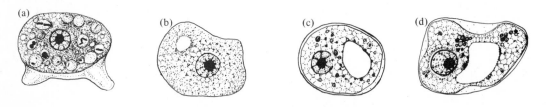

Iodamoeba bütschlii. (a) Trophozoite; (b) precystic form; (c) and (d) cysts.

[Simple double circles represent the size of red cells.]

PROTOZOA IN FECES (× 2000)*

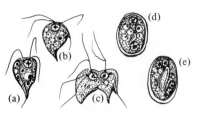

Enteromonas hominis. (a, b, c) Trophozoites; (d) and (e) cysts.

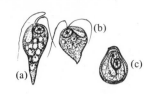

Embadomonas intestinalis. (a) and (b) trophozoites; (c) cyst.

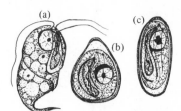

Chilomastix mesnili. (a) Trophozoite; (b) and (c) cysts.

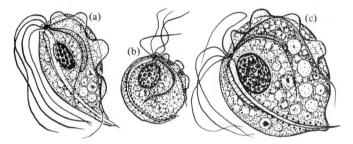

Trichomonas vaginalis. (a) Normal trophozoite; (b) round form after division; (c) common round form.

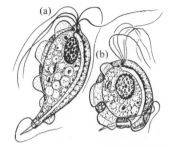

Trichomonas hominis. (a) Normal and (b) round forms of trophozoites.

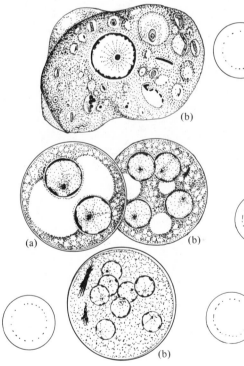

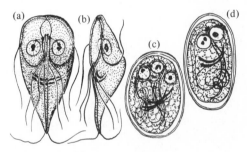

Giardia intestinalis. (a) Face and (b) profile of vegetative forms; (c) and (d) cysts.

Entamoeba coli. (a) Trophozoite with vacuoles and inclusions; (b) cysts with 2, 4, and 8 nuclei.

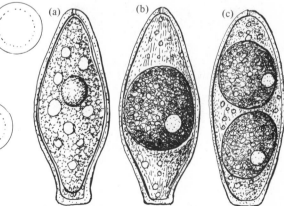

Isospora hominis. (a) Degenerate oocyst; (b) unsegmented oocyst; (c) oocyst segmented into 2 sporoblasts after passage into feces.

[Simple double circles represent the size of red cells.]

*_Trichomonas vaginalis_ is found in vaginal and prostatic secretions.

PROTOZOA IN FECES (× 2000)

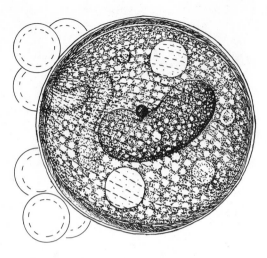

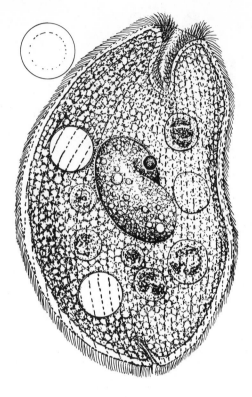

Balantidium coli. **Right**: Trophozoite. **Above**: Cyst.

PROTOZOA IN BLOOD AND TISSUES (× 2000)

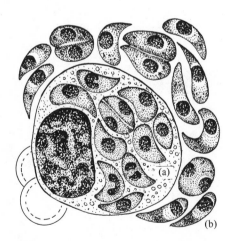

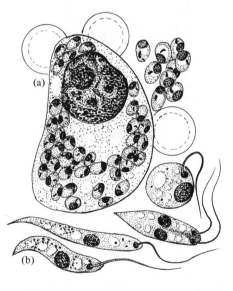

Toxoplasma gondii. (a) In large mononuclear cells; (b) free in blood.

Leishmania donovani. (a) Large reticuloendothelial cell of spleen with Leishman–Donovan bodies. (b) Flagellate forms as seen in sandfly or culture.

[Simple double circles represent the size of red cells.]

PROTOZOA IN BLOOD (× 1700)

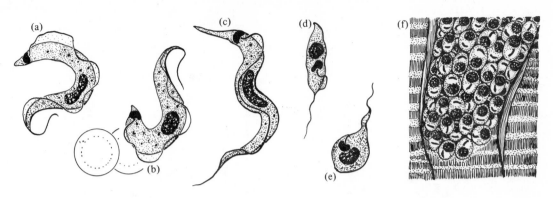

Trypanosoma cruzi. (a, b, c) Blood forms; (d) leptomonad; (e) crithidial forms; (f) in heart muscle.

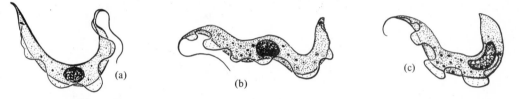

Trypanosoma gambiense (or *T rhodesiense*, indistinguishable in practice). (a, b) Blood forms; (c) crithidial form (intermediate type; kinetoplast not yet anterior to nucleus), found only in tsetse fly, Glossina sp.

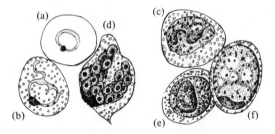

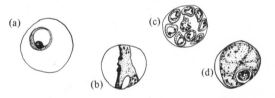

Plasmodium vivax. (a) Young signet ring trophozoite; (b) ameboid trophozoite; (c) mature trophozoite; (d) mature schizont; (e) microgametocyte; (f) macrogametocyte.

Plasmodium malariae. (a) Developing ring form of trophozoite; (b) band form of trophozoite (note absence of granules); (c) mature schizont in "rosette" with 8 merozoites; (d) mature gametocyte.

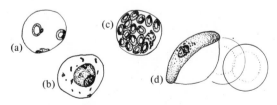

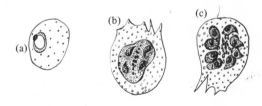

Plasmodium falciparum. (a) Young trophozoites (triple infection); (b) mature trophozoite showing clumped pigment in cytoplasm and Maurer's dots in erythrocyte; (c) mature schizont; (d) mature gametocyte.

Plasmodium ovale. (a) Young signet-ring trophozoite and Schüffner's dots; (b) ameboid trophozoite developing in fimbriated erythrocyte; (c) mature schizont showing 8 merozoites.

[Simple double circles represent the size of red cells.]

MICROFILARIAE (× 600)

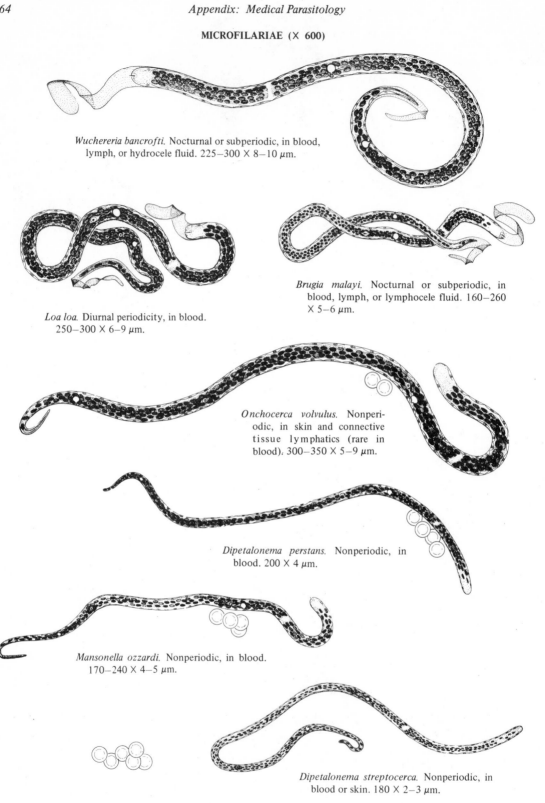

Wuchereria bancrofti. Nocturnal or subperiodic, in blood,
lymph, or hydrocele fluid. 225–300 × 8–10 µm.

Brugia malayi. Nocturnal or subperiodic, in
blood, lymph, or lymphocele fluid. 160–260
× 5–6 µm.

Loa loa. Diurnal periodicity, in blood.
250–300 × 6–9 µm.

Onchocerca volvulus. Nonperiodic, in skin and connective
tissue lymphatics (rare in
blood). 300–350 × 5–9 µm.

Dipetalonema perstans. Nonperiodic, in
blood. 200 × 4 µm.

Mansonella ozzardi. Nonperiodic, in blood.
170–240 × 4–5 µm.

Dipetalonema streptocerca. Nonperiodic, in
blood or skin. 180 × 2–3 µm.

[Simple double circles represent the size of red cells.]

OVA OF TREMATODES (X 400)

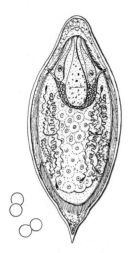

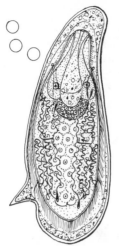

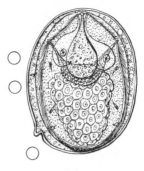

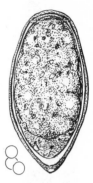

Schistosoma japonicum. Ovum containing miracidium.

Paragonimus wester- mani. Unembryo- nated operculated ovum.

Schistosoma haematobium. Ovum containing miracidium.

Schistosoma mansoni. Ovum containing miracidium.

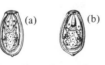

Clonorchis sinensis. Small operculated and em- bryonated ovum.

Heterophyes heterophyes (a) or *Metagonimus yokogawai* (b)

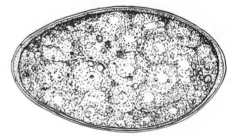

Fasciola hepatica or *Fasciolopsis buski.* Unem- bryonated operculated ovum. Operculum of ovum of *Fasciolopsis buski* is smaller than that of *Fasciola hepatica.*

OVA OF NEMATODES (X 400)

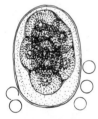

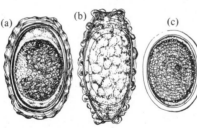

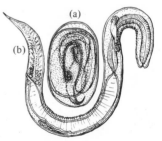

Ancylostoma duode- nale or *Necator americanus*

Ascaris lumbricoides. (a) Fertilized unem- bryonated ovum; (b) unfertilized ovum; (c) fertilized decorticated ovum.

Strongyloides stercoralis. (a) Embryonated ovum (rarely seen); (b) larva encountered in feces.

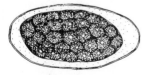

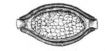

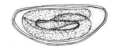

Trichostrongylus orientalis. Unembryonated ovum.

Trichuris trichiura. Unembryo- nated double-plug ovum.

Enterobius vermicularis. Em- bryonated ovum with char- acteristic flattening on one side.

[Simple circles represent the size of red cells.]

TREMATODES

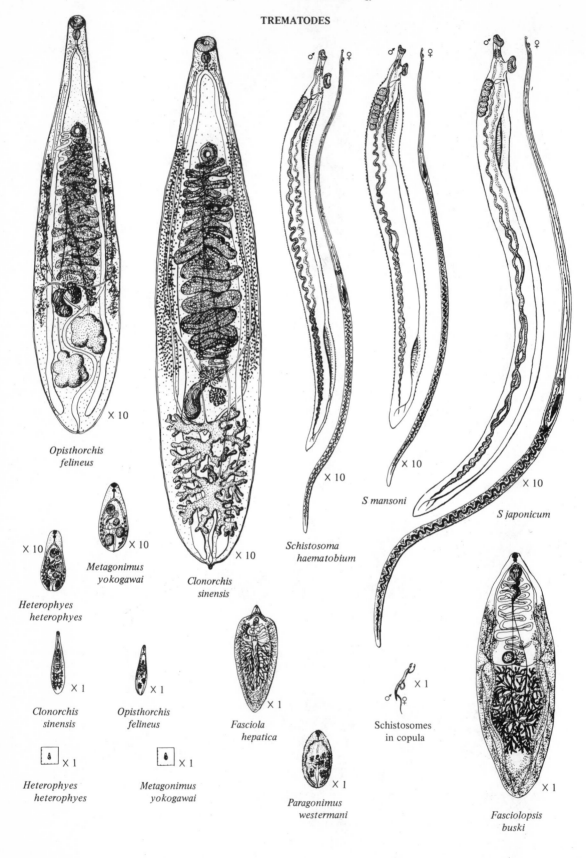

Opisthorchis
felineus

× 10

Heterophyes
heterophyes

× 10

Metagonimus
yokogawai

× 10

Clonorchis
sinensis

× 10

Schistosoma
haematobium

× 10

S mansoni

× 10

S japonicum

× 10

Clonorchis
sinensis

× 1

Opisthorchis
felineus

× 1

Fasciola
hepatica

× 1

Schistosomes
in copula

× 1

Heterophyes
heterophyes

× 1

Metagonimus
yokogawai

× 1

Paragonimus
westermani

× 1

Fasciolopsis
buski

× 1

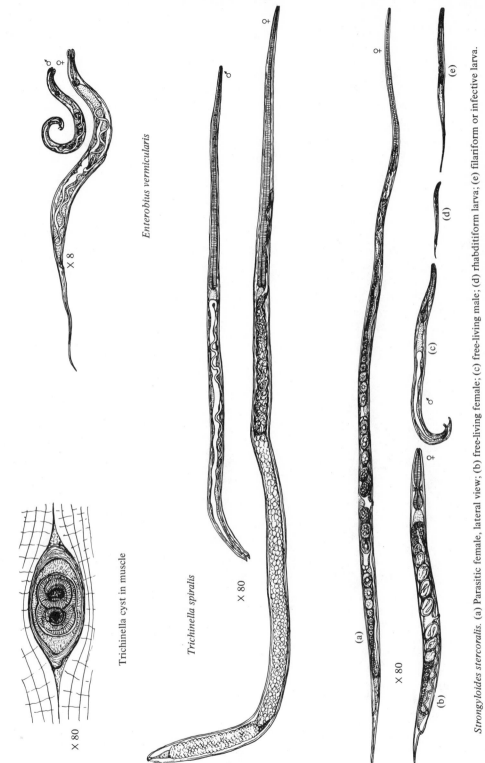

NEMATODES

×8

Enterobius vermicularis

×80

Trichinella cyst in muscle

Trichinella spiralis

×80

×80

(a) (b) (c) (d) (e)

Strongyloides stercoralis. (a) Parasitic female, lateral view; (b) free-living female; (c) free-living male; (d) rhabditiform larva; (e) filariform or infective larva.

NEMATODES

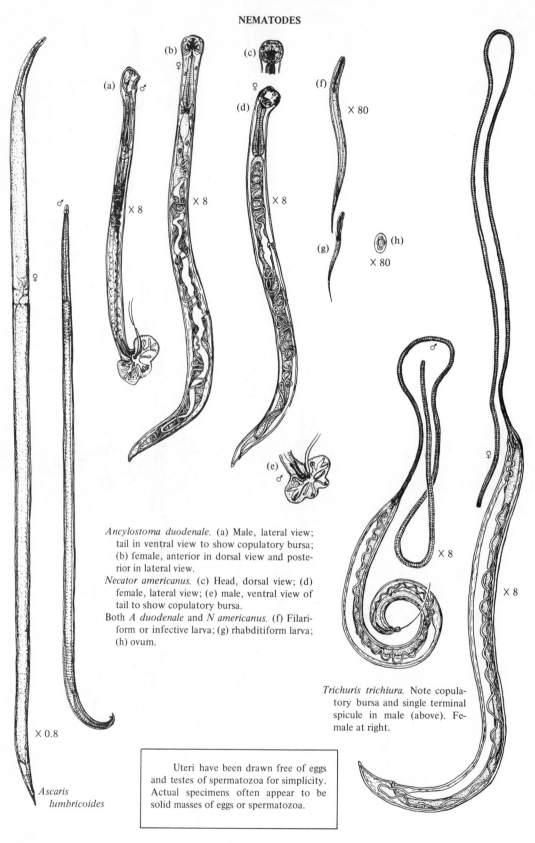

Ancylostoma duodenale. (a) Male, lateral view; tail in ventral view to show copulatory bursa; (b) female, anterior in dorsal view and posterior in lateral view.

Necator americanus. (c) Head, dorsal view; (d) female, lateral view; (e) male, ventral view of tail to show copulatory bursa.

Both *A duodenale* and *N americanus.* (f) Filariform or infective larva; (g) rhabditiform larva; (h) ovum.

Trichuris trichiura. Note copulatory bursa and single terminal spicule in male (above). Female at right.

Uteri have been drawn free of eggs and testes of spermatozoa for simplicity. Actual specimens often appear to be solid masses of eggs or spermatozoa.

Ascaris lumbricoides

CESTODES (TAPEWORMS)

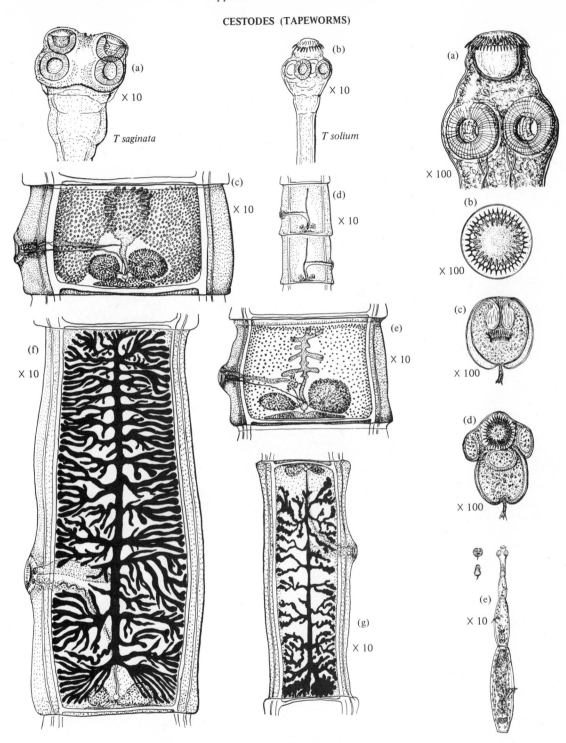

Taenia saginata and *T solium.* (a) Scolex of *T saginata;* (b) scolex of *T solium* with beginning of strobila; (c) mature proglottid of *T saginata;* (d) immature proglottids of *T solium;* (e) mature proglottid of *T solium;* (f) gravid proglottid of *T saginata* with much more numerous uterine ramifications than in *T solium* (see at right); (g) gravid proglottid of *T solium.*

Echinococcus granulosus. (a) Scolex of adult; (b) end view of rostellum, showing arrangement of 2 hook rows; (c) larva from hydatid fluid, invaginated; (d) same, evaginated; (e) entire adult worm.

CESTODES

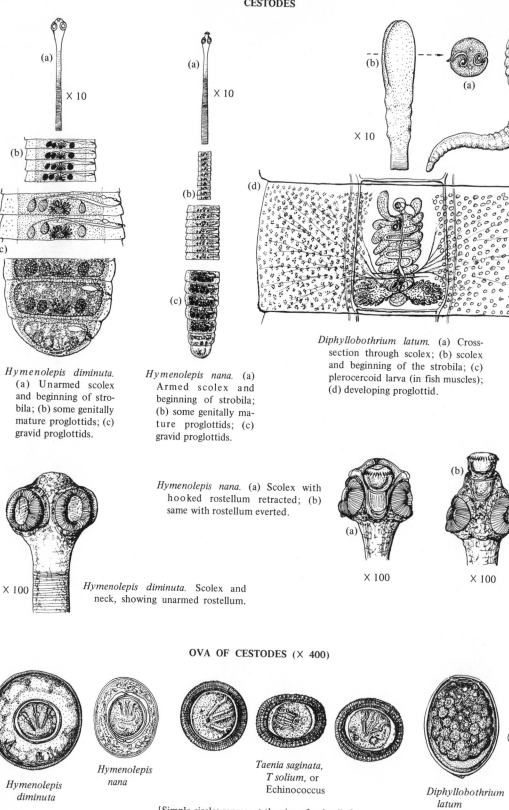

Hymenolepis diminuta.
(a) Unarmed scolex
and beginning of stro-
bila; (b) some genitally
mature proglottids; (c)
gravid proglottids.

Hymenolepis nana. (a)
Armed scolex and
beginning of strobila;
(b) some genitally ma-
ture proglottids; (c)
gravid proglottids.

Diphyllobothrium latum. (a) Cross-
section through scolex; (b) scolex
and beginning of the strobila; (c)
plerocercoid larva (in fish muscles);
(d) developing proglottid.

Hymenolepis nana. (a) Scolex with
hooked rostellum retracted; (b)
same with rostellum everted.

Hymenolepis diminuta. Scolex and
neck, showing unarmed rostellum.

OVA OF CESTODES (X 400)

*Hymenolepis
diminuta*

*Hymenolepis
nana*

*Taenia saginata,
T solium,* or
Echinococcus

*Diphyllobothrium
latum*

[Simple circles represent the size of red cells.]

Index